MRCP Part 2

450 BOFs

SECOND EDITION

CW00953069

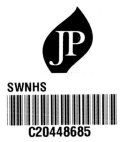

MRCP Part 2

450 BOFs

SECOND EDITION

Heather Lewis MBChB MD(Res) FRCP
Consultant Hepatologist
Imperial College NHS Healthcare Trust
London, UK

Ravi Menon MBBS MRCP MD
Honorary Clinical Lecturer
Newham University Hospital
Barts Health NHS Trust
London, UK

Luke Moore FRCPath MRCP(Inf DIs) PhD MSc MPH DTMH MBChB
Consultant in Infectious Diseases and Microbiology
Chelsea and Westminster NHS Foundation Trust
London, UK

George Greenhall MBChB BSc MRCP(Neph)
Specialist Registrar in Nephrology
Royal London Hospital
Barts Health NHS Trust
London, UK

Katherine Stockton BSc(Hons) MSc MBBS MRCP(Neuro)
Specialist Registrar in Neurology
Chelsea and Westminster Hospital
London, UK

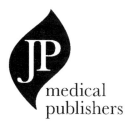

JP
medical
publishers

London • Panama City • New Delhi

ISBN: 978-1-909836-84-6

British Library Cataloguing in Publication Data
A catalogue record for this book is available from the British Library

Library of Congress Cataloging in Publication Data
A catalog record for this book is available from the Library of Congress

Commissioning Editor: Steffan Clements
Editorial Assistants: Adam Rajah, Katie Pattullo
Design: Designers Collective Ltd

Preface

Passing the MRCP examination is a challenging task for trainee physicians, who have to balance the acquisition of medical knowledge, clinical aptitude and communication skills with work, family and social life.

The second edition of *MRCP Part 2: 450 BOFs* is designed to help you prepare for the MRCP Part 2 written examination by providing comprehensive coverage of the curriculum through 450 practice best-of-five questions. The book is designed for the trainee physician who is looking for a broad, evidence-based review of major topics in each specialty. It has been written by experts in the field who have passed the exam themselves relatively recently and who are involved in teaching. All the specialties covered in the MRCP exam are included, with the numbers of questions proportional to the coverage in the exam. Each chapter encompasses a wide range of topics within its specialty, offering a variety of clinical scenarios. Each answer is referenced and based on the most up-to-date evidence and specialty guidelines, and gives a comprehensive explanation which will expand your knowledge of the subject. As in the examination itself, some questions are easier than others and some are more challenging.

Medicine is a constantly changing field and so the book has been completely revised for this new edition. Every question and answer has been reviewed and updated in line with the latest evidence, and 50 questions have been replaced across the book to reflect significant updates to guidelines and changes in best practice.

By passing the MRCP Part 1 you have already demonstrated your knowledge of the basic medical sciences; the MRCP Part 2 examination is designed to test the practical application of that knowledge in clinical situations. We hope this book will provide a useful aid to your revision and a reference for many years to come in your future medical careers. Good luck!

Heather Lewis, Ravi Menon, Luke Moore,
George Greenhall, Katherine Stockton
October 2018

Contents

Exam revision advice

Format

The MRCP(UK) exam consists of three elements. Part 1 is a written exam, whereas Part 2 is split into a written exam and a clinical exam (PACES). Part 2 can be attempted only by candidates who have passed Part 1 within the previous 7 years. The Part 2 written exam and PACES can be attempted in either order. Part 2 tests the candidate's ability to make clinical judgements, apply clinical understanding, plan investigations and make a management plan.

The MRCP(UK) Part 2 written exam has a two-paper format. Each paper lasts 3 hours and consists of 100 multiple choice questions. The examination lasts 1 day. As in the Part 1 exam, questions take a best of five (BOF) approach, where the most appropriate answer must be selected from a choice of five possibilities, with questions covering the full range of medical specialties. However, one major difference between the two exams is that a proportion of Part 2 questions are illustrated with a medical image (e.g. ECG, radiograph, CT, MRI, blood film, photograph of a clinical finding), interpretation of which is key to correctly answering the question. The composition of the papers is demonstrated in **Table 1**.

There is no specific syllabus for the MRCP(UK) Part 2 examination, but the Royal Colleges recommend that candidates refer to the *Specialty Training Curriculum for General Internal Medicine*, prepared by the Joint Royal Colleges of Physicians Training Board.

Table 1 Composition of the MRCP Part 2 exam	
Specialty	**Number of questions***
Cardiology	19
Dermatology	9
Endocrinology and metabolic medicine	19
Gastroenterology	19
Haematology, immunology	9
Infectious diseases and genitourinary medicine	19
Neurology, ophthalmology, psychiatry	23
Oncology and palliative medicine	9
Renal medicine	19
Respiratory medicine	19
Rheumatology	9
Therapeutics and toxicology	18
Geriatric medicine	9
Total	**200**

*Figures should be taken as an indication of the likely number of questions – the actual number may vary by up to 2%. A proportion of the questions will be on adolescent medicine and medicine for elderly people.

The MRCP(UK) Part 2 exam is now marked using a process called equating. This means that rather than being given a percentage overall score, candidates will instead be given an 'overall scaled score'. This is a number between 0 and 999, which is calculated from the number of questions a candidate has answered correctly (out of the maximum possible) and takes into account the relative difficulty of the exam. Since no two exams contain the same questions, some papers may be slightly easier or harder than others. Equating is a statistical process that addresses this. At present, the equated score required to pass MRCP(UK) Part 2 is 454.

Candidates are strongly advised to visit the MRCP(UK) website for further details of the exam.

How to prepare for MRCP(UK) Part 2
Here are some general tips to help prepare for the exam:
- Discuss with your supervisor regarding timing of the examination and whether they think you are ready
- Start early – it is advisable to start revision at least 3 months before the exam date
- Approach revision specialty by specialty
- Cover all topics and read widely, particularly focusing on the topics from which a greater number of questions will be drawn
- Ensure you are familiar with the key UK guidelines including NICE and SIGN, and the main Specialty Society guidelines
- Remember to think laterally when revising – for example, a question on vasculitis could appear in the renal, rheumatology, respiratory, neurology or dermatology sections
- Tackle the questions as you would in the exam, by reading the rubric carefully and thinking of what the correct answer might be before reading the A–E options. Next, select which of the options best fits the answer that you were thinking of
- There are no 'trick' questions, but there are definitely questions that are not as straightforward as they initially appear. Read the question very carefully. In this book only the minimum relevant information necessary to get the correct answer is provided. In the actual exam the questions may be longer but the information given may not necessarily be useful
- Use the information in the answer to confirm and expand upon what you already know, or to help understand and remember why a certain answer is more appropriate than others
- As a large part of the exam is on the practical application of knowledge, you will be expected to know the current guidelines of the various medical societies, which can be found on their websites. Review these before the exam

Medical Society websites
Association of British Neurologists – http://www.theabn.org
British Association of Dermatologists – http://www.bad.org.uk
British Cardiovascular Society – http://www.bcs.com
British Infection Association – http://www.britishinfection.org
British Society of Gastroenterology – http://www.bsg.org.uk
British Society for Haematology – http://www.b-s-h.org.uk
British Society for Rheumatology – http://www.rheumatology.org.uk

British Thoracic Society – http://www.brit-thoracic.org.uk
European Federation of Neurological Societies – http://www.efns.org
European Association for the Study of the Liver - http://www.easl.eu
National Institute for Health and Clinical Excellence (NICE) – http://www.nice.org.uk
Renal Association – http://www.renal.org
Society for Endocrinology – http://www.endocrinology.org

Acknowledgements

We would like to acknowledge the support of their family and friends in writing this book.

We would also like to thank Carolyn Allen, Suzanne Forbes and David Hunt for their contributions to the first edition and Aruna Dias and Eric Beck for editing the first edition.

HL, RM, LM, GG, KS

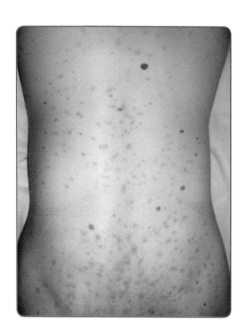

Figure 2.1

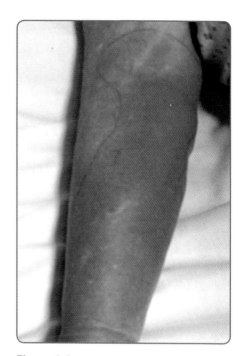

Figure 2.2

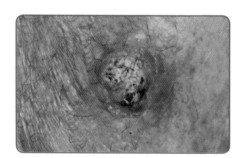

Figure 2.3

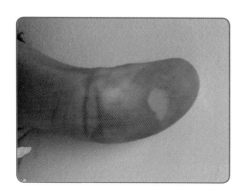

Figure 2.5

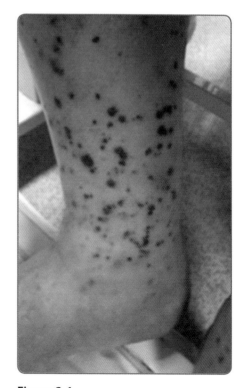

Figure 2.4

Plate 2

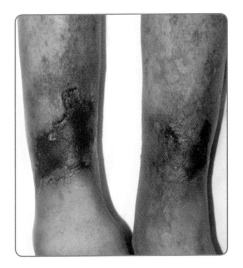

Figure 2.6

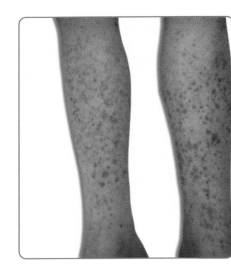

Figure 2.7

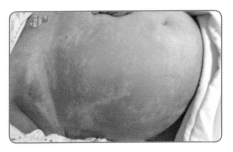

Figure 2.8

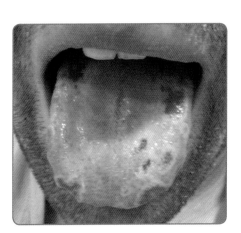

Figure 2.9

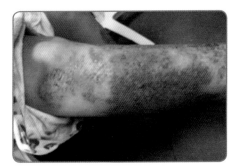

Figure 2.10

Plate 3

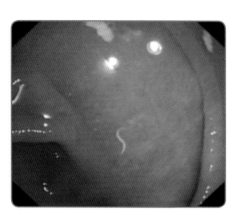

Figure 4.1

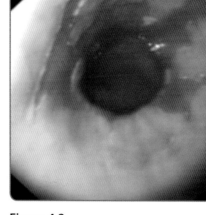

Figure 4.2

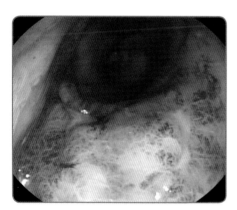

Figure 4.4

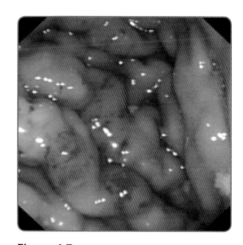

Figure 4.7

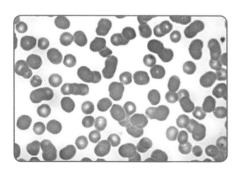

Figure 5.1

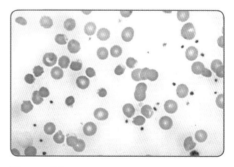

Figure 5.3

Plate 4

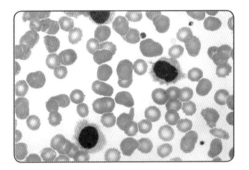

Figure 5.4

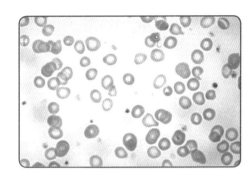

Figure 5.5

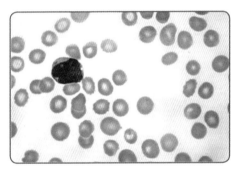

Figure 5.6

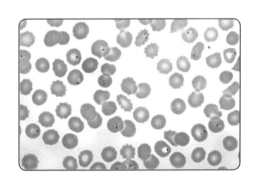

Figure 5.7

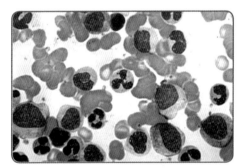

Figure 5.8

Plate 5

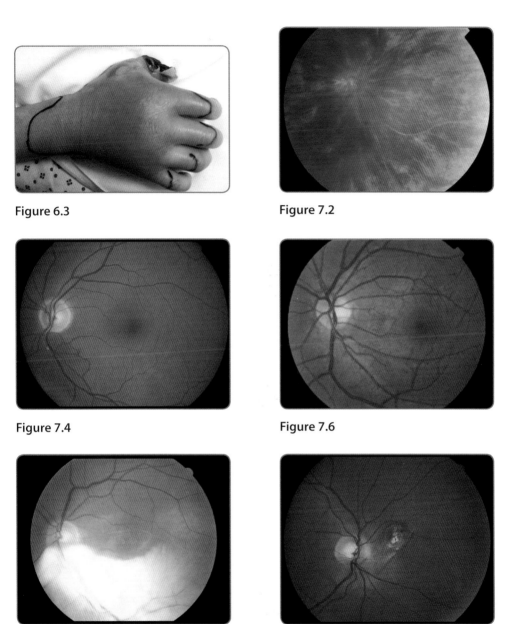

Figure 6.3

Figure 7.2

Figure 7.4

Figure 7.6

Figure 7.8

Figure 7.10

Plate 6

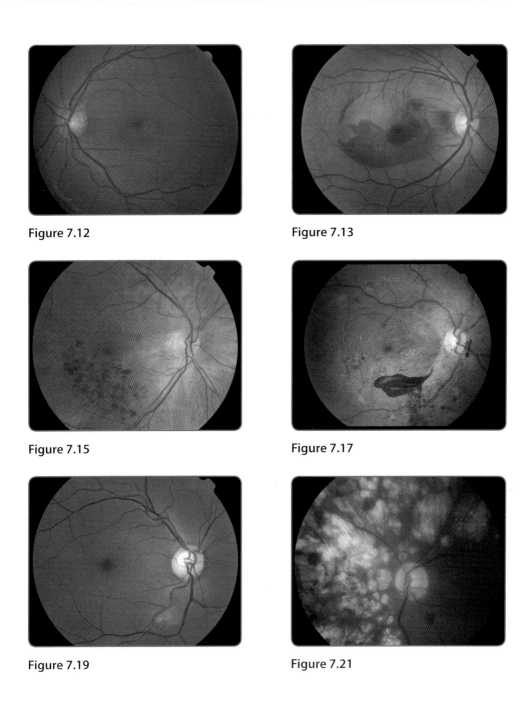

Figure 7.12

Figure 7.13

Figure 7.15

Figure 7.17

Figure 7.19

Figure 7.21

Plate 7

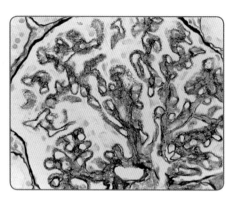

Figure 9.1

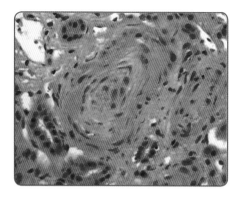

Figure 9.2

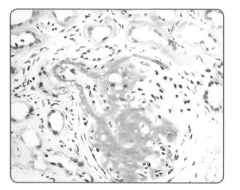

Figure 9.5

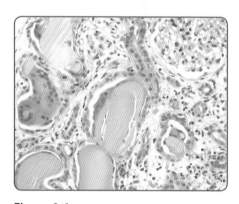

Figure 9.6

Chapter 1

Cardiology

Questions

1. A 34-year-old man presented with a history of acute-onset chest pain lasting 30 minutes. The pain was central and was described as stabbing and of 6/10 severity but had since gone down to a dull ache. He worked as a swimming instructor and had no symptoms prior to this. He had no significant past medical history. His father had had a myocardial infarction aged 52 years and his mother had suffered from angina since the age of 56.

   On examination, his body mass index was 29 kg/m², pulse 98 beats per minute, blood pressure 130/90 mmHg and respiratory rate 34 breaths per minute. Heart sounds were normal and rest of the physical examination was non-contributory.

   Investigations:

haemoglobin 129 g/L (130–180)	creatinine 88 μmol/L (60–110)
white cell count 8 × 10⁹/L (4–11)	albumin 38 g/L (37–49)
neutrophil 6 × 10⁹/L (1.5–7.0)	alanine transaminase 32 U/L (5–35)
sodium 139 mmol/L (135–145)	alkaline phosphatase 67 U/L (45–105)
potassium 4.4 mmol/L (3.5–5.0)	bilirubin 4 mmol/L (1–22)

   Chest X-ray: normal

   Electrocardiogram: see **Figure 1.1**

   What is the most appropriate next step in management?

   A Aspirin, clopidogrel, low molecular weight heparin, intravenous morphine, high flow oxygen and transfer for primary percutaneous coronary intervention
   B Aspirin, sublingual nitrates, bisoprolol, statin and ramipril, and put on the list for coronary angiogram for the next day
   C Therapeutic dose of low molecular weight heparin and order a CT pulmonary angiogram
   D No acute treatment needed but monitor vital signs, repeat ECG and await 6-hour troponin results
   E Echocardiogram to look for the presence of pericardial effusion

2. A 59-year-old man was admitted to hospital with acute onset chest pain which had lasted more than an hour. He was pale, sweaty and clammy.

   On examination, his pulse rate was 100 beats per minute and regular, blood pressure 86/50 mmHg and respiratory rate 24 breaths per minute. Jugular venous pressure was +10 cm. On auscultation, a third heart sound was heard in the left 4th intercostal area close to the sternum. Chest auscultation revealed vesicular breath sounds only. The ECG tracing is shown in **Figure 1.2** [the precordial leads (V1–V6) are right sided].

What is the most appropriate next step in management?

A   Dopamine infusion
B   Intravenous glyceryl trinitrate infusion
C   Intravenous normal (0.9%) saline
D   Levosimendan infusion
E   Noradrenaline infusion

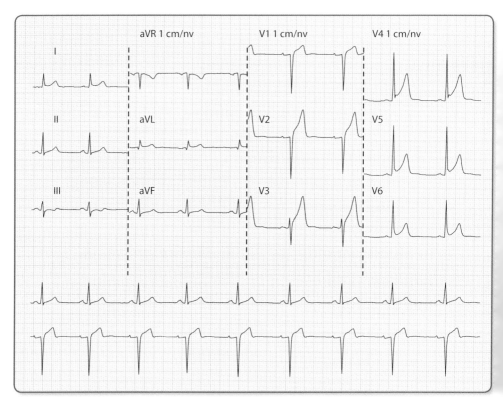

Figure 1.1

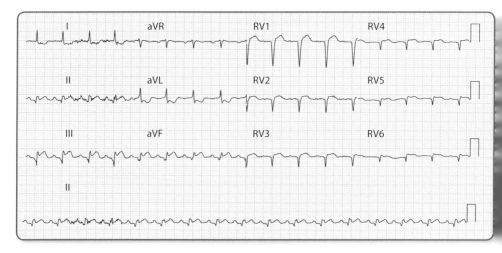

Figure 1.2

3. A 47-year-old man was admitted with peripheral oedema, cough, hoarseness of voice and shortness of breath. He had a history of hypertension and was on bendroflumethiazide 2.5 mg once daily. The only other past history of note was a treated sexually transmitted disease 25 years ago.

    On examination, his pulse was 96 beats per minute and regular, blood pressure 160/40 mmHg and respiratory rate 26 breaths per minute. There was a long, high pitched, decrescendo diastolic murmur in the left third intercostal space, close to the sternum, which was equally well heard in the right 3rd intercostal space.

    Investigations:

    > Chest X-ray:
    > cardiomegaly
    > pulmonary venous congestion

    What is the most appropriate test to confirm the diagnosis?
    A   Antiacetylcholine esterase antibodies
    B   High resolution CT of the chest followed by biopsy
    C   IgG antibodies against *Borrelia burgdorferi*
    D   Rapid plasma reagin test
    E   Video-assisted thoracoscopic biopsy (VATS)

4. A 33-year-old man of Turkish origin was seen in the emergency department with a history of fever, malaise and shortness of breath for the last 15 days. He had no significant past history of note. He had travelled to Turkey several times over the last few years. He did not have any pets or any other contact with animals.

    On examination, his temperature was 39.1°C, pulse 110 beats per minute and regular, blood pressure 110/40 mmHg and respiratory rate 22 breaths per minute. Auscultation revealed a systolic murmur at the apex radiating to the left axilla.

    Investigations:

haemoglobin 112 g/L (130–180)	lymphocytes 4×10^9/L (1.5–4.0)
white cell count 9×10^9/L (4–11)	sodium 139 mmol/L (135–145)
platelets 248×10^9/L (150–400)	potassium 4.5 mmol/L (3.5–5.0)
neutrophils 4×10^9/L (1.5–7.0)	creatinine 98 µmol/L (60–110)

    Urine dipstick: protein 1+, white blood cells 1+, red blood cells 1+

    Echocardiogram:
    moderate mitral regurgitation
    vegetation (2 mm × 2 mm) on the anterior mitral valve leaflet
    billowing of anterior mitral valve leaflet

    Blood cultures (three samples): negative after 5 days

    He was started on benzylpenicillin and gentamicin with no clinical improvement. What is the most appropriate next diagnostic test?
    A   *Bartonella* antibodies
    B   *Brucella* antibodies
    C   Fungal cultures
    D   Surgical biopsy and culture of the vegetation
    E   Transoesophageal echocardiogram to look for root abscess

5. A 38-year-old man was admitted to hospital with a 3-week history of leg swelling, decreased appetite, increased abdominal girth, tiredness and shortness of breath. He had no significant past medical or family history. He had no recent contact with pets and his only travel history of note was to South Africa, 3 years ago.

   On examination, his pulse was 108 beats per minute and regular, blood pressure 110/60 mmHg and respiratory rate 24 breaths per minute. His jugular venous pressure was elevated at +12 cm with sharp x and y descents. There was a sustained inspiratory rise in mean jugular venous pressure (Kussmaul's sign). Cardiac auscultation was normal and abdominal examination revealed shifting dullness and slight hepatosplenomegaly.

Investigations:

haemoglobin 120 g/L (130–180)	sodium 137 mmol/L (135–145)
white cell count 8 × 10⁹/L (4–11)	potassium 4.2 mmol/L (3.5–5.0)
neutrophils 4 × 10⁹/L (1.5–7.0)	creatinine 97 μmol/L (60–110)
lymphocytes 4 × 10⁹/L (1.5–4.0)	brain natriuretic peptide 110 ng/L (<100)
platelets 234 × 10⁹/L (150–400)	N-terminal pro-brain natriuretic peptide 376 pg/mL (N <300)

Abdominal ultrasound:

mild hepatosplenomegaly and ascites

liver echogenicity was mildly increased

Echocardiogram:

normal left ventricular function and size with ejection fraction of 65% (normal >55%)

pulmonary artery systolic pressure 30 mmHg (15–30)

interventricular septum shift to left on inspiration tissue

Doppler echocardiography showed normal early relaxation velocity

Cardiac catheterisation:

equalised right and left ventricular diastolic pressures at 50 mmHg

there was a 'dip and plateau' (square root) pattern of the ventricular pressures

right atrial pressure 18 mmHg (0–8)

What is the most likely diagnosis?

A   Arrhythmogenic right ventricular cardiomyopathy
B   Cardiac amyloidosis
C   Constrictive pericarditis
D   Haemochromatosis
E   Restrictive cardiomyopathy

6. A 46-year-old woman was referred to the cardiology clinic with a history of shortness of breath on exertion for the last 6 months. The only significant past history was a febrile illness in childhood with joint pains. She was originally from Pakistan but had recently emigrated to the UK.

   On examination, her pulse rate was 88 beats per minute, irregularly irregular, blood pressure 110/68 mmHg and respiratory rate 16 breaths per minute. She had a 2/6 mid-diastolic murmur at the apex and mild pitting pedal oedema.

Investigations:

Echocardiography:

enlarged left atrium (3.2 cm × 4.0 cm)

mitral valve stenosis with transvalvar gradient 15 mmHg (normal) and valve area of 1.3 cm² (4–6) with commissural fusion and only minimal calcification

trace mitral regurgitation

pulmonary artery systolic pressure (PASP) 50 mmHg (15–30)

What is the most appropriate next step in the management?

A   Echocardiographic surveillance with surgery if PASP rises to >60 mmHg
B   Mitral valve repair
C   Mitral valve replacement
D   Percutaneous balloon mitral commissurotomy
E   Surgical mitral valvotomy

7.   A 63-year-old man was referred to the cardiology clinic after an annual health evaluation at work showed T-wave inversion in the lateral leads of his ECG. His past medical history included type 2 diabetes, hypertension and asthma. He was on metformin, gliclazide, ramipril and salbutamol inhaler.

On examination, his pulse was 82 beats per minute and regular, blood pressure 110/70 mmHg and respiratory rate 14 breaths per minute. The rest of the physical examination was normal apart from a left carotid bruit.

Blood tests were normal apart from a serum creatinine level of 130 μmol/L (60–110). His eGFR was 51 mL/min/1.73 m².

Exercise tolerance test using modified Bruce protocol showed a 1-mm ST depression in the anterior leads, which recovered after 2 minutes.

Investigations:

Coronary angiography:
85% stenosis in the proximal left anterior descending (LAD) artery
90% stenosis in the right coronary artery (RCA)
60% stenosis of the left main stem (LMS)
65% stenosis of the left circumflex artery (LCx)
Ejection Fraction 50% (normal >55%)

What is the most appropriate next step in management?

A   Coronary artery bypass graft (CABG) surgery
B   Maximise medical therapy by adding a statin and starting insulin
C   Maximise medical therapy by adding high-dose statin and nicorandil
D   Percutaneous coronary intervention with stents to the RCA and LAD
E   Percutaneous coronary intervention with stents to the RCA, LAD and LCx

8.   A 72-year-old woman was admitted with shortness of breath on exertion for the last week. She had also had palpitations during this period. She had hypertension, for which she was on ramipril 5 mg once daily. On examination, her pulse rate was 140 beats per minute and irregular, blood pressure 130/70 mmHg, respiratory rate 24 breaths per minute and temperature 37.3°C. Pulse oximetry showed oxygen saturation on air of 96%. Heart sounds were normal and chest was clear to auscultation.

Investigations:

sodium 141 mmol/L (135–145)	haemoglobin 120 g/L (115–165)
potassium 4.5 mmol/L (3.5–5.0)	white cell count 8 × 10⁹/L (4–11)
urea 9 mmol/L (2.5–7.5)	platelets 135 × 10⁹/L (150–400)
creatinine 90 μmol/L (45–90)	

Chest X-ray: normal

Electrocardiogram: see **Figure 1.3**

    C   Implantable cardioverter defibrillator (ICD)
    D   Initiate beta-blocker therapy
    E   Septal myomectomy

12. A 59-year-old man presented with shortness of breath. He had breathlessness on minimal exertion but no chest pain; there was some swelling of his feet. Past history included ischaemic heart disease with two previous myocardial infarctions and a coronary artery bypass graft (CABG). He also had a history of hypertension and hyperlipidaemia.

    He had been under the care of the heart failure clinic for 8 months and was on ramipril 5 mg once daily, bisoprolol 7.5 mg once daily, simvastatin 40 mg once daily, aspirin 75 mg once daily, spironolactone 12.5 mg once daily and furosemide 40 mg twice daily.

    On examination, his temperature was 37.2°C, pulse rate 56 beats per minute and regular, blood pressure 104/50 mmHg and respiratory rate 18 breaths per minute. He had pitting pedal and ankle oedema. Jugular venous pressure was +9 cm, the apex was displaced laterally but the hearts sounds were normal. ECG showed sinus rhythm with a PR interval of 180 ms, intraventricular conduction block with QRS duration of 160 ms and poor R-wave progression in the anterior chest leads.

    Stress echocardiogram revealed an akinetic segment in the anterior wall of the left ventricle (LV), dilated LV with an ejection fraction of 30% (normal >55%) and mild mitral regurgitation. There was no evidence of reversible ischaemia.

What is the most appropriate therapeutic option?

    A   Amiodarone
    B   Biventricular pacemaker–defibrillator
    C   Coronary angiogram with percutaneous coronary intervention to any blocked vessels detected
    D   Dual-chamber pacemaker
    E   Implantable cardioverter defibrillator

13. A 39-year-old woman was admitted with upper abdominal pain and a small amount of haematemesis. She was known to have a cardiac murmur. She was treated with proton pump inhibitors and was scheduled to have an upper gastrointestinal endoscopy. She had been under cardiology follow-up for the cardiac murmur and had an echocardiogram 2 months ago. She was asymptomatic from the cardiac point of view.

Investigations:

Echocardiogram:
mitral valve prolapse with moderate mitral regurgitation
LV end-diastolic diameter 42 mm (39–53)
LV ejection fraction 65% (>55%)
pulmonary artery systolic pressure 32 mmHg (15–30)
other valves normal

Electrocardiogram: sinus rhythm and no abnormalities

What is the most appropriate course of action?

    A   Chlorhexidine mouthwash for infective endocarditis prophylaxis prior to endoscopy
    B   Intravenous amoxicillin 2 g (30–60 minutes) prior to endoscopy
    C   No infective endocarditis prophylaxis required
    D   Oral amoxicillin 2 g (30–60 minutes) prior to endoscopy
    E   Postpone endoscopy until a stress echocardiogram can be arranged

14. A 56-year-old man was seen in the clinic after being diagnosed with hypertension and was put on amlodipine 5 mg once daily. There was no other significant past history. He smoked five cigarettes per day and had a small glass of wine most days. On examination, his pulse was 88 beats per minute, blood pressure 156/88 mmHg and respiratory rate 14 breaths per minute. Heart sounds were normal and chest was clear. On abdominal examination, a pulsatile mass was felt in the upper abdomen.

    Ultrasound of the abdomen showed a 4.2 cm diameter suprarenal abdominal aortic aneurysm. Watchful waiting was initiated and an ultrasound 6 months later showed a 5.3 cm aneurysm.

    What is the next most appropriate step in management?

    A   Aggressive medical management with blood pressure target of <125/75 mmHg and statin therapy, monitor every 6 months and repair if aneurysm size >6 cm
    B   Perform a MR angiogram for wall characteristics and operate if high risk of rupture
    C   Endovascular/open surgical repair of the aneurysm
    D   Repeat ultrasound or CT in 3 months' time and advise repair if aneurysm diameter exceeds 5.5 cm
    E   Repeat ultrasound or CT in 6 months' time and advise repair if aneurysm diameter exceeds 5.5 cm

15. A 71-year-old man was referred to the emergency department with a history of central chest pain at rest. It lasted 15 minutes and had resolved by the time he reached the emergency department. He had had chest pain on and off for the last week. Episodes lasted 15–20 minutes and were often relieved by sublingual glyceryl trinitrate spray. He had a history of medically treated angina for the last 8 years. His other past medical history included hypertension and hypercholesterolaemia. He was on atenolol 50 mg once daily, ramipril 2.5 mg once daily, simvastatin 40 mg once daily and aspirin 75 mg once daily.

    On examination, his pulse was 68 beats per minute, blood pressure 106/66 mmHg and respiratory rate 22 breaths per minute. JVP was not elevated and chest was clear. He was started on enoxaparin and clopidogrel 300 mg followed by 75 mg once daily. The rest of the medications were continued.

    Investigations:

    creatinine 98 µmol (60–110)   troponin 10.9 µg/L (<0.04)

    Electrocardiogram: see **Figure 1.5**

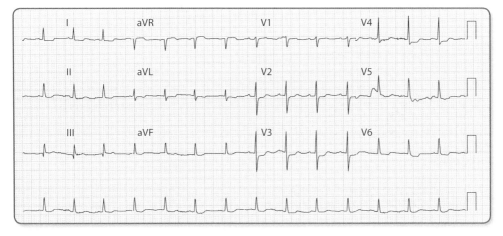

Figure 1.5

What is the most appropriate next step in management?

A   Add glycoprotein IIb/IIIa inhibitor
B   Immediate left heart catheterisation
C   Maximise medical therapy by adding nicorandil and substituting simvastatin with atorvastatin 80 mg once daily
D   Plan left heart catheterisation within the next 24 hours
E   Plan left heart catheterisation within next 72 hours

16. A 17-year-old boy was referred to the emergency department after suffering from palpitations and shortness of breath at a party. He had no past history of note apart from asthma for which he was on salbutamol and budesonide inhalers. He had one previous admission to an intensive treatment unit because of acute severe asthma. He admitted to taking an unknown substance that his friends gave him during the party. There was no previous history of illicit drug use.
    On examination, his pulse was 200 beats per minute and regular, blood pressure 104/54 mmHg, respiratory rate 24 breaths per minute and oxygen saturation 96% on air.
    ECG: see **Figure 1.6**.

What is the next most appropriate step in management?

A   Adenosine 6 mg intravenous bolus followed by saline bolus
B   Amiodarone 150 mg intravenously over 10 minutes
C   DC cardioversion with 100 J energy
D   Metoprolol 5 mg intravenously over 1 minute
E   Verapamil 2.5 mg intravenously over 2.5 minutes

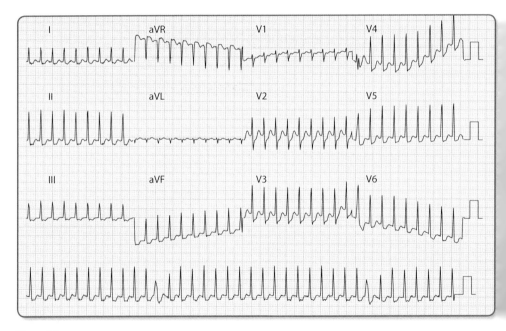

Figure 1.6

17. A 60-year-old man was seen at a screening visit for a community-based research trial on diet and lifestyle modification to prevent diabetes. He had no significant past medical history and was not on any medications. He was found to have an irregular heart beat and a subsequent ECG showed atrial fibrillation at a rate of 110 beats per minute.

Blood tests, including urea and electrolytes, full blood count, thyroid and liver function tests, were normal.

His general practitioner started him on bisoprolol 2.5 mg once daily and referred him for an echocardiogram which showed normal atrial dimensions and good left ventricular function. Considering that he was asymptomatic and due to patient preference, rate control was accepted as the management strategy.

What is the next most appropriate step in management?

A   Low-molecular-weight heparin followed by oral anticoagulation
B   No anti-coagulation/anti-platelet therapy
C   Oral aspirin 75 mg once daily
D   Oral aspirin 75 mg once daily and dipyridamole 200 mg twice daily
E   Start on oral anticoagulation

18. An 86-year-old man was brought to the emergency department following an episode of chest pain. It is 8/10 in severity. He also had an episode of brief loss of consciousness a few weeks ago. On closer questioning he mentioned that he had been finding it increasingly difficult to do activities such as shopping and gardening. He had shortness of breath when walking more than 10–15 metres. His other past medical history included osteoarthritis of the hips, for which he had a right hip replacement 10 years ago. He used one stick and was unable to cook or shop for himself.

On examination, his pulse was 86 beats per minute, blood pressure 110/85 mmHg, and respiratory rate 18 breaths per minute. He had a weak pulse, heaving apex and an ejection systolic murmur loudest at the aortic area and radiating to the carotids.

Investigations:

> Electrocardiogram: sinus rhythm and left ventricular (LV) hypertrophy
>
> ---
>
> Echocardiogram:
> mild LV dilatation with LV hypertrophy
> LV ejection fraction 50% (>55%)
> calcified aortic valve with valve area of 0.8 cm^2 (3–4)
> transvalvar gradient 55 mmHg (0)
> mitral valve normal E/A (early to late ratio) 0.9 (0.98–2.78)
> pulmonary valve normal
> mild tricuspid regurgitation
> pulmonary artery systolic pressure 32 mmHg (15–30)

What is the most appropriate next step in management?

A   Arrange social and palliative care
B   Balloon aortic valvotomy
C   Medical management including high-dose statins
D   Open aortic valve replacement
E   Transcatheter aortic valve implantation

19. A 45-year-old woman was referred to the clinic with a history of shortness of breath for the past 6 months. She had progressive exertional breathlessness and now could walk only a few hundred metres. She also had one episode of loss of consciousness. She had noticed swelling of her ankles for the last 3 weeks. Her only past medical history was of hay fever in childhood. She was a non-smoker and only drank 3–4 units of alcohol a week. She was not on any medication. Her general practitioner had started her on salbutamol and beclomethasone inhaler with no improvement.

On examination, her pulse was 88 beats per minute, blood pressure 140/86 mmHg, respiratory rate 24 breaths per minute and oxygen saturation 94% on room air.

Investigations:

Full blood count, urea and electrolytes, liver function test: normal
Autoantibody screen: negative
Chest X-ray: clear lung fields, normal cardiac size

Lung function tests:
forced expiratory volume in 1 second 2.9 L (120% predicted)
forced vital capacity 3.5 L (130% predicted)
total lung capacity 5.8 L (120% predicted)
carbon monoxide diffusion in the lung 92%

Echocardiogram:
left ventricle size normal
LV (left ventricular) ejection fraction 64% (>55)
normal aortic and pulmonary valves
right ventricle dilated, mild tricuspid regurgitation
pulmonary artery systolic pressure – 60 mmHg

CT of the chest: normal
Ventilation–perfusion (/) scan: low probability for thromboembolic disease

What is the most appropriate next investigation?

A   Bronchoalveolar lavage
B   Cardiac catheterisation
C   CT-guided lung biopsy
D   CT pulmonary angiography
E   Sweat chloride testing

20. A 28-year-old woman was admitted with shortness of breath on minimal exertion and pedal oedema. She had a Caesarean section 2 months ago following failure of induction with pessary and oxytocin at term. During the pregnancy she had gestational hypertension but no evidence of pre-eclampsia. Her previous two deliveries were normal. She was a non-smoker and did not drink any alcohol.

On examination, her pulse was 94 beats per minute and regular, blood pressure 100/50 mmHg, respiratory rate 20 breaths per minute and temperature 36.7°C. Jugular venous pressure was elevated at 12 cm, first and second heart sounds were normal, and there was a left ventricular third heart sound as well as a long systolic murmur at the apex.

Investigations:

sodium 139 mmol/L (135–145)	creatinine 96 µmol/L (45–90)
potassium 4.3 mmol/L (3.5–5.0)	troponin I 0.9 µg/L (<0.04)
urea 9 mmol/L (2.5–7.5)	

NTpBNP (N-terminal pro-brain natriuretic peptide) 1860 pg/mL (N <300)
Thyroid function test: normal
Serology for cytomegalovirus, Coxsackievirus and HIV: negative
Antinuclear antibody: negative

Chest X-ray:
cardiomegaly with upper lobe venous dilatation
small bilateral pleural effusions

Contd...

> Electrocardiogram: sinus tachycardia, left axis deviation, P mitrale and tall R waves in V4–V6
>
> ---
>
> Echocardiogram:
> dilated left ventricle with end-diastolic diameter 5.7 cm
> LV ejection fraction 35%
> mild mitral and tricuspid regurgitation
> dilated left atrium
> pulmonary artery systolic pressure 35 mmHg (15–30)

What is the most likely diagnosis?

A   Cor pulmonale due to pulmonary thromboembolism
B   Hypertensive heart failure
C   Idiopathic dilated cardiomyopathy unmasked by pregnancy
D   Myocardial infarction related to coronary vasculitis
E   Peripartum cardiomyopathy

21. A 56-year-old man presented to the emergency department with sudden severe pain in the central chest and back that occurred while he was playing tennis. He had a past history of hypertension for which he was on amlodipine 5 mg once daily. He was an ex-smoker. The pain was 7/10 in severity and associated with mild sweating and nausea.

     On general examination, he was 188 cm tall and weighed 82 kg. Heart rate was 98 beats per minute and regular, blood pressure 190/98 mmHg, respiratory rate 20 breaths per minute and oxygen saturation on air 96%. Heart sounds were normal but there was a short early diastolic murmur at the third left intercostal space.

Investigations:

> Electrocardiogram: sinus tachycardia and chest X-ray was normal

What would be the most appropriate next investigation?

A   Cardiac troponin
B   CT aortogram
C   CT pulmonary angiogram
D   Transthoracic echocardiogram (TTE)
E   Ventilation–perfusion scan after D-dimer

22. A 57-year-old woman was admitted with a history of progressive shortness of breath. She did not have any chest pain. She had a past history of hypertension (for which she was on ramipril 10 mg once daily and amlodipine 2.5 mg once daily), hypercholesterolaemia (on simvastatin 20 mg nocte) and had had breast carcinoma, which was resected 10 years ago.

     On examination, her pulse was 98 beats per minute and regular, blood pressure 106/58 mmHg, respiratory rate 24 breaths per minute and oxygen saturation on air 95%. Jugular venous pressure was elevated with an inspiratory increase in pressure. Heart sounds were normal. Chest was clear to auscultation. Abdominal examination showed an enlarged tender liver and moderate ascites. There was pitting oedema up to mid-shin level. There was an inspiratory decrease in blood pressure of 15 mmHg.

Investigations:

> Chest X-ray: enlarged cardiac silhouette with normal lung
> ---
> Echocardiogram:
> pericardial effusion with 1.4 cm fluid between pericardium and right ventricle
> right atrial collapse during diastole
> right ventricular collapse in early diastole
> LV ejection fraction 62% (>55)

What is the next most appropriate step in the management?

A   Abdominal ultrasound
B   Cardiac MRI
C   CT of the chest, abdomen and pelvis
D   Diagnostic pericardiocentesis
E   Therapeutic pericardiocentesis

23. A 27-year-old woman was seen in the clinic with a history of progressive shortness of breath for the past 3 weeks. She was 16 weeks pregnant and was awaiting an antenatal clinic appointment. She had no significant past medical history. However, her mother mentioned that she had a heart murmur at birth but she had been subsequently lost to follow-up.

   On examination, her pulse was 98 beats per minute, blood pressure 106/58 mmHg, respiratory rate 18 breaths per minute and oxygen saturation on air 95%. The first heart sound was soft and there was wide fixed split of the second with accentuation of P2. There was a parasternal heave. There was a 2/6 ejection systolic murmur at the second left intercostal space and a 2/6 pansystolic murmur at the apex.

Investigations:

> Electrocardiogram: first-degree heart block and left axis deviation

What is the most likely diagnosis?

A   Ostium primum atrial septal defect
B   Ostium secundum atrial septal defect
C   Patent foramen ovale
D   Trilogy of Fallot
E   Ventricular septal defect

24. A 54-year-old man was admitted to the coronary care unit with central chest heaviness and shortness of breath of 2 hours' duration. ECG showed ST elevation in V3–V6 and I and aVL, and he subsequently underwent primary percutaneous coronary intervention with stenting to the left circumflex artery.

   He was discharged from the hospital on the fourth day after admission on aspirin, clopidogrel, ramipril, atorvastatin and bisoprolol. There was no significant past medical history.

   Two weeks later he came to the emergency department with recurrent chest pain, malaise, tiredness and diffuse joint aches. He described the chest pain as sharp, over the precordium and left chest, and radiating to the left shoulder.

Investigations:

haemoglobin 138 g/L (130–180)	sodium 141 mmol/L (135–145)
white cell count 16×10^9/L (4–11)	potassium 3.9 mmol/L (3.5–5.0)
platelets 375×10^9/L (150–400)	urea 8 mmol/L (2.5–7.5)
erythrocyte sedimentation rate 80 mm/1st h (0–20)	creatinine 102 µmol/L (60–110)
C-reactive protein 145 mg/L (<5)	troponin I 0.45 µg/L (<0.04)
neutrophils 12×10^9/L (1.5–7.0)	bilirubin 5 mmol/L (1–22)
lymphocytes 3×10^9/L (1.5–4.0)	albumin 40 g/L (37–49)
monocytes 1×10^9/L (0–0.8)	alanine aminotransferase 45 U/L (5–35)
	alkaline phosphatase 68 U/L (45–105)

Electrocardiogram: concave upwards ST elevation in leads I, II, aVL, aVF and V2–V6

Chest X-ray: normal cardiac contour and a small left pleural effusion

Pleural tap: protein 43 g/L (30)
white cell count 20 x 10^9/L (<1)

lactate dehydrogenase (LDH) 150 U/L = [plasma LDH 120 U/L (10–250)]
(normal pleural fluid to serum ratio 0.6)
no malignant cells or culture
Gram and acid-fast bacillus stain and cultures: negative

Echocardiogram:
dilated left ventricle with end-diastolic diameter 5.7 cm
LV ejection fraction – 35% (>55)
mild mitral and tricuspid regurgitation
dilated left atrium
pulmonary artery systolic pressure 35 mmHg (15–30)

On examination, his temperature was 38.9°C, pulse 70 beats per minute, blood pressure 110/60 mmHg and respiratory rate 18 breaths per minute. There was mild pitting pedal oedema. Jugular venous pressure was not elevated and cardiac auscultation revealed normal heart sounds and a scratchy sound, best heard in the left lower sternal edge on leaning forward. There was reduced air entry in the left lower lobe with dullness to percussion

What is the most appropriate next step in management?

A   Aspirin 300 mg four times daily
B   Blood cultures and start ceftriaxone and gentamicin intravenously
C   Pleural biopsy
D   Urgent coronary angiogram
E   Viral serology for Coxsackievirus, cytomegalovirus, HIV and Epstein–Barr virus

25. A 24-year-old man was seen in the clinic with gradual shortness of breath on exertion. He was from Burkina Faso originally and had been in the UK for the last 2 years. He had had these symptoms for the past few years, but now his exercise tolerance was reduced to 400 metres on the flat; he could manage only one flight of stairs.

His past history was of recurrent respiratory illnesses and two bouts of malaria. His mother who had accompanied him said that he used to have episodes of shortness of breath with blue lips in childhood which was relieved by squatting down.

On examination, his temperature was 37.5°C, pulse 98 beats per minute, blood pressure 104/65 mmHg, respiratory rate 18 breaths per minute and oxygen saturation 92% on room air.

He had finger clubbing and central and peripheral cyanosis. The apex beat was undisplaced but there was a parasternal heave. There was a normal first heart sound, a single second sound, best heard in the right 2nd intercostal space and an ejection systolic murmur in the left second intercostal space.

ECG: see **Figure 1.7**.

What is most likely diagnosis?

A   Atrial septal defect with reversal of shunt
B   Eisenmenger's disease
C   Fallot's tetralogy
D   Noonan's syndrome
E   Patent ductus arteriosus with reversal of shunt

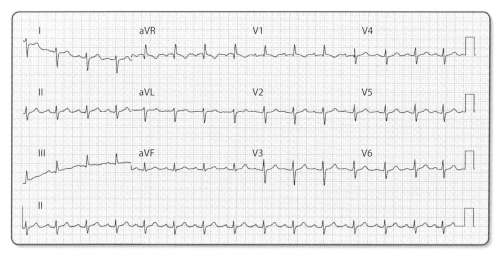

Figure 1.7

26. A 48-year-old man was seen in the emergency department with shortness of breath for the last few days. He was an ex-smoker and had been diagnosed with chronic obstructive pulmonary disease previously. He was on salbutamol, ipratropium, fluticasone and tiotropium inhalers. There was no other past history of note.

On examination, his temperature was 37.4°C, pulse 152 beats per minute, blood pressure 110/60 mmHg, respiratory rate 30 breaths per minute and oxygen saturation 90% on air. Chest auscultation revealed bilateral polyphonic wheeze, but no crepitations and equal air entry.

He was given hydrocortisone 100 mg intravenously, salbutamol and ipratropium nebulisers, and started on oxygen 4 L/min.

ECG: see **Figure 1.8**.

What is the most appropriate next step in management?

A   Adenosine 6 mg rapid intravenously
B   DC cardioversion
C   Digoxin 500 µg intravenously
D   Flecainide 300 mg orally
E   Verapamil 5 mg intravenously

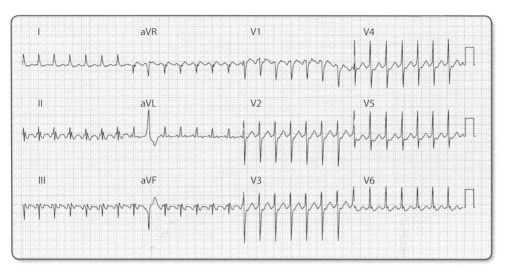

Figure 1.8

27. A 56-year-old man was admitted with congestive cardiac failure. On the third day after admission he collapsed in the ward. The initial rhythm was asystole. Cardiopulmonary resuscitation (CPR) was initiated with chest compression and the airway was secured.

What is the most appropriate next step in management?

A DC cardioversion biphasic 150 J × 1
B Intravenous adrenaline 10 mL of 1 in 10,000 solution (1 mg/10 mL)
C Intravenous adrenaline 10 mL of 1 in 1000 solution (1 mg/mL)
D Intravenous atropine 3 mg single dose
E Intravenous calcium gluconate 10 mL

28. A 68-year old woman was admitted with a history of chest pain of 2 hours' duration, which woke her up from sleep. Her ECG showed ST elevation in the lateral leads as well as T inversion. She had been referred 2 months earlier to a rapid access chest pain clinic and had been discharged after having a normal exercise tolerance test. On closer questioning she had had episodes of chest pain lasting up to 15–20 minutes for the last year. She could not recall any specific triggering factors. Her only other past medical history was of osteoarthritis affecting her knees, hips and fingers. She was on diclofenac and a paracetamol–codeine combination for pain relief.

Troponin I was positive at 1.8 µg/L (<0.04). She was started on aspirin, clopidogrel, bisoprolol, ramipril and simvastatin.

She underwent a left heart catheterisation on the day of admission, which showed only minor <50% blockages in the coronary arteries. Left ventricular size and function were within normal limits. Clopidogrel was discontinued. Serial ECGs showed resolution of the previous ST depression.

What is the most appropriate next step in management?

A Optimise the dose of non-steroidal anti-inflammatories and opiates for pain relief
B Repeat coronary angiogram and do flow studies across the area of blockage
C Stop all medications and follow up as an outpatient
D Stop beta-blockers and start diltiazem and nitrates
E Titrate beta-blockers and add nitrates if episodes of chest pain persist

29. A 57-year-old man was referred by the general practitioner for shortness of breath on exertion. There was no chest discomfort or coughing. He had a past history of type 2 diabetes and hypertension. He had been on holiday in Spain 2 months ago where he had some chest discomfort and shortness of breath for 2 days, which he attributed to the heat and humidity. After coming back, he had progressive shortness of breath which took him to the general practitioner.

On examination, his temperature was 37.2°C, pulse 100 beats per minute, blood pressure 100/60 mmHg and oxygen saturation 94% on room air. Jugular venous pressure was +12 cm, his apex was difficult to locate, and he had a left-sided third heart sound (S3). There were some basal crackles in his lungs.

ECG: see **Figure 1.9**.

What is the most likely cause of his symptoms?

A   Acute anterior ST segment elevation myocardial infarction with left ventricular failure (LVF)
B   Brugada's syndrome
C   Left main stem artery stenosis with recurrent angina and LVF
D   Previous anterior myocardial infarction with left ventricular aneurysm and LVF
E   Previous anterior myocardial infarction with LVF and papillary muscle dysfunction

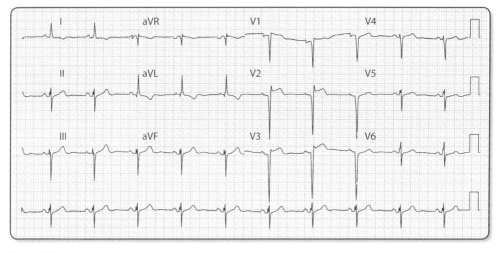

Figure 1.9

30. A 79-year-old man was admitted with two episodes of syncope. Over the last 3 months, he had had episodes of dizziness and had lost consciousness twice. There were no seizures and he was not disoriented after regaining consciousness. He was on amlodipine for hypertension and simvastatin for high cholesterol. There was no other relevant past medical history.

ECG: see **Figure 1.10**.

What is the most likely diagnosis?

A   First-degree heart block
B   Sinus bradycardia with sinus pause
C   Complete heart block
D   Trifascicular block
E   2:1 second-degree heart block

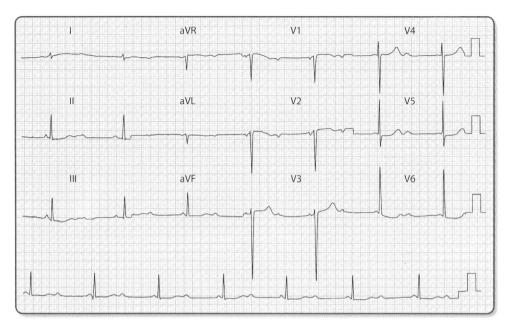

Figure 1.10

31. A 78-year-old woman was admitted with weakness in her right arm and difficulty in speaking which started the day before. On admission, her temperature was 37.3°C, pulse 92 beats per minute, blood pressure 160/100 mmHg and oxygen saturation 96% on air. Her chest was clear, heart sounds were normal and there was right hemiparesis.

She later had a short run of non-sustained ventricular tachycardia (NSVT) on the monitor. A subsequent CT of the head confirmed an infarct in the left middle cerebral artery territory. She was started on antiplatelet agents.

ECG: see **Figure 1.11.**

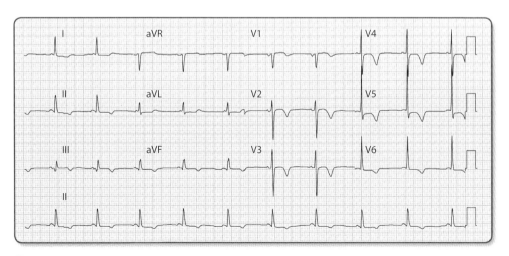

Figure 1.11

What is the next most appropriate management?

A   Start amiodarone and evaluate for implantable cardioverter defibrillator (ICD) implantation, once acute phase resolves
B   Start antiplatelet agents and beta-blockers; monitor cardiac markers and serial ECGs
C   Arrange for percutaneous coronary intervention in the next 2–3 days
D   Arrange urgent echocardiogram
E   Consider thrombolysis or primary percutaneous intervention urgently

32. A 28-year-old man was admitted with acute-onset shortness of breath and chest pain. He had a non-productive cough. He had just flown back to London from a trip to Shanghai. His immunisations were up to date and he reported no night sweats or myalgia. He had no significant past history of illnesses apart from childhood asthma and was not on any medication. He did not smoke.

   On examination, his temperature was 37.6°C, pulse 110 beats per minute, blood pressure 100/50 mmHg, respiratory rate 20 breaths per minute and oxygen saturation 91% on air. He had a pleural rub and some crackles in the left lower zone; a third heart sound was heard in the left lower sternal edge.

   ECG: see **Figure 1.12**.

What is the most appropriate diagnostic investigation?

A   CT angiogram for aortic dissection
B   CT pulmonary angiogram
C   D-dimer assay
D   Echocardiogram
E   Peak flow assessment

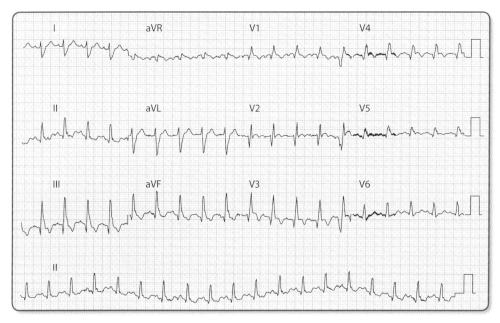

Figure 1.12

33. A 46-year-old man was admitted with history of abdominal pain, diarrhoea and dizzy spells. CT of the abdomen had revealed a mass in the head of the pancreas 2.3 × 1.2 cm in size. There was no lymph node enlargement or other lesions on the CT. He was awaiting the results of a gut hormone panel and was being investigated for a neuroendocrine tumour, and a CT-guided biopsy of the mass was planned. He did not have any significant past medical history and was not on any medications.

The next morning, he collapsed with sudden onset of severe right-sided chest pain. His pulse was 140 beats per minute, blood pressure 70/40 mmHg, respiratory rate 34 breaths per minute and oxygen saturation 87% on air. ECG showed sinus tachycardia and a partial right bundle-branch block (RBBB) pattern.

Despite being resuscitated with intravenous fluids, oxygen, heparin and inotropes, after 10 minutes the blood pressure was still 60 mmHg systolic and oxygen saturation 88% on 15 L O_2/min.

What is the most appropriate next step in management?

A   Coronary angiography and stenting
B   CT pulmonary angiogram
C   Emergency echocardiogram
D   Start clopidogrel and abciximab
E   Start intravenous alteplase

34. A 26-year-old man was admitted with shortness of breath on walking 200 metres. He had progressive shortness of breath over the past year. He was a heavy smoker but had cut down in the last year. He had no significant past history apart from being told that he had a heart murmur as a child. He was taking no medication.

On examination, there was no central cyanosis but he had clubbing of his toes and a systolic murmur at the left upper sternal edge radiating to the left infraclavicular region.

What is the most likely cause?

A   Patent ductus arteriosus with reversal of shunt
B   Rupture of sinus of Valsalva into the right ventricle
C   Tetralogy of Fallot
D   Total anomalous pulmonary venous return
E   Ventricular septal defect with reversal of shunt

35. A 54-year-old woman was seen in the clinic with a history of fever, night sweats and malaise. She also had shortness of breath on brisk walking and climbing stairs. She had no significant past history of illnesses, no recent travel history and no relevant family history. She was not on any medications apart from paracetamol taken on an as required basis.

On examination, her temperature was 38.9°C, pulse 88 beats per minute, blood pressure 110/60 mmHg and oxygen saturation 94% on room air. Her chest was clear but there was a mid-diastolic murmur with an added sound which was variable on position.

Investigations:

Electrocardiogram: sinus rhythm and P mitrale

Echocardiogram:
4 mm structure attached to the atrial septum and prolapsing into the left ventricle with a trans-mitral valve mean gradient of 14 mmHg (normal 0).

What is the most likely diagnosis?

A   Left atrial myxoma
B   Leiomyosarcoma of the interatrial septum

    C   Mitral regurgitation with infective endocarditis
    D   Mitral stenosis with infective endocarditis
    E   Mitral valve prolapse with infective endocarditis

36. A 59-year-old man was admitted with a 2-day history of chest pain and shortness of breath. He had a past history of type 2 diabetes controlled with metformin and pioglitazone. He was also on ramipril for hypertension.

    He was admitted and started on aspirin, clopidogrel, fondaparinux and subcutaneous twice daily mixed insulin. He had a coronary angiogram and insertion of two stents to the posterior descending artery and left circumflex artery.

    On the third day of admission, his shortness of breath was more severe with a pulse rate of 98 beats per minute and blood pressure 110/70 mmHg. On examination, jugular venous pressure was elevated at 10 cm and auscultation revealed a gallop rhythm and a grade 3 systolic murmur, heard best at the apex and radiating to the base. There was no radiation to the axilla. There were crackles at both lung bases.

What is the most likely diagnosis?

    A   Dressler's syndrome
    B   Left ventricular free wall rupture
    C   Mitral regurgitation due to anterolateral papillary muscle rupture
    D   Mitral regurgitation due to posteromedial chordal rupture
    E   Ventricular septal rupture

37. A 26-year-old man of Romanian origin was admitted with history of shortness of breath. He had had fever with rigors and chills intermittently for the last week. For the past day he had had weakness and pain in the left arm. He did not have any significant past medical history and denied any recreational drug use.

    On examination, his temperature was 39.4°C, pulse 112 beats per minute, blood pressure 92/50 mmHg, respiratory rate 24 breaths per minute and oxygen saturation 94% on air. Jugular venous pressure was elevated +6 cm and there was an early diastolic murmur best heard in the 3rd left intercostal space in expiration. Auscultation of the lungs revealed bi-basal crackles. There was some weakness in the left hand.

Investigations:

haemoglobin 102 g/L (130–180)	lymphocytes 3×10^9/L (1.5–4.0)
mean corpuscular volume 84 fL (80–96)	sodium 138 mmol/L (135–145)
white cell count 26×10^9/L (4–11)	potassium 5.0 mmol/L (3.5–5.0)
platelets 349×10^9/L (150–400)	urea 8 mmol/L (2.5–7.5)
neutrophils 23×10^9/L (1.5–7.0)	creatinine 114 µmol/L (60–110)

Urinalysis: protein 2+, blood 2+, leukocytes +, nitrites negative

Electrocardiogram: sinus tachycardia

Transoesophageal echocardiogram:
normal left ventricular size with hyperdynamic systolic function
left ventricular (LV) ejection fraction 60% (>55)
aortic valve bicuspid with three masses on the leaflets as well as leaflet disruption
largest mass 7 mm in size
moderate aortic regurgitation with high LV end-diastolic pressure
fluid present around the aortic annulus

Ultrasound: infarct of left kidney

What is the most appropriate next step in management?

A   Immediate aortic valve surgery under antibiotic cover
B   Start antibiotics and monitor clinical condition
C   Start antibiotics and plan aortic valve replacement after 48 hours of antibiotics
D   Start antibiotics, unfractionated heparin and monitor
E   Start antibiotics, warfarin and monitor

38. A 50-year-old woman was admitted with a history of shortness of breath, swelling of her ankles, poor appetite, bruising and constipation. She could only walk 200 metres on the flat. She had noticed that she had bruises on her chest and around her eyes, but there was no history of any trauma. She did not have any significant past medical history and denied any recreational drug use.

On examination, her temperature was 36.9°C, pulse 92 beats per minute, blood pressure 112/50 mmHg, respiratory rate 18 breaths per minute and oxygen saturation 94% on air. There was no pallor, cyanosis or jaundice.

Ecchymotic patches were present around the eyes and on the trunk. Macroglossia was present with teeth marks around the edges of the tongue. Jugular venous pressure was elevated +6 cm and there was a left ventricular third heart sound (S3). Chest auscultation revealed bi-basal crackles.

Investigations:

haemoglobin 102 g/L (115–165)	lymphocytes 3×10^9/L (1.5–4.0)
mean corpuscular volume 82 fL (80–96)	sodium 138 mmol/L (135–145)
white cell count 9×10^9/L (4–11)	potassium 5.1 mmol/L (3.5–5.0)
platelets 210×10^9/L (150–400)	urea 8.1 mmol/L (2.5–7.5)
neutrophils 6×10^9/L (1.5–7.0)	creatinine 134 µmol/L (45–90)

Urinalysis: protein 2+

Electrocardiogram: sinus rhythm, low-voltage complexes

Echocardiogram:
left atrium enlarged at 5.2 cm
LV (Left ventricular) mild enlargement
LV ejection fraction 40% (>55)
moderate LV hypertrophy with LV septal thickness of 2.0 cm (0.6–0.9)
posterior wall thickness of 1.7 cm (0.6–0.9)
LV diastolic dysfunction present
myocardium had a 'ground-glass' appearance

What is the most appropriate diagnostic investigation?

A   Abdominal fat pad aspiration
B   Left heart catheterisation
C   Serum angiotensin-converting enzyme level
D   Serum ferritin level
E   Urine metanephrines

39. A 23-year-old woman was referred by her GP after being noted to have a heart rate of 40 beats per minute. She works as a part-time geologist and is a competitive swimmer. She does not smoke, take recreational drugs or have any significant past medical history. Her blood pressure is 102/66 mmHg and her physical examination is normal. There is no history of syncope or pre-syncope. She is booked to go to Australia for a swimming tournament next week.

Investigations:

> ECG: sinus rhythm with a PR interval of 118 ms, QRS duration of 80 ms
>
> 24-hour Holter monitor: nocturnal heart rate of 38 beats per minute and occasional pauses as long as 2.5 seconds

What would you advise?

A   Implant an 'implantable loop recorder' device for recording cardiac electrical activity
B   No further follow-up is needed, and she may travel and compete
C   Obtain a 48-hour Holter monitor tracing
D   Perform electrophysiologic evaluation for a pacemaker
E   She should not compete and will need a tilt-table test

40. A 62-year-old man with longstanding hypertension and poorly-controlled diabetes was referred to the cardiology clinic with a history of several months of breathlessness on exertion, episodes of breathlessness in the middle of the night, and significant leg and ankle swelling. On examination, he had an elevated jugular venous pulse and fourth heart sound (LVS4) on auscultation.

Investigations:

> ECG: sinus rhythm and P mitrale
>
> Echocardiogram: a left ventricular ejection fraction of 55% with a large left atrium
>
> *N*-terminal pro-brain natriuretic peptide (NT pro-BNP): elevated

Which drugs would have a beneficial effect in lowering his mortality?

A   Ramipril
B   Bisoprolol
C   Spironolactone
D   Digoxin
E   None of the above

41. A 32-year-old junior doctor with no significant past medical history came to the emergency department with shortness of breath and fatigue. He mentioned that he had 'flu-like' symptoms for the last week, but had worked his usual shifts in the hospital and had only taken paracetamol for symptom control. He had a pulse rate of 120 beats per minute and a blood pressure of 75/52 mmHg. His capillary refill was 4 seconds and jugular venous pulse was elevated. Cardiac auscultation showed quiet heart sounds and a systolic murmur at the apex.

Investigations:

> Echocardiogram:
>
> no pericardial effusionleft ventricle (LV) nondilated
>
> LV ejection fraction 25% (55–65)
>
> mild–moderate mitral regurgitation

What is the most appropriate treatment?

A   Immediate implantation of a left ventricular assist device and listing for cardiac transplantation
B   Listing for cardiac transplant immediately as studies show <10% survival without urgent transplantation
C   Urgent cardiac MRI, endomyocardial biopsy and anti-viral agents such as oseltamivir

    D   Urgent high-dose steroid therapy with intravenous methylprednisolone followed by steroid sparing immunosuppressants later

    E   Urgent inotropic support and possibly temporary mechanical circulatory support in the intensive care unit

42. A 74-year-old woman with a history of diabetes, hyperlipidaemia and knee ostoarthritis had primary percutaneous coronary intervention to an acutely occluded left anterior descending artery 3 weeks ago, having presented with anterior STEMI. An everolimus-eluting stent was inserted and she was discharged after 4 days on aspirin, clopidogrel, atorvastatin, bisoprolol, ramipril, gliclazide, metformin and insulin glargine.

    She developed significant right knee pain and was referred to an orthopaedic surgeon. Given significant mobility issues and pain, the surgeon suggested a total knee replacement. The surgeon wrote to the cardiology clinic asking for options regarding stopping anti-platelet therapy.

What is the most appropriate advice?

    A   Continue on dual anti-platelet therapy indefinitely and then proceed towards surgery with careful planning to minimise bleeding

    B   Postpone surgery for at least 6 months or even 12 months and then have surgery off clopidogrel

    C   Stop aspirin, continue clopidogrel and proceed with knee surgery

    D   Stop both aspirin and clopidogrel and proceed with knee surgery

    E   Stop clopidogrel, continue aspirin, and proceed with knee surgery

Answers

1. D No acute treatment needed but monitor vital signs, repeat ECG and await 6-hour troponin results

The ECG trace is suggestive of early repolarisation syndrome. There is a J wave present (elevation of the QRS complex – ST segment junction) in at least two leads (V4, V5 and V6 here) and concave upward elevation of the ST segment. Inferolateral leads are most commonly involved. If the right precordial leads (V1–V3) are involved, Brugada's syndrome and arrhythmogenic right ventricular cardiomyopathy (ARVC) must be ruled out.

Early repolarisation has been long considered a benign variant and is easily obliterated by exercise. However, attention has been focused on its possible relationship with sudden cardiac death.

Answers A and B are essentially treatment of ST elevation myocardial infarction and unstable angina, and is not appropriate in this instance.

Although the ECG pattern is suggestive of early repolarisation, it does not preclude underlying cardiac disease especially if there is a family history of premature ischaemic heart disease, and hence monitoring and checking a 6-hour troponin is appropriate. Newer troponin assays can give an answer in 3 hours, but are not available in all centres.

The history and ECG pattern are not suggestive of pulmonary embolism or pericarditis and hence answers C and E are incorrect. The most common ECG abnormality in pulmonary embolism is tachycardia with occasionally incomplete or complete right bundle-branch block and other signs of right ventricular strain. Widespread concave upward elevation of the ST segment is observed in pericarditis, but J point elevation is not a characteristic pattern.

Haissaguerre M, et al. Sudden cardiac arrest associated with early repolarization. N Engl J Med 2008; 358:2016–2023.

2. C Intravenous normal (0.9%) saline

The ECG shows inferior ST elevation myocardial infarction (MI) with right ventricular involvement. Those with inferior MI often tend to have right ventricular involvement as well. The best lead to assess right ventricular involvement is right-sided V4. To detect right ventricular myocardial infarction (RVMI), an ECG with right precordial leads should be done at admission for those presenting with inferior MI.

Right ventricular involvement classically results in a triad of low blood pressure; elevated jugular venous pressure (JVP) and absence of signs of pulmonary oedema (i.e. clear lung fields on auscultation). Right ventricular third heart sound is often heard.

RVMI usually occurs along with left ventricular myocardial infarction (LVMI) and not in isolation. It mostly occurs in conjunction with inferior wall MI. Thin wall, lower pressures and good collaterals with lower oxygen requirements mean that RVMI is relatively rare. RVMIs are more often complicated by all types of arrhythmias compared with 'simple' inferior or anterior wall LVMIs.

RVMI leads to poor contractility of right ventricle leading to increased right atrial pressure, elevated JVP and venous congestion resulting in peripheral oedema. Furthermore, flow into the pulmonary artery is reduced, resulting in reduced left ventricular preload and hence low systolic blood pressure.

Volume expansion with 0.9% saline is the first step in order to increase the left ventricular preload and systolic pressure. Once adequate volume expansion has been achieved (e.g. with one litre of normal saline) and if haemodynamic instability persists then dobutamine infusion or dobutamine with noradrenaline infusion may be tried. Dopamine use results in increased mortality in cardiogenic shock.

Glyceryl trinitrate would further reduce the left ventricular preload and is contraindicated in this situation. RV assist devices have also been used.

Ondrus T, Kanovsky J, Novotny T, Andrsova I, Spinar J, Kala P. Right ventricular myocardial infarction: From pathophysiology to prognosis. Experimental & Clinical Cardiology. 2013;18(1):27–30.

Buerke M, et al. Pathophysiology, diagnosis, and treatment of infarction-related cardiogenic shock. Herz 2011; 36(2):73–83.

3. D Rapid plasma reagin test

The clinical features are suggestive of severe aortic regurgitation because of widening of the aortic root (aortic root aneurysm). Given the previous history of sexually transmitted infection, tertiary syphilis with cardiovascular manifestations must be considered. In advanced cases, aortic root aneurysm leads to severe volume overload of the left ventricle with gross left ventricular hypertrophy and dilatation (cor bovinum or bovine heart). Cough and hoarseness of voice may be due to compression of the bronchus and the left recurrent laryngeal nerve by the enlarged aortic root.

The standard serological test for syphilis consists of the rapid plasma reagin test or the VDRL (Venereal Disease Reference Laboratory) test (98% sensitive in tertiary syphilis) followed by a confirmatory test such as the FTA-Abs (fluorescent treponemal antibody – absorption) test.

Antiacetylcholine esterase antibodies are positive in myasthenia gravis (which may be associated with thymoma causing mediastinal widening). In this case symptoms are not suggestive of myasthenia.

Borrelia burgdorferi causes Lyme disease which may lead to a myocarditis or cardiac conduction blocks, but not aortic root widening.

Video-assisted thorascoscopic surgery biopsy and CT-guided biopsy are not indicated in cases of aortic root widening.

4. B *Brucella* antibodies

The clinical and echocardiographic features point to infective endocarditis. The lack of neutrophilia and relative lymphocytosis, in the presence of fever, points towards unusual or fastidious organisms. There is no history to suggest an immunocompromised status. This, combined with the travel history, leads to the possibility of *Brucella* endocarditis. Endocarditis is a rare feature in brucellosis; however, travel in the endemic area and typical presentation of culture-negative endocarditis should raise the suspicion. Brucellosis can be acquired by ingestion of unpasteurised milk.

Bartonella causes trench fever and cat scratch disease. The patient has no history suggestive of contact with cats. Although fungal cultures should be asked for in culture-negative endocarditis, there is no specific history here that would raise the suspicion of fungal endocarditis.

Although aortic root abscess is a possibility when the clinical condition does not improve after appropriate antibiotics, the situation here is of culture-negative endocarditis with relative lymphocytosis. Transoesophageal echocardiogram (TOE) is helpful especially in cases where transthoracic echocardiogram (TTE) is negative.

Treatment is usually with a combination of doxycycline, rifampicin and co-trimoxazole for up to 3 months. Other drugs include fluoroquinolones and streptomycin. Often surgical treatment is required as well. Treatment is monitored by looking at the antibody titres. *Brucella melitensis* results in more severe infection compared with *Brucella abortus*.

Andriopoulos P, Antoniou C, Manolakou P, Vasilopoulos A, Assimakopoulos G, Tsironi M. Brucella endocarditis as a late onset complication of brucellosis. Case Rep Infect Dis 2015; 2015:836826.

5. C Constrictive pericarditis

The clinical picture is suggestive of right heart failure. Rapid x and y descents and elevated jugular venous pressure on inspiration (Kussmaul's sign) suggest either restrictive cardiomyopathy or constrictive pericarditis (cardiac tamponade would lead to distended neck veins with absent y descent and paradoxical pulse). The interventricular septal shift on inspiration again suggests a constrictive physiology rather than restrictive. The normal tissue Doppler (early relaxation myocardial velocity) suggests that myocardial relaxation was normal and hence right ventricular cardiomyopathy was less likely.

Cardiac catheterisation in constrictive pericarditis classically shows:
1. Elevated right atrial pressure
2. Relative equalisation of left and right ventricular diastolic pressures which are usually elevated
3. Kussmaul's pattern (elevation of right atrial and ventricular pressures on inspiration)

4. Elevated right ventricular systolic pressure
5. Exaggerated x and y descents in the right atrial pressure pattern
6. Dip and plateau pattern (square root sign) of the right or left ventricular pressures

Brain natriuretic peptide values, which are near normal, also support constrictive over restrictive physiology.

Correlation of these signs with the clinical symptoms and signs is essential. In many cases pericardial thickening is not evident on echocardiography. This is better seen with a high-resolution CT (HRCT) of the chest or MRI. However, the pericardium may not be thickened in constrictive pericarditis and thickened pericardium by itself does not prove constrictive physiology. Calcification of the pericardium is usually seen with tuberculosis.

Given the travel history, tuberculous constrictive pericarditis is a possibility here. However, many cases of pericarditis are idiopathic (thought to be due to past viral infections, e.g. with Coxsackievirus, adeno- or hepatitis viruses). The three dominant aetiologies reported now in North America and Europe are idiopathic, prior cardiac surgery, and radiation therapy.

Cardiac amyloidosis results in a restrictive pattern of heart failure.

Welch TD, Oh JK. Constrictive Pericarditis. Cardiol Clin 2017; 35:539–549.

6.   D Percutaneous balloon mitral commissurotomy

The history and echocardiographic findings are suggestive of rheumatic mitral stenosis. Rheumatic mitral valve involvement is associated with leaflet thickening, calcification, chordal fusion and fusion of the commissures. Normal mitral valve area is 4–5 cm^2; however, symptoms of mitral stenosis start developing when the valve area drops below 1.5 cm^2. Symptoms can develop with exercise even when the valve area is between 1.5 and 2.5 cm^2.

Mitral stenosis results in left atrial dilatation and pulmonary hypertension. Severity of mitral stenosis is graded based on the valve area, pressure gradient across the valve and pulmonary systolic pressure (see **Table 1.1**).

Table 1.1 Assessment of severity of mitral stenosis			
Severity	Valve area (cm^2)	Mean transvalvar gradient (mmHg)	Pulmonary artery systolic pressure (mmHg)
Mild	>1.5	<5	<30
Moderate	1–1.5	5–10	30–50
Severe	<1	>10	>50

This classification has now been revised by the American Heart Association (AHA)/American College of Cardiology (ACC) and the new guidelines issued in 2014 divide severity into:

- **At risk** – echocardiography shows mitral valve doming
- **Progressive mitral stenosis** - commissural fusion and diastolic doming is present but the planimeteric mitral valve area (MVA) is still >1.5 cm^2, diastolic pressure half time (T1/2) is >150 ms and there is only mild to moderate left atrial enlargement with normal pulmonary pressures. Patient is asymptomatic.
- **Asymptomatic severe mitral stenosis** – valve features of mitral stenosis; MVA < 1.5 cm^2; MVA <1 cm^2 (very severe mitral stenosis); T1/2 >150 ms; severe left atrial enlargement and elevated pulmonary artery systolic pressure (PASP) > 30 mmHg.
- **Symptomatic severe mitral stenosis** – same features as above but with decreased exercise tolerance or exertional dyspnoea.

Treatment depends on symptoms and severity of the valve stenosis. It also depends on the presence of associated valvular lesions such as mitral regurgitation or aortic lesions. Atrial fibrillation is common due to left atrial dilatation and would need anticoagulation and rate control. Patients with asymptomatic mild mitral stenosis should be monitored yearly in clinic and have an ECG and chest X-ray done. Echocardiography should be repeated if disease progression is suspected. No specific intervention or treatment is required.

In asymptomatic patients with moderate mitral stenosis, exercise evaluation should be performed, and if it shows low capacity they should be offered percutaneous mitral commisurotomy (PMV), sometimes called percutaneous balloon mitral commissurotomy (PBMC) if suitable, or surgical options. If exercise evaluation shows normal capacity, but has any of the high-risk features, PBV or surgical options must still be considered.

Patients with symptoms and severe mitral stenosis, and those with significant pulmonary hypertension (>50 mmHg systolic) should be offered PBMC. However, people with significant mitral regurgitation, severe calcification of the leaflets or significant sub-valvar thickening and calcification are not suitable for balloon valvotomy and are best treated with open valvotomy or mitral valve replacement.

Contraindications for PBMC are LA thrombus, more than mild MR, severe or bi-commissural calcification, absence of commissural fusion, severe concomitant aortic valve disease/severe combined tricuspid stenosis and regurgitation requiring surgery and concomitant coronary artery disease requiring CABG.

Nishimura RA, et al. American College of Cardiology/American Heart Association Task Force on Practice Guidelines. 2014 AHA/ACC guideline for the management of patients with valvular heart disease: executive summary: a report of the American College of Cardiology/American Heart Association Task Force on Practice Guidelines. J Am Coll Cardiol 2014; 63:2438–2488.
Baumgartner H, et al. ESC Scientific Document Group. 2017 ESC/EACTS Guidelines for the management of valvular heart disease. Eur Heart J 2017; 38:2739–2791.

7. A Coronary artery bypass graft (CABG) surgery

This patient has diabetes and multi-vessel coronary artery disease. In such a setting, the outcomes with CABG are better. This is especially true with left internal mammary artery grafts to left anterior descending artery. His other indications for CABG as opposed to percutaneous coronary intervention (PCI) are three-vessel disease, left main stem involvement and mildly depressed left ventricular systolic function.

An additional point is the presence of a left carotid bruit, which needs to be resolved prior to surgery. Carotid Doppler should be followed by a decision to treat/not treat based on symptoms and degree of stenosis.

PCI is being increasingly used to treat patients with multi-vessel disease as well as in patients with left main stem disease, especially those who are not fit for surgery. There are no clear contra-indications for surgery in this patient and hence the best option here is CABG.

Maximising medical therapy by adding a statin and antianginal therapy is a logical decision in this patient. However, answer B is not correct as there are no clear grounds to switch to insulin with the information given in the question. Switching to insulin is a decision dependent on the overall glycaemic control and success with the current regimen. There is insufficient information here to make the decision.

Intensive glucose lowering with insulin–dextrose infusion did bring down mortality in acute ST elevation myocardial infarction (STEMI) in the DIGAMI 1 trial. However, subsequent trials have failed to yield the same benefit. Current guidelines only give it as a class II recommendation due to insufficient evidence. In this case, the patient does not have acute STEMI and hence the guidelines do not apply.

Answer C is also not the preferred one here as the angiographic picture is best treated by CABG.

Fihn SD, Blankenship JC, Alexander KP, et al. 2014 ACC/AHA/AATS/PCNA/SCAI/STS focused update of the guideline for the diagnosis and management of patients with stable ischemic heart disease: a report of the American College of Cardiology/American Heart Association Task Force on Practice Guidelines, and the American Association for Thoracic Surgery, Preventive Cardiovascular Nurses Association, Society for Cardiovascular Angiography and Interventions, and Society of Thoracic Surgeons. Circulation 2014; 130:1749–1767.

8.   D Oral metoprolol and enoxaparin therapeutic dose

The ECG shows atrial fibrillation at a rate of 130 beats per minute. There are also some T-wave changes in the lateral leads.

The patient is haemodynamically stable and from the history it is likely that she developed the atrial fibrillation in the last week. Hence, there is no indication for DC cardioversion at present. Chemical or DC cardioversion should only be attempted after an adequate period of anticoagulation to prevent thromboembolism, since it is >48 hours after onset. If facilities for transoesophageal echocardiography (TOE) are available at short notice, then TOE can be used to look for the presence of left atrial thrombus and if absent, cardioversion can be carried out under heparin cover.

In this clinical scenario (haemodynamically stable atrial fibrillation 48 hours after onset) rhythm control and anti-coagulation are preferred.

She does not have any contra indications for beta-blocker therapy from the history and examination and she is clinically stable; hence, beta blockers would be the drug of choice. Enoxaparin followed by warfarin is also indicated in a 72-year-old with history of hypertension and no other contra-indication for anti-coagulation.

To determine the need for anti-coagulation, CHA2DS2-VASc scoring is used (**Table 1.2**). A score of >2 suggest the need for anti-coagulation. If the patient's CHA2DS2-VASc score is 'low risk' (i.e. 0 in men or 1 in women), anticoagulant therapy is not recommended. In males with one stroke risk factor (i.e. a CHA2DS2-VASc score of 1), antithrombotic therapy with oral anti-coagulant may be considered, and patients' values and preferences should be considered.

Table 1.2 CHADS2-VAS score		
	Condition	**Points**
C	Congestive heart failure (or left ventricular systolic dysfunction)	1
H	Hypertension: blood pressure consistently above 140/90 mmHg (or treated hypertension on medication)	1
A2	Age ≥75 years	2
D	Diabetes mellitus	1
S2	Prior stroke or TIA or thromboembolism	2
V	Vascular disease (e.g. peripheral artery disease, myocardial infarction, aortic plaque)	1
A	Age 65–74 years	1
Sc	Sex category (female/male)	1

Several bleeding scores are also used to assess risk of bleeding on anticoagulants such as HAS-BLED [hypertension, abnormal renal/liver function (1 point each), stroke, bleeding history or predisposition, labile INR, elderly (>65 years), drugs/alcohol concomitantly (1 point each)]. A high bleeding risk score should generally not result in withholding OAC. Rather, bleeding risk factors should be identified and treatable factors corrected.

Verapamil and diltiazem are the other first-line agents in cases where beta-blockers are contra indicated. However, she is clinically stable, so there is no clear indication for intravenous verapamil.

Digoxin is no longer recommended as the first-line agent in atrial fibrillation but is used as a second line agent.

After rate control and anti-coagulation, she should be considered for rhythm control depending on echocardiographic and other features.

Kirchhof P, Benussi S, Kotecha D, et al. 2016 ESC Guidelines for the management of atrial fibrillation developed in collaboration with EACTS. Eur J Cardiothorac Surg 2016; 50:e1–e88.

9. D No medical therapy

The ECG shows Wolff–Parkinson–White (WPW) syndrome. Characteristics of WPW syndrome in an ECG are:

1. Short PR interval <120 ms
2. Wide QRS complex >120 ms with slurred (slowed) initial deflection of the QRS complex (delta wave)
3. ST-T changes

These features, when associated with an episode of tachycardia, are called WPW syndrome.

WPW syndrome is due to the presence of an abnormal conduction pathway between the atria and ventricles (bundle of Kent or accessory pathway). Apart from the atrioventricular (AV) node and the His–Purkinje fibres, the atria and ventricles are electrically isolated from each other. The bundle of Kent offers another pathway via the ventricular musculature for the electrical impulses to reach the ventricles from the atria. Impulses passing through this accessory pathway (AP) produce a wider, 'fusion' QRS complex as the ventricular muscle is activated first, as represented by the initial delta wave, followed by activation of the His–Purkinje system occurring via the normal conduction pathway. On the other hand, this accessory pathway bypasses the normal AV nodal delay, thus resulting in the shorter PR interval (pre-excitation). Concealed WPW syndrome occurs when the AP conducts retrogradely only from ventricles to atria and hence normal sinus beats show a narrow QRS complex with normal PR interval.

Typically, the AP has more rapid conduction but a longer refractory period compared with the AV node. The most common arrhythmia in WPW syndrome is narrow complex AV re-entry tachycardia. The second most common is atrial fibrillation (AF), which occurs in about half of people with WPW syndrome. In individuals who have rapid conduction from the atria to the ventricles via the AP, the AP can conduct without the associated AV nodal delay resulting in rapid ventricular rates. This can result in shock and can lead to ventricular fibrillation (VF). QRS complexes are often wide in this instance and can change from beat to beat, especially if there are fusion beats from the conduction through the AV node as well.

In cases of AF with WPW syndrome and complexes showing pre-excitation, drugs that inhibit the AV node such as digoxin and verapamil are contraindicated. Hence digoxin, beta-blockers (apart from sotalol) and non-dihydropyridine calcium channel blockers such as verapamil and diltiazem should be only cautiously used in WPW syndrome with pre-excitation AF as they may increase the conduction through the AP. Digoxin and verapamil given intravenously tend to shorten the refractory interval of the AP, resulting in faster ventricular rates and may increase the risk of AF. When there is no haemodynamic compromise, procainamide, amiodarone or ibutilide can be used. If the patient is haemodynamically unstable, DC cardioversion should be used. There are, however, some reports stating that amiodarone could induce ventricular fibrillation in pre-excitation AF.

In tachyarrhythmias without the pre-excitation, AV nodal slowing can be used. For long-term therapy, the best option is electrophysiological evaluation and ablation of the AP. For narrow complex tachycardias, beta-blockers and calcium channel blockers can be used. In this patient who presented with wide complex AF with haemodynamic compromise and ECG after cardioversion, showing classical features of WPW syndrome, the best treatment would be catheter ablation which has over 90% success rate, regardless of age. If medical therapy is preferred for whatever reason, especially where ablation has failed or arrhythmias have recurred, class Ia, Ic or III drugs such as quinidine, flecainide, amiodarone and propafenone are preferred as they increase the refractoriness and slow the conduction rate of the AP.

Kirchhof P, Benussi S, Kotecha D, et al. 2016 ESC Guidelines for the management of atrial fibrillation developed in collaboration with EACTS. Eur J Cardiothorac Surg 2016; 50:e1–e88.
Fengler BT, Brady WJ, Plautz CU. Atrial fibrillation in the Wolff–Parkinson–White syndrome: ECG recognition and treatment in the ED. Am J Emerg Med 2007; 25(5):576–583.
Thanavaro JL, Thanavaro S. Clinical presentation and treatment of atrial fibrillation in Wolff–Parkinson–White syndrome. Heart Lung 2010; 39(2):131–136.

10. B Bisoprolol

Cocaine blocks the re-uptake of noradrenaline and dopamine at the presynaptic adrenergic terminals, causing an accumulation of catecholamines at the postsynaptic terminal and is hence a powerful sympathomimetic. Cocaine can induce coronary ischaemia via arterial spasm as well as by increasing myocardial oxygen demand (increased heart rate and contraction because of adrenergic stimulation). Cocaine is also known to increase platelet adhesion and enhance thrombosis.

Coronary spasm is due to vasoconstriction via α-adrenergic stimulation as well as by increasing endothelin-1, which is a powerful vasoconstrictor. Aspirin would therefore be indicated since cocaine has effects on platelet adhesion. Benzodiazepines are also indicated especially in acute cocaine intoxication.

Angiotensin-converting enzyme inhibitors are also not contraindicated as they do not have much effect on the sympathetic system. Nitroglycerin is a vasodilator and is useful in reducing the high blood pressure induced by cocaine and also in relieving vasospasm.

Calcium channel blockers such as diltiazem and nitroglycerin are the first line agents for treatment of cocaine-associated chest pain.

Beta blockers, on the other hand, can cause unopposed α-adrenergic stimulation and hence can enhance vasospasm and increase blood pressure. Hence, they are to be used with caution in acute cocaine intoxication. There are very few randomised control trials on the use of betablockers in this population. Observational and retrospective studies indicate that they may not cause harm and may help with refractory tachycardia and hypertension in this group.

Finkel JB, Marhefka GD. Rethinking cocaine-associated chest pain and acute coronary syndromes. Mayo Clin Proc 2011; 86:1198–207.

11. C Implantable cardioverter defibrillator

The echocardiographic findings suggest hypertrophic cardiomyopathy (HCM). It should be noted that cardiac MRI (CMR) is being increasing used in the diagnosis of HCM and may identify pre-diagnostic spectrum of HCM changes. CMR helps distinguish between hypertrophy of different types and HCM. Late gadolinium enhancement, non-contrast-enhanced T1 mapping and equilibrium contrast enhancement CMR are helpful techniques in this regard.

Although there is systolic anterior motion of the anterior mitral valve leaflet, the mitral regurgitation is mild. The left ventricular outflow tract (LVOT) gradient is 20 mmHg and this, along with the absence of other symptoms, suggests that he does not need septal ablation or myomectomy. Although dual chamber pacing would improve the outflow tract obstruction, in isolation it is not indicated here. Sudden cardiac death is a very real threat in the case of hypertrophic cardiomyopathy and risk stratification is important. Approximately 6% of non-diagnosed cases of HCM can result in SCD. ICD is recommended as secondary prevention in people with previous sustained VT and cardiac arrest. In terms of primary prevention, the following factors are considered.

The risk of sudden cardiac death is higher if:
- There is family history of sudden cardiac death related to HCM
- One or more unexplained recent syncopal episodes
- Significant LV hypertrophy with wall thickness >30 mmHg
- Non-sustained ventricular tachycardia (NSVT) on ambulatory ECG monitoring
- Attenuated or hypotensive blood pressure response to exercise.

In those aged 18–50 years, the presence of one or more of these risk factors would merit consideration for an implantable cardioverter defibrillator (ICD) implantation. In those aged 65 years or more, a stronger risk factor profile needs to be present prior to ICD implantation.

There are other secondary risk factors to be considered as well, such as: LVOT gradient >30 mmHg, LV apical aneurysm, certain genetic mutations such as double sarcomere mutations and *LAMP2*, late gadolinium enhancement in cardiac MRI and end-stage phase with widespread scarring.

Management of HCM is dependent on obstructive versus non-obstructive phenotype in HCM. Left ventricular outflow tract (LVOT) obstruction (gradient >30 mm Hg) may occur at rest or may be provoked with physical activity and is evident in the majority of patients with HCM. In comparison with obstructive HCM, non-obstructive HCM is associated with lower annual rate of progression to advanced, NYHA three or four heart failure symptoms.

For patients with symptomatic, obstructive HCM, initial management includes medications that increase diastolic ventricular filling time (preload) and reduce contractility – beta-blockers, non-dihydropyridine calcium channel antagonists and disopyramide. If these are no longer effective – surgical myomectomy is the first line treatment. Alcohol septal ablation has lower effectiveness. Mitral valve repair for SAM (systolic anterior motion) is also used for symptom management.

In this case, this young man has a strong family history of sudden cardiac death and episodes of NSVT in Holter monitoring, as well as a recent episode of unexplained syncope. Even in the absence of significant abnormalities in exercise testing, he would be a strong candidate for ICD implantation.

Fraiche A, Wang A. Hypertrophic cardiomyopathy: new evidence since the 2011 American Cardiology of Cardiology Foundation and American Heart Association Guideline. Curr Cardiol Rep 2016; 18:70.
Marron BJ. Contemporary insights and strategies for risk stratification and prevention of sudden death in hypertrophic cardiomyopathy. Circulation 2010; 121:445–456.

12. B Biventricular pacemaker–defibrillator

This person has New York Heart Association (NYHA) class 4 symptoms. He is already under the care of the heart failure (HF) clinic and is on optimised medical therapy. His ECG shows a widened QRS complex, his echocardiogram shows an ejection fraction less than 35% and there is no reversible ischaemia.

Under these circumstances he has a significant risk of death due to arrhythmia. However, a single chamber ICD would not do anything for his symptoms.

A biventricular pacemaker–defibrillator, on the other hand, would allow for resynchronisation of right and left ventricles [cardiac resynchronisation therapy (CRT)] and might result in symptomatic improvement.

CRT should be considered in chronic HF patients and LVEF ≤35% who remain in NYHA class II, III and ambulatory IV despite adequate medical treatment and who have non-LBBB with QRS duration >150 ms. If QRS duration is 120–150 ms, the benefits are uncertain. CRT in patients with chronic HF with QRS duration <120 ms is not recommended.

Brignole M, Auricchio A, et al. 2013 ESC Guidelines on cardiac pacing and cardiac resynchronization therapy: The Task Force on cardiac pacing and resynchronization therapy of the European Society of Cardiology (ESC). Developed in collaboration with the European Heart Rhythm Association (EHRA). Eur Heart J 2013; 34:2281–2329.

13. C No infective endocarditis prophylaxis required

There have been changes in the recent guidelines for infective endocarditis (IE) prophylaxis since it has been recognised that there is no firm evidence to suggest that routine IE prophylaxis is of any benefit. Some harm may be present due to the potential for anaphylaxis.

The National Institute of Health and Care Excellence and the European Society of Cardiology recommend that infective endocarditis prophylaxis be given to those at the highest risk of IE and only for the most infection-prone procedures. Currently only people with prosthetic heart valves, previous IE and certain congenital heart diseases are recommended to have IE prophylaxis.

Most dental procedures, upper and lower gastrointestinal endoscopy, bronchoscopy, and obstetric and urological procedures need not be accompanied by IE prophylaxis.

Antibiotic prophylaxis must be limited to patients with the highest risk of IE undergoing the highest risk dental procedures (i.e. procedures requiring manipulation of the gingival or periapical region of the teeth, or perforation of the oral mucosa). According to current European Society of Cardiology guidelines, prophylaxis would be indicated in:
a. Patients with a prosthetic valve, including transcatheter valve
b. Patients with previous IE

c.   Patients with congenital heart disease:
    –   any cyanotic congenital heart disease
    –   congenital heart disease repaired with prosthetic material

Good oral hygiene and regular dental review are more important than antibiotic prophylaxis to reduce the risk of IE. Aseptic measures are mandatory during venous catheter manipulation and during any invasive procedures in order to reduce the rate of health care-associated IE.

Habib G, Lancellotti P, Antunes MJ, et al. 2015 ESC Guidelines for the management of infective endocarditis: The Task Force for the Management of Infective Endocarditis of the European Society of Cardiology (ESC). Endorsed by: European Association for Cardio-Thoracic Surgery (EACTS), the European Association of Nuclear Medicine (EANM). Eur Heart J 2015; 36:3075–3128.

14. C Endovascular/open surgical repair of the aneurysm

The important question here is the rate of growth. In general, the larger the aneurysm diameter, the higher the risk of rupture. For size 4.0–5.4 cm the risk of rupture is between 0.5 and 5%.

Symptomatic aneurysms warrant repair. In asymptomatic aneurysms, ultrasound/CT monitoring is advised. The interval depends on size. If it is less than 4 cm, monitoring every 2–3 years is advised. The frequency is increased to 6 monthly when size exceeds 4 cm and if it exceeds 5 cm 3 monthly.

The American College of Cardiology (ACC) criteria suggest that aneurysm repair should be contemplated when the diameter exceeds 5.5 cm. However, the rate of expansion is also important. In this case, the aneurysm grew by 1.1 cm over a period of 6 months. If the rate of growth exceeds 0.5 cm every 6 months, then repair has to be considered.

Medical therapy would consist of good blood pressure control and a target of 125/75 mmHg. Beta-blockers have been tried with equivocal results. Statin therapy improves overall mortality but not aneurysm expansion. Smoking increases the rate of expansion.

About 60% of all abdominal aortic aneurysms (AAA) are suitable for endovascular therapy. In randomised controlled studies endovascular aortic repair (EVAR) reduced mortality. But long-term results were similar due to high re-intervention rates.

Current European Society of Cardiology recommendations are:
•   AAA repair is indicated if AAA diameter exceeds 55 mm
•   If the anatomy is suitable for EVAR, either open or endovascular aortic repair is recommended
•   If the aneurysm is anatomically not suitable for EVAR, open endovascular aortic surgery is recommended

While MR angiography is useful, it does not add to clinical decision making in this instance.

Erbel R, Aboyans V, Boileau C, et al. 2014 ESC Guidelines on the diagnosis and treatment of aortic diseases: Document covering acute and chronic aortic diseases of the thoracic and abdominal aorta of the adult. The Task Force for the Diagnosis and Treatment of Aortic Diseases of the European Society of Cardiology (ESC). Eur Heart J 2014;35:2873–2926.

15. D Plan left heart catheterisation within the next 24 hours

This patient presented with symptoms suggestive of unstable angina and has had a positive troponin, hence he has a non-ST elevation myocardial infarction (NSTEMI). ECG shows ST–T changes suggestive of NSTE-ACS (non ST elevation acute coronary syndrome).

The initial management of NSTE-ACS is as suggested: continue aspirin if already on it; if not load with 300 mg aspirin and continue at 75 mg once daily. The second antiplatelet agent of choice is P2 Y12 inhibitor, such as clopidogrel or ticagrelor. The next step depends on the patient's risk status.

Very high risk patients
•   Haemodynamic instability
•   Life-threatening arrhythmias or cardiac arrest
•   Recurrent or on-going ischaemia (e.g. chest pain refractory to medical treatment) or recurrent dynamic ST segment and/or T wave changes, particularly with

High risk patients
- Rise and/or fall in troponin level consistent with myocardial infarction
- Dynamic episode of ST segment and/or T wave changes with or without symptoms
- Global Registry of Acute Coronary Events (GRACE) score >140

Intermediate risk patients
- Diabetes mellitus
- Renal insufficiency (glomerular filtration rate <60 mL/min/1.73 m^2)
- Left ventricular ejection fraction ≤40%
- Prior revascularisation
- GRACE score >10^9 and <140

Low risk patients
- Patients with NSTE-ACS who have both of:
  - no recurrent symptoms
  - no risk criteria (as listed above)

Reperfusion therapy
Patients with confirmed (i.e. elevated troponin levels) intermediate, high and very high risk NSTE-ACS (except patients with type 2 myocardial infarction) should have angiography with coronary revascularisation [i.e. percutaneous coronary intervention (PCI) or coronary artery bypass grafting where appropriate].
Recommended intervention times vary according to the level of risk:
- Very high risk NSTE-ACS: within 2 hours
- High risk NSTE-ACS: within 24 hours
- Intermediate risk NSTE-ACS: within 72 hours
- Low risk NSTE-ACS (no recurrent symptoms and no risk criteria): selective invasive strategy guided by provocative testing for inducible ischaemia

This man has high-risk NSTEMI, given his ECG changes and troponin rise, so he requires PCI within the next 24 hours. His GRACE score is 135, but the decision in this instance can be made without GRACE scoring.

Roffi M, Patrono C, Collet JP, et al. 2015 ESC Guidelines for the management of acute coronary syndromes in patients presenting without persistent ST-segment elevation: Task Force for the Management of Acute Coronary Syndromes in Patients Presenting without Persistent ST-Segment Elevation of the European Society of Cardiology (ESC). Eur Heart J 2016; 37:267–315.

16. E Verapamil 2.5 mg intravenous over 2.5 minutes

His ECG is suggestive of narrow complex tachycardia at a rate of 210 beats per minute. Closer analysis suggests that it is probably AV re-entry tachycardia (AVRT) as evidenced by retrograde P waves visible in some leads with PR interval <70 ms.

Clinically there is no evidence of haemodynamic compromise; hence vagal manoeuvres should be tried first. However, that has not been given as an option in this question. In the absence of haemodynamic compromise, DC cardioversion is not immediately indicated.

Given that the patient has asthma, with a previous intensive therapy unit admission with severe asthma, adenosine is relatively contraindicated. Although the literature suggests that asthma is a relative contraindication and adenosine has been successfully used in people with asthma, the probability of a severe episode of asthma could be considered as a contra-indication. This applies to metoprolol as well.

Digoxin is not beneficial in AVRT or AVNRT. Due to its side-effect profile and slow onset of action, amiodarone is not preferred in this instance. Verapamil has a longer duration of action and is well tolerated in asthma. In recent studies, verapamil 2.5–5.0 mg given at a rate of 1 mg/min intravenously has shown good results.

Page RL, Joglar JA, Caldwell MA, et al. 2015 ACC/AHA/HRS guideline for the management of adult patients with supraventricular tachycardia: a report of the American College of Cardiology/American Heart Association Task Force on Clinical Practice Guidelines and the Heart Rhythm Society. J Am Coll Cardiol. 2016; 67:e27-e115.

17. B No anti-coagulation/anti-platelet therapy

To determine the need for anti-coagulation, CHA2DS2-VASc scoring is used (**Table 1.2**). A score of >2 suggests the need for anti-coagulation.

If the patient's CHA2DS2-VASc score is 'low risk' (i.e. 0 in males or 1 in females), no anticoagulant therapy is recommended. In males with one stroke risk factor (i.e. a score of 1), antithrombotic therapy with oral anti-coagulants may be considered, and patients' values and preferences should be considered.

This man has no risk factors (his score is 0), so no anticoagulant or anti-platelet therapy is recommended. However, given permanent atrial fibrillation, this should be reviewed annually.

Kirchhof P, Benussi S, Kotecha D, et al. 2016 ESC Guidelines for the management of atrial fibrillation developed in collaboration with EACTS. Eur J Cardiothorac Surg 2016; 50:e1–e88.

18. D Open aortic valve replacement

This 86-year-old has severe aortic valve stenosis as evidenced by a valve area <1 cm^2 and a transvalvar gradient of >50 mmHg (**Table 1.3**). The stenosis is probably more than this since there is left ventricular (LV) dilatation and reduction in LV ejection fraction.

Table 1.3 American College of Cardiology and American Heart Association classification of aortic valve lesion severity			
Severity	Valve area (cm^2)	Mean transvalvar gradient (mmHg)	Peak jet velocity (m/s)
Mild	>1.5	<25	<3
Moderate	1.0–1.5	25–40	3.0–4.0
Severe	<1.0	>40	>4.0

In this circumstance, the best option is aortic valve replacement. Balloon aortic valvotomy has a high complication rate and recurrence is common. Furthermore, the survival advantage is not greater than no intervention at all.

Transcatheter aortic valve implantation (TAVI) is currently recommended for those who are a very poor surgical risk. This patient was independent prior to hospital admission and had no significant past medical history apart from osteoarthritis. His surgical risk would primarily be from his age and slightly diminished LV function, so he would not fall into the very high-risk group (EUROSCORE – 7 with a perioperative mortality rate of around 7–8%).

Medical management of aortic stenosis is limited because it is primarily a mechanical issue. Statins have no convincing evidence to suggest regression or indeed reduction in progression of the stenosis.

19. B Cardiac catheterisation

The blood tests and echocardiogram, along with the negative CT and V/Q scan, suggest a diagnosis of idiopathic pulmonary arterial hypertension (IPAH), previously called primary pulmonary hypertension.

Presentation with progressive exertional breathlessness, syncope and haemoptysis is commonly seen in IPAH. Physical examination might show a loud P2 (pulmonary second heart sound). Eventually pulmonary and tricuspid regurgitant murmurs may be heard. Similarly, elevated jugular venous pressure, enlarged liver and ascites with peripheral oedema may be seen as a consequence of right heart failure in later stages.

IPAH is more common among women. Other causes of pulmonary hypertension, such as congenital or acquired cardiac lesions, chronic obstructive lung disease, other lung pathology, pulmonary thromboembolic disease and vasculitides, should be screened for and excluded.

Other rare aetiologies include HIV, anorexic drugs such as fenfluramine and dexfenfluramine and recreational drugs such as methamphetamine and cocaine. Haemoglobinopathies such as sickle cell disease, homozygous β-thalassaemia and hereditary spherocytosis have been associated with pulmonary hypertension as well.

The gold standard for diagnosis of IPAH is right heart catheterisation (RHC). Echocardiography is a good screening test, but confirmation requires right heart catheterisation. RHC allows for measurement of oxygen saturation in the veins and in the chambers of the heart, and allows for accurate measurement of right atrial, ventricular and pulmonary artery pressures. It also allows for the measurement of pulmonary capillary wedge pressures, pulmonary vascular resistance and, importantly for treatment, response to acute vasodilators. The definition of pulmonary hypertension includes a mean pulmonary artery pressure >25 mmHg, pulmonary artery wedge pressure ≤15 mmHg and pulmonary vascular resistance >3 Wood units.

McLaughlin VV, et al. ACCF/AHA 2009 expert consensus document on pulmonary hypertension: a report of the American College of Cardiology Foundation Task Force on Expert Consensus Documents and the American Heart Association: developed in collaboration with the American College of Chest Physicians, American Thoracic Society, Inc., and the Pulmonary Hypertension Association. Circulation 2009; 119:2250–2252.

20. E Peripartum cardiomyopathy

Peripartum cardiomyopathy usually presents between the last trimester of pregnancy and 5 months after delivery. The most common time of diagnosis is between the last month of pregnancy and the first 2 months postpartum. Left ventricular (LV) dilatation is common and the left ventricular ejection fraction (LVEF) is usually less than 45%.

The cause is unknown but genetic, immunological, viral and pregnancy-related haemodynamic factors have all been postulated. Peripartum cardiomyopathy appears to be a disease caused by unbalanced oxidative stress, impaired cardioprotective and pro-angiogenic signalling, and high expression of anti-angiogenic factors. 16 kDa prolactin has been implicated in the pathology and recently bromocriptine has been used in treatment of peripartum cardiomyopathy.

Factors that predispose to this condition include: multi-parity, family history, smoking, diabetes, hypertension, ethnicity, malnutrition, pre-eclampsia, advanced maternal age and teenage pregnancy. It is defined as non-genetic, non-familial heart failure in pregnancy.

It is a diagnosis of exclusion, and alcohol, thyroid disease, phaeochromocytoma, cocaine, valvular heart disease and pulmonary thromboembolism need to be excluded. Some studies have shown that people who develop peripartum cardiomyopathy are carriers of mutations associated with familial dilated cardiomyopathic forms, and a higher incidence has been noted in people of African ancestry, hence it is often difficult to distinguish familial forms of cardiomyopathy from peripartum cardiomyopathy, so a thorough family history must be taken. Idiopathic dilated cardiomyopathy is usually unmasked in the first two trimesters rather than in the post-partum period.

In this instance the patient only had gestational hypertension, but not pre-existing severe hypertension, and hence hypertensive heart failure is unlikely. Pre-eclampsia can affect the heart and lead to diastolic heart dysfunction, and can occasionally cause systolic heart failure as well, therefore heart failure prior to delivery can be difficult to distinguish. However, pre-eclampsia-related cardiac problems resolve after delivery whereas peripartum cardiomyopathy would require treatment even after delivery.

Her history is not suggestive of myocardial infarction (MI) and the electrocardiogram (ECG) did not show evidence of MI. Echocardiogram did not show any hypo- or akinetic regions.

While pulmonary embolism-related heart failure remains a possibility, her echocardiogram does not show right heart dilatation or hypertrophy.

Spontaneous recovery is common in peri-partum cardiomyopathy, and up to 70% of women recover to LVEF>50%. The recurrence rate in subsequent pregnancies is 30–50%, therefore in women who have not recovered ventricular function fully, subsequent pregnancies must be discouraged. Even when the ejection fraction has normalised, counselling should be advised due to the incidence of recurrence. However, in many instances, subsequent pregnancies have been tolerated well, especially when left ventricular function has normalised. Heart failure treatment and bromocriptine has shown good effect in subsequent pregnancies.

Hilfiker-Kleiner D, Haghikia A, Nonhoff J, Bauersachs J. Peripartum cardiomyopathy: current management and future perspectives. Eur Heart J 2015; 36; 1090–1097.

21. B CT aortogram

The clinical picture of sudden severe central chest pain during activity in a middle-aged ex-smoker with a history of hypertension is suggestive of thoracic aortic dissection.

The ECG may show only non-specific ST–T changes. Chest X-ray may be normal or show mediastinal widening, small pleural effusion, abnormal aortic contour or the displacement of calcium in the aortic arch. Although pulmonary embolism is the other differential diagnosis, the history of sudden sharp chest pain with back pain, normal oxygen saturation and significant hypertension on admission, points much more towards aortic dissection. He has no predisposing conditions for pulmonary embolism.

The investigation of choice would be a CT angiogram. A transthoracic echocardiogram (TTE) does not have sufficient sensitivity; a transoesophageal echocardiogram (TOE) offers better sensitivity, but is not an option in this question. Cardiac troponin would be elevated in aortic dissection, pulmonary embolism and myocardial infarction. D-dimer would be elevated in both dissection and embolism and would be helpful only to rule out both conditions when pre-test probability is low.

V/Q scan is not useful in aortic dissection.

22. E Therapeutic pericardiocentesis

The clinical features suggest cardiac tamponade – especially the inspiratory drop of 15 mmHg pressure (paradoxical pulse).

The echocardiographic picture of right atrial and ventricular collapse supports the diagnosis of cardiac tamponade.

Given that the patient is symptomatic and that the clinical picture points towards tamponade, therapeutic pericardiocentesis is the urgent intervention of choice.

The other investigations would delineate the aetiology of pericardial effusion, especially as this is likely to be a malignant effusion related to the previous breast cancer. However, the immediate intervention here would be to aspirate the effusion.

23. A Ostium primum atrial septal defect

The physical examination features such as the fixed wide split of the second sound are suggestive of an atrial septal defect (ASD). There are several types of ASD. A common one is the ostium secundum ASD in which there is a failure of closure of the embryonic ostium secundum. The ejection systolic murmur at the pulmonary area is due to increased flow across the valve in ASD. This situation is exacerbated by pregnancy. In adults, features of pulmonary hypertension often include a loud P2 (pulmonary component of second heart sound) and a parasternal heave. This is due to the increased blood flow through the pulmonary circulation.

This woman has also has a pansystolic murmur at the apex. This is suggestive of mitral regurgitation. In ostium primum ASD, there is an atrioventricular valve cleft which has, in this case, resulted in an additional finding of mitral regurgitation. Often in these cases there is also a tricuspid valve incompetency.

Trilogy of Fallot consists of pulmonary valve stenosis, right ventricular hypertrophy and atrial septal defect [tetralogy of Fallot has ventricular septal defect (VSD) with over-riding aorta instead of the ASD]. Here again, the apical pansystolic murmur would not be present. Patent foramen ovale is usually clinically difficult to detect and VSD would give rise to a pansystolic murmur at the left sternal edge but not at the apex. Sometimes these VSDs affect the musculature and have multiple holes so as to resemble a Swiss cheese and these are difficult to close.

Given the constellation of clinical findings, the diagnostic possibility strongly favours ostium primum ASD.

24. A Aspirin 300 mg four times daily

This patient has developed low-grade fever, malaise, tiredness, chest pain and arthralgia, a few weeks after admission for acute myocardial infarction and percutaneous insertion of a coronary stent. Physical examination reveals a pericardial rub and left pleural effusion. Investigations show a pericarditic ECG (ST elevation in non-classic distribution), an acute inflammatory picture (raised leucocytosis with leftward shift, raised C-reactive protein and erythrocyte sedimentation rate), signs of cardiac injury (raised troponin) and an exudative pleural fluid. There is no definite evidence of infection or cardiac failure.

This picture, developing a few weeks after an acute myocardial infarction and percutaneous coronary intervention, is suggestive of postcardiac injury syndrome or Dressler's syndrome.

The provoking cardiac injury of postcardiac injury syndrome or Dressler's syndrome ranges from myocardial necrosis (postmyocardial infarction pericarditis), cardiac surgery (postpericardiotomy syndrome) to minor, often unrecognised iatrogenic breaches of the pericardium (complicating the course of percutaneous coronary intervention), or percutaneous intracardiac interventions, such as pacemaker lead insertion, or radiofrequency ablation. Anti-heart antibodies may be seen in high titre. Following injury to the heart, autoantigens are exposed which subsequently leads to the formation of autoantibodies and an immunological reaction.

In the era before thrombolysis and primary percutaneous coronary intervention, Dressler's syndrome was much more common. However, whether due to reduced extent of myocardial damage resulting from early intervention or due to the multiple drugs such as angiotensin-converting enzyme inhibitors, antiplatelet agents and statins, all of which have anti-inflammatory actions, this syndrome is much less common in the modern era.

Treatment is mainly by anti-inflammatory agents such as non-steroidal anti-inflammatories and colchicine. European guidelines suggest ibuprofen whereas the American ones suggest aspirin. In general, in ischaemic heart disease aspirin might be the better choice. Corticosteroids may be used in small doses when aspirin and NSAIDs are contraindicated. Colchicine may prevent post cardiac injury syndrome.

Imazio M, Hoit BD. Post-cardiac injury syndromes. An emerging cause of pericardial diseases. Int J Cardiol 2013; 168:648–652.

25. C Fallot's tetralogy

This patient has all the four components of Fallot's tetralogy:
1. Large ventricular septal defect (VSD)
2. Overriding aorta, i.e. aorta overrides the VSD and straddles both left and right ventricular outflow tracts
3. RV outflow tract (RVOT) obstruction/pulmonary valve stenosis
4. Right ventricular hypertrophy.

Since there is a VSD with pulmonary stenosis and overriding aorta, the blood ejected from the RV also goes into the aorta, giving rise to a cyanotic congenital heart disease. The severity depends on the degree of RVOT obstruction. This determines the degree to which deoxygenated blood enters the systemic circulation.

Squatting increases systemic vascular resistance and hence forces the blood away from the systemic circulation towards the pulmonary circulation, relieving the dyspnoeic spells. Due to reduced blood flow through the RVOT, the pulmonary component of the second heart sound is usually soft or inaudible, leaving a single loud A2.

The ejection systolic murmur is due to turbulent blood flow in the RVOT. Often there is an ejection sound due to either stenotic pulmonary valve or overriding aorta, but not in this particular patient.

ECG usually shows right ventricular hypertrophy, with no p pulmonale and often a rightward QRS axis, as in this instance.

In atrial septal defect with reversal of shunt and Eisenmenger's syndrome, cyanosis is not likely to manifest in early childhood. Noonan's syndrome is associated with pulmonary stenosis, which is not a cyanotic disease. PDA (patend ductus arteriosus) with reversal of shunt again does not cause early cyanosis and once reversal of shunt occurs, produces differential clubbing.

Perloff JK, Child JS. Congenital heart disease in adults, 2nd edn. Philadelphia, PA: Saunders, 1998.

26. E Verapamil 5 mg intravenous

This patient with chronic obstructive pulmonary disease has an atrial flutter with a ventricular rate of 150 beats per minute on the ECG. The atrial rate is 300 beats per minute with 2:1 block due to the high atrial rate. The usual dictum is to rule out an atrial flutter when the ventricular rate is 150 beats per minute.

Management of atrial flutter is very similar to that of atrial fibrillation (AF) and studies have shown that it increases the risk of thromboembolism, but less so compared with AF. Atrial flutters also have a tendency to convert to AF, reflected by the common usage flutter–fibrillation.

Management strategy depends on time of onset (</> than 48 hours), risk of thromboembolism (as decided by the CHA2DS2-VASc score) and haemodynamic instability. Haemodynamic instability would suggest the need for DC cardioversion immediately followed by anticoagulation.

Adenosine is ineffective as with AF. An atrial flutter of new onset (<48 hours) can be cardioverted either chemically or electrically. DC cardioversion is mostly done when the patient is unstable cardiovascularly and requires less energy than AF. Chemical cardioversion can be achieved using amiodarone, flecainide (pill-in-pocket approach for recurrent atrial flutters), ibutilide, dronedarone, etc.

However, in this instance we do not know the time of onset of atrial flutter, hence rhythm control is not appropriate prior to anticoagulation for 3–4 weeks. The appropriate treatment here would be ventricular rate control. The drug of choice would be a beta-blocker such as esmolol or metoprolol. However, this person has widespread wheeze and hence beta-blockers might not be appropriate. Hence verapamil, which is a calcium channel blocker with negative chronotropic properties, would be the drug of choice. Digoxin could be used but is not a first-line drug, in this instance.

Once good rate control has been achieved and anticoagulation started, he could then have an elective DC cardioversion.

Stiell IG, Macle L; CCS Atrial Fibrillation Guidelines Committee. Canadian Cardiovascular Society atrial fibrillation guidelines 2010: management of recent-onset atrial fibrillation and flutter in the emergency department. Can J Cardiol 2011; 27(1):38–46.

27. B Intravenous adrenaline 10 mL of 1 in 10,000 solution (1 mg/10 mL)

This question hinges on the management of asystole in a cardiac arrest situation. According to the Resuscitation Council guidelines, the management of asystole is to maintain proper cardiopulmonary resuscitation (CPR) and to give intravenous adrenaline every 4 minutes (3–5 minutes). Atropine is no longer recommended for asystole and pulseless electrical activity (PEA); 1 mg of (intravenous) adrenaline is used, most commonly as 10 mL of 1 in 10,000 solution (1 mg/10 mL).

Though there is good cause to suspect hyperkalaemia in this instance, given that the patient is on both ramipril and spironolactone, the immediate priority is intravenous adrenaline. DC cardioversion is not recommended for asystole.

Resuscitation Council (UK). Guidelines for Adult Advanced Life Support. London: Resuscitation Council, 2010.

28. D Stop beta-blockers and start diltiazem and nitrates

This woman most likely has variant angina or Prinzmetal's angina. This is primarily due to coronary vasospasm, which non-steroidal anti-inflammatories can often worsen by blocking cyclo-oxygenase. Characteristically, the attacks often occur at rest and bear no relationship to exertion or food intake. Often the attacks occur at night.

Classically, chest pain is accompanied by ST elevation and minimal coronary artery disease on angiography. The ECG changes and symptoms are not in proportion to the angiography findings. Certain ethnic groups such as the Japanese have a higher incidence of variant angina.

Diagnosis depends on a typical history with ECG findings. In some cases, the diagnosis is made on changes in Holter recordings. Provocative agents such as acetylcholine or ergonovine during coronary angiography are also used to make the diagnosis.

Beta-blockers, especially unselective ones, may worsen the vasospasm. However, people with significant concurrent atherosclerotic lesions may benefit from the negative chronotropic and inotropic actions. In general, beta-blockers are better avoided in variant angina.

The main drugs used for treatment are calcium channel blockers, such as diltiazem, and long-acting nitrates. In patients who have significant life-threatening arrhythmic episodes with vasospastic episodes, an implantable cardioverter defibrillator may be of benefit.

JCS Joint Working Group. Guidelines for diagnosis and treatment of patients with vasospastic angina (coronary spastic angina) (JCS 2013). Circ J. 2014;78(11):2779–801.

29. D Previous anterior myocardial infarction with left ventricular aneurysm and LVF

The ECG shows ST elevation in anteroseptal leads with QS complexes suggestive of a previous myocardial infarction. His symptoms began 2 months ago and lasted 2 days initially. This was followed by progressive shortness of breath. The physical examination findings suggest left ventricular failure and diffuse apex with persistent ST elevation suggests left ventricular aneurysm. Persistence of ST elevation in the presence of Q waves and for several weeks after the onset of symptoms suggests a left ventricular aneurysm.

The onset of symptoms several weeks ago does not suggest acute anterior ST segment elevation myocardial infarction. Brugada's syndrome presents with episodes of syncope or presyncope and palpitations. It can also result in sudden cardiac death. ECG findings include ST elevation in V1 and V2 as well as partial right bundle-branch block pattern. Left main stem stenosis with recurrent angina would present with recurrent episodes of chest pain or its equivalent.

Papillary muscle dysfunction should not present with persistent ST elevation. Investigations in this instance should include an echocardiogram and coronary angiogram. Treatment would depend on the findings of the investigations but would include secondary prevention in the form of statins, angiotensin-converting enzyme inhibitors, beta-blockers and aspirin.

Left ventricular aneurysm (LVA) is an area of abnormal left ventricular shape with systolic paradoxical bulge, i.e. systolic dyskinesia. The usual cause is myocardial infarction. Other rare causes include hypertrophic cardiomyopathy, sarcoidosis and unknown (idiopathic). Differentials include LV pseudoaneurysm (which is often a contained rupture), which has a more serious prognosis and is more likely to rupture. Post-myocardial infarction, both aneurysm and pseudoaneurysm, is likely to develop. Complications of LVA include thromboembolism, refractory angina, congestive cardiac failure, arrhythmias and, rarely, rupture. Treatment depends on the size of the aneurysm, thromboembolic potential and likelihood of rupture. Anticoagulation with warfarin and treatment of heart failure are generally accepted; surgical treatment with left ventricular repair would depend on the factors outlined.

Makkuni P, Kotler MN, Figueredo VM. Diverticular and aneurysmal structures of the left ventricle in adults: report of a case within the context of a literature review. Tex Heart Inst J 2010; 37:699–705.

30. E 2:1 second-degree heart block

The ECG clearly shows one P wave with a normally conducted QRS complex and the second P wave which is not conducted. The heart rate is around 20 beats per minute. This is a 2:1 second-degree heart block; however, the distinction between Mobitz type I block and Mobitz type II block cannot be made from the ECG when a 2:1 block is present. In this situation, every other beat is not conducted and there is no opportunity to observe for possible PR prolongation that is characteristic of a Mobitz type I AV block. A long rhythm strip should be obtained or a previous ECG examined to try to find evidence of PR prolongation with non-conducted beats in a pattern other than 2:1.

Given the age, absence of any contributing factors and slowness of the heart rate, this is more likely to be Mobitz type II than type I.

Treatment depends on identifying and correcting reversible causes of slowed conduction such as myocardial ischaemia, increased vagal tone and drugs that depress conduction. There is a high likelihood of progression to complete heart block and hence a permanent pacemaker is indicated.

European Society of Cardiology (ESC); European Heart Rhythm Association (EHRA), Brignole M, Auricchio A, Baron-Esquivias G, Bordachar P, et al. 2013 ESC guidelines on cardiac pacing and cardiac resynchronization therapy: the task force on cardiac pacing and resynchronization therapy of the European Society of Cardiology (ESC). Developed in collaboration with the European Heart Rhythm Association (EHRA). Europace 2013; 15:1070–118.

31. B Start on anti-platelet agents and beta-blockers; monitor cardiac markers and serial ECGs

This woman has presented with a stroke affecting the right middle cerebral artery (MCA) territory. ECG changes are well known to be associated with central nervous system (CNS) events such as subarachnoid haemorrhage, thromboembolic stroke, subdural haemorrhage or intracerebral haemorrhage.

The common ECG abnormalities associated with these conditions include alterations in the repolarisation patterns such as ST–T segment changes, deeply inverted symmetrical T waves or peaked T waves and QT interval prolongation. These appear soon after the event or can evolve over several days. Cardiac arrhythmias such as ectopic ventricular beats, ventricular tachycardia and bradycardia can also be seen. Atrial fibrillation was the most common arrhythmia (16%). Ventricular arrhythmias were rarer (2.6%). The incidence of arrhythmia was highest in the first 24 hours.

Pathogenesis is commonly attributed to adrenergic surge due to central nervous system trauma. Involvement of insular cortex is shown to cause surge of noradrenaline resulting in ECG changes, arrhythmias and occasionally death. Autonomic imbalance is also seen in acute stroke, which may contribute.

Symmetrical T-wave inversions can be seen in the ECG shown. This pattern is commonly associated with coronary artery stenosis, but in the setting of an acute stroke this pattern can be seen without any coronary disease. An echocardiogram in these patients can show regional wall motion abnormalities and in many instances a rise in serum cardiac markers can follow.

In many cases, these changes revert, the ECG normalises and long-term echocardiographic changes are not seen. Since the risk factors of acute ischaemic stroke and myocardial ischaemia are similar, myocardial perfusion imaging may be indicated in some individuals during the recovery period. However, at present there is no routine indication for proceeding to a coronary angiogram directly in this setting. Cardioprotection in this setting may be achieved by beta-blockers and angiotensin-converting enzyme inhibitors/angiotensin receptor blockers.

Since the patient was seen beyond the window for thrombolysis for the acute stroke, the management would be to initiate antiplatelet agents. Since she also had a short run of non-sustained ventricular tachycardia, adding a beta-blocker would be appropriate to control the adrenergic surge. She should be monitored in an intensive care/high dependency care setting. Serial ECG and cardiac markers would also be appropriate so that a decision on further evaluation of the coronary artery status can be made if the abnormalities persist.

Ruthirago D, Julayanont P, Tantrachoti P, et al. Cardiac arrhythmias and abnormal electrocardiograms after acute stroke. Am J Med Sci 2016; 351:112–118.
Jauch EC. Acute management of stroke. Medscape: Neurology 2017.
Sharma JC, et al. Cardio-protection in acute stroke. Int J Stroke 2007; 2:288–290.

32. B CT pulmonary angiogram

The electrocardiogram shows sinus tachycardia, S1Q3T3 pattern (deep S waves in I, Q waves in III and T-wave inversion in III) and partial right bundle-branch block. This combined with a history of recent long-haul flight, chest pain and shortness of breath as well as the pleural rub, reduced saturations and right ventricular S3 suggests pulmonary embolism.

A D-dimer assay is not needed when the clinical suspicion of pulmonary embolism is very high. Among the options given, a CT pulmonary angiogram is the most appropriate investigation. The other option would be a ventilation–perfusion scan, which is not among the options given.

Konstantinides SV, Torbicki A, Agnelli G, et al. and the Task Force for the Diagnosis and Management of Acute Pulmonary Embolism of the European Society of Cardiology (ESC). 2014 ESC guidelines on the diagnosis and management of acute pulmonary embolism. Eur Heart J 2014; 35:3033–3069.

33. E Start intravenous alteplase

This patient has had a massive pulmonary embolism (PE) with haemodynamic compromise. Despite being on low-molecular-weight heparin, inotropes and fluids, he is heading for a pulseless electrical activity (PEA) cardiac arrest. The strongest predictor of poor outcome in a pulmonary embolism is low systolic pressure. It also indicates massive pulmonary embolism. The tumour in his pancreas and the hospital stay were probably instrumental reasons for developing the PE.

Acute right ventricular failure with resulting low systemic output is the leading cause of death in patients with high-risk PE. Therefore, supportive treatment is vital in patients with PE and RV failure. Aggressive volume expansion may worsen RV failure. Modest volume expansion with a 500 mL fluid challenge may be attempted. Use of vasopressors is often necessary, while waiting for pharmacological, surgical, or interventional reperfusion treatment. Noradrenaline, in hypotensive patients appears to improve RV function via a direct positive inotropic effect, while also improving RV coronary perfusion by peripheral vascular alpha-receptor stimulation and the increase in systemic blood pressure. Adrenaline and dobutamine have also been used.

The major interventions to be considered at this stage are (a) thrombolysis of the pulmonary embolus with intravenous alteplase/streptokinase/tenecteplase or (b) pulmonary artery catheterisation and either direct thrombolysis or embolectomy. At this level of haemodynamic compromise, arranging a surgical thrombectomy is unlikely to be practical.

Similarly, catheter-based interventions may also not be practical for this patient unless experienced operators are available immediately and a catheter lab is also ready to receive the patient and is located close by.

Several regimens are available for thrombolysis of massive PE – outcomes with streptokinase and alteplase are similar. A 2-hour bolus of alteplase at a dose of 100 mg is commonly considered. In imminent collapse, as in this patient, a 0.6 mg/kg bolus at a maximum dose of 50 mg over 15 minutes is another alternative.

If thrombolysis fails, catheter-based intervention should be considered.

Surgical embolectomy is indicated for high-risk PE, and also for selected patients with intermediate-high-risk PE, particularly if thrombolysis is contraindicated or has failed.

Konstantinides SV, Torbicki A, Agnelli G, et al. and the Task Force for the Diagnosis and Management of Acute Pulmonary Embolism of the European Society of Cardiology (ESC). 2014 ESC guidelines on the diagnosis and management of acute pulmonary embolism. Eur Heart J. 2014; 35:3033–3069.
Marshall PS, et al. Diagnosis and management of life-threatening pulmonary embolism. J Intensive Care Med 2011; 26: 275–294.

34. A Patent ductus arteriosus with reversal of shunt

This patient has differential clubbing, i.e. clubbing of toes but not hands (there is likely to be differential cyanosis as well, but not mentioned in the case report). This, along with the murmur, suggests patent ductus arteriosus with reversal of shunt.

The most common location of ductus arteriosus is just below the origin of the left subclavian artery. Hence when there is a right-to-left shunt, the pulmonary arterial blood from the ductus is directed distal to the left subclavian artery origin.

This means that the toes are cyanosed and clubbed whereas the fingers are not – so-called differential cyanosis and clubbing.

The murmur radiating to the clavicle is characteristic of PDA and is continuous (systolo-diastolic) prior to reversal, but often confined to the systole after the reversal of the shunt.

35. A Left atrial myxoma

Myxomas are predominantly seen in women and 90% are sporadic. They can present with systemic symptoms such as fever, weight loss, malaise, night sweats, cachexia, rash, arthralgia, clubbing, Raynaud's disease, anaemia, leucocytosis, elevated erythrocyte sedimentation ratio (ESR) and thrombocytosis.

The characteristic tumour 'plop' sound is often heard early to mid-systole and is often variable with position. Because of obstruction to the mitral valve, symptoms and signs akin to mitral stenosis are often seen.

41. E Urgent inotropic support and possibly temporary mechanical circulatory support in intensive care unit

This patient has fulminant viral myocarditis with rapidly developing heart failure and cardiogenic shock. A small number of patients present with fulminant myocarditis, with rapid progression from flu like illness to severe cardiac failure with subsequent multi-organ failure.

These individuals need early intensive treatment with often, inotropic support and mechanical circulatory support such as intra-aortic balloon pump, ventricular assist devices or extra-corporeal membrane oxygenation. More than half survive with reasonably preserved LV function. The ejection fraction function of these patients often recovers to near-normal, although residual diastolic dysfunction may limit exercise for some. Long-term survival is good, if they survive the acute phase. There is currently no specific therapy recommended during any stage of viral myocarditis.

Several trials of immunosuppressive therapy for viral myocarditis have been unsuccessful. Two studies did prove benefit in 'virus negative' chronic myocarditis. Cardiac MRI and endomyocardial biopsy are very useful tools in diagnosing acute myocarditis, however anti-viral agents such as oseltamivir are not currently recommended in fulminant myocarditis, though their role in chronic myocarditis is currently being investigated. There have been case reports of beneficial effect in H1N1-associated myocarditis, but robust trials are lacking.

Fung G, Luo H, Qiu Y, et al. Myocarditis. Circ Res 2016; 118:496–514.
Shauer A, Gotsman I, Keren A, et al. Acute viral myocarditis: current concepts in diagnosis and treatment. Isr Med Assoc J 2013; 15:180–185.

42. B Postpone surgery for at least 6 months or even 12 months and then have surgery off clopidogrel

The patient has had a drug eluting stent inserted. There is a significant risk of instent thrombosis off dual anti-platelet therapy. The current US recommendations are for 12 months of dual anti-platelet therapy (DAPT), however the European guidelines recommend 6–12 months of therapy especially with the second-generation drug-eluting stents. Since this is an elective procedure, the best course of action would be to wait and do the surgery in 6–12 months' time.

Helft G. Dual antiplatelet therapy duration after drug-eluting stents: how long? J Thorac Dis 2016; 8:E844-E846.

Chapter 2

Dermatology

Questions

1. A 54-year-old woman presented with symptoms of muscle weakness and myalgia. She had also noticed some stiffness and pain in the small joints of her fingers. She had recently been diagnosed with hypercholesterolaemia and started simvastatin 3 weeks ago. She had no other past medical history of note and took no other medication.

   On examination, she had an erythematous rash on her upper eyelids, some mild tenderness of the muscles in her upper limbs and a violaceous erythema over the extensor surface of her fingers. The rest of her examination was unremarkable.

   Investigations:

haemoglobin 132 g/L (115–165)	creatine kinase 564 U/L (35–170)
white cell count 5.4 × 10⁹/L (4–11)	C-reactive protein 45 mg/L (<10)
platelets 168 × 10⁹/L (150–400)	

antinuclear antibody 1/160 (negative)
anti-Jo-1 antibody positive (negative)

   What is the most likely diagnosis?

   A   Cutaneous T-cell lymphoma
   B   Dermatomyositis
   C   Systemic lupus erythematosus
   D   Systemic sclerosis
   E   Trichinosis

2. A 19-year-old woman presented with fever, pain, and skin breakdown in her right popliteal fossa. She had a long history of atopic dermatitis which she had been treating with a topical steroid and emollients.

   On examination her temperature was 38.2°C, pulse 110 beats per minute and blood pressure 115/70 mmHg. Her left popliteal fossa is excoriated, with dry skin, and is red, hot, tender, and multiple vesicles are visible, some of which have been de-roofed. On further examination of the rest of her skin there were no other rashes, but there was evidence of atopic dermatitis on other flexural surfaces.

   What is the most likely diagnosis?

   A   Primary varicella
   B   Herpes zoster
   C   Eczema herpeticum
   D   Guttate psoriasis
   E   Psoriasis herpeticum

3. A 70-year-old woman presented with blistering on her arms and legs which was preceded by itching. She had a past medical history of ischaemic heart disease and was recently admitted to hospital with congestive cardiac failure. Her current medication included aspirin, simvastatin, ramipril and furosemide.

On examination, she appeared well. There were no oral or mucosal lesions. She had tense blisters on the flexor aspects of her elbows and knees.

What is the most likely diagnosis?

A   Bullous pemphigoid
B   Cicatricial pemphigoid
C   Dermatitis herpetiformis
D   Epidermolysis bullosa
E   Pemphigus vulgaris

4. A 48-year-old businessman presented with a non-pruritic rash. He was otherwise well. He had no past medical history and took no regular medications. He had travelled to New York 2 weeks ago and Thailand 2 months ago.

On examination, he had a diffuse erythematous rash over his torso and limbs extending to his palms. The lesions were not ulcerated and there was no exudate. Inspection of his oropharynx revealed broad, flat, whitish lesions on his mucosal surface. Otherwise examination was normal.

Investigations:

haemoglobin 145 g/L (130–180)	C-reactive protein 31 mg/L (<5)
white cell count 9.8 × 10⁹/L (4–11)	erythrocyte sedimentation rate 89 mm/1st h (0–20)
platelets 389 × 10⁹/L (150–400)	

What is the most likely diagnosis?

A   Coxsackievirus
B   *Coxiella*
C   Dengue
D   Hand, foot and mouth disease
E   Syphilis

5. A 24-year-old woman presented with a pruritic rash. She had no significant past medical history and took no regular or new medications. She first noticed a few lesions on her abdomen which spread over 3 days to cover her trunk, all of her limbs and her face (see **Figure 2.1**).

Which one of the following is not associated with the aetiology of this condition?

A   Atenolol
B   Lithium
C   Streptococcal throat infection
D   Viral infection
E   Vitamin D deficiency

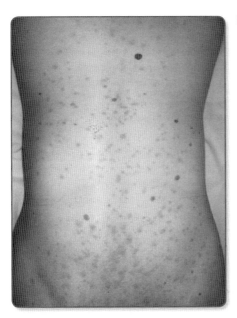

Figure 2.1 *See colour plate section.*

6. A 63-year-old woman presented with a 48-hour history of pain in the palm of her right hand and a spreading rash. She was a keen gardener and also had many cats. She reported a fever and rigors over the last 24 hours. She had experienced some palpitations earlier that same day.

   On examination, her temperature was 37.2°C, pulse 63 beats per minute, blood pressure 124/78 mmHg, respiratory rate 18 breaths per minute and oxygen saturation 99% on air. There was a non-confluent rash that extended across her torso and left leg (see **Figure 2.2**).

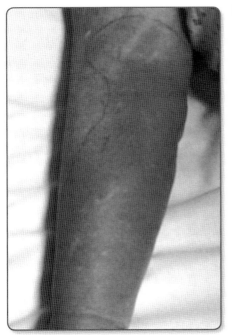

Figure 2.2 *See colour plate section.*

Investigations:

haemoglobin 118 g/L (115–165)	platelets 435×10^9/L (150–400)
white cell count 12.9×10^9/L (4–11)	C-reactive protein 286 mg/L (<5)
neutrophils 10.8×10^9/L (1.5–7.0)	erythrocyte sedimentation rate 45 mm/1st h (0–30)

Electrocardiogram: PR interval 300 ms with premature ventricular ectopics

What is the most likely diagnosis?

A   Bullous pemphigoid
B   Cat scratch fever (bartonellosis)
C   Cellulitis
D   Cutaneous diphtheria
E   Wegener's granulomatosis

7. A 19-year-old female student presented with a slowly creeping skin eruption on her foot that was intensely pruritic. It had been present for the last 7 days and had extended from the initial 1 cm at which she first noticed it to now being 4–5 cm long. She had no other past medical history and reported no recent travel.

On examination, she was apyrexial and systemic examination was normal. On the lateral plantar aspect of her left foot there was a 5-cm serpiginous tract with overlying excoriations but little surrounding erythema. The rest of her cutaneous examination showed no other lesions.

Investigations:

haemoglobin 128 g/L (115–165)	platelets 178×10^9/L (150–400)
white cell count 4.5×10^9/L (4–11)	C-reactive protein 2 mg/L (<5)
neutrophils 2.9×10^9/L (1.5–7.0)	creatine kinase 54 U/L (35–170)
eosinophils 0.7×10^9/L (0.04–0.4)	

What is the most likely diagnosis?

A   Cutaneous larva migrans
B   Filariasis
C   *Loa loa* filariasis
D   Schistosomiasis
E   Strongyloidiasis

8. A 53-year-old man presented for investigation of a lesion he had noticed on his right lower leg. He had received a renal transplant 15 years ago for IgA nephropathy. His regular medications included ciclosporin, azathioprine and low-dose prednisolone.

On examination, he was generally well. There was a lesion on his right leg (see **Figure 2.3**).

Figure 2.3 *See colour plate section.*

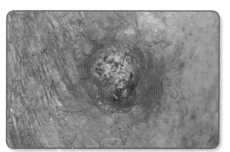

Which one of the following is not considered a risk factor for the development of this condition?

A   Age at transplantation
B   Azathioprine
C   Human papillomavirus
D   Keratotic skin lesions
E   Sirolimus

9.   A 55-year-old man with known hepatitis C presented with cough, pleuritic chest pain and breathlessness. He also complained of a rash over his lower legs.

On examination, his pulse was 89 beats per minute, blood pressure 110/75 mmHg, respiratory rate 24 breaths per minute and oxygen saturation 92% on air. Auscultation of his chest revealed fine inspiratory crackles in both lung fields. Abdominal examination was normal. Inspection of his legs revealed an erythematous rash (see **Figure 2.4**).

Investigations:

haemoglobin 102 g/L (130–180)	creatinine 125 µmol/L (135–145)
white cell count 8.9 × 10⁹/L (4–11)	bilirubin 23 mmol/L (1–22)
platelets 78 × 10⁹/L (150–400)	albumin 28 g/L (37–49)
erythrocyte sedimentation rate 88 mm/1st h (0–20)	alanine transaminase 135 U/L (5–35)
urea 6.7 mmol/L (2.5–7.5)	alkaline phosphatase 198 U/L (45–105)

What is the most likely diagnosis?

A   Livedo reticularis
B   Livedoid vasculitis

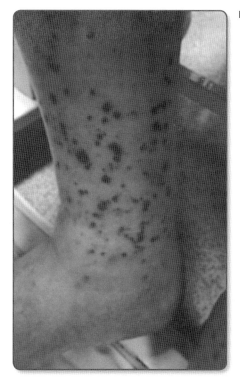

Figure 2.4 *See colour plate section.*

      C Mixed cryoglobulinaemia
      D Polyarteritis nodosa
      E Systemic lupus erythematosus

10. A 24-year-old male healthcare worker presented with a painful lesion on the pulp of his thumb. This had arisen over the last 24 hours with no history of trauma. He had no past medical history and took no regular medication.

      On examination, he was otherwise well. There was a painful lesion on his thumb (see **Figure 2.5**).

What is the most likely diagnosis?

      A Behçet's disease
      B Chancroid
      C Disseminated gonococcal infection
      D Herpes simplex
      E Syphilis

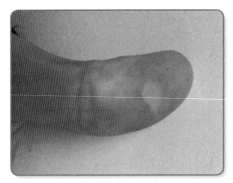

Figure 2.5 *See colour plate section.*

11. A 54-year-old woman presented with blisters on the back of her hands, forearms and face. She had noticed that the skin of the backs of her hands had become very fragile. She had also developed increased facial hair. She had a past medical history of chronic hepatitis C virus. She was not taking any current medication and had no other medical problems.

      On examination, she had bullae and erosions on the backs of her hands, forearms and face associated with scarring and pigmentary change. There was increased facial hair particularly around the temple and malar regions. She had no oral or genital lesions. The rest of the examination was normal.

What is the most likely diagnosis?

      A Bullous pemphigoid
      B Cicatricial pemphigoid
      C Epidermolysis bullosa
      D Pemphigus vulgaris
      E Porphyria cutanea tarda

12. A 52-year-man presented with painful lesions on both legs. He first noticed it about 3 weeks ago. He had type 1 diabetes with diabetic nephropathy and was a long-standing renal replacement patient, currently undergoing haemodialysis three times a week via a left brachiocephalic fistula. He had a history of atrial fibrillation with embolic stroke and took warfarin. He often missed dialysis sessions and was non-compliant with his medications which included calcium supplements, alfacalcidol, atorvastatin and novomix insulin. He has been otherwise well and had had no recent procedures or changes to his medications.

      On examination, he was systemically well. On both legs there were painful lesions (see **Figure 2.6**).

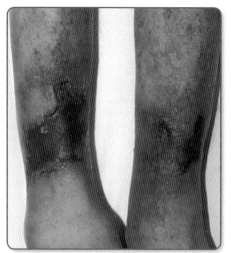

Figure 2.6 *See colour plate section.*

Investigations:

haemoglobin 98 g/L (aim 110–120 in dialysis)	phosphate 1.95 mmol/L (1.13–1.78 in CKD stage 5)
platelets 169 × 10⁹ L (150–400)	
international normalised ratio 2.2	parathyroid hormone 153 pmol/L (16.5–33.0 in CKD stage 5)
corrected calcium 2.71 mmol/L [2.1–2.37 in chronic kidney disease (CKD) stage 5]	

What is the most likely diagnosis?

A   Calciphylaxis
B   Cholesterol emboli
C   Disseminated intravascular coagulopathy
D   Malignant melanoma
E   Vasculitis

13. A 25-year-old woman who is 14 weeks' pregnant presented with a diffuse, macular rash over her torso and face. It was non-blanching. She was otherwise well.

On examination, she was apyrexial with normal chest examination. Abdominal examination revealed a palpable smooth mass arising from her pelvis. There was a fine macular rash covering her torso. There was no neck stiffness.

Investigations:

haemoglobin 101 g/L (115–165)	neutrophils 4.9 × 10⁹/L (1.5–7.0)
mean corpuscular volume 77 fL (80–96)	platelets 345 × 10⁹/L (150–400)
white cell count 5.7 × 10⁹/L (4–11)	C-reactive protein 13 mg/L (<5)

Urine dipstick: negative

Urine β-human chorionic gonadotrophin: positive

What is the next most appropriate management step?

A   Intravenous aciclovir
B   Intravenous ceftriaxone
C   Intravenous immunoglobulin
D   Send rubella and parvovirus serology
E   Send varicella-zoster serology

14. A 65-year-old woman was admitted with left-sided abdominal pain and vomiting that was diagnosed as acute diverticulitis. She had a history of chronic cryptogenic cirrhosis and known diverticular disease.

On admission, she was hypotensive and septic, and developed both an acute liver and acute kidney injury. She was treated empirically with piperacillin-tazobactam and gentamicin. Ten days later, she had a mildly pruritic, erythematous, maculopapular rash on both lower limbs (see **Figure 2.7**).

Investigations:

IgA 1.0 g/L (0.8–3.0)	C3 1.9 g/L (0.65–1.9)
IgG 8.0 g/L (6–13)	C4 0.18 g/L (0.15–0.5)
IgM 1.6 g/L (0.4–2.5)	

Antineutrophil cytoplasmic antibody: negative
Urine dipstick: negative
Hepatitis B and C serology: negative

What is the most likely cause of the rash?

A   Cryoglobulinaemia
B   Granulomatosis with polyangiitis (GPA) (Wegener's granulomatosis)
C   Henoch–Schönlein syndrome
D   Piperacillin-tazobactam
E   Toxic shock syndrome

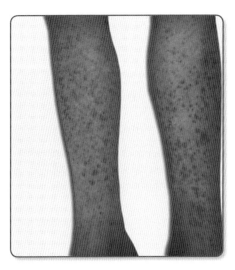

Figure 2.7 *See colour plate section.*

15. A 34-year-old woman with severe psoriasis undergoing infliximab therapy presented with breathlessness. Her last infliximab infusion had been 7 days prior. On examination her temperature was 38°C, respiratory rate 32 breaths per minute, oxygen saturation 85% on air, heart rate 115 beats per minute and blood pressure 125/75 mmHg. Respiratory examination was unremarkable.

> haemoglobin 119 g/L (115–165)
> white cell count 1.2×10^9/L (4–11)
> neutrophils 0.8×10^9/L (1.5–7.0)
> lymphocytes 0.1×10^9/L (1.5–4.0)
> C-reactive protein 56 mg/L (<5)
>
> Chest X-ray: bilateral infiltrates
>
> Peak expiratory flow rate: 380 L/min (normal range 420–480)

What is the most likely diagnosis?

A   *Streptococcus pneumoniae* pneumonia
B   *Pneumocystis jirovecii* pneumonia
C   Infliximab-induced pneumonitis
D   Asthma
E   Acute respiratory distress syndrome

16. A 69-year-old man presented unwell with a rash. This had progressed over the last 12 hours after he received his first erythropoietin injection the day before. He had a past medical history of diabetes mellitus and chronic kidney disease.

    His temperature was 35.6°C, pulse 125 beats per minute, blood pressure 85/52 mmHg and oxygen saturation 99% on air. Systemic examination was normal. He had a generalised, erythematous skin rash (see **Figure 2.8**).

Investigations:

> haemoglobin 89 g/L (130–180)   C-reactive protein 13 mg/L (<5)
> white cell count 16.9×10^9/L (4–11)   urea 2.9 mmol/L (2.5–7.5)
> platelets 568×10^9/L (150–400)   creatinine 348 µmol/L (60–110)

What is the most appropriate next step in management?

A   Intravenous flucloxacillin
B   Intravenous fluids

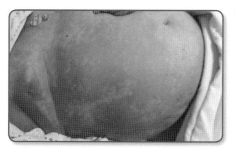

Figure 2.8 *See colour plate section.*

    C   Intravenous methylprednisolone
    D   Oral methotrexate
    E   Topical steroids

17. A 34-year-old South African woman presented for investigation of a mole on her neck which had recently become darker and seemed to bleed after minor trauma. She had an urgent biopsy which confirmed the diagnosis of malignant melanoma.

Which one of the following is most appropriate concerning the patient's prognosis?

    A   Nodal status at diagnosis is the most important factor in prognosis
    B   Non-ulcerated tumours have a worse prognosis than ulcerated ones of the same Breslow thickness
    C   Stage I disease confers a 75% 5-year survival rate
    D   Stage III disease confers a 10% 5-year survival rate
    E   Tumours on the head and neck carry a better prognosis than on the limbs

18. A 19-year-old man presented with a 5-day history of malaise, fatigue, odynophagia and a low-grade fever. A course of amoxicillin from his general practitioner did not improve his symptoms.

    His temperature was 38.1°C, blood pressure 124/72 mmHg, pulse 86 beats per minute and regular, and respiratory rate 16 breaths per minute. There was cervical lymphadenopathy, a tender palpable liver edge and a fine maculopapular rash over his trunk. Examination of his oropharynx revealed the following appearance which was painless (see **Figure 2.9**).

Investigations:

haemoglobin 131 g/L (130–180)	bilirubin 7 mmol/L (1–22)
white cell count 10.6 × 10⁹/L (4–11)	alanine transaminase 56 U/L (5–35)
neutrophils 8.9 × 10⁹/L (1.5–7.0)	aspartate transaminase 76 U/L (1–31)
lymphocytes 0.2 × 10⁹/L (1.5–4.0)	alkaline phosphatase 156 U/L (45–105)
platelets 179 × 10⁹/L (150–400)	albumin 38 g/L (37–49)
Monospot: negative	
Paul Bunnell test: positive	

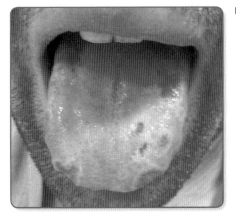

Figure 2.9 *See colour plate section.*

What is the most likely diagnosis?

A   Behçet's disease
B   Cytomegalovirus infection
C   Epstein–Barr virus infection
D   HIV seroconversion
E   Systemic lupus erythematosus

19. A 63-year-old woman was referred with a 2-year history of an ulcerating lesion over her right leg. She had received multiple courses of antimicrobials with little effect. Except for some constipation, she had no other complaints and no past medical history.

On examination, she was well and general examination was normal. There was an obvious rash over her right leg (see **Figure 2.10**).

Investigations:

haemoglobin 97 g/L (115–165)	alanine aminotransferase 31 U/L (5–35)
white cell count 7.4 × 10⁹/L (4–11)	alkaline phosphatase 10⁹ U/L (45–105)
platelets 587 × 10⁹/L (150–400)	total protein 95
urea 5.8 mmol/L (2.5–7.5)	albumin 31 g/L (37–49)
creatinine 189 µmol/L (60–110)	corrected calcium 2.9 mmol/L (2.2–2.6)
bilirubin 5 mmol/L (1–22)	

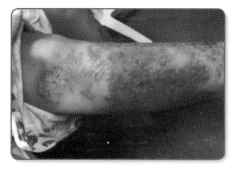

Figure 2.10 *See colour plate section.*

What is the most appropriate next step in management?

A   Colonoscopy
B   Oral co-amoxiclav for 2 weeks
C   Oral prednisolone
D   Protein electrophoresis and urinary Bence Jones protein
E   Skin biopsy

20. A 28-year-old woman presented with a 3-week history of a pruritic rash on her left shin that had not responded to over-the-counter topical emollients. She was otherwise well and on no regular medications. She reported that her boyfriend had a similar lesion on his calf.

On examination, there was a roughly circular scaly lesion with a leading edge. It was approximately 5 cm in diameter with obvious excoriations. Otherwise examination was normal.

Investigations:

haemoglobin 129 g/L (115–165)	platelets 389 × 10^9/L (150–400)
white cell count 4.8 × 10^9/L (4–11)	C-reactive protein <5 mg/L (<5)
Urea and electrolysis and liver function test: normal	

What is the most likely diagnosis?
A   Cellulitis
B   Cutaneous larva migrans
C   Erysipelas
D   Larva currens
E   Tinea pedis

21. A 48-year-old woman with known human immunodeficiency virus presented with extensive redness and desquamation. She also complained of odynophagia. There had been no recent changes in medication and she had an exemplary CD4$^+$ count of greater than 700 and fully suppressed viral load. She reported having a respiratory tract infection 2 weeks ago.
    On examination, she had a temperature of 37.8°C, heart rate of 135 beats per minute, and a blood pressure of 95/68 mmHg. Skin examination demonstrated sheets of epidermis being shed and necrosis of areas of her lower limbs. There were erosions on her buccal and genital mucosae.

Mycoplasma serology: IgG 1: 128

What is the most likely diagnosis?

A   Erythroderma
B   Scleroderma
C   Staphlococcal scalded skin syndrome
D   Toxic epidermal necrolysis
E   Toxic shock syndrome

22. A 56-year-old woman presented with blistering lesions on her face, scalp and back. She also had painful ulcers of her buccal mucosa for the past 6 weeks which had not healed. She had no other past medical history of note and took no medication.
    On examination, she had flaccid blisters and erosions on the areas mentioned as well as multiple oral ulcers. Nikolsky's sign was positive.
    Direct immunofluorescence showed IgG deposits on the surface of keratinocytes.

What is the most likely diagnosis?

A   Behçet's disease
B   Bullous pemphigoid
C   Dermatitis herpetiformis
D   Epidermolysis bullosa
E   Pemphigus vulgaris

Answers

1. B Dermatomyositis

Dermatomyositis is a disorder that consists of characteristic skin manifestations and an inflammatory myopathy. The peak age of onset is 50 years, and women are affected twice as commonly as men. The characteristic cutaneous manifestations are a heliotrope rash, which manifests as an oedematous erythema on the upper eyelids, and Gottron's papules – a red/violaceous scaly eruption on the extensor surface of the fingers. Other characteristic features include a photosensitive eruption, particularly over the malar region of the face, V of the neck and a violaceous erythema on the extensor surfaces, as well as periungual changes. Criteria for the diagnosis of dermatomyositis include the presence of the characteristic cutaneous findings in association with three or four of the following: proximal muscle weakness, elevated serum creatine kinase, myopathic changes on electromyography or pathological findings compatible with inflammatory myositis. Underlying malignancy should be considered in patients with dermatomyositis. A positive antinuclear antibody is common in patients with dermatomyositis; anti-Jo-1 antibodies are often positive in polymyositis. The rash classically seen in systemic lupus erythematosus is a butterfly rash across the bridge of the nose and cheeks. Systemic sclerosis causes sclerosis of the skin rather than the rash described here. Cutaneous T-cell lymphoma causes cutaneous lesions that are not photodistributed, as in this case. Trichinosis usually causes an urticarial rash.

Dalakas MC. Inflammatory muscle diseases. N Engl J Med 2015;372:1734–1747.

2. C Eczema herpeticum

This patient has flexural surface dermatitis, most in keeping with eczema rather than psoriasis (the latter predominantly affecting extensor surfaces). Eczema, or atopic dermatitis, is a particularly common skin complaint prevalent in children and adults. Treatment focuses on maintaining the barrier function of the epidermis through use of emollients, and where necessary, topical steroids. Super-infection of eczematous areas of skin are frequent. These infections are usually bacterial in origin (*Staphylococcus aureus* or *Streptococcus* spp.) necessitating antimicrobial therapy. Less common, but with similar potential for severity, is viral super-infection, including with herpes simplex. The resulting eczema herpeticum can cause intense local pain and inflammation, with local vesicular/herpetiform lesions visible. Treatment is with antiviral agents (such as aciclovir), and may need to be parenteral initially.

Psoriasis can also become superinfected with herpes simplex but again, the cutaneous distribution typically follows the classical psoriatic (extensor surface) pattern. Guttate psoriasis typically manifests as drop like small lesions scattered across the skin, often being triggered by streptococcal pharyngitis, although some childhood viral infections (including varicella and rubella) can also act as triggers. Varicella zoster virus causes cutaneous manifestations in primary disease with an all over cropping vesicular rash (chicken pox), and in later life through dermotomal reactivation (shingles).

Weidinger S, Novak N. Atopic dermatitis. Lancet 2016;387:1109–1122.

3. A Bullous pemphigoid

Bullous pemphigoid is an autoimmune subepidermal blistering disorder with autoantibodies directed against the basement membrane zone of the skin. It presents with tense blisters which can have a generalised pattern of distribution with a predilection towards the flexural areas of the skin. The bullae can appear on normal skin as well as on skin affected by urticaria. Mucous membranes are less commonly involved than in pemphigus. It is usually a disease of elderly people. Pathological findings demonstrate a subepidermal blister with a mixed dermal inflammatory infiltrate with prominent eosinophils. It may be precipitated by drugs such as furosemide.

Revised American Joint Committee on Cancer staging in 2010 categorises the disease into four stages, with several subcategories. In keeping with other staging systems, it is based on the depth of the tumour (T), the presence and number of lymph nodes (N), and the presence of metastases (M):

Stage I refers to patients with melanomas (T1a through T2a), without evidence of lymph node involvement and without regional or distant metastases. Stage I is subdivided into stages IA and IB, based upon the thickness of the melanoma (<2 mm), its mitotic rate, and the absence (a) or presence (b) of ulceration. The 5-year survival rate is >90%.

Stage II refers to tumours that have a higher risk of recurrence (T2b through T4b), but do not have any evidence of lymph node involvement or metastases. Stage II is subdivided into stages IIA, IIB, and IIC, depending upon tumour thickness (>1 mm) and the absence (a) or presence (b) of ulceration. It has a 5-year survival rate of 50–80%.

Stage III refers to tumours where there is involvement of regional lymph nodes or the presence of satellite metastases and no primary tumour is found (N1–N3). Patients with stage III disease are subdivided as having stage IIIA, IIIB or IIIC disease, depending upon the number of regional lymph nodes involved. The 5-year-survival rate is 40–70%.

Stage IV refers to the presence of distant metastases (M1a–M1c). There are no subgroups and prognosis is poor with 5-year survival <20%.

Tumours on the head and neck or trunk are associated with a worse survival than those on the limbs owing to their lymphatic drainage.

Gershenwald JE, et al. Melanoma staging: Evidence-based changes in the American Joint Committee on Cancer 8th edition, cancer staging manual. CA Cancer J Clin 2017; 67(6):472–492.

18. C Epstein–Barr virus infection

The oropharynx shows red patches on the surface of the tongue bordered with greyish-white areas. This can be differentiated from oral thrush as the white areas cannot be scraped off with a tongue depressor and form oral hairy leukoplakia, as they manifest over the ventral surface as well as the sides of the tongue. Geographic tongue is most commonly painless, whereas the ulcers of Behçet's disease are painful. Geographic tongue itself is not pathognomonic of any particular disease process and occurs in up to 2% of the population during periods of physiological stress.

Lymphadenopathy, mild hepatitis, lymphopenia and rash following amoxicillin are typical of infectious mononucleosis, the causative agent of which is Epstein–Barr virus (EBV). Cytomegalovirus can cause an infectious mononucleosis-like illness but the monospot and Paul Bunnell tests are usually negative. In this case the differential positivity in the heterophile tests is probably due to being tested early in the course of this illness. A repeat test in several weeks' time should return as both monospot and Paul Bunnell positive if this were EBV. It should be noted that all five of the answers listed can cause a false-positive heterophile test, but that the definitive laboratory investigation would be serology for EBV with a raised IgM a confirmed diagnosis.

Odumade OA, Hogquist KA, Balfour HH Jr. Progress and problems in understanding and managing primary Epstein-Barr virus infections. Clin Microbiol Rev 2011; 24(1):193–209.

19. D Protein electrophoresis and urinary Bence Jones protein

This woman has pyoderma gangrenosum, an ulcerating necrotic process that most frequently affects the legs, although atypical forms that affect the hands and arms and also a peristomal form can occur. Pyoderma gangrenosum is commonly mistaken for other infective or vascular causes of ulcers on the lower limbs but does not resolve with antimicrobials and vascular studies are frequently normal. The pyoderma gangrenosum itself can cause pain and disfiguration but rarely causes greater morbidity. The condition is associated with various other conditions, however, and when pyoderma gangrenosum is diagnosed further investigation for these may be indicated. These associated conditions include:

- Gastroenterological: ulcerative colitis, Crohn's disease, chronic active hepatitis
- Rheumatological: rheumatoid arthritis, Wegener's granulomatosis
- Haematological: multiple myeloma

The constipation mentioned in this case with the raised plasma globulins (note the marked difference between the total protein and albumin), thrombocythaemia and hypercalcaemia make multiple myeloma a distinct possibility. As a malignant condition, investigations for this, with protein electrophoresis and Bence Jones protein, should be carried out promptly. Colonoscopy is not indicated in this case, but if pyoderma gangrenosum is diagnosed in the context of symptoms consistent with inflammatory bowel disease then this would be the next step. The diagnosis of pyoderma gangrenosum is typically a clinical one although if confirmation is required a skin biopsy may show a neutrophilic inflammatory infiltrate which is not always present. Further antimicrobials are not indicated – the clinical picture shows no signs of super added infection around the ulcer. Empirical steroids are not yet indicated in this case until diagnosis of any underlying condition has been made.

Alavi A, et al. Pyoderma gangrenosum: an update on pathophysiology, diagnosis and treatment. Am J Clin Dermatol 2017; 18:355–372.

20. E Tinea pedis

This woman presents with a pruritic, contagious, lower limb rash typical of a fungal skin infection – tinea pedis in this case. This is a common presentation in those who visit the gym or public swimming pools and can be passed within households through direct contact and fomites. Clinical presentation is with a pruritic, circumscribed, erythematous, often scaly lesion that is often nearly circular in nature. In the toe web spaces it may appear as just an erythematous discoloration, sometimes with an exudate or flaky scaling. The causative organisms vary in their antifungal sensitivities and so skin scrapings for culture are advisable. Empirical therapy can then be trialled while cultures incubate – topical agents such as miconazole or clotrimazole are appropriate first-line agents. In some cases oral terbinafine or itraconazole is necessary.

Bacterial causes of this rash such as cellulitis and erysipelas are unlikely given the more indolent presentation over several weeks and the absence of a C-reactive protein or white cell response. Cutaneous larva migrans is acquired through environmental exposure to canine hookworm and cannot be transmitted from human to human. It leaves a serpiginous trail that slowly progresses over several weeks. Larva currens is the term used to describe the cutaneous manifestations of strongyloides and presents as intensely pruritic lesions anywhere on the body which appear, track for several centimetres and disappear again, all within several hours.

Kaushik N, Pujalte GG, Reese ST. Superficial fungal infections. Prim Care 2015;42(4):501–16.

21. D Toxic epidermal necrolysis

Toxic epidermal necrolysis (TEN), or Stevens–Johnson syndrome, is a life-threatening dermatological emergency. It can be triggered by a range of drugs including antimicrobials, anticonvulsants, antiretrovirals and methotrexate, among others. It can also be triggered, as in this case, by a preceding *Mycoplasma pneumoniae* infection, and patients living with human immunodeficiency virus are at particular risk. Certain human leukocyte antigen (HLA) types also predispose to TEN. Clinical presentation is with marked skin blistering and desquamation – often in large sheets and often associated with areas of necrosis. There is involvement of the mucosa. Diagnosis is by biopsy and histology. Management is predominantly supportive, with intravenous immunoglobulin, steroids and other immunosuppressive agents such as tumour necrosis factor inhibitors (e.g. etanercept) possibly being used by dermatology specialists.

Staphylococcal infections can frequently be associated with exotoxin-mediated complications; widespread desquamation (but not in sheets and not involving mucosa) in scalded skin syndrome and toxic shock syndrome (rarely skin desquamation, but severe shock and clotting derangement) are two such conditions. Scleroderma is a more chronic autoimmune condition which is associated with marked changes to soft tissue appearance, but not widespread desquamation. Erythroderma causes widespread skin erythema and desquamation, but not in sheets and with no areas of soft tissue necrosis.

Schneider JA, Cohen PR. Stevens–Johnson syndrome and toxic epidermal necrolysis: a concise review with a comprehensive summary of therapeutic interventions emphasizing supportive measures. Adv Ther 2017;34(6):1235–1244.

22. E Pemphigus vulgaris

Pemphigus vulgaris is an autoimmune blistering disease which is caused by autoantibodies directed against antigens on keratinocytes, leading to the formation of blisters within the epidermis. It typically presents with oral lesions followed by cutaneous blisters, which are usually distributed on the face, scalp and upper torso. The blisters are usually flaccid and rupture easily. Affected skin is often painful. Oral lesions present as persistent oral mucosal ulceration. Nikolsky's sign is positive – this is characterised by gentle rubbing of the skin surface producing erosion. Under direct immunofluorescence IgG deposits can be seen on the surface of keratinocytes. Behçet's disease is suspected when oral ulceration is seen in the presence of two of the following: genital ulceration, skin lesions (papulo-pustules), ocular inflammation or a positive pathergy reaction. Bullous pemphigoid presents with tense blisters and rarely affects the oral cavity. Dermatitis herpetiformis presents as a papular, vesicular eruption and epidermolysis bullosa is an inherited blistering disorder where blisters often form at sites of mechanical trauma.

Sinha AA, Hoffman MB, Janicke EC. Pemphigus vulgaris: approach to treatment. Eur J Dermatol 2015; 25:103–113.

Chapter 3

Endocrinology

Questions

1. A 20-year-old woman presented to the emergency department with lethargy and vomiting. She was 8 weeks pregnant and had severe vomiting, with >15 episodes every day. She had been unable to keep food and fluids down and had been losing weight. She had been transferred to the early pregnancy unit and subsequently admitted and given intravenous fluids and antiemetics.

   The next evening, the obstetric registrar calls you to ask advice about her thyroid function tests, which are given below. He reported that the woman has a small goitre, which is soft and smooth. Her pulse rate was 126 beats per minute and blood pressure 100/62 mmHg. She has been receiving to receive intravenous fluids and antiemetics and can now keep food and fluids down.

   Investigations:

   > thyroid stimulating hormone <0.01 (0.4–5 mU/L)
   > free thyroxine (FT4) 35.8 (10–25 pmol/L)
   > thyroid stimulating hormone receptor antibodies (TRAb) - negative
   >
   > ECG: sinus tachycardia

   What is the most appropriate next step?

   A Request US examination of pelvis and repeat thyroid function tests
   B Start carbimazole 10 mg twice daily and propranolol 10 mg three times daily
   C Start propranolol 20 mg three times daily and withhold anti-thyroid drugs until second trimester
   D Start propylthiouracil 50 mg three times daily and propranolol 20 mg three times daily
   E Start propylthiouracil 50 mg three times daily and switch to carbimazole in the second trimester

2. A 69-year-old woman was seen in the emergency department complaining of tiredness and dizziness. She gave a history of increased thirst and polyuria.

   On examination, her pulse was 110 beats per minute and regular, blood pressure 90/60 mmHg and respiratory rate 24 breaths per minute. Examination of her chest revealed dullness in the right mid-zone and reduced air entry in the same area.

   Investigations:

   > sodium 137 mmol/L (135–145)   corrected calcium 3.9 mmol/L (2.2–2.6)
   > potassium 4.2 mmol/L (3.5–5.0)   phosphate 0.8 mmol/L (0.8–1.4)
   > urea 15 mmol/L (2.5–7.5)   albumin 40 g/L (37–49)
   > creatinine 190 µmol/L (45–90)
   >
   > Chest X-ray: mass lesion in right mid-zone

What is the next most appropriate management step?

A   Calcitonin
B   Furosemide
C   Intravenous fluids
D   Pamidronate
E   Prednisolone

3.   A 43-year-old woman was seen in the clinic with a history of a neck lump. She did not have any symptoms and the lump was pointed out by her friend. There was no relevant past medical history or family history. She was not on any medications.
     Examination revealed a palpable nodule in the right lobe of the thyroid gland. Clinically she was euthyroid.

Investigations:

thyroid-stimulating hormone 3.85 mU/L (0.4–5.0)	corrected calcium 2.45 mmol/L (2.2–2.6)
free thyroxine (FT4) 15.8 pmol/L (10–25)	
Ultrasound: 1.5 × 1.75 cm solid lesion in the right lobe of thyroid with microcalcifications (U3)	

What is the next most appropriate management step?

A   Fine-needle aspiration cytology
B   Radio-iodine uptake scan
C   Right lobectomy with removal of isthmus
D   Serum calcitonin estimation
E   Serum thyroglobulin estimation

4.   A 52-year-old man with type 2 diabetes and hyperlipidaemia had his annual review. He had no other medical problems. He is currently on metformin, gliclazide and atorvastatin.
     Physical examination was unremarkable except that he had a body mass index of $32 \, kg/m^2$ and his blood pressure was 140/90 mmHg.

Investigations:

total cholesterol 4.9 mmol/L (3–5)	potassium 3.5 mmol/L (3.5–5.0)
low-density lipoprotein-cholesterol 2.6 mmol/L (2–3)	urea 5.5 mmol/L (2.5–7.5)
	creatinine 102 µmol/L (60–110)
triglyceride 2.9 mmol/L (0.6–1.69)	HbA1c 62 mmol/mol (18–37 mmol/mol)
sodium 135 mmol/L (135–145)	

He was started on ramipril and exenatide (glucagon-like peptide-1 analogue) injections for better hypertension and diabetic control. To improve his lipid control, he was started on bezafibrate in addition to atorvastatin. Three weeks later he was admitted to the emergency department with epigastric pain and vomiting.

sodium 139 mmol/L (135–145)	creatinine 152 µmol/L (60–110)
potassium 3.9 mmol/L (3.5–5.0)	amylase 380 U/L (60–180)
urea 12 mmol/L (2.5–7.5)	creatine kinase 348 U/L (25–195)

What is the most likely cause of his symptoms?

A   Acute kidney injury due to dehydration and ramipril/bezafibrate
B   Acute pancreatitis resulting from hypertriglyceridaemia

C Acute peptic ulcer induced by bezafibrate
D Acute rhabdomyolysis due to bezafibrate and atorvastatin combination
E Exenatide-induced acute pancreatitis

5. A 53-year-old man was referred by his general practitioner with a 2-month history of decreased libido and erectile dysfunction. He had a past history of type 2 diabetes mellitus and depression and was on metformin, ramipril, fluoxetine and simvastatin. He has had diabetes for the last 5 years and did not have any evidence of diabetic nephropathy, retinopathy or neuropathy.

　　Physical examination was unremarkable and he had normal testicular volume.

Investigations:

sodium 139 mmol/L (135–145)	serum testosterone 8 nmol/L (9–30)
potassium 4.2 mmol/L (3.5–5.0)	luteinising hormone (LH) 4 IU/mL (1–9)
urea 4.4 mmol/L (2.5–7.5)	follicle-stimulating hormone (FSH) 3 IU/mL (1–13)
creatinine 78 µmol/L (60–110)	prolactin 1890 mU/L (<360)
Pituitary MRI: normal	

What is the most likely cause of his symptoms?

A Depression-related erectile dysfunction
B Diabetes-related erectile dysfunction
C Fluoxetine-induced hyperprolactinaemia
D Hypergonadotropic hypogonadism
E Metformin-induced hyperprolactinaemia

6. A 39-year-old woman was referred with a history of weight gain, secondary amenorrhoea and weakness on getting up from a sitting position. There was no significant past medical history. She was on the combined oral contraceptive pill.

　　On examination, she was obese, had proximal muscle weakness and central fat distribution with a rounded face. Pulse was 90 beats per minute and blood pressure 150/90 mmHg.

Investigations:

sodium 142 mmol/L (135–145)	thyroid-stimulating hormone 2.0 mU/L (0.4–5.0)
potassium 3.3 mmol/L (3.5–5.0)	free thyroxine 12 pmol/L (10–25)
urea 5.0 mmol/L (2.5–7.5)	corrected calcium 2.32 mmol/L (2.2–2.6)
creatinine 76 µmol/L (60–110)	

What is the most appropriate diagnostic investigation?

A High-dose dexamethasone suppression test
B Insulin tolerance test
C Plasma adrenocorticotrophic hormone (ACTH) level
D Two 24-hour urine collections for free cortisol
E Short Synacthen test

7. A 35-year-old woman was bought into the emergency department with reduced consciousness. While in the emergency department she had a seizure and was found to have a glucose level of 1.5 mmol/L. She was treated with intravenous dextrose.

　　She had no past history of note and was not on any medications. Her mother died of a medullary thyroid cancer and her father was diabetic.

Investigations:

plasma insulin 140 pmol/L (fasting 20–140)	C-peptide 5 pmol/L (30–75, dependent on the value of insulin)

What is the most likely diagnosis?

A   Exogenous insulin use
B   Insulinoma
C   Liver dysfunction
D   Neuroendocrine tumour
E   Sulphonylurea abuse

8. A 52-year-old man was referred with a history of headaches, decreased libido, malaise and obstructive sleep apnoea. His wife mentioned that her husband's appearance had changed from family photos and that now his chin and eyebrows are prominent. He was being treated with ramipril 10 mg and amlodipine 10 mg once daily for hypertension, but the blood pressure control was poor.
    On examination, he had prominent supraorbital ridges and large hands.

Investigations:

sodium 138 mmol/L (135–145)	creatinine 97 µmol/L (45-90)
potassium 4.3 mmol/L (3.5–5.0)	fasting glucose 6.3 mmol/L (4–6)
urea 5.8 mmol/L (2.5–7.5)	

What is the most appropriate diagnostic investigation?

A   Growth hormone level
B   Insulin tolerance test
C   Low-dose dexamethasone suppression test
D   Oral glucose tolerance test with growth hormone levels
E   Pituitary MRI

9. A 45-year-old man was seen in the emergency department after having fainted. He also gave a history of general tiredness, malaise, decreased libido and increased weight. He did not have any significant past medical history apart from an admission to the intensive care unit 5 years ago with head injury because of a road traffic accident.
    His general practitioner had recently diagnosed hypothyroidism and had started 50 µg levothyroxine 2 weeks ago. On examination, his pulse was 70 beats per minute and regular, blood pressure 96/50 mmHg and respiratory rate 24 breaths per minute.
    He had slight pallor and delayed relaxation of ankle reflexes.

Investigations:

sodium 138 mmol/L (135–145)	creatinine 97 µmol/L (45-90)
potassium 4.3 mmol/L (3.5–5.0)	fasting glucose 6.3 mmol/L (4–6)
urea 5.8 mmol/L (2.5–7.5)	

What is the most appropriate next step in management?

A   Insulin–dextrose infusion (8 units of regular insulin with 50 mL 50% dextrose over 30 minutes)
B   Intravenous dextrose (50 mL of 25% dextrose)

C   Intravenous hydrocortisone (100 mg every 8 hours)
D   Intravenous levothyroxine (500 mg loading dose then 50–100 mg daily)
E   Intravenous liothyronine (25 mg every 8 hours)

10. A 23-year-old woman was involved in a road traffic accident. Subsequently she had a subdural
     haematoma evacuated. She had a basal skull fracture as well. Postoperatively she had been doing
     well but 48 hours later developed nausea, headache and vomiting.
         On examination, her temperature was 37.6°C, pulse 110 beats per minute and regular, blood
     pressure 130/85 mmHg, and respiratory rate 18 breaths per minute.
         Her total fluid intake was 3 L during the past 24 hours and output was 1.2 L.

     Investigations:

sodium 123 mmol/L (135–145)	creatinine 69 µmol/L (45–90)
potassium 3.5 mmol/L (3.5–5.0)	plasma osmolality 258 mosmol/kg (275–295)
urea 4.3 mmol/L (2.5–7.5)	urine osmolality 450 mosmol/kg (50–1400)

     What is the most appropriate next step in management?

     A   Aldosterone
     B   Carbamazepine
     C   Demeclocycline
     D   Desmopressin
     E   Fluid restriction

11. A 56-year-old man with type 2 diabetes was seen in the clinic for annual review. He was on
     12 units of lispro (short-acting analogue) insulin three times a day and on 24 units of NPH (neutral
     protamine Hagedorn) insulin at bedtime. He was also on metformin 850 mg twice a day. His other
     medications included ramipril 5 mg once daily and simvastatin 40 mg at night. He did not report
     any hypoglycaemic events but said that occasionally, on waking up, the bed sheets were drenched
     in sweat and that he had headaches in the morning.
         Home glucose monitoring showed (normal random glucose 4.0–7.8 mmol/L).

     Investigations:

Pre-breakfast: 8–11 mmol/L	Pre-bedtime: 4.5–6.0 mmol/L
Pre-lunch: 5–6 mmol/L	2-hour post-lunch: 8–11 mmol/L
Pre-evening meal: 4.5–7.0 mmol/L	HbA1c 52 mmol/mol (18–37)

     What is the most appropriate next step in management?

     A   Increase lunchtime regular insulin
     B   Increase metformin to 850 mg three times daily
     C   Increase morning regular insulin
     D   Increase night-time NPH insulin
     E   Reduce night-time NPH insulin

12. A 45-year-old woman was admitted with nausea and vomiting. Two months prior to admission,
     she had undergone a Roux-en-Y gastric bypass operation for obesity. Her postoperative period
     was uneventful and she was discharged with nutritional advice. She had lost about 20 kg of body
     weight postoperatively.
         She was treated on admission with intravenous 0.9% saline and dextrose. On the second
     day of admission, the nurses noticed that she was confused and unsteady on her feet. She also
     complained of tingling and numbness in her legs.

On examination, her temperature was 37.2°C, pulse 94 beats per minute and regular, blood pressure 110/70 mmHg and respiratory rate 18 breaths per minute. She was alert but confused in time and place. Neurological examination revealed horizontal nystagmus and reduced fine touch and joint position sense in her legs.

Investigations:

sodium 139 mmol/L (135–145)	haemoglobin 120 g/L (115–165)
potassium 3.8 mmol/L (3.5–5.0)	white cell count 10×10^9/L (4–11)
urea 10 mmol/L (2.5–7.5)	platelets 156×10^9/L (150–400)
creatinine 102 µmol/L (45–90)	
Chest X-ray: normal	

What is the most appropriate next step in management?

A   Intramuscular hydroxocobalamin supplementation
B   Intravenous magnesium supplementation
C   Intravenous niacin supplementation
D   Intravenous thiamine supplementation
E   Oral zinc supplementation

13. A 59-year-old man was referred with a 2-year history of difficult-to-control hypertension. He was on amlodipine 10 mg once daily, ramipril 10 mg once daily and doxazosin 4 mg once daily. However, clinic and home readings were still in the range of 160/90 mmHg. He did not give any significant past medical history apart from hypertension.
     On examination, his pulse was 78 beats per minute and regular, blood pressure 172/88 mmHg and respiratory rate 14 breaths per minute. His body mass index was 24.8 kg/m² (20–25), body habitus normal; heart sounds normal and there were no bruits.

Investigations:

sodium 138 mmol/L (135–145)	haemoglobin 128 g/L (130–180)
potassium 3.4 mmol/L (3.5–5.0)	white cell count 9×10^9/L (4–11)
urea 7 mmol/L (2.5–7.5)	platelets 126×10^9/L (150–400)
creatinine 124 µmol/L (45-90)	
Chest X-ray: normal	

What is the most appropriate next investigation?

A   CT of the adrenals
B   Meta-iodobenzylguanidine (MIBG) scan
C   Plasma aldosterone:renin ratio
D   Plasma metanephrine level
E   Plasma renin activity

14. A 56-year-old man was admitted with increasing lethargy, weight gain and constipation. He had been diagnosed with hypothyroidism 2 years ago, but had not been taking the levothyroxine regularly. He also complained of loss of libido.
     On examination, his body mass index was 34 kg/m². He had coarse skin, scalp alopecia, loss of the lateral third of the eyebrows and gynaecomastia. His temperature was 36.4°C, pulse 58 beats per minute, blood pressure 170/104 mmHg and respiratory rate 14 breaths per minute.

Investigations:

haemoglobin 102 g/L (130–180)	thyroid-stimulating hormone 98 mU/L (0.4–5.0)
mean corpuscular volume 88 fL (80–96)	free thyroxine (FT4) 1.2 pmol/L (10–25)
white cell count 10×10^9/L (4–11)	free triidothyronine (FT3) 0.2 pmol/L (5–10)
platelets 162×10^9/L (150–400)	9 am cortisol 200 nmol/L (200–700)
sodium 135 mmol/L (135–145)	prolactin 1597 U/L (75–375)
potassium 5 mmol/L (3.5–5.0)	luteinising hormone 3 U/L (1–9)
creatinine 112 µmol/L (60–110)	

Chest X–ray: mass lesion in right mid–zone

What is the most appropriate management?

A Oral levothyroxine and oral bromocriptine
B Oral levothyroxine replacement
C Oral levothyroxine, intravenous hydrocortisone and intravenous triiodothyronine
D Triiodothyronine intravenously with fluids and hydrocortisone
E Triiodothyronine intravenously and oral bromocriptine

15. A 50-year-old man was referred to the hypertension clinic with a 5-year history of hypertension that was difficult to control. He was on ramipril 10 mg once daily, bendrofluazide 2.5 mg once daily, amlodipine 10 mg once daily and doxazosin 8 mg twice daily. There was no other past history or family history of note. He denied excessive salt intake and had made dietary and lifestyle adjustments.

On examination, his temperature was 37.2°C, pulse 90 beats per minute and regular, blood pressure 180/100 mmHg with no significant difference between the arms, and respiratory rate 14 breaths per minute. The rest of the physical examination was unremarkable.

After withdrawing and substituting the interfering drugs, the following tests were done:

Investigations:

sodium 145 mmol/L (135–145)	haemoglobin 148 g/L (130–180)
potassium 3.8 mmol/L (3.5–5.0)	white cell count 6×10^9/L (4–11)
urea 8 mmol/L (2.5–7.5)	platelets 150×10^9/L (150–400)
creatinine 97 µmol/L (45-90)	

Echocardiogram: left ventricular hypertrophy

urine free metanephrines: normal
plasma aldosterone 90 pmol/L (aldosterone 90 – 700)
direct plasma renin 0.1 nmol/L/h (0.5-3.5)
aldosterone:renin ratio 900 (aldosterone:renin ratio <800)
9 am cortisol after overnight 1 mg dexamethasone 40 mmol/L (<50)

CT of the abdomen: no abnormalities detected

What is the next step in management?

A Add spironolactone
B High-dose dexamethasone suppression test
C Meta-iodobenzylguanidine (MIBG) scan
D Pituitary MRI
E Selective adrenal vein sampling

16. A 43-year-old man was referred to the emergency department after a fall. He sustained a fracture–dislocation of his left ankle, but could not remember how the fall had happened. In the past he had had a few episodes of palpitations. The dislocation was reduced under opiate analgesia. His only other significant past medical history was hypertension for which he was on amlodipine 10 mg once daily.

On examination, his pulse was 80 beats per minute, blood pressure 150/90 mmHg and respiratory rate 16 breaths per minute. The rest of the physical examination was normal.

Investigations:

haemoglobin 134 g/L (130–180)	sodium 141 mmol/L (135–145)
white cell count 8 × 10⁹/L (4–11)	potassium 4.5 mmol/L (3.5–5.0)
neutrophils 5 × 10⁹/L (1.5–7.0)	urea 9 mmol/L (2.5–7.5)
platelets 295 × 10⁹/L (150–400)	creatinine 78 µmol/L (60–110)

Electrocardiogram: left ventricular hypertrophy and sinus rhythm

Later on in the evening, he was taken to the theatre for an open reduction and internal fixation of the fracture. However, on induction of anaesthesia, his blood pressure rose up to 280/150 mmHg and the operation was abandoned.

What is the most appropriate next investigation?

A   24-hour urine free cortisol
B   24-hour urine metanephrines
C   Plasma aldosterone:renin ratio
D   Thyroid function tests
E   Urine porphobilinogen

17. A 39-year-old woman was referred for suspected hyperthyroidism. 4 weeks ago, she had a sore neck with difficulty in swallowing. This subsided, but was followed by palpitations, excessive sweating, diarrhoea and heat intolerance. She had also lost weight. She went to her general practitioner who ordered thyroid function tests which showed:

Investigations:

free thyroxine (FT4) 37.4 pmol/L (10–25)	thyroid stimulating hormone 0.01 mU/L (0.4–5.0)
C-reactive protein 30 mg/L (<5)	

She was started on carbimazole 20 mg daily and propranolol 10 mg three times a day by her general practitioner. 3 weeks after starting the drugs she was seen in the clinic where she said that her symptoms had subsided and her weight had steadily increased.

Physical examination showed a pulse of 70 beats per minute and regular, and she was clinically euthyroid. There was a small smooth firm goitre with no bruit.

Repeat blood tests showed:

free thyroxine (FT4) 8 pmol/L (10–25)	thyroid peroxidase antibodies 4 IU/mL (<50)
thyroid stimulating hormone 10 mU/L (0.4–5.0)	thyroid stimulating hormone receptor antibodies 0.1 U/L (<0.4)

What is the most appropriate next step in management?

A   Reduce propranolol to 5 mg three times a day and carbimazole to 5 mg daily and recheck thyroid function

B   Stop carbimazole and propranolol and monitor thyroid function tests in 6 weeks
C   Stop carbimazole and propranolol and order thyroid ultrasound to assess the goitre
D   Stop carbimazole and propranolol and start levothyroxine replacement at 25 mg daily
E   Stop propranolol and reduce carbimazole to 10 mg daily and monitor thyroid function tests

18. A 45-year-woman was seen in the clinic for a follow-up visit. She had been diagnosed with hyperparathyroidism secondary to parathyroid hyperplasia and had had a parathyroidectomy 2 years ago. She was maintained on calcium and α-calcidiol. During the clinic visit she complained of severe, burning abdominal pain as well as diarrhoea and occasionally she passed large amounts of foul-smelling faeces which floated in the toilet. She was troubled by severe episodes of reflux at night.
      Physical examination was normal apart from mild epigastric tenderness. Steatorrhoea was confirmed by Sudan III staining of the stool.

Investigations:

Gastroscopy: two small gastric ulcers and severe oesophagitis

What is the next most appropriate investigation?

A   D-xylose test
B   Faecal elastase and chymotrypsin
C   Fasting gastrin and chromogranin A level in serum
D   24-hour urinary 5–hydroxyindoleacetic acid (5-HIAA)
E   Vasoactive intestinal peptide (VIP) (serum)

19. A 46-year-old woman was seen in the clinic with a history of palpitations and weight loss. She had been diagnosed with hyperthyroidism and started on carbimazole which was titrated accordingly. After 6 months, she complained of grittiness in the eyes and watering.
      On examination, she had exophthalmos, diplopia and corneal ulceration with oedema of the optic discs.

Investigations:

free thyroxine (FT4) 11 pmol/L (10–25)	thyroid-stimulating hormone (TSH) 4.9 mU/L (0.4–5.0)
free triiodothyronine (FT3) 4 pmol/L (5–10)	
Chest X–ray: mass lesion in right mid–zone	

What would be the most appropriate treatment?

A   Ablation of thyroid gland with radio-iodine [131]I
B   Increase the dose of carbimazole
C   Radiotherapy to the eye
D   Systemic steroids
E   Total thyroidectomy

20. A 49-year-old woman was being reviewed at the clinic for primary hypothyroidism. Blood tests at the time showed that she was euthyroid. However, her corrected serum calcium was 2.7 mmol/L.
      Further questioning showed that she did not have a history of renal stones, depression, constipation, back pain, other mental health problems or abdominal pain. She did not have any recent history of fractures.

Investigations:

sodium 134 mmol/L (135–145)	corrected calcium 2.71 mmol/L (2.2–2.6)
potassium 5.4 mmol/L (3.5–5.0)	phosphate 0.7 mmol/L (0.8–1.4)
urea 6 mmol/L (2.5–7.5)	parathyroid hormone 8.2 pmol/L (0.9–5.4)
creatinine 86 µmol/L (45–90)	25 (OH)vitamin $D_2 + D_3$ 70 nmol/L (75–150)
Urine calcium:creatinine clearance ratio 0.008 (>0.01)	

What is the next step in management?

A   CT of the neck
B   DXA (dual-energy X-ray absorptiometry) scan for bone mineral density
C   Reassure the patient
D   Refer for parathyroid surgery
E ^{99m}Tc-sestamibi scan for parathyroid

21. A 49-year-old man was seen in the diabetes clinic for his annual review. He has had type 2 diabetes for the past 6 years and was on metformin 1000 mg twice daily and gliclazide 160 mg twice daily. He was also on simvastatin 40 mg once daily and ramipril 5 mg once daily. He did not report any hypoglycaemic episodes. His home blood sugar monitoring showed the following levels (normal random glucose level 4.0–7.8 mmol/L). His body mass index was 28 kg/m² and blood pressure 132/84 mmHg.

Investigations:

pre-meal glucose level (mmol/L) to 2-h post-meal level (mmol/L):	breakfast 7.8–14.1
	lunch 7.1–10.1
	dinner 8.1–15.1
HbA1c 84 mmol/mol (18-37)	creatinine 86 µmol/L (60–11045-90)
haemoglobin 135 g/L (130–180)	total cholesterol 3.8 mmol/L (3–5)
sodium 138 mmol/L (135–145)	low-density lipoprotein 1.6 mmol/L (<3)
potassium 3.6 mmol/L (3.5–5.0)	
Urine dipstick: normal	

What is the most appropriate next step in management?

A   Add basal insulin glargine in the morning
B   Add exenatide 10 µg twice daily
C   Add mixed insulin (short and intermediate acting) twice a day
D   Add pioglitazone 15 mg once daily
E   Add sitagliptin 100 mg once daily

22. A 42-year-old man was admitted with severe central abdominal pain, worse on lying down. He also had episodes of vomiting. His only past medical history was of inguinal hernia repair at the age of 28 years.
    On examination, his temperature was 37.8°C, pulse 110 beats per minute, blood pressure 160/96 mmHg and respiratory rate 24 breaths per minute. Abdominal examination revealed tenderness in the epigastric region. CT showed evidence of acute pancreatitis for which he was treated conservatively and discharged a week later.

On the subsequent outpatient visit 3 months later, fasting blood tests showed the following picture:

Investigations:

haemoglobin 145 g/L (130–180)	corrected calcium 2.56 mmol/L (2.2–2.6)
white cell count 8.5×10^9/L (4–11)	phosphate 0.8 mmol/L (0.8–1.4)
neutrophils 5×10^9/L (1.5–7.0)	fasting glucose 6.2 mmol/L (4–6)
platelets 213×10^9/L (150–400)	HbA1c 41 mmol/mol (18-37)
sodium 135 mmol/L (135–145)	cholesterol 9.5 mmol/L (3–5)
potassium 3.6 mmol/L (3.5–5.0)	high-density lipoprotein 1.2 mmol/L (>1)
urea 4 mmol/L (2.5–7.5)	triglycerides 7.5 mmol/L (0.6–1.69)
creatinine 77 µmol/L (45-90)	

What would be the most appropriate treatment?

A   Bezafibrate
B   Nicotinic acid
C   Pamidronate
D   Rosuvastatin
E   Simvastatin

23. A 56-year-old Caucasian man was recently found to have type 2 diabetes on an incidental blood test and was started on metformin 1000 mg twice daily.

6 months later, on review, his blood tests were:

HbA1c 54 mmol/mol (18-37)	low-density lipoprotein-cholesterol
haemoglobin 142 g/L (130–180)	3.1 mmol/L (<3)
creatinine 78 µmol/L (45-90)	triglycerides 1.4 mmol/L (0.6–1.69)
total cholesterol 4.9 mmol/L (3–5)	bilirubin 3 mmol/L (1–22)
high-density lipoprotein-cholesterol	alanine transaminase 38 U/L (5–35)
1.0 mmol/L (>1)	alkaline phosphatase 65 U/L (45–105)

He was started on simvastatin 40 mg at night. 2 months later, he came back with diffuse muscle aches, especially in the thighs and upper arms.

Repeat investigations showed:

creatine kinase (CK) 1628 U/L (25–195)

What is the most appropriate next step in management?

A   Continue simvastatin and monitor CK levels and symptoms after 4 weeks
B   Continue simvastatin and start coenzyme Q supplementation
C   Stop simvastatin and later switch to bezafibrate
D   Stop simvastatin and later switch to ezetimibe
E   Stop simvastatin and later switch to a lower dose of a more potent statin

24. A 34-year-old man of Taiwanese origin presented to the emergency department with severe weakness of all four limbs of 6 hours' duration.
    On further questioning, he has had some muscle aches over the past 2 days. The day of presentation, he had woken up with muscle aches, especially in the thigh and around the

shoulders. By midday he found it difficult walking or climbing stairs and could not get up from the chair and called the ambulance. He had no visual, sensory or bladder/bowel symptoms. He did, however, give a history of increased sweating, tremulousness, anxiety and palpitations over the last 2 months. He had no significant past history of note and was not on any medications.

On examination, he had hypotonia, grade 3 power proximally and grade 4 power distally with reduced reflexes in all four limbs. Sensory examination was normal and plantar reflex was flexor.

Investigations:

sodium 138 mmol/L (135–145)	bilirubin 4 mmol/L (1–22)
potassium 2.8 mmol/L (3.5–5.0)	alanine aminotransferase 21 U/L (5–35)
urea 4 mmol/L (2.5–7.5)	aspartate transaminase 32 U/L (5–35)
creatinine 76 µmol/L (45-90)	corrected calcium 2.39 mmol/L (2.2–2.6)
albumin 43 g/L (37–49)	creatine kinase 155 U/L (25–195)

He was started on potassium infusion and his symptoms improved.

Which test would confirm the diagnosis?

A   HIV serology
B   Lumbar puncture and protein analysis with microscopy
C   MRI of cervical spine
D   Nerve conduction studies
E   Thyroid function tests

25. A 19-year-old woman with type 1 diabetes and recently diagnosed hypothyroidism was seen in the clinic. Normally her glycaemic control was good with HbA1c between 48 and 53 mmol/mol and very few hypoglycaemic episodes. She was maintained on a basal bolus regimen with rapid-acting analogue insulin and the basal insulin glargine. She was also on levothyroxine 50 mg daily. However, recently she had been having several episodes of hypoglycaemia along with increased fatigue.

Examination was normal.

What is the most appropriate diagnostic investigation?

A   C-peptide level
B   Nocturnal oxygen saturations
C   Serum calcium, vitamin D and parathyroid hormone level
D   Serum vitamin B_{12} level
E   Short Synacthen test

26. A 45-year-old woman of Middle Eastern origin was referred to the clinic because of a fractured right humerus after minimal trauma. She mentioned that she had had diffuse body aches for several years. She also had noticed difficulty in getting up from sitting position as well as climbing stairs. She did not exercise much and seldom went out, other than for shopping. She took no supplements and had no other significant past history.

Dual-energy X-ray absorptiometry (DXA) scan showed T-scores of –3 in the vertebrae and –2.5 in the femur (> –1).

Investigations:

corrected calcium 2.06 mmol/L (2.2–2.6)	parathyroid hormone 11.8 pmol/L (0.9–5.4)
phosphate 0.5 mmol/L (0.8–1.4)	25(OH)-vitamin D_2 + vitamin D_3 10 nmol/L (50-150)
alkaline phosphatase 585 U/L (45–105)	creatinine 75 µmol/L (45-90)

What would be the most appropriate next step in management?

A   Parathyroidectomy
B   Start cholecalciferol/ergocalciferol supplementation
C   Start cinacalcet
D   Start metyrapone
E   Start pamidronate therapy

27. A 38-year-old man went to the general practitioner with a history of burning sensation while passing urine. Physical examination was unremarkable. His body mass index was 21 kg/m². Urine analysis was positive for glucose, nitrites and white blood cells.

He was treated with antibiotics and later an oral glucose tolerance test showed a fasting glucose of 9.2 mmol/L and 2-hour postprandial glucose of 16 mmol/L. HbA1c was 70 mmol/mol (18-37). He was started on gliclazide 40 mg once daily with variable control. This was later increased to 80 mg twice daily. HbA1c measured 6 months later was 74 mmol/mol (8.9%).

What is the most appropriate next step in management?

A   Add metformin 500 mg twice daily
B   Add pioglitazone 15 mg once daily
C   Increase gliclazide to 160 mg twice daily
D   Measure fructosamine levels
E   Measure glutamic acid decarboxylase (GAD) antibodies

28. A 24-year-old woman was referred with a history of secondary amenorrhoea, 6 months after stopping the oral contraceptive pill. She also complained of occasional headache and that she stumbled occasionally when climbing stairs. She had no other significant past medical history. She was not on any medications. She had noticed that her blouses were slightly damp.

On examination, milk could be expressed from her breasts. Visual field examination showed a field defect in the upper outer quadrants of both eyes.

Investigations:

haemoglobin 110 g/L (115–165)	prolactin 1080 mU/L (normal <360) (serial dilutions done)
white cell count 4 × 10⁹/L (4–11)	
platelets 125 × 10⁹/L (150–400)	follicle-stimulating hormone 0.1 U/mL (1–13)
sodium 138 mmol/L (135–145)	luteinising hormone 0.2 U/mL (1–9)
potassium 3.9 mmol/L (3.5–5.0)	thyroid stimulating hormone 0.1 mU/L (0.4–5.0)
urea 3.9 mmol/L (2.5–7.5)	free thyroxine (FT4) 8 pmol/L (10–25)
creatinine 67 µmol/L (45–90)	9 am cortisol 22 nmol/L (200–700)
	insulin-like growth factor 1 (IGF-1) 186 ng/mL (110–360)

Pituitary MRI: 3-cm pituitary mass with a slight tenting of the optic chiasma
No evidence of parasellar extension

What is the most appropriate next step in management?

A   Bromocriptine
B   Octreotide
C   Stereotactic radiosurgery
D   Transcranial hypophysectomy
E   Trans-sphenoidal surgery

29. A 28-year-old woman was seen in the clinic for a review of type 1 diabetes. She has had type 1 diabetes for the last 16 years and was on a basal bolus regimen with a long-acting analogue insulin glargine and short-acting insulin analogue lispro. Her only other medication was occasional paracetamol for headaches.

Over the past few months, she has had three hypoglycaemic episodes, one of which required external assistance. On looking at her glucose diary, there were several readings between 3 and 4 mmol/L during which she was asymptomatic. She had recently started a fitness regime. She did not have any other past medical history. For the last 7 years she has had good glycaemic control with HbA1c between 42 and 48 mmol/mol. She tested blood sugars four times a day and took regular exercise.

On examination, her body mass index was 21 kg/m² and blood pressure 140/85 mmHg.

Investigations:

fasting glucose 4.1 mmol/L (4–6)	low-density lipoprotein 2.5 mmol/L (<3)
HbA1c 43 mmol/mol (18–37)	high-density lipoprotein 1.3 mmol/L (>1.3)
cholesterol 4.5 mmol/L (3–5)	

What is the most appropriate next step in management?

A   Add ramipril 5 mg once daily and titrate the dose to target blood pressure of <130/80 mmHg
B   Add simvastatin 40 mg at night
C   Reduce basal insulin and pre-exercise rapid-acting insulin and avoid hypoglycaemia for the next 2 months
D   Switch from basal bolus to continuous subcutaneous insulin infusion therapy (insulin pump)
E   Switch from once daily glargine to twice daily detemir to improve glycaemic control

30. A 21-year-old woman was referred to the clinic with acne and hirsuitism. She had menarche at the age of 11 years and had occasional irregular periods. She had noticed increasing hirsuitism over the last few years. There was no other relevant history or family history.

On examination, her body mass index was 28 kg/m², pulse 76 beats per minute and blood pressure 130/85 mmHg.

She had hirsutism and acanthosis nigricans. Breast development was normal. Vaginal examination was normal apart from mild clitoromegaly.

Blood tests taken on the fifth day after menstruation showed:

Investigations:

oestradiol 300 pmol/L (early follicular <300)	luteinising hormone 4 U/L (1–9)
17OH-progesterone 20 nmol/L (<10)	follicle-stimulating hormone 3 U/L (1–13)
free testosterone 3 nmol/L (<3)	cortisol (9 am) 150 nmol/L (200–700)

What is the single most useful diagnostic test?

A   CT of the adrenals
B   Karyotyping
C   MRI of the pituitary
D   Short Synacthen test
E   Ultrasound of the pelvis

31. A 58-year-old man was referred because of watery diarrhoea and 6-kg weight loss over the past 2 months. There was no history of bleeding or abdominal pain. He also felt weak and lethargic, and had increased thirst and reduced urine output. He had a previous history of hypertension for which he was taking ramipril. There was no relevant family history.

On examination, he looked thin and mildly dehydrated. The rest of the examination was normal.

Investigations:

sodium 139 mmol/L (135–145)	pH 7.20 (7.34–7.44)
potassium 2.6 mmol/L (3.5–5.0)	bicarbonate 18 mmol/L (18–24)
creatinine 135 µmol/L (45-90)	urinary 5HIAA (5-hydroxyindoleacetic acid) – normal
corrected calcium 2.75 mmol/L (2.2–2.6)	
fasting glucose 6.5 mmol/L (4–6)	faecal fat 2 g/24 h (<7 g/24 h)
	stool volume 1.5 L/24 h

Stool culture: no ova, cysts or pathogens isolated

What is the most useful diagnostic test?

A   Glucagon
B   Faecal elastase
C   Plasma vasoactive intestinal peptide (VIP)
D   Secretin stimulation test
E   Somatostatin test

32. A 67-year-old man was seen in the neurology clinic with a 6-month history of severe pain in the right thigh. He also had difficulty getting up from squatting position and had noticed wasting in the legs. Pain was more severe at night. He had a past history of type 2 diabetes for 11 years and hypertension for 14 years. He was on metformin and gliclazide for diabetes and lisinopril for hypertension. He was also on simvastatin and ezetimibe for hyperlipidemia.

On examination, he was haemodynamically stable. Neurological examination of the lower limbs showed quadriceps wasting bilaterally with weakness in knee extension bilaterally and absent knee reflexes. Plantar reflex was flexor bilaterally. Sensations were intact.

Investigations:

haemoglobin 128 g/L (130–180)	potassium 4.5 mmol/L (3.5–5.0)
white cell count 9×10^9/L (4–11)	urea 7 mmol/L (2.5–7.5)
neutrophils 6×10^9/L (1.5–7.0)	creatinine 98 µmol/L (60–110)
platelets 178×10^9/L (150–400)	HbA1c 72 mmol/mol (18–37)
sodium 137 mmol/L (135–145)	

Chest X-ray: normal

Cerebrospinal fluid: clear, protein 0.52 g/L (0.2–0.4), white cell count 2×10^9/L (lymphocytes only)

What is the most likely diagnosis?

A   Amyotrophic lateral sclerosis
B   Diabetic lumbosacral plexopathy
C   Guillain–Barré syndrome
D   Meralgia paraesthetica
E   Mononeuritis multiplex

33. A 55-year-old man was admitted with a history of nausea and vomiting. He had a past history of diabetes for which he was on gliclazide 160 mg twice daily and metformin 850 mg three times daily. His last HbA1c was 73 mmol/mol (18–37) He was also on simvastatin 40 mg at night and ramipril 10 mg once daily.

On examination, he was haemodynamically stable and had some epigastric tenderness. He also had eruptive xanthomas on his trunk and upper arms.

Investigations:

haemoglobin 131 g/L (130–180)	bilirubin 3 mmol/L (1–22)
mean corpuscular volume 82 fL (80–96)	albumin 45 g/L (37–49)
white cell count 12 × 10⁹/L (4–11)	alanine transaminase 78 U/L (5–35)
platelets 180 × 10⁹/L (150–400)	alkaline phosphatase 290 U/L (45–105)
sodium 140 mmol/L (135–145)	total cholesterol 17 mmol/L (3–5)
potassium 3.8 mmol/L (3.5–5.0)	triglycerides 22 mmol/L (0.6–1.69)
creatinine 110 µmol/L (60–110)	high-density lipoprotein 1.2 mmol/L (>1.0)
glucose 21 mmol/L (4.0–7.8)	

What is the most appropriate next step in management?

A   Atorvastatin
B   Dextrose–insulin infusion
C   Gemfibrozil
D   Heparin infusion
E   Niacin

34. A 65-year-old woman was admitted with chest pain, cough and fever. She had a past history of diabetes for which she was on metformin 850 mg twice daily. She was also on simvastatin 40 mg at night and ramipril 10 mg once daily.

    Chest X-ray showed left lower lobe consolidation and she was started on intravenous amoxicillin and gentamicin.

    Blood tests 3 days after admission showed:

Investigations:

haemoglobin 131 g/L (115–165)	glucose 15 mmol/L (4–7.8)
mean corpuscular volume 82 fL (80–96)	bilirubin 3 mmol/L (1–22)
white cell count 21 × 10⁹/L (4–11)	albumin 35 g/L (37–49)
neutrophils 16 × 10⁹/L (1.5–7.0)	alanine transaminase 45 U/L (5–35)
platelets 180 × 10⁹/L (150–400)	alkaline phosphatase 110 U/L (45–105)
sodium 140 mmol/L (135–145)	thyroid-stimulating hormone 0.6 mU/L (0.4–5.0)
potassium 3.8 mmol/L (3.5–5.0)	free thyroxine (FT4) 9.1 pmol/L (10–25)
creatinine 110 µmol/L (45–90)	free triiodothyronine (FT3) 2.3 pmol/L (5–10)
estimated glomerular filtration rate 46 mL/min (>90)	

What is the most appropriate investigation?

A   Radio-iodine uptake scan
B   Repeat thyroid function tests in a week and then in 2–3 months
C   Thyroid-binding globulin measurement
D   Thyroid peroxidase antibody measurement
E   Thyroid ultrasound

35. A 38-year-old man with a 2-year history of type 2 diabetes had his annual review. He was taking metformin and pioglitazone.

    His blood pressure was 145/88 mmHg on ramipril.

Investigations:

HbA1c 55 mmolmol (18-37)	total cholesterol 5.3 mmol/L (3–5)
creatinine 97 µmol/L (60–110)	high-density lipoprotein 0.9 mmol/L (>1.0)
estimated glomerular filtration rate (eGFR)	low-density lipoprotein 3 mmol/L (2–3)
80 mL/min (>90)	triglycerides 2.8 mmol/L (0.6–1.69)
alanine transaminase 45 U/L (5–35)	

Urine albumin: creatinine ratio 0.9 (<2.5)

What is the most appropriate management?

A   Lifestyle advice and recheck in 3 months
B   Start bezafibrate
C   Start nicotinic acid
D   Start omega 3 fatty acids
E   Start simvastatin

36. A 65-year-old man with a 12-year history of type 2 diabetes was seen for an annual review. He was on metformin, gliclazide and pioglitazone, along with ramipril for hypertension and microalbuminuria. He had previous proliferative retinopathy treated with laser photocoagulation. He also mentioned that he had a deep aching pain in his left forefoot.

On examination, the left foot was hot to touch and there was swelling and redness over the left forefoot, but no tenderness over the tarsal bones. He also had bilateral peripheral sensory neuropathy up to the mid-shin level.

Investigations:

haemoglobin 129 g/L (130–180)	creatinine 107 µmol/L (60–110)
white cell count 8.2 × 10⁹/L (4–11)	estimated glomerular filtration rate (eGFR)
C-reactive protein 10 mg/L (<10)	58 mL/min (>90)
erythrocyte sedimentation rate 32 mm/1st h (0–20)	alanine transaminase 45 U/L (5–35)
	uric acid 0.28 mmol/L (0.23–0.46)

Urine albumin:creatinine ratio – 21.9 (<2.5)

X-ray of left foot: soft tissue oedema over the tarsal bones as well as joint space widening

MRI of left foot: soft tissue swelling and stretching of ligaments

What is the most likely diagnosis?

A   Cellulitis due to diabetic foot
B   Charcot's foot affecting the forefoot bones
C   Diffuse interstitial skeletal hyperostosis (DISH) of diabetes
D   Gouty arthritis
E   Osteomyelitis of the forefoot

37. A 17-year-old girl was referred to the clinic with a history of primary amenorrhoea. She had always been athletic and had attributed this amenorrhoea to her lifestyle. There was no family history of delayed menarche.

On examination, she had normal breasts with pale areolae and scanty pubic hair development. Pelvic examination revealed that the vagina was short and ended blindly.

Karyotyping showed XY genotype.

What is the most appropriate next step in management?

A   Day 21 progesterone measurement
B   Gonadotrophin-releasing hormone therapy
C   Human chorionic gonadotrophin (hCG) therapy
D   Orchidectomy
E   Transvaginal ultrasound

38. A 57-year-old woman was referred to the clinic with a history of fatigue, decreased libido and malaise. She was diagnosed with hypothyroidism 3 years ago by her general practitioner and was on levothyroxine 75 µg daily. However, despite thyroxine replacement, her symptoms did not subside. She had her menopause 5 years ago. She took her medicines regularly. There was no other past history of significance.

Investigations:

haemoglobin 10⁹ g/L (115–165)	potassium 5.5 mmol/L (3.5–5.0)
white cell count 5.4 × 10⁹/L (4–11)	creatinine 65 µmol/L (45–90)
platelets 158 × 10⁹/L (150–400)	thyroid-stimulating hormone 0.3 mU/L (0.4–5.0)
mean corpuscular volume 82 fL (80–96)	free thyroxine (FT4) 15.8 pmol/L (10–25)
sodium 132 mmol/L (135–145)	free triiodothyronine (FT3) 5.1 pmol/L (5–10)

What is the most appropriate investigation?

A   Assay for interfering antibodies to thyroid-stimulating hormone (TSH)
B   Iodine-131 uptake scan
C   Insulin tolerance test
D   Serum thyroid-binding globulin measurement
E   Thyroid-stimulating hormone receptor-stimulating antibody measurement

39. A 32-year-old man was seen in the clinic along with his wife for primary infertility. She previously has had one child and had a gynaecology review which was normal.
    He had no significant past medical history and was a non-smoker. Alcohol intake was <10 units/week and he did not report any recreational drug use. He had normal onset of puberty. However, he had a 'weak' libido. On questioning he shaved only once a week.
    On examination: height 183 cm, weight 81 kg, heart rate 69 beats per minute, blood pressure 108/66 mmHg, temperature 37.1°C. He had mild gynaecomastia. Testicular volume was 4 mL (15–25).

Investigations:

testosterone 5 nmol/L (10–28)	oestradiol 350 pmol/l (<250)
luteinising hormone (LH) 20 U/L (1–9)	thyroid-stimulating hormone 2 mU/L (0.4–5.0)
sex hormone-binding globulin 28 nmol/L (20–40)	cortisol (9 am) 390 nmol/L (200–700)
follicle-stimulating hormone (FSH) 14 U/L (1–13)	prolactin 140 mU/L (<360)

What is the most useful diagnostic investigation?

A   CT of the adrenal gland
B   Karyotyping

    C   MRI pituitary
    D   Short Synacthen test
    E   Testicular ultrasound

40. A 20-year-old student was referred by her university general practice to the local endocrinology clinic for management of panhypopituitarism which had developed after surgery for craniopharyngioma in her childhood. She reported that she would usually take her medications regularly but would occasionally forget. However, she felt generally well. She was taking levothyroxine 125 µg once daily, oestrogen + progesterone patch twice weekly, and hydrocortisone 10 mg at 8 am, 5 mg at 1300 and 5 mg at 5 pm daily. She stopped growth hormone at the age of 18 years and did not want to restart. Physical examination, including visual fields, were normal.

9 am blood tests forwarded by the general practitioner showed:

haemoglobin 119 g/L (115–165)	potassium 5.5 mmol/L (3.5–5.0)
white cell count 4.4 × 10⁹/L (4–11)	creatinine 65 µmol/L (45–90)
platelets 188 × 10⁹/L (150–400)	thyroid-stimulating hormone 0.01 mU/L (0.4–5.0)
mean corpuscular volume 82 fL (80–96)	
sodium 132 mmol/L (135–145)	

Which of the following is the next most appropriate action?

    A   Arrange MRI pituitary
    B   Arrange thyroid uptake scan
    C   Check FT4 level
    D   Reassure and arrange follow-up next year
    E   Reduce levothyroxine to 75 µg once daily and recheck in 3 months

41. A 38-year-old woman presented to the emergency department a week ago with a headache. She had a head MRI which was normal apart from an incidental empty sella with a small rim of pituitary tissue. The radiology report suggested clinical correlation. She was discharged from the emergency department and was referred to the endocrinology clinic. Her headache resolved, and she has no complaints apart from occasional fatigue. Physical examination, including fundoscopy and visual fields, on perimetry was normal. Her body mass index was 24 kg/m² and she had no significant past medical history and was not on any drugs.

What is the next appropriate step in the management?

    A   Obtain 9 am pituitary function tests and arrange yearly follow-up
    B   Reassure her and repeat MRI pituitary in 6 months
    C   Repeat MRI – MRI pituitary with contrast
    D   She is asymptomatic – discharge from the endocrinology clinic
    E   This may represent idiopathic intracranial hypertension (IIH), therefore refer to neurology clinic for lumbar puncture.

42. A 45-year-old woman presented to her general practitioner with increasing fatigue, weight gain and constipation. She had seen a gynaecologist for heavy periods and had had a levonorgestrel-releasing intrauterine system (Mirena coil) inserted, which resulted in resolution of the menorrhagia and was given ferrous sulphate tablets. She had a past medical history of stable asthma and hypothyroidism since her early twenties, and she was on levothyroxine 100 µg daily and salbutamol inhaler as required for several years. Physical examination showed pulse rate of 60 beats per minute and blood pressure 165/100 mmHg, and the rest of the examination was normal.

Investigations:

haemoglobin 138 g/L (115–165)	corrected calcium 2.32 mmol/L (2.2–2.6)
sodium 142 mmol/L (135–145)	bilirubin 8 mmol/L (1–22)
potassium 3.9 mmol/L (3.5–5.0)	albumin 45 g/L (37–49)
urea 5.0 (2.5–7.5 mmol/L)	alanine aminotransferase 45 U/L (5–35)
creatinine 75 µmol/L (60–110)	alkaline phosphatase 45 U/L (45–105)
thyroid-stimulating hormone 22.0 mU/L (0.4–5.0)	total cholesterol 7.9 mmol/L (3–5)
free thyroxine (FT4) 8 (10–25 pmol/L)	low-density lipoprotein 5.6 mmol/L (2–3)
	triglyceride 2.9 mmol/L (0.6–1.69)

What is next appropriate step in management?

A   Advise her regarding the importance of taking thyroid tablets regularly as well as lifestyle advice for hypercholesterolemia and hypertension, and recheck in 3 months

B   Check 9 am pituitary function tests and consider pituitary MRI

C   Increase levothyroxine to 125 µg once daily and give lifestyle advice for hypercholesterolemia and hypertension, and recheck in 6 months

D   Increase levothyroxine to 125 µg once daily and start atorvastatin 20 mg nocte and ramipril 2.5 mg once daily, and recheck in 6 months

E   Stop ferrous sulphate and recheck thyroid function, blood pressure and lipid profile in 3 months

43. A 55-year-old man was brought into the emergency department with chest pain and confusion. His blood pressure was 240/130 mmHg and the emergency consultant concerned about aortic dissection, ordered a CT aortogram. This revealed a 4 cm left adrenal mass with a heterogenous texture.

    Phaeochromocytoma was suspected and he was transferred to the high dependency unit (HDU). In the HDU, he was noted to be confused with a Glasgow Coma Scale score of 14/15, pulse rate of 130 beats per minute and blood pressure of 220/140 mmHg, and fundoscopy showed papilloedema. A plasma sample was sent for measurement of the metanephrine level. Renal function remained stable.

What is the next step in his management?

A   Alert the surgeons and prepare for unilateral adrenalectomy immediately with intravenous labetalol to lower blood pressure

B   Salt and fluid restrict and start oral doxazosin at 4 mg twice daily dose. Start bisoprolol once the patient is established on doxazosin. Plan surgery in the next few months

C   Start intravenous glycery trinitrate to lower blood pressure, initiate oral amlodipine and doxazosin. Plan for a left adrenalectomy in 24–48 hours

D   Start intravenous phentolamine and initiate low dose oral phenoxybenzamine. Plan for an adrenalectomy when blood pressure <160/100 mmHg. Start bisoprolol once established on phenoxybenzamine for tachycardia

E   Start oral phenoxybenzamine at 30 mg three times daily and titrate dose depending on blood pressure. Start bisoprolol once established on phenoxybenzamine for tachycardia. Plan for surgery in the next 2–3 months

44. A 17-year-old boy with type 1 diabetes was admitted to the emergency department with vomiting and diarrhoea for several days and progressive fatigue. He usually is on insulin glargine 20 units once daily and insulin lispro at meal times but he had been off insulin because he was not eating. An examination showed pulse rate 130 beats per minute, blood pressure 95/60 mmHg, respiratory rate 40/min and temperature 37 °C. He was lethargic and had dry mucosa. He had mild epigastric tenderness and his chest was clear.

Investigations:

haemoglobin 158 g/L (130–180)	urea 14.0 × 10⁹/L (2.5–7)
white cell count 12.5 × 10⁹/L (4–11)	creatinine 130 µmol/L (60–110)
neutrophils 9 × 10⁹/L (1.5–7)	glucose 36 mmol/L (4 – 7.8)
platelets 513 × 10⁹/L (150–400)	amylase 233 U/L (60–180)
sodium 128 mmol/L (135–145)	
potassium 2.8 mmol/L (3.5–5.0)	

Arterial blood gases on air:

pH 7.1 (7.34–7.44)

PaO_2 13 кРа (10–13)

$PaCO_2$ 2.2 кРа (4.4–5.9)

bicarbonate 9 mmol/L (18–24)

serum ketones 4.7 mmol/L (<0.6)

He was moved to the high dependency unit and started on intravenous normal saline at a rate of 1 litre per hour.

What is the next most appropriate step in his management?

A   Start potassium chloride 20 mmol/L in 1 litre normal saline and give over 2 hours, recheck potassium and initiate insulin infusion only after potassium >3.3 mmol/L

B   Start fixed dose insulin infusion (FRII) at 0.05 U/kg, and add potassium chloride 40 mmol to the next litre of normal saline and infuse over 4 hours

C   Start fixed dose insulin infusion (FRII) at 0.1 U/kg, and add potassium chloride 40 mmol to next litre of normal saline and infuse over 4 hours

D   Start fixed dose insulin infusion (FRII) at 0.1 U/kg and 1.26% sodium bicarbonate 500 mL over 4 hours. Give 1 L normal saline with 40 mmol of potassium chloride over 2 hours

E   Start fixed dose insulin infusion (FRII) at 0.1 U/kg and add potassium chloride 40 mmol to the next litre of normal saline and infuse over 4 hours

Answers

1.   A   Request US examination of pelvis and repeat thyroid function tests

This woman has hyperemesis gravidarum (HG). HG is defined as persistent nausea and vomiting in the first trimester of pregnancy, resulting in greater than 5% weight loss, ketonuria, dehydration liver and electrolyte abnormalities, and is reported to occur in 0.3 to 1.0% of pregnancies. The onset of nausea is at 4–6 week's gestation, and it worsens at 7–9 weeks' gestation. In 60% of cases, it resolves by the end of the first trimester, and in the vast majority of women, complete resolution is by 20 weeks.

Hyperemesis is associated with high hCG levels in early first trimester, but the exact cause remains uncertain. 30–60% of patients with HG have elevated free thyroxine (FT4) concentrations and a suppressed TSH level. The aetiology of excessive thyroid stimulation is considered to be hCG (or derivatives of hCG) directly stimulating thyroid cells by binding to the TSH receptor. Severity of the emesis correlates positively with the serum free T_4 and hCG levels, and inversely with the degree of TSH suppression.

Differentiation from Graves' thyrotoxicosis may be difficult, because vomiting is a presenting symptom in both. The diagnosis of transient hyperthyroidism of hyperemesis gravidarum should be considered in women with severe vomiting, no clinical manifestations of Graves' disease, and biochemical evidence of hyperthyroidism. The presence of thyroid receptor antibodies favours the diagnosis of Graves' hyperthyroidism.

Trophoblastic diseases, partial and complete hydatidiform moles, and choriocarcinoma are the causes of hyperthyroidism early in pregnancy. Patients may present without symptoms in spite of chemical hyperthyroidism, or with various degrees of severity, including congestive heart failure.

Evacuation of the mole eliminates the source of the excessive hCG and reverses the clinical and biochemical features of hyperthyroidism.

Twin or multiple pregnancy can result in higher hCG levels and hence higher incidence of hyperemesis with consequent abnormal thyroid picture.

Given the importance of excluding trophoblastic disease, ultrasound would be the next step in managing this patient. Management of hyperthyroidism in hyperemesis gravidarum relies on fluid replacement and anti-emetics. Once vomiting subsides and hCG comes down, the thyrotoxicosis subsides. Beta-blockers such as propranolol can be used transiently but they have the potential to cause intrauterine growth restriction.

Very rarely, anti-thyroid drugs may be needed, but most cases resolve with the administration of fluids, and once the pregnancy advances and the hCG levels fall.

Cooper DS, Laurberg P. Hyperthyroidism in pregnancy. Lancet Diabetes Endocrinol 2013;1:238–249.

2.   C   Intravenous fluids

The clinical picture is suggestive of a lung cancer with hypercalcaemia. Her symptoms are primarily due to hypercalcaemia; a calcium level >3.5 mmol/L suggest severe hypercalcaemia. Symptoms of severe hypercalcaemia include polyuria, polydipsia, dehydration, nausea, vomiting, pancreatitis and cardiac arrhythmias. The ECG changes include a shortened QT interval and a widened T wave.

Initial treatment is adequate fluid replacement. This alone may be enough to bring the calcium level down. After adequate fluid replacement, diuresis with loop diuretics may enhance calcium excretion. For cancer-related hypercalcaemia, bisphosphonates such as pamidronate or zoledronate would be the next step, though the effect on calcium levels is usually a delayed one. Denosumab has also been trialled. Glucocorticoids such as prednisolone can be also used in the treatment of hypercalcaemia.

Mechanism of hypercalcaemia, in this instance, is most likely to be paraneoplastic secretion of PTHrP (parathyroid hormone-related peptide) by the carcinoma. Parathyroid hormone levels would be low or undetectable in this instance. The other mechanism of hypercalcaemia in this case could be lytic metastases in the bones.

Demshar R, Vanek R, Mazanec P. Oncologic emergencies: new decade, new perspectives. AACN Adv Crit Care 2011; 22:337–348.

3.   A Fine-needle aspiration cytology

This question concerns the management of a single nodule in the thyroid. She is clinically and biochemically euthyroid and the ultrasound reveals some microcalcifications which point towards a neoplastic process.

Sonographically suggestive features are microcalcifications, hypoechoic solid lesions, irregular margins, increased vascularity within nodule and signs of extracapsular spread. The ultrasound 'U' classification of thyroid nodules was developed by the British Thyroid Association as part of their 2014 guidelines on the management of thyroid cancer:

U1 (normal – no nodule)
U2 (benign)
U3 (indeterminate)
U4 (suspicious)
U5 (malignant)

In this instance, since ultrasound shows a U3 nodule, the first step would be ultrasound-guided FNA of the nodule.

The histology determines further management. The Royal College of Pathologists' classification is used for thyroid FNA reporting and is:

- Thy1, Thy1c (non-diagnostic)
    - Cystic fluid specimens without abundant colloid/epithelial cells. Can be considered benign, if radiology correlates – consider multi-disciplinary discussion.
- Thy2, Thy2c (non-neoplastic)
- Thy3 (neoplasm possible)
- Thy3a – atypiaThy3f follicular neoplasm. Possibilities include hyperplastic or other cellular but non-neoplastic nodules, as well as neoplasms, including follicular adenomas and follicular carcinomas
- Thy4 (suspicion of malignancy)
- Thy5 (malignant)

Perros P, Boelaert K, Colley S, et al. British Thyroid Association guidelines for the management of thyroid cancer. Clin Endocrin 2014;81: 1–122.
The Royal College of Pathologists (RCP). Guidance on the reporting of thyroid cytology (G089). London: RCP, 2016.

4.   E Exenatide-induced acute pancreatitis

Exenatide, a GLP-1 (glucagon-like peptide-1) analogue, is known to increase the risk of developing acute pancreatitis. The risk, however, is low, and diabetes itself increases the risk of pancreatitis. The risk is also increased if the person has hypertriglyceridaemia or a previous history of pancreatitis. On starting exenatide injections, patients are warned to contact their doctor and stop exenatide if they develop abdominal pain.

Exenatide is often given as a second- or third-line agent in type 2 diabetes prior to insulin therapy. It tends to produce some weight loss as well, which is advantageous in a person with high body mass index. GLP-1 is an incretin hormone which is produced by the gut in response to food intake and increases food-related insulin release.

Although hypertriglyceridaemia can induce acute pancreatitis this is mainly seen in severe cases with triglyceride levels >11.3 mmol/L. Bezafibrate does not increase the incidence of or worsen the symptoms of peptic ulcer disease.

Combination therapy with a fibrate and a statin is known to increase the incidence of myalgia and rhabdomyolysis. However, the creatine kinase level is only modestly elevated whereas in rhabdomyolysis it is usually elevated 5 times above the upper limit. Also, hyperkalaemia is a feature of rhabdomyolysis which is not seen here.

Acute kidney injury can be worsened by ramipril; however, the symptoms and elevated amylase level in this case points towards pancreatitis rather than renal injury as the cause.

Li L, Shen J, Bala MM, et al. Incretin treatment and risk of pancreatitis in patients with type 2 diabetes mellitus: systematic review and meta-analysis of randomised and non-randomised studies. BMJ 2014; 348:g2366.

5.   C Fluoxetine-induced hyperprolactinaemia

Selective serotonin reuptake inhibitors (SSRIs), such as fluoxetine, activate serotoninergic pathways (via type 2A serotonin receptors) and stimulate prolactin release. They are associated with an approximate eight-fold increased risk of development of galactorrhoea compared with other antidepressants.

While depression and diabetes can cause erectile dysfunction, given the high prolactin level, this has to be considered as the most important factor.

Follicle-stimulating hormone and luteinising hormone levels are both normal and hence the patient does not have hypogonadotrophic hypogonadism. Metformin does not cause hyperprolactinaemia.

Treatment of SSRI-related sexual dysfunction consists of switching the drug (in consultation with a psychiatrist), adding small amounts of dopamine agonist (such as bromocriptine) cautiously, phosphodiesterase-5 inhibitors and other drugs.

Rizvi SJ1, Kennedy SH. Management strategies for SSRI-induced sexual dysfunction. J Psychiatry Neurosci. 2013; 38:E27–8.
Papakostas GI, et al. Serum prolactin levels among outpatients with major depressive disorder during the acute phase of treatment with fluoxetine. J Clin Psychiatry 2006; 67:952–957.

6.   D Two 24-hour urine collections for free cortisol

The history and physical examination is suggestive of Cushing's syndrome. The next step is a screening test for Cushing's syndrome. The currently acceptable screening tests for Cushing's syndrome are: overnight 1 mg dexamethasone suppression test, urinary free cortisol levels and salivary cortisol level. Of these, because she is on combined oral contraceptive pills, urine collection for free cortisol is more appropriate because oestrogen can interfere with the overnight suppression test, unless it is stopped a few weeks prior to the test.

The low-dose dexamethasone suppression test is often used as a screening test in those with high pretest probability of Cushing's syndrome and also to confirm the diagnosis.

The high-dose dexamethasone suppression test is used to identify the source of the cortisol hypersecretion. Late night cortisol and salivary cortisol may also be used.

Insulin tolerance testing is used to diagnose ACTH/cortisol and growth hormone reserve and short Synacthen test is for hypoadrenalism.

Plasma adrenocorticotrophic hormone (ACTH) levels are useful for identifying the source of hypercortisolism. High ACTH levels suggest either pituitary or ectopic ACTH secretion and low levels suggest primary adrenal hypersecretion. However, ACTH levels are not useful as a screening test.

Guignat L, Bertherat J. The diagnosis of Cushing's syndrome: an Endocrine Society Clinical Practice Guideline: commentary from a European perspective. Eur J Endocrinol 2010; 163:9–13.
Nieman LK, et al. The diagnosis of Cushing's syndrome: an Endocrine Society Clinical Practice Guideline. J Clin Endocrinol Metab 2008; 93:1526–1540.

7.   A Exogenous insulin use

The combination of reduced blood sugar, low C-peptide and high insulin level suggests exogenous insulin use. In the case of both insulinoma and sulphonylurea abuse, C-peptide levels would be high. A blood or urine screen for sulphonylurea would clarify the diagnosis in that case.

The insulin mRNA is translated as a single chain precursor called pre-proinsulin, and removal of its signal peptide during insertion into the endoplasmic reticulum generates proinsulin. Within the endoplasmic reticulum, proinsulin is cleaved by endopeptidases into insulin and C-peptide. Insulin and free C-peptide are stored in secretory granules within the cytoplasm. When the beta cell is stimulated, insulin and C-peptide are secreted into the islet capillary blood.

Hence both sulphonylurea compounds, which stimulate insulin release and insulinoma (which oversecretes insulin), produce elevated insulin and C-peptide levels. Insulinoma is a type of neuroendocrine tumour.

In liver dysfunction with hypoglycaemia, the insulin level would not be high with a suppressed C-peptide level.

Cryer PE, et al. Evaluation and management of adult hypoglycemic disorders: an Endocrine Society Clinical Practice Guideline. J Clin Endocrinol Metab 2009; 94(3):709–728.

8. D Oral glucose tolerance test with growth hormone levels

The clinical scenario described is suggestive of acromegaly. This is strengthened by the difficult to control hypertension and impaired glucose tolerance.

To screen for the presence of acromegaly, IGF-1 (insulin-like growth factor-1) level can be used and, to confirm, an oral glucose tolerance test with serial measurement of growth hormone is commonly used.

Isolated growth hormone levels are less useful as the secretion tends to be episodic. IGF-1 levels are more useful for screening. Measurement of IGF-1 should be followed by an oral glucose tolerance test. Serial measurement of glucose and growth hormone levels are done 30, 60 and 120 minutes after a 75 g oral glucose load. In normal people growth hormone level will be suppressed to <1 ng/mL after a 75 g oral glucose load. If there is still doubt then a thyroid-stimulating hormone-releasing hormone test may be useful.

Pituitary MRI is done after biochemical confirmation of acromegaly as incidental pituitary masses are seen in approximately 10% of normal volunteers.

The low-dose dexamethasone suppression test is used in Cushing's syndrome and the insulin tolerance test in hypoadrenalism.

Hall WA. Pituitary magnetic resonance imaging in normal human volunteers: occult adenomas in the general population. Ann Intern Med 1994; 120(10):817–820.

9. C Intravenous hydrocortisone (100 mg every 8 hours)

The history of possible previous traumatic brain injury followed by malaise, decreased libido and increased weight suggest the development of hypopituitarism due to head injury. Traumatic brain injury can cause pituitary dysfunction in up to a third of cases. Most commonly this is manifested acutely as diabetes insipidus. However, later on panhypopituitarism may develop insidiously.

Supplementing thyroxine alone in this situation may precipitate an adrenal crisis since thyroxine can accelerate the catabolism of cortisol. Treatment of adrenal crisis is primarily fluid replacement, hydrocortisone and treatment of the precipitating condition such as an infection. Before starting treatment blood sample for cortisol and adrenocorticotrophic hormone estimation are sent off. Once the crisis is over, tests of pituitary reserve are carried out such as short Synacthen test, luteinising hormone or follicle-stimulating hormone levels, thyroid function tests, testosterone, prolactin and insulin-like growth factor-1 levels. Urine and plasma osmolality should be measured to assess posterior pituitary function.

Schneider M, et al. Anterior pituitary hormone abnormalities following traumatic brain injury. J Neurotrauma 2005; 22(9):937–46.
Behan LA, Agha A. Endocrine consequences of adult traumatic brain injury. Horm Res 2007; 68(5):18–21.

10. E Fluid restriction

The clinical picture is suggestive of the syndrome of inappropriate antidiuretic hormone (SIADH) release due to release of stored vasopressin from the hypothalamopituitary axons because of neural trauma from the basal skull fracture. The released vasopressin causes excess retention of free water, especially if fluids are administered, as in this case. This leads to plasma hypo-osmolality and urine hyperosmolality; hyponatraemia may also result.

The initial management is fluid restriction. Demeclocycline can be tried if fluid restriction is not effective. In severe cases hyponatraemia may lead to convulsions and altered state of consciousness. Treatment in severe cases is with hypertonic saline, but this must be used very cautiously. Serum sodium must be monitored carefully and rate of rise of sodium must be slow.

Tolvaptan and other Vasopressin V2 receptor antagonists have a role. Injury to the pituitary stalk produces a classic triphasic response – an initial phase of reduced vasopressin secretion leading to diabetes insipidus, followed by a phase of release of stored vasopressin leading to SIADH; this is followed by a phase of diabetes insipidus again while the neural damage recovers. The final phase of diabetes insipidus may result in only partial or no recovery.

11. E Reduce night-time NPH insulin

The history of night sweats and headache points towards nocturnal hypoglycaemia. The pre-bed glucose levels are low which again points towards nocturnal hypoglycaemia. The high morning glucose levels point towards 'Somogyi's effect' – i.e. nocturnal hypoglycaemia causes anti-insulin hormones such as cortisol, glucagon and adrenaline to be secreted, which drives the blood sugar up. This results in nocturnal hypoglycaemic episodes followed by early morning hyperglycaemia.

Since the neutral protamine Hagedorn (NPH) insulin given at bedtime is the most likely cause of the nocturnal hypoglycaemia, dose reduction is the most logical step. Furthermore, as pre-bed blood glucose values are low normal, depending on when the evening meals are, the evening dose of regular insulin might also need to be reduced.

It is vital to consider possible 'Somogyi's effects' prior to increasing the night-time insulin dose. Nocturnal hypoglycaemia is often asymptomatic but can result in night sweats, nightmares, headache and sudden death (increased risk of cardiac arrhythmias). A 2 am capillary blood glucose levels often helps to diagnose this problem. Continuous blood glucose monitoring may also be helpful. This should be contrasted with the 'Dawn effect' where there is a morning rise in blood sugar in response to waning insulin and a growth hormone surge which antagonises the action of insulin.

12. D Intravenous thiamine supplementation

Thiamine is a water-soluble vitamin with low body stores that can be depleted in around 10–20 days. Its active metabolite is thiamine pyrophosphate, which is important for carbohydrate metabolism.

Prolonged starvation leads to thiamine depletion. In such a situation, sudden carbohydrate load without accompanying thiamine would lead to Wernicke's encephalopathy (WE) and peripheral neuropathy (dry beri-beri).

The classic triad of WE is confusion, ocular problems and ataxia. Delirium, ophthalmoplegia and nystagmus are the common manifestations. Peripheral neuropathy is also seen. Chronic alcoholism is the most common cause due to reduced intake of thiamine and reduced absorption from the gut.

Diagnosis is by measuring thiamine levels in blood or red cell transketolase activity. Both are difficult to perform and are not entirely specific. Other methods that have recently come into play include measuring thiamine and its metabolites in red cells by high-performance liquid chromatography.

MRI is specific but not sensitive. Typically, there is involvement of periventricular areas bilaterally. These include the medial aspect of the thalamus, hypothalamus and mamillary bodies, the periaqueductal region and the floor of the fourth ventricle where an increased T2 signal is seen.

Korsakoff's syndrome with loss of short-term memory and variable cognitive problems may develop subacutely, often after WE.

Treatment is intravenous thiamine. This should be done upon suspecting the condition and should not wait for biochemical or radiological confirmation. In this case rapid weight loss due to bariatric surgery and vomiting followed by intravenous dextrose precipitated the condition. Recently more than 200 cases of WE have been reported after bariatric surgery.

Post-bariatric surgery, patients are also prone to vitamin B$_{12}$, zinc, vitamin D and magnesium deficiencies, and hence these should also be monitored. Here the clinical picture is clearly that of WE.

Sechi G, Serra A. Wernicke's encephalopathy: new clinical settings and recent advances in diagnosis and management. Lancet Neurol 2007; 6:442–455.

13. C Plasma aldosterone:renin ratio

In the presence of difficult to control hypertension, a low potassium concentration in the serum (despite being on ramipril) should raise the suspicion of primary hyperaldosteronism (PA). It must be remembered that only a minority of patients with PA (9 to 37%) has hypokalemia and therefore absence of hypokalaemia does not exclude PA. The screening test for this is plasma aldosterone:renin ratio. The ratio is more sensitive than plasma renin activity or plasma aldosterone levels on their own.

Many drugs, especially spironolactone, amiloride, diuretics and angiotensin-converting enzyme inhibitors, affect the test. Most guidelines recommend a morning (2 hours after waking up and after 15–30 minutes rest) plasma aldosterone:renin ratio measurement (off spironolactone and diuretics) as a screening test, followed by a confirmatory test.

One of four confirmatory tests used involves measuring plasma aldosterone after doing one of the following:
1. Oral salt load
2. Saline infusion
3. After fludrocortisone suppression
4. Captopril challenge test

Once biochemically confirmed, then a CT/MRI of the adrenals would be helpful to distinguish between adenoma (Conn's syndrome) and hyperplasia. If there is still any doubt, selective adrenal vein sampling may be required.

[11]C-metomidate, a potent inhibitor of the enzyme 11-β hydroxylase, which is over-expressed in adrenocortical adenomas, has recently been used as a radiotracer in positron emission tomography (PET) and shows good specificity for aldosterone secreting adrenal adenomas.

Plasma metanephrine level and meta-iodobenzylguanidine scan are used to diagnose phaeochromocytomas rather than primary hyperaldosteronism.

Funder JW, Carey RM, Mantero F, et al. The management of primary aldosteronism: case detection, diagnosis, and treatment: an Endocrine Society Clinical Practice guideline. J Clin Endocrinol Metab. 2016; 101:1889–916.

14. B Oral levothyroxine replacement

The clinical features and the lab data are suggestive of severe primary hypothyroidism with low free thyroxine and free triiodothyronine and high thyroid-stimulating hormone. There is also the history of poor concordance with medication. The clinical features are not suggestive of myxoedema coma, and so intravenous triiodothyronine is not necessary in this instance. Oral levothyroxine therapy is sufficient.

Severe hypothyroidism by itself causes hyperprolactinaemia. Bromocriptine is not necessary; correction of the hypothyroidism would bring the level of prolactin down.

Severe hypothyroidism can occasionally result in significant thyrotroph, hyperplasia, causing a secondary thyrotroph adenoma in the pituitary. This thyrotroph hyperplasia usually resolves with thyroxine replacement.

Hekimsoy Z, Kafesçiler S, Güçlü, et al. The prevalence of hyperprolactinaemia in overt and subclinical hypothyroidism. Endocr J 2010; 57:1011–1015.

15. A Add spironolactone

Though the aldosterone:renin ratio is high, both aldosterone and renin levels are low in this instance. In this case effective treatment would be to add a small dose of spironolactone.

Given the low aldosterone level the suspicion of primary aldosteronism (Conn's syndrome and other causes of high aldosterone level) is less here. The most likely diagnosis is low renin essential hypertension and, given that the patient is already on bendrofluazide, the best course is adding a mineralocorticoid antagonist such as spironolactone. The other possibilities are extremely rare such as Liddle's syndrome, rare mutations in steroidogenesis pathway and congenital adrenal hyperplasia (CAH). Another rare cause is excessive liquorice ingestion. These possibilities are entertained if spironolactone fails to control the blood pressure.

Selective adrenal vein sampling is the current gold standard for Conn's syndrome and, as described above, is not indicated here.

The urine metanephrine level was normal twice and hence there is no need to do an meta-iodobenzylguaridine (MIBG) scan. Similarly, pituitary MRI and high-dose dexamethasone suppression tests are not indicated here, since the screening test (overnight dexamethasone suppression test) is negative and the index of suspicion is low.

Low renin hypertension can be seen in significant proportion (up to 30%) of hypertensives and does respond to diuretics and mineralocorticoid antagonists. There is a higher incidence in the black population. The exact cause of low renin with normal or low aldosterone level is not known. Several putative causes are currently being investigated.

There is an emerging view that in many cases low-renin hypertension represents occult primary aldosteronism and hence why mineralocorticoid antagonists are very effective.

Funder JW. Primary aldosteronism: new answers, new questions. Horm Metab Res 2015; 47:935–40.
Mulatero P, et al. Diagnosis and treatment of low-renin hypertension. Clin Endocrinol 2007; 67: 324–334.

16. B 24-hour urine metanephrines

His past history of hypertension, palpitations, left ventricular hypertrophy (LVH) on the ECG and syncopal episodes, together with the hypertensive episode on anaesthesia, is suggestive of phaeochromocytoma, and hence a 24-hour urine metanephrine is the best investigation among the options. The other screening test would be plasma metanephrine level.

While primary aldosteronism would result in hypertension and LVH on the ECG, a hypertensive crisis with anaesthesia is not common. Furthermore, serum potassium was normal, which does not exclude primary aldosteronism but makes it less likely. Similarly, Cushing's syndrome does not commonly produce crisis on anaesthesia induction.

Although hypertension is known to occur with a thyroid storm, and surgery on the thyroid can precipitate it, the symptom complex here favours a catecholamine-related tumour rather than thyroid dysfunction. Though there is history of episodic palpitations, other history suggestive of thyrotoxicosis, such as fever, diarrhoea and weight loss, is absent. Resting ECG did not show sinus tachycardia or abnormal rhythms and physical examination did not reveal any signs of thyrotoxicosis.

Acute intermittent porphyria presents more with abdominal pain and neuropsychiatric symptoms rather than syncopal episodes.

Terzolo M, et al. AME position statement on adrenal incidentaloma. Eur J Endocrinol 2011; 164:851–870.
Chen H, et al. The North American Neuroendocrine Tumor Society consensus guideline for the diagnosis and management of neuroendocrine tumors: pheochromocytoma, paraganglioma, and medullary thyroid cancer. Pancreas 2010; 39:775–783.

17. B Stop carbimazole and propranolol and monitor thyroid function tests in 6 weeks

The clinical and biochemical picture is suggestive of subacute thyroiditis (de Quervain's thyroiditis). The aetiology is unknown, but immune alteration following a viral illness in susceptible individuals is suspected.

Initial presentation is with sore throat and flu-like symptoms, followed by transient hyperthyroidism (because of release of preformed thyroid hormones from follicles due to follicular disruption). Four to 6 weeks later, there may be a phase of hypothyroidism (because of glandular destruction) in about 25% of those affected followed by return of normal thyroid function (due to regeneration from the edges of the areas of destruction). In the initial phase a thyroid gland is often enlarged and tender.

Treatment is mainly supportive. For pain and sore throat non-steroidal anti-inflammatory drugs can be used. For the hyperthyroid phase propranolol is useful for symptomatic control. In severe cases, prednisolone may be useful once acute bacterial or suppurative thyroiditis has been ruled out. Recurrences are common.

Watchful monitoring is all that is required during the hypothyroid phase. In 10% of cases hypothyroidism may be prolonged and require levothyroxine supplementation.

Carbimazole is not useful as the primary pathology is not overproduction of thyroid hormones but release of preformed hormones from follicular disruption. During the recovery process, there may be a marked but transient increase in the 24-hour radioactive iodine uptake which can reach levels typical of Graves' disease but thyrotoxicosis is not simultaneously present.

Propranolol can be stopped as she does not have any hyperthyroid symptoms.

Thyroid ultrasound is not indicated as the clinical and biochemical picture is suggestive of subacute thyroiditis. An iodine-131 uptake scan during the hyperthyroid phase may be useful as it would show decreased uptake of iodine [whereas Graves' disease or thyroid nodule causing hyperthyroidism would show increased uptake either diffusely (Graves' disease) or as a hot spot (nodule)].

Other causes of sub-acute thyroiditis include interferon-α therapy, radiation, renal cell carcinoma (paraneoplastic) and amiodarone.

Bindra A, Braunstein GD. Thyroiditis. Am Fam Physician 2006; 73:1769–1776.

18. C Fasting gastrin and chromogranin A level in serum

The clinical picture described here is suggestive of multiple endocrine neoplasia 1 (MEN1) or Wermer's syndrome. This comes from a history of parathyroid involvement (nearly all of those with MEN1 develop hyperparathyroidism by the age of 50) and gastrinoma, which is suggested by the gastric ulcers. Up to 40% of those with MEN1 may develop gastrinoma. Gastrinoma is the second most common endocrine tumour and is the most common cause of severe symptoms and signs in MEN1. Zolliger–Ellison syndrome (ZES) is the manifestation of excess gastric acid due to gastrinoma. Twenty-five per cent of cases of ZES are due to MEN1. Less commonly, insulinomas and glucagonomas may develop.

In MEN1 this is more likely to be due to multiple intraduodenal tumours rather than a pancreatic tumour. These are also more likely to be malignant than the sporadic tumours and more likely to metastasise. The presence of steatorrhoea in this case suggests inactivation of pancreatic lipase due to the high gastrin and acid levels. In the case of neuroendocrine tumours, chromogranin A, a storage vesicle protein, is a good marker and can be elevated in up to 46% of cases of gastrinoma. Fasting gastrin level is usually elevated in gastrinomas. Care must be taken to exclude conditions which cause hypergastrinaemia such as atrophic gastritis and PPI (proton pump inhibitor) treatment.

As mentioned, MEN1 presents with parathyroid, pancreatic and pituitary tumours. Prolactinomas and growth hormone-secreting adenomas are the common pituitary lesions. Monitoring consists of measuring serum calcium, prolactin, insulin-like growth factor-1 and chromogranin A levels periodically. Somatostatin receptor scintigraphy is used to image the neuroendocrine tumours such as gastrinomas.

Surgical management is difficult in gastrinoma due to MEN 1 and total cure is virtually zero with surgical methods due to the multiplicity of tumours. Hence medical treatment with proton pump inhibitors and H_2 receptor blockers such as ranitidine is often employed. The somatostatin analogue octreotide inhibits partially the secretion of both gastrin and gastric acid. This is currently being trialled.

Marx SJ. Wells Jr SA. Chapter 39. Multiple endocrine neoplasia. In: Melmed S, Polonsky KP, Larsen R, Kronenberg H. Williams Textbook of Endocrinology (13th ed). Elsevier, 2016.

19. D Systemic steroids

Graves' ophthalmopathy can develop before or after the thyroid disease manifests. Management is dependent on the severity of the disease. Many classifications, including the scoring system NOSPECS, have been used for assessing the severity of Graves' disease. Most also look at the level of inflammatory activity.

The treatment depends on the severity and activity. This patient is euthyroid after antithyroid drug therapy. At this point in time neither radio-iodine nor surgery would be the treatments of choice. There are reports that radio-iodine treatment in patients with active hyperthyroidism can worsen the eye disease. Smoking can also worsen eye disease in Graves' disease.

For mild eye disease, observation is the best policy supplemented by artificial tears.

Moderate to severe orbitopathy

Medical treatment is likely to be beneficial in patients with active Graves' orbitopathy (GO), with florid signs and symptoms of inflammation, recent onset extraocular muscle dysfunction and recent progression of the ocular abnormalities as a whole. In longstanding GO, with chronic proptosis and residual, stable diplopia and/or strabismus, but no evidence of inflammation, surgery has more benefit. Orbital radiotherapy is the other option. The rationale for its use and the indications are quite similar to those of glucocorticoids. Rituximab has been used successfully in GO.

Dysthyroid optic neuropathy, the most severe expression of the orbitopathy, is a sight-threatening emergency, which requires immediate treatment. If there is no response to medical treatment (high-dose intravenous glucocorticoids), orbital decompression is warranted. Other important indications for decompressive surgery are corneal damage due to eyeball exposure in patients with marked proptosis, or recurrent subluxation of the globe, which may stretch the optic nerve and cause sight loss.

In this instance, with euthyroid status achieved by antithyroid drugs, the best therapeutic option would be pulsed intravenous steroid therapy. If that does not work, decompression is warranted given corneal ulceration and oedema of optic discs.

Soeters MR, van Zeijl CJ, Boelen A, et al. Optimal management of Graves' orbitopathy: a multidisciplinary approach. Neth J Med 2011; 69(7):302–308.

20. C Reassure the patient

This person has mildly elevated serum calcium and parathyroid hormone (PTH) levels. She also has a normal phosphate and vitamin D levels. However, the urine calcium:creatinine clearance ratio is reduced, suggesting that she has relative hypocalciuria in the presence of hypercalcaemia. PTH is also not suppressed in the presence of hypercalcaemia. The combination of these suggests familial hypocalciuric hypercalcaemia (FHH). In primary hyperparathyroidism, the urine calcium:creatinine clearance ratio would be higher than 0.01, suggesting that urine calcium excretion in normal or increased.

Most of FHH is caused by autosomal dominant loss-of-function mutations in the calcium-sensing receptor (*CaSR*) gene, which encodes the CaSR. Elevations in serum calcium concentration stimulate the CaSR, which promotes calcitonin production and urinary calcium excretion while suppressing the synthesis and secretion of PTH, thereby lowering the calcium concentration. Mutations in *CaSR* impair the feedback inhibition of PTH with rising serum calcium. Hence higher than normal serum calcium levels are needed to inhibit the release of PTH, thus leading to either a normal or slightly elevated PTH level, despite hypercalcaemia. The degree of hypercalcaemia depends on how severely the mutation affects the function of the CaSR molecule. In effect the mutation resets the calcium homeostasis to a slightly higher serum calcium level.

In the kidneys, CaSR is involved in the feedback inhibition of PTH-independent calcium reabsorption. Mutations in the CaSR gene prevent this feedback inhibition of calcium which helps lower serum calcium in the presence of hypercalcaemia. Since calcium is reabsorbed despite hypercalcaemia, the calcium concentration in the urine is low despite high serum calcium (relative hypocalciuria).

FHH is a benign disorder and does not usually need treatment. Genetic testing for mutations in CaSR can be carried out to confirm the diagnosis. More than 200 different mutations in CaSR have been identified to date.

Rarely there is an autoimmune version of this with autoantibodies against CaSR.

Varghese J, Rich T, Jimenez C. Benign familial hypocalciuric hypercalcemia. Endocr Pract 2010: 1–16.

21. C Add mixed insulin (short and intermediate acting) twice a day

This patient has significant hyperglycaemia with high, fasting, postprandial, blood sugar levels and a very high HbA1c. In particular, his postprandial blood sugars are high. The target HbA1c in this individual is 7% (or lower, if it can be safely achieved without hypoglycaemic episodes).

Addition of pioglitazone and sitagliptin would each only bring the HbA1c down by < 1%. Addition of a glucagon-like peptide-1 (GLP-1) agonist such as exenatide would bring the HbA1c down by 1–1.7% and in addition would benefit the weight. However, in this instance the HbA1c is >9% and there is significant hyperglycaemia. Insulin therapy is usually initiated in type 2 diabetes mellitus when combination oral agent therapy, with or without GLP-1 receptor agonist therapy, fails to achieve the glycaemic goal or when a patient, whether drug naïve or on a treatment regimen, presents with a HbA1c level >9.0% and symptomatic hyperglycaemia.

Since the HbA1c is 9.8% and the person is already on metformin and gliclazide, only the addition of insulin would bring about adequate control. The ideal regimen would be a basal bolus one, since his home monitoring indicates both pre-meal and post-meal hyperglycaemia. The options given here are basal insulin and twice a day insulin. Of these, basal insulin is unlikely to do be fully effective, especially for the postprandial hyperglycaemia, and hence the most effective technique among the options would be twice a day mixed insulin. Once the insulin regimen has been established, insulin secretagogues such as sulphonylureas should ideally be tapered and stopped. Guidelines on the optimal drug to be used and optimal time to start each class of drugs as well as optimal combinations of various drugs are evolving.

22. A Bezafibrate

This patient has pre-diabetes and hypertriglyceridaemia. Though type 2 diabetes itself can lead to hypertriglyceridaemia, in this instance one has to think about other conditions that raise triglyceride levels as well, such as familial hypertriglyceridaemia (FHT). High levels of triglycerides are seen in uncontrolled diabetes, especially in conditions of insulin deficiency. However, it is unlikely that pre-diabetes would lead to such high levels of triglycerides in the absence of another abnormality in the lipid metabolism.

It is likely that the hypertriglyceridaemia itself induced the acute pancreatitis. FHT is relatively common with an incidence of 1 in 500. Aetiology is unknown and it causes an elevated VLDL (very-low-density lipoprotein) level.

Complications include acute pancreatitis and premature coronary heart disease.

Treatment includes dietary fat restriction, alcohol restriction. Statins also lower the triglyceride level, but to a much lesser extent than fibrates or nicotinic acid. The drug of choice in this instance would be fibrates. Nicotinic acid, even in the long-acting formulations, has a high rate of producing flushing and diarrhoea. It also worsens glycaemic control, and therefore fibrates would be the drug of choice. Orlistat may have a modest effect.

Treatment with fibrates does lead to an increase in incidence of abnormalities in the liver function tests. Hence monitoring the liver function is important. The other issue with fibrates is increased incidence of muscle aches (myalgia) and rarely myositis and rhabdomyolysis. Statins have the same adverse effect and if combined, there is a higher risk of myalgia and myositis.

The other therapy that has been shown to be effective is omega-3 fatty acids.

The treatment options for severe hypertriglyceridemia with pancreatitis include insulin/dextrose infusion and therapeutic apheresis. Heparin is another option. Dietary fat restriction works well also.

Filippatos TD, Elisaf MS. Recommendations for severe hypertriglyceridemia treatment, are there new strategies? Curr Vasc Pharmacol. 2014; 12:598–616.

23. E Stop simvastatin and later switch to a lower dose of a more potent statin

Statin therapy has been associated with myalgia, myositis and rhabdomyolysis. Often cases of myositis are not accompanied by creatine kinase (CK) elevations. In most instances, however, symptomatic myalgias are accompanied by CK elevation. The mechanism of myalgia/myositis with statins has not been fully elucidated. Complicating this picture are studies suggesting that CK levels vary widely within the population and with activity and exercise. CK levels also have ethnic variations. Many centres suggest obtaining a baseline CK level prior to starting statins to reduce the effect of this variability. Some guidelines do not recommend this for the general population but do so for ethnic minorities and people at risk of myopathy. Routine later monitoring of statins is not recommended. Measure CK levels later only if the patient is symptomatic.

Always rule out hepatic problems, alcoholism and hypothyroidism because all of these can increase the incidence of statin-induced muscle damage.

Strategies to manage statin-related myopathies generally suggest:
- If asymptomatic and CK elevations <5–10 times the upper limit then continue the statin and monitor.
- If symptomatic (mild muscle aches and tolerable symptoms) and CK levels <5–10 times the upper limit, then continue statin at same or reduced dose and monitor.
- If tolerable symptoms and CK levels >5 times upper limit then stop statin and allow time for muscle to recover. Then alternative strategies for restarting statins – see below.
- If significant symptoms/rhabdomyolysis develops then stop statin and carefully consider the risk of restarting statins. Think of alternatives to statins.

Alternative strategies:
1. Use a lower dose of a more potent statin, e.g. atorvastatin or rosuvastatin
2. Use a statin with less impact on cytochrome P450 such as pravastatin or fluvastatin
3. Use alternate-day dosage of longer-acting statin such as atorvastatin
4. Use combination of lower-dose statin with ezetimibe.

In general, combining fibrates with statins increases the risk of myopathy. Ezetimibe by itself does not have clinical trial evidence to indicate lower cardiovascular risk. Coenzyme Q has been shown in some trials to mitigate the effect of statin-induced myopathy; however, larger trials have failed to replicate the effect.

Hence, in this instance, the correct strategy would be to stop simvastatin and allow time for recovery and then switch to a lower dose of a more potent statin.

Although not given as options in the question, evolocumab and alirocumab (the two PCSK9 inhibitors) are now approved for treating hyperlipidaemia in statin intolerant patients.

Arca M, Pigna G. Treating statin-intolerant patients. Diabetes Metab Syndr Obes 2011; 4:155–166.
McKenney JM, Davidson MH, Jacobson TA, et al. Final conclusions and recommendations of the National Lipid Association Statin Safety Assessment Task Force. Am J Cardiol 2006; 97:89C–94C.

24. E Thyroid function tests

The presentation is suggestive of hypokalaemic periodic paralysis. The features are hypotonia, reduced power and reflexes as well as intact sensorium, allied with a low potassium and improvement with potassium supplementation. Patients also have muscle cramps and aches.

The main differential diagnosis here would be Guillain–Barré syndrome and transverse myelitis apart from myasthenia gravis and polymyositis. However, the low potassium level would suggest that the diagnosis is hypokalaemic periodic paralysis. Most cases of hypokalaemic periodic paralysis are familial. In males of Chinese and Latin American origin, hyperthyroidism can lead to hypokalaemic periodic paralysis.

In thyrotoxic periodic paralysis, the hypokalaemia is due to an intracellular shift of potassium rather than absolute deficiency. Other causes of potassium depletion such as diarrhoea must be ruled out first. Heavy physical activity and stress can precipitate the attack, as can carbohydrate-rich meals.

There are two aspects to the treatment: immediate restoration of normal serum potassium level and later attainment of euthyroid status.

Oral or intravenous potassium can be used. However, it is important to remember that the hypokalaemia is due to intracellular shift. Hence aggressive treatment could lead to hyperkalaemia. Beta-blockers can be effective in preventing episodes.

Once the acute treatment is done, attaining euthyroid status would be important in preventing future episodes.

Pothiwala P, Levine SN. Analytic review: thyrotoxic periodic paralysis: a review. J Intensive Care Med 2010; 25:71–77.

25. E Short Synacthen test

A person with a history of multiple autoimmune problems (type 1 diabetes and hypothyroidism) is at risk of developing other autoimmune problems and should raise the suspicion of polyglandular autoimmune syndrome (PAI) type 2.

The symptoms of fatigue and recurrent hypoglycaemia in a person with type 1 diabetes should raise the suspicion of Addison's disease. In the presence of Addison's disease, adding levothyroxine without replacing hydrocortisone could potentially exacerbate the symptoms.

PAI type 2 is characterised by Addison's disease plus one of the other autoimmune diseases such as type 1 diabetes, hypothyroidism, pernicious anaemia and myasthenia gravis.

Women have a higher risk than men. Polygenic inheritance associated with HLA-DR3 and HLA-DR4 and non-HLA genes (MICA5.1, PTPN22, CTLA4, VNTR).

The standard diagnostic test for hypoadrenalism is the short Synacthen test.

Michels AW, Gottlieb PA. Autoimmune polyglandular syndromes. Nat Rev Endocrinol 2010; 6:270–277.

26. B Start cholecalciferol/ergocalciferol supplementation

The most likely explanation of this woman's symptoms is severe vitamin D deficiency. Prolonged vitamin D deficiency would result in persistent hypocalcaemia and raised parathyroid hormone (PTH). This rise in PTH is called secondary hyperparathyroidism.

The initial therapy would be replacement of vitamin D either as cholecalciferol/ergocalciferol or as calcitriol. She should also be evaluated for malabsorption syndromes such as coeliac disease, though in this case lack of adequate sun exposure is more likely to the reason.

Proximal myopathy is very common in severe vitamin D deficiency.

Fraser WD. Hyperparathyroidism. Lancet 2009; 374:145–158.

27. E Measure glutamic acid decarboxylase (GAD) antibodies

The clinical picture of normal body mass index (BMI), young age and difficult to control blood sugars with oral hypoglycaemic agents soon after diagnosis points towards 'latent autoimmune diabetes of adulthood' (LADA).

In this instance a positive GAD antibody result would suggest that the person probably has LADA. A C-peptide level would also give additional information regarding β-cell reserve.

However, there is controversy on the management of LADA; some authorities advocate early insulin therapy whereas others prefer oral agents first and insulin later.

Given his BMI, metformin may not be the first choice here. Pioglitazone has shown some benefit in small clinical trials; however, early insulin therapy in LADA is known to preserve β- cell function better. Immunomodulatory agents are undergoing trials in LADA.

Fructosamine levels are measured in instances where HbA1c results may not be reliable – for instance in anaemia, pregnancy, haemoglobinopathies.

Cernea S, et al. Beta-cell protection and therapy for latent autoimmune diabetes in adults. Diabetes Care 2009; 32(2):S246–S252.

28. E Trans-sphenoidal surgery

Trans-sphenoidal removal of the adenoma is appropriate for a non-functioning macroadenoma resulting in visual field defects. The raised prolactin level is most probably due to stalk compression and subsequent reduction in dopamine reaching the pituitary. Lack of dopamine results in disinhibition of the pituitary lactotrophs, resulting in hyperprolactinaemia.

The symptoms are suggestive of hyperprolactinaemia with galactorrhoea and amenorrhoea. Her visual field symptoms are suggestive of optic chiasma involvement.

Pituitary MRI shows a 3-cm lesion which suggests that it is a macroadenoma (>1 cm). Prolactin-secreting macroadenomas (macroprolactinomas) generally secrete large quantities of prolactin – usually >8000 mU/mL. Since the prolactin level is <2000 mU/mL, it is more likely that the prolactin secretion is from disinhibition rather than from the adenoma itself. Treatment for a prolactinoma is medical therapy initially with dopamine agonists such as bromocriptine or cabergoline.

Octreotide is useful as medical therapy in acromegaly to reduce growth hormone levels. Stereotactic radiosurgery is useful in situations where surgery is contraindicated or if there is residual tumour after surgery. Transcranial surgery is generally reserved for large tumours where full resection may not be possible with trans-sphenoidal approach.

Melmed S, Casanueva FF, Hoffman AR, et al. Diagnosis and treatment of hyperprolactinemia: an Endocrine Society clinical practice guideline. J Clin Endocrinol Metab 2011; 96:273–288.

29. C Reduce basal insulin and pre-exercise rapid-acting insulin and avoid hypoglycaemia for the next 2 months

This young woman had very good glycaemic control with low HbA1c. Since she started her exercise regimen without altering her insulin doses, she has had several episodes of severe hypoglycaemia. More worryingly, she has hypoglycaemia unawareness with several hypoglycaemic episodes being asymptomatic. In general, hypoglycaemia tends to provoke hypoglycaemia unawareness, with the threshold of blood sugar at which symptoms arise getting lower with prolonged low blood sugar levels. Restoration of hypoglycaemia awareness is best brought about by avoiding hypoglycaemia for 6–8 weeks. Conversely prolonged hyperglycaemia would lead to symptoms occurring at higher blood sugar levels.

At the age of 28 years there is no compelling rationale to start simvastatin with a single raised cholesterol level. Dietary and lifestyle adjustment would be the first step. Similarly, for high blood pressure, the reading should be interpreted cautiously and the test repeated. Again initial management would be lifestyle modification, but the drug of choice, if that does not work, would be ramipril. In the child-bearing age group, warning must be given about the teratogenic potential.

Although an insulin pump would alleviate the recurrent hypoglycaemia, simpler measures should be tried first. Similarly, whereas twice a day detemir might offer some beneficial effect, advice on exercise and a modification of the current regimen should be tried first.

Bakatselos SO. Hypoglycemia unawareness. Diabetes Res Clin Pract 2011; 93:S92–96.

30. D Short Synacthen test

This woman has features of hyperandrogenism such as acne and hirsuitism as well as high levels of 17OH-progesterone. The combination would suggest 'non-classic' congenital adrenal hyperplasia (CAH).

Congenital adrenal hyperplasia is most commonly due to mutations in 21-hydroxylase (cytochrome P450 CYP21A2) enzyme. This is an important enzyme in the steroid biosynthetic pathway which mediates the conversion of 17OH-progesterone to 11-deoxycortisol (precursor of cortisol) and of progesterone to deoxycorticosterone (precursor of aldosterone). If there is loss of function of this enzyme, cortisol production is affected, the adrenocorticotrophic hormone (ACTH) level goes up due to lack of feedback and hence there is over-stimulation of the adrenal cortex with excess production of cortisol precursors. These precursors are then diverted into sex hormone synthesis. This may lead to androgen excess and ambiguous genitalia in girls. Aldosterone deficiency may lead to salt wasting, hypovolaemia and shock. Approximately, 90% of CAH is due to mutations in this enzyme. The phenotype varies depending on the severity of the deletion/mutation. Rarer forms of CAH are associated with mutations in 11β-hydroxylase and 3β-steroid dehydrogenase.

Classically there are three phenotypes with CYP21A2 involvement: classic type with either salt wasting or simple virilising without aldosterone deficiency and non-classic. Classic salt wasting CAH is apparent in the neonatal period with failure to thrive, hypovolaemia and shock. The simple virilising form may present with ambiguous genitalia in girls.

Non-classic CAH is often asymptomatic and only may be apparent in adulthood with androgen excess. In late childhood, it may present with premature pubarche, accelerated bone age and acne. In women, this may present with hirsutism, oligomenorrhoea, subfertility and acne, and can be mistaken for polycystic ovarian syndrome.

Non-classic CAH usually presents with signs of hyperandrogenism such as acne and hirsuitism. Some women also have irregular cycles and subfertility.

In the classic forms, basal 17OH-progesterone levels are high; in non-classic CAH, the elevation in 17OH-progesterone level may be modest and hence a more confirmatory test is needed. This is the Synacthen test, performed by measuring 17OH-progesterone prior to and 60 minutes after 250 mg synthetic adrenocorticotrophic hormone (ACTH). Stimulated values are elevated in patients with classic and non-classic varieties (in excess of 35 nmol/L usually).

In adult women with non-classic CAH, glucocorticoid treatment does not bring additional benefit for hyperandrogenism. Hirsuitism in these individuals can be treated with eflornithine locally, spironolactone, cyproterone acetate and oral contraceptives systemically.

Subfertility, however, may benefit from glucocorticoid therapy to reduce ACTH levels. Similarly, men with non-classic CAH require treatment only in cases of sub-fertility.

31. C Plasma vasoactive intestinal peptide (VIP)

Symptoms of large-volume watery diarrhoea, metabolic acidosis and hypokalaemia suggest a VIPoma. A serum VIP level >200 pmol/L would establish the diagnosis. It is also called WDHA (watery diarrhoea, hypokalaemia and achlorhydria) syndrome. Hypercalcaemia can be seen with this presentation. Raised creatinine is most likely because of the dehydration. Hyperglycaemia is seen in a third of cases because of increased glycogenolysis in liver.

Localisation of the tumour can be achieved by CT of the abdomen and for small tumours by endoscopic ultrasound and radiolabelled octreotide scanning. The last can also be used for looking for local recurrence and metastases. Most of these tumours are located in the pancreas. VIP is involved in smooth muscle relaxation, secretion of water and bicarbonate from the intestine and pancreas, and also inhibits gastric acid secretion and colonic reabsorption of potassium.

Immediate treatment is to correct the fluid loss, hypokalaemia and metabolic acidosis. Somatostatin analogues such as octreotide are effective in controlling the diarrhoea. Surgical resection is the only curative treatment. Debate persists as to whether somatostatin analogues can shrink the tumour.

With gastrinomas, abdominal pain, heart burn and diarrhoea are the common symptoms. Diarrhoea is partly due to the fat malabsorption because of lack of pancreatic lipase (degraded by the excess gastric acid) and partly due to small bowel inflammation. Very high serum gastrin level and gastric acid hypersecretion would clinch the diagnosis. In cases of intermediate gastrin levels, a secretin stimulation test should be performed.

Song S, Shi R, Li B, Liu Y. Diagnosis and treatment of pancreatic vasoactive intestinal peptide endocrine tumors. Pancreas 2009; 38:811–814.
Batcher E, Madaj P, Gianoukakis AG. Pancreatic neuroendocrine tumors. Endocr Res 2011; 36:35–43.

32. B Diabetic lumbosaccral plexopathy

The clinical picture of severe pain in the proximal legs with wasting, weakness and loss of knee jerk, and minimal sensory involvement is typical of diabetic lumbosacral plexopathy or diabetic amyotrophy.

It is usually seen with poorly controlled diabetes and the aetiology has not been fully elucidated. It is thought to be an immune-mediated vascular radiculopathy.

Treatment is essentially symptomatic, with physiotherapy and occupational therapy. Good control of diabetes is essential. Intravenous immunoglobulin and pulse glucocorticoid such as methylprednisolone have been tried, but neither has an extensive evidence base.

Tricyclic antidepressants may improve the pain as do pregabalin and gabapentin.

Little AA, Edwards JL, Feldman EL. Diabetic neuropathies. Pract Neurol 2007; 7:82–92.

33. B Dextrose–insulin infusion

This patient has severe triglyceridaemia, probably due to insulin deficiency from longstanding, poorly controlled diabetes and diet/alcohol and genetic factors. Both very-low-density lipoprotein (VLDL) and chylomicrons would be raised. At such high triglyceride (TG) levels, the VLDL and chylomicron removal mechanisms would be saturated.

The priority here would be to get the triglyceride level under control to avoid complications such as pancreatitis.

Though niacin and gemfibrozil would bring the TG level under control, in such an acute setting a better option needs to be adopted. Heparin has the issue that, although it causes the release of endothelial lipoprotein lipase (LPL) early on, later the LPL level decreases, so monotherapy with heparin is not advocated.

Insulin–dextrose infusion would correct the insulin deficiency, which brought this on as well as reduce the triglyceride level. It will also provide calories for the patient and allow him to remain nil by mouth, reducing the dietary lipids temporarily.

Once the TG level comes down, gemfibrozil or other alternatives may be considered. A low-fat diet should also be advised.

Ewald N, Hardt PD, Kloer HU. Severe hypertriglyceridemia and pancreatitis: presentation and management. Curr Opin Lipidol 2009; 20:497–504.

34. B Repeat thyroid function tests in a week and then in 2–3 months

This patient has sick euthyroid syndrome (non-thyroidal illness syndrome). In this condition, the thyroid function tests may be variable. No treatment or investigations are required at this stage. Once she has recovered from the acute illness, the thyroid function can be reassessed. The thyroid function should be monitored during the illness and 1–2 months after recovery.

The conditions to exclude include primary thyroid illness, other medications affecting the thyroid and pituitary–hypothalamic illness. Drugs that affect the thyroid include glucocorticoids, dobutamine, amiodarone, salicylates, beta-blockers and anticonvulsants.

Adler SM, Wartofsky L. The nonthyroidal illness syndrome. Endocrinol Metab Clin North Am 2007; 36:657–672.

35. E Start simvastatin

The patient has risk factors for coronary vessel disease: nearly 40 years old, 2-year history of type 2 diabetes, hypertension, and total cholesterol and low-density lipoprotein (LDL) are high. The National Institute for Health and Clinical Excellence (NICE) recommends simvastatin for those with type 2 diabetes and aged above 40 years. For people below 40 years, if cardiovascular disease risk is high then statins are recommended. Since he has significant risk, statin is the best initial therapy.

If the triglycerides continue to be high despite optimal statin therapy then addition of a fibrate may be considered especially when other factors such as alcohol, liver disease and poor control are ruled out. Given his raised LDL, omega-3 fatty acids may not be the best choice.

Though lifestyle advice may be given, the high-risk profile means that, in addition to lifestyle changes, pharmaceuticals may be needed.

36. B Charcot's foot affecting the forefoot bones

This presentation is typical of Charcot's foot (neuropathic arthropathy). This patient has diabetes and peripheral neuropathy. He has non-tender swelling over the forefoot with increased temperature and redness. Erythrocyte sedimentation rate is elevated but C-reactive protein and white cell count are normal.

Charcot's foot develops over a background of neurological impairment in the foot. There are two main contributors: the neuropathy results in increased likelihood of trauma and sympathetic denervation results in increased blood supply. This hyperaemia increases bone resorption and renders the foot more vulnerable to micro- and macro-fractures during weight bearing. Normal walking may result in micro-fractures and dislocations, and these fail to heal properly eventually resulting in architectural changes in the foot. Continued walking would result in abnormal weight bearing, leading to ulcers and other complications. The most common areas affected are the mid- and forefoot.

The condition is self-limiting with treatment mainly consisting of avoiding weight bearing on the foot. This usually means an air-cast boot initially with consideration of total contact cast, which would be the gold standard. Disease activity may take weeks to months to abate.

Rogers LC, Frykberg RG, Armstrong DG, et al. The Charcot foot in diabetes. Diabetes Care 2011; 34:2123–2129.

37. D Orchidectomy

Karyotyping shows a XY genotype, but phenotypically she is female from birth with well-developed secondary sexual characteristics.

This suggests androgen insensitivity syndrome (AIS), previously called testicular feminisation syndrome (this term was considered pejorative and is no longer used).

AIS is a diverse syndrome of many causes and has many phenotypes, ranging from mild to partial to complete.

This girl probably has complete AIS. In partial AIS, the external genitalia are not fully feminised and, in mild AIS, the external genitalia are those of a male.

In AIS due to androgen receptor mutations, the tissues are insensitive to the androgens and hence Wolffian duct structures do not develop. In the absence of testosterone action on tissues, oestrogen causes unopposed development of female external genitalia. However, the testes still produce anti-müllerian hormone which inhibits the development of müllerian duct structures such as the uterus and the fallopian tubes. Hence in complete AIS, the vagina ends blindly.

The other conditions resembling AIS with an XY genotype are:
- 3β-hydroxysteroid dehydrogenase 2 deficiency
- Leydig cell hypoplasia or aplasia
- Smith–Lemli–Opitz syndrome (associated with learning disability)
- Lipoid congenital adrenal hyperplasia
- Swyer's syndrome
- 5α-reductase deficiency
- Luteinising hormone receptor mutations
- 17α-hydroxylase deficiency
- 17,20-lyase deficiency
- 7β-hydroxysteroid dehydrogenase deficiency

Other lab findings in complete AIS include elevated testosterone levels; genetic sequencing of the androgen receptor gene can identify the mutation responsible.

In complete AIS, since the testes could be found in the labia, inguinal ring or intra-abdominally, the incidence of testicular malignancy is high (4–9%) and hence, after attaining puberty, the testes should be removed. Since the testes are genetically normal, the rate of malignancy prior to puberty is very low. However, they should be removed earlier if there are concerns about carcinoma in situ and puberty induced hormonally.

Oakes MB, Eyvazzadeh AD, Quint E, Smith YR. Complete androgen insensitivity syndrome – a review. J Pediatr Adolesc Gynecol 2008; 21:305–310.

38. C Insulin tolerance test

This woman has been adequately replaced with thyroxine (T$_4$) as indicated by the free T4 and triiodothyronine (T3) levels. Additional measurement of thyroid-binding globulins is not necessary since the free hormone levels are already given. Her symptoms are not suggestive of thyrotoxicosis; hence radio-iodine uptake scan and thyroid-stimulating hormone (TSH) receptor antibody measurement are not required. Her symptoms are persistent, hence hypopituitarism should be ruled out first.

In the set of options given, insulin tolerance test showing failure of growth hormone and cortisol levels to increase with hypoglycaemia would suggest hypopituitarism. Indeed, a low TSH level in the presence of low thyroid hormone levels (normal in this case due to supplementation) should raise suspicion of a pituitary problem.

Luteinising hormone and follicle-stimulating hormone should be high in postmenopausal women; absence of this or reduction in adrenocorticotrophic hormone level or TSH-releasing hormone stimulation test could also be used to diagnose hypopituitarism.

39. B Karyotyping

Klinefelter's syndrome (KS) is one of the most common genetic forms of male hypogonadism affecting up to 1 in 600 adult males. This is classically because of meiotic non-disjunction. The phenotype becomes clear only after puberty. In the early years of life, the gonadal function as well as the pituitary function is normal and the phenotype is not apparent. However, during puberty, the follicle-stimulating hormone and luteinising hormone levels rise whereas the inhibin B concentrations become undetectable. Testosterone levels do not rise much and, typically in adulthood, the testosterone levels are low or low–normal. Oestradiol levels are high–normal or high. The reason for hypogonadism in KS is likely to be abnormalities in the steroidogenic enzyme pathway or due to elevated oestradiol levels within the testes.

Adults with KS show a varying degree of androgenisation with androgen deficiency and hypergonadotrophism. Testes show extensive fibrosis and hyalinisation of the seminiferous tubules and hyperplasia of the interstitium. The tubules show scanty areas of preserved spermatogenesis.

Typically adults with KS have hypergonadotrophic hypogonadism with small testes, increased height, gynaecomastia, narrow shoulders, broad hips, and a tendency towards insulin resistance and metabolic syndrome. If not treated adequately, there may be loss of muscle mass, redistribution of body fat and osteoporosis. However, it must be emphasised that the phenotype is widely variable and men with KS may be completely asymptomatic and commonly have no intellectual impairment.

These individuals have a higher than normal incidence of autoimmune disorders.

Karyotyping will show the extra X chromosome and will confirm the diagnosis. 80–90% patients are the non-mosaic 47 XXY genotype; 5–10% have a mosaic form, the most common being 47 XXY/46 XY mosaicism. The rest are due to 48 XXXY, 48 XXYY and 49 XXXXY abnormalities.

Androgen replacement is the treatment of choice to maintain muscle mass, prevent metabolic complications and restore libido.

Men with KS generally have azoospermia; however, some individuals, especially those with mosaicism, may have areas of spermatogenesis and have occasionally been found to have spermatozoa in the ejaculate, and rare cases of spontaneous fertility have been described. Fertility can be restored in up to 50% of these individuals especially in mosaicism with intracytoplasmic sperm injection (ICSI) when spermatozoa can be retrieved by testicular exploration (TESE – testicular sperm extraction).

Children with KS have preserved spermatogonia which undergo massive apoptosis around the early pubertal stage. Cryopreservation of sperm in adolescence is therefore of importance.

Aksglaede L, Juul A. Testicular function and fertility in men with Klinefelter syndrome: a review. Eur J Endocrinol. 2013; 168:R67–76.

40. C Check FT4 level

The patient has long standing panhypopituitarism, so her thyroid-stimulating hormone (TSH) production is always going to be low. In her case, the levothyroxine dose adjustment is predicated on FT4 level rather than TSH levels. The current recommendation is to maintain TSH in the upper half of the normal range taking into account symptoms. There is no evidence of recurrent disease clinically; therefore MRI is not useful. She is unlikely to have primary thyroid disease, and FT4 level are not available, so thyroid uptake scan is not indicated at this time.

41. A Obtain 9 am pituitary function tests and arrange yearly follow-up

Empty sella is often an incidental MRI finding. Empty sella could be primary (idiopathic) or secondary. Secondary causes include surgical treatment of pituitary adenoma, auto-infarction or haemorrhage of pituitary adenoma, head trauma, cranial radiotherapy and idiopathic intracranial hypertension (IIH). In many cases of primary idiopathic empty sella, a defect in diagphragma sellae has been identified. The rim of tissue identified is likely to give her full pituitary function, especially as she is asymptomatic. However, an empty sella may signal the onset of hypopituitarism, and 9 am pituitary function should be monitored closely.

Hyperprolactinemia has been reported in empty sella syndrome. The patient should be advised about symptoms of hypopituitarism and idiopathic intracranial hyperstension, and asked to come back earlier, if she is symptomatic. Unless her clinical situation changes, a repeat MRI is not indicated. While a dedicated pituitary MRI with contrast would give better definition, in the absence of any other abnormality, this is not warranted. Infarction or haemorrhage of a large pituitary adenoma would result in empty sella eventually, but in this instance the history is only a week long and hence this is unlikely. A single episode of a headache which resolved spontaneously and with normal fundoscopy and perimetry does not suggest significant intracranial hypertension.

De Marinis L, Bonadonna S, Bianchi A, et al. Primary empty sella. J Clin Endocrinol Metab. 2005; 90:5471–7.
Saindane AM, Lim PP, Aiken A, et al. Factors determining the clinical significance of an empty sella turcica. AJR Am J Roentgenol. 2013;200:1125–31.

42. E Stop ferrous sulphate and recheck thyroid function, blood pressure and lipid profile in 3 months

This patient has had stable hypothyroidism for several years, but now her thyroid-stimulating hormone concentration has gone up considerably with a drop in free thyroxine T4 levels. This suggests either an issue with concordance with medications or malabsorption or interaction with other drugs affecting absorption or clearance. Given that her disease has been stable previously, non-concordance is less likely. Her history does not show anything that might suggest, malabsorption, such as coeliac disease or small bowel surgery, and her albumin level is stable. Iron tablets such as ferrous sulphate (and other drugs such as calcium, proton pump inhibitors, statins, oestrogen and cholestyramine) can interfere with absorption of levothyroxine. Drugs that interfere with clearance include carbamazepine, phenytoin and amiodarone (which has multiple effects on thyroid).

Given significant hypothyroidism which can of course result in hypertension and hyperlipidemia, the best course of action would be to recheck blood pressure and lipid profile once thyroid function is back to normal.

Irving SA, Vadiveloo T, Leese GP. Drugs that interact with levothyroxine: an observational study from the Thyroid Epidemiology, Audit and Research Study (TEARS). Clin Endocrinol 2015; 82:136–41.

43. D Start intravenous phentolamine and initiate low dose oral phenoxybenzamine. Plan for an adrenalectomy when blood pressure <160/100 mmHg. Start bisoprolol once established on phenoxybenzamine for tachycardia

This is a hypertensive crisis with encephalopathy and papilloedema. The aim should be to lower blood pressure by around 20% over the initial 24-hour period. Phentolamine is a reversible non-selective α-adrenergic antagonist and is indicated in hypertensive emergencies due to phaeochromocytoma. Intravenous boluses of 2.5–5 mg repeated every 5 minutes or an intravenous infusion is used to achieve blood pressure control. Nitroglycerine and nitroprusside can also be used.

Once acute hypertensive crisis has abated, use oral α-blockers such as phenoxybenzamine, which is a non-selective, irreversible $α_1$ and $α_2$ blocker. Doxazosin, an $α_1$-selective alpha blocker can also be used, but most centres prefer phenoxybenzamine. Start phenoxybenzamine at 10 mg three times daily and titrate up, to achieve a blood pressure of <160/100 mmHg. Beta-blockers can be started once patient is established on alpha blockade, especially for persistent tachycardia. Salt and fluids should be replaced as often patients are significantly fluid depleted. If patients are still significantly hypertensive on a good dose of alpha blockers, then calcium channel blockers, angiotensin converting enzyme blockers or angiotensin receptor blockers may be used.

Surgery is the definitive treatment but it is imperative that good alpha blockade and blood pressure control is achieved prior to surgery to prevent perioperative mortality and morbidity. Volume expansion is also recommended prior to surgery. Most institutions suggest a target blood pressure of 130/80 mmHg sitting and >90 mmHg systolic blood pressure on standing, prior to surgery.

Lenders JW, Duh QY, Eisenhofer G, et al. Endocrine Society. Pheochromocytoma and paraganglioma: an endocrine society clinical practice guideline. J Clin Endocrinol Metab 2014;99:1915–42.

44. A Start potassium chloride 20 mmol/L in 1 litre normal saline and give over 2 hours, recheck potassium and initiate insulin infusion only after potassium >3.3 mmol/L

Patients with diabetic ketoacidosis (DKA) who had severe vomiting or had been on diuretics may present with significant hypokalaemia. In such cases, potassium replacement should begin with fluid therapy, and insulin treatment should be postponed until potassium concentration becomes >3.3 mmol/L in order to prevent arrhythmias and respiratory muscle weakness.

Hypokalaemia on presentation is indicator of severity of DKA and these patients should be managed in intensive care setting where higher concentrations on potassium can be used intravenously. The recommended potassium use with peripheral lines is a maximum of 10 mmol of potassium chloride per hour.

There is a slight divergence in the UK and US guidelines on DKA, however both agree that if there is initial hypokalaemia, it should be corrected prior to insulin infusion.

Kitabchi AE, Umpierrez GE, Miles JM, Fisher JN. Hyperglycemic crises in adult patients with diabetes. Diabetes Care. 2009; 32:1335–1343.
Dhatariya, K, Savage, M, Claydon, A, et al. Joint British Diabetes Societies Inpatient Care Group. The management of diabetic ketoacidosis in adults (2nd edn). London: Joint British Diabetes Societies Inpatient Care Group (Diabetes UK), 2013.

Chapter 4

Gastroenterology

Questions

1. A 56-year-old man with a history of chronic pancreatitis presented to the emergency department with epigastric pain. Five weeks ago, he had suffered from a very severe episode of epigastric pain that lasted for 2 days, which had been precipitated by an alcohol binge. After the initial episode the pain reduced, but over the past 4 weeks had been gradually increasing in severity. His appetite had been reduced and he had early satiety and nausea. He had lost 3 kg in weight.

    On examination, he had a body mass index of 23 kg/m^2 and looked comfortable at rest. He was not icteric. His cardiovascular and respiratory examinations were normal but he had a tender epigastric mass. Murphy's sign was negative.

    Investigations:

haemoglobin 136 g/L (130–180)	alkaline phosphatase 168 U/L (45–105)
white cell count 12.1 × 10^9/L (4–11)	alanine transaminase 26 U/L (5–35)
platelets 187 × 10^9/L (150–400)	albumin 34 g/L (37–49)
bilirubin 15 mmol/L (1–22)	amylase 220 U/L (60–180)

    What is the most likely diagnosis?

    A   Adenocarcinoma of the pancreas
    B   Biliary stricture
    C   Intraductal papillary mucinous neoplasm
    D   Pancreatic pseudocyst
    E   Splenic vein thrombosis

2. A 54-year-old woman was referred by her general practitioner with a 6-week history of gradual onset abdominal pain and distension. She had no previous medical history, did not drink alcohol and was not taking any medication.

    On abdominal examination, she had tender hepatomegaly and shifting dullness. The rest of her physical examination was normal.

    Investigations:

haemoglobin 173 g/L (115–165)	bilirubin 37 mmol/L (1–22)
white cell count 5.8 × 10^9/L (4–11)	alkaline phosphatase 138 U/L (45–105)
platelets 362 × 10^9/L (150–400)	alanine transaminase 120 U/L (5–35)
haematocrit 74% (36–46)	albumin 29 g/L (37–49)
international normalised ratio 1.6 (<1.4)	

What is the most likely diagnosis?

A   Budd–Chiari syndrome
B   Constrictive pericarditis
C   Hepatocellular carcinoma
D   Portal vein thrombosis
E   Tricuspid regurgitation

3.   A 38-year-old man presented with a 6-hour history of haematemesis and melaena. He had been diagnosed with alcohol-related cirrhosis 3 years ago, but had been lost to follow-up. He had no other past medical history, and currently took no medications.
On examination, he was agitated with a Glasgow Coma Scale score of 14/15, pulse 114 beats per minute and blood pressure 83/40 mmHg. He had pale conjunctivae, icteric sclera and asterixis. There were multiple spider naevi on his anterior chest wall, moderate ascites and splenomegaly.
He was resuscitated with blood products and an upper gastrointestinal endoscopy was requested.

Investigations:

haemoglobin 76 g/L (130–180)	urea 16 mmol/L (2.5–7.5)
white cell count 7 × 10⁹/L (4–11)	creatinine 76 µmol/L (60–110)
platelets 101 × 10⁹/L (150–400)	bilirubin 86 mmol/L (1–22)
international normalised ratio 1.9 (<1.4)	alkaline phosphatase 453 U/L (45–105)
sodium 132 mmol/L (135–145)	alanine transaminase 44 U/L (5–35)
potassium 4.2 mmol/L (3.5–5.0)	albumin 28 g/L (37–49)

What is the appropriate first-line pharmacological therapy prior to endoscopy?

A   Antibiotics, propranolol and terlipressin
B   Antibiotics and terlipressin
C   Antibiotics, propranolol and octreotide
D   Propranolol and octreotide
E   Propranolol and terlipressin

4.   A 56-year-old homeless and alcohol-dependent man was admitted to hospital with 48 hours of persistent vomiting and haematemesis at a weekend. He was kept nil by mouth while awaiting an endoscopy. He had his endoscopy on his third day of admission.
Endoscopy revealed erosive gastritis. Following the endoscopy he was allowed to eat but the next day he still felt unwell.

Investigations:

haemoglobin 132 g/L (130–180)	urea 6.9 mmol/L (2.5–7.5)
white cell count 6 × 10⁹/L (4–11)	creatinine 76 µmol/L (60–110)
platelets 189 × 10⁹/L (150–400)	glucose 4.2 mmol/L (3.0–6.0)
sodium 138 mmol/L (135–145)	phosphate 0.23 mmol/L (0.8–1.4)
potassium 3.1 mmol/L (3.5–5.0)	magnesium 0.5 mmol/L (0.75–1.05)

What is the most appropriate next step in management?

A   Replace magnesium
B   Replace potassium
C   Replace phosphate
D   Start nasogastric (NG) feeding at a reduced rate
E   Thiamine administration

5. A 54-year-old woman was referred to the hepatology clinic with positive antimitochondrial antibodies (AMAs). She complained of fatigue but had no other symptoms.

   On examination she was not icteric and had no peripheral stigmata of chronic liver disease. Further investigations were performed.

   Investigations:

haemoglobin 140 g/L (115–165)	cholesterol 5.6 (mmol/L (<5.2 mmol/L)
white cell count 7 × 10⁹/L (4–11)	IgA 2.4 g/L (0.8-3.0 g/L)
platelets 178 × 10⁹/L (150–400)	IgG 7.9 g/L (6.0-13.0 g/L)
bilirubin 15 mmol/L (1–22)	IgM 3.6 g/L (0.4-2.5 g/L)
alkaline phosphatase 94 U/L (45–105)	ANA: negative
alanine transaminase 31 U/L (5–35)	SMA: negative
GGT 27 U/L (4-35 U/L)	Anti-LKM1: negative
albumin 40 g/L (37–49)	AMA: positive 1:160
Fibroscan: 4.5 kPa	US scan liver: normal

   What is the most appropriate next step in management?

   A   Start ursodeoxycholic acid at a dose of 13–15 mg/kg
   B   Start obeticholic acid 5 mg once daily
   C   Monitor LFTs and serological markers yearly
   D   Perform a liver biopsy
   E   Start prednisolone 40 mg once daily

6. A 29-year-old woman was referred for colonoscopic screening for a hereditary polyposis syndrome. Her maternal grandfather was diagnosed with colorectal cancer at the age of 65 years, and her maternal aunt was diagnosed with colorectal cancer at the age of 52 years. Her mother was diagnosed with endometrial cancer at the age of 48 years.

   DNA testing had shown a mutation in the mismatch repair (MMR) gene. Her colonoscopy showed colonic polyps.

   What is the most likely syndrome?

   A   Familial adenomatous polyposis (FAP)
   B   Juvenile polyposis
   C   Lynch's syndrome (hereditary non-polyposis colorectal cancer)
   D   MUTYH-associated polyposis
   E   Peutz–Jeghers syndrome

7. A 54-year-old woman presented with a longstanding history of diarrhoea. This was not associated with bleeding but she had recently suffered some weight loss and pruritus ani.

   Examination was normal.

   Colonoscopy: the following was seen (see **Figure 4.1**).

   What is the most appropriate management?

   A   Endoscopic removal
   B   Ivermectin
   C   Mebendazole
   D   Praziquantel
   E   Steroids and albendazole

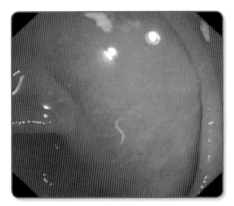

Figure 4.1 *See colour plate section.*

8. A 76-year-old man was due to have a colonoscopy with random colonic biopsies to investigate diarrhoea and rectal bleeding. He had a history of a NSTEMI in 2015 for which he had an angiogram and drug-eluting stent. He was taking clopidogrel, ramipril, atorvastatin and bisoprolol.

   What should the management of his clopidogrel be prior to his colonoscopy?

   A Stop clopidogrel for 5 days prior to the procedure
   B Continue with clopidogrel
   C Discuss management of clopidogrel with a cardiologist
   D Stop clopidogrel and start aspirin 5 days prior to the procedure
   E Stop clopidogrel 5 days prior to the procedure and start low molecular weight heparin

9. A 35-year-old man presented to the hepatology clinic with a new diagnosis of hepatitis B virus infection.

Hepatitis B surface antigen (HBsAg): positive
Hepatitis B e antigen (HBeAg): negative
Hepatitis B e antibody (HBeAb): positive

HBV DNA 564 IU/mL	alanine transaminase 18 U/L (5–35)

   What is the most appropriate management?

   A Entecavir
   B Lamivudine
   C Pegylated interferon-α
   D Tenofovir
   E Watch and wait

10. A 25-year-old man was referred to the gastroenterology clinic with abnormal liver function tests and right upper quadrant pain. He had a 2-month history of intermittent diarrhoea, associated with episodes of rectal bleeding. He had no past medical history and took no medications. He drank occasional alcohol.

Investigations:

haemoglobin 120 g/L (130–180)	bilirubin 35 mmol/L (1–22)
white cell count 7 × 10⁹/L (4–11)	alkaline phosphatase 280 U/L (45–105)
platelets 167 × 10⁹/L (150–400)	alanine transaminase 23 U/L (5–35)
ferritin 56 g/L (15–300)	albumin 36 g/L (37–49)

Hepatitis B and C serology: negative
HIV: negative
Antimitochondrial antibodies: negative
Antinuclear antibodies: negative

Perinuclear antineutrophil cytoplasmic antibodies (pANCAs) 1:160 (<5)

Ultrasound of abdomen: normal

What is the most appropriate next investigation?

A   Endoscopic retrograde cholangiopancreatography (ERCP)
B   Fibroscan
C   Liver biopsy
D   Magnetic resonance cholangiopancreatography (MRCP)
E   Triple-phase CT of the liver

11. A 64-year-old woman presented with symptoms of pain on swallowing over the last 2 weeks. There was no history of dysphagia or reflux. She had a history of type 2 diabetes for which she took metformin. She took no other medications.
    Examination was normal.

What is the most likely diagnosis?

A   Cytomegalovirus
B   Eosinophilic oesophagitis
C   Oesophageal candidiasis
D   Oesophageal carcinoma
E   Achalasia

12. A 44-year-old man presented with abnormal liver function tests. He had diet-controlled type 2 diabetes. He drank 40 units of alcohol per week. He was on no medication.

On examination he had a 3-cm hepatomegaly but no other signs of chronic liver disease.

Investigations:

haemoglobin 143 g/L (130–180)	alanine transaminase 58 U/L (5–35)
white cell count 6.8 × 10⁹/L (4–11)	albumin 35 g/L (37–49)
platelets 189 × 10⁹/L (150–400)	ferritin 467 g/L (15–300)
mean cell volume 84 fl (80-96 fl)	transferrin saturation 21% (20–50)
bilirubin 18 mmol/L (1–22)	random glucose 8.1 mmol/L (3.0–6.0)
alkaline phosphatase 134 U/L (45–105)	

Hepatitis C virus IgG: positive   Hepatitis C virus RNA 0 IU/mL

Liver ultrasound: mild hepatomegaly with bright echotexture.

Liver biopsy: haemosiderosis

What is the most likely cause of his iron overload?

A   Alcohol-related fatty liver disease
B   Non-alcoholic fatty liver disease (NAFLD)
C   Hepatitis C virus
D   Hereditary haemochromatosis
E   Thalassaemia

13. A 54-year-old man presented with a 6-month history of loose stools, 12-kg weight loss and non-specific abdominal pain. There was no blood or mucus in the stools. Six years ago, he was investigated by the rheumatologists for arthralgia affecting a number of joints. He had no other past medical or surgical history. There was no family history of note. He attended with his son who was concerned that his personality had changed and he had become more forgetful recently.

On examination, he was thin. He had angular stomatitis. Neurological, cardiovascular and respiratory examinations were normal. His Mini-Mental State Examination score was 16/30.

Investigations:

haemoglobin 112 g/L (130–180)	platelets 567 × 10⁹/L (150–400)
white cell count 5.6 × 109/L (4–11)	C-reactive protein 13 mg/L (<10)

Chest X-ray: normal

Duodenal biopsies: non-specific granulomas

What is the most likely diagnosis?

A   Abdominal tuberculosis
B   Crohn's disease
C   Sarcoidosis with small bowel involvement
D   Small intestinal lymphoma
E   Whipple's disease

14. A 60-year-old woman was referred with symptoms of fatigue, right upper quadrant pain, pruritus and abnormal liver function tests. She was generally fit and well, but had been treated for Graves' disease 10 years ago. Her current medications were thyroxine and hormone replacement therapy.
    On examination, she had a 3-cm tender hepatomegaly.

Investigations:

bilirubin 9 mmol/L (1–22)	alanine transaminase 350 U/L (5–35)
alkaline phosphatase 100 U/L (45–105)	albumin 37 g/L (37–49)
Antinuclear antibody 1: 160	
Anti-smooth muscle 1: 80	
Anti-LKM1: negative	
Anti-mitochondrial antibody: negative	
IgA 2.3 g/L (0.8–3.0)	IgM 1.2 g/L (0.4–2.5)
IgG 34 g/L (6.0–13.0)	

Histology:
interface hepatitis and portal plasma cell infiltration, with bridging necrosis
normal biliary histology

What is the most appropriate first line treatment?

A   Azathioprine
B   Ciclosporin
C   Methotrexate
D   Prednisolone and azathioprine
E   Ursodeoxycholic acid

15. A 57-year-old woman presented with a 6-month history of worsening abdominal pain that occurred after eating. The pain had been so severe that she had not wanted to eat and she had lost around 4 kg in weight. She had no history of dysphagia, early satiety, nausea or vomiting. Her past medical history included a transient ischaemic attack, hypertension and hypercholesterolaemia. Her current medications were simvastatin, ramipril, aspirin and dipyridamole. There was no relevant family history.
    She had a regular pulse rate of 68 beats per minute and a blood pressure of 146/84 mmHg. Her cardiovascular and respiratory examinations were normal. On abdominal examination, she had mild central abdominal tenderness, with no abdominal masses or organomegaly.

What is the most likely diagnosis?

A   Biliary colic
B   Chronic mesenteric ischaemia
C   Duodenal ulcer
D   Gastric carcinoma
E   Gastric ulcer

16. A 34-year-old woman presented 4 days after an intentional paracetamol overdose, with jaundice and vomiting. On admission, she was confused and drowsy.

    On examination she was deeply jaundiced. Her Glasgow Coma Scale score was 11/15 (eyes 2, verbal 4, movement 5). Her capillary refill time was 4 seconds. Her blood pressure was 74/45 mmHg with a mean arterial pressure of 50 mmHg. Her heart rate was 124 beats per minute. Her respiratory rate was 28 breaths per minute. Her oxygen saturation was 90% on room air. She had asterixis and bipedal peripheral oedema. Her respiratory and cardiovascular examinations were normal. On abdominal examination, ascites and hepatomegaly were present.

    Investigations:

haemoglobin 104 g/L (115–165)	bilirubin 250 mmol/L (1–22)
white cell count 5 × 10⁹/L (4–11)	alkaline phosphatase 280 U/L (45–105)
platelets 489 × 10⁹/L (150–400)	alanine transaminase 13,567 U/L (5–35)
	aspartate aminotransferase 15,932 U/L (1-31 U/L)
sodium 136 mmol/L (135–145)	albumin 31 g/L (37–49)
potassium 6.2 mmol/L (3.5–5.0)	
urea 26 mmol/L (2.5–7.5)	
creatinine 419 µmol/L (60–110)	lactate 6.8 mmol/L (0.6–1.8 mmol/L)

    Fluid resuscitation with colloid was initiated, *N*-acetylcysteine infusion was commenced. The local liver transplant centre was contacted and accepted the patient and the intensive care unit registrar was contacted to review the patient. The patient's blood pressure remained low despite adequate fluid resuscitation. The intensive care unit registrar recommended commencing cardiovascular support.

    Which cardiovascular support should be started?

    A   Epinephrine
    B   Vasopressin
    C   Norepinephrine
    D   Dobutamine
    E   Hydrocortisone

17. A 28-year-old man with known ulcerative colitis was admitted to hospital with symptoms of bloody diarrhoea and abdominal pain for the preceding 4 days. He was opening his bowels 16 times per day, including 3–4 times at night, and complained of severe central abdominal pain. His ulcerative colitis was normally well controlled on 5-aminosalicylate treatment.

    On examination, he was pale and had a pulse of 100 beats per minute and blood pressure of 118/68 mmHg. Abdominal examination revealed a generally tender abdomen, with no guarding or rigidity.

    Investigations:

haemoglobin 104 g/L (130–180)	urea 9 mmol/L (2.5–7.5)
white cell count 5 × 10⁹/L (4–11)	creatinine 110 µmol/L (60–110)
platelets 489 × 10⁹/L (150–400)	erythrocyte sedimentation rate 68 mm/1st h (0–20)
sodium 136 mmol/L (135–145)	
potassium 4 mmol/L (3.5–5.0)	C-reactive protein 36 mg/L (<10)

    Abdominal X-ray: large bowel diameter within normal limits

What is the next most appropriate step in management?

A   Ciclosporin, intravenous hydrocortisone, subcutaneous heparin and calcium supplementation

B   Intravenous hydrocortisone 100 mg four times daily, oral metronidazole, subcutaneous heparin, calcium supplementation

C   Intravenous hydrocortisone 100 mg four times daily, subcutaneous heparin, calcium supplementation

D   Oral prednisolone 40 mg once daily, calcium supplementation, oral metronidazole

E   Oral prednisolone 40 mg once daily, calcium supplementation and mesalazine enemas

18. A 45-year-old man was admitted to hospital with confusion and jaundice. He had a history of alcohol dependence, and drank 10 cans of strong lager per day. He had developed vomiting and diarrhoea 2 days ago and had been unable to eat or drink anything since. He had no other medical history and no relevant family history.

On examination, he was icteric and had palmar erythema. Temperature was 38.0°C. There was no asterixis. Abdominal examination revealed tender 4-cm hepatomegaly, with no splenomegaly or ascites.

Investigations:

haemoglobin 132 g/L (130–180)	urea 9.7 mmol/L (2.5–7.5)
white cell count 14.5 × 10⁹/L (4–11)	creatinine 136 µmol/L (60–110)
platelets 156 × 10⁹/L (150–400)	bilirubin 256 mmol/L (1–22)
prothrombin time 18 s (11.5–13)	alkaline phosphatase 189 U/L (45–105)
sodium 143 mmol/L (135–145)	alanine transaminase 67 U/L (5–35)
potassium 3.3 mmol/L (3.3–5.0)	albumin 34 g/L (37–49)

Maddrey discriminant function: 38
Chest X-ray, blood cultures and urine cultures were negative

What is the most appropriate treatment?

A   *N*-Acetylcysteine
B   Nutritional supplementation
C   Pentoxifylline
D   Prednisolone
E   Supportive care

19. A 57-year-old woman with known ulcerative colitis attended the outpatient clinic. Her ulcerative colitis had previously been refractory to steroids but since starting azathioprine 6 months ago her symptoms had been well controlled and she was opening her bowels two times per day with no blood and no abdominal pain.

On examination, she was thin and abdominal examination was unremarkable.

Investigations:

Flexible sigmoidoscopy: quiescent colitis

Histology: quiescent ulcerative colitis with inclusion cell bodies
C-reactive protein 5 (<10 mg/L)

Serum cytomegalovirus IgG: positive
Serum cytomegalovirus DNA: positive

What is the next most appropriate step in management?

A   Continue current treatment
B   Intravenous ganciclovir for 3 weeks
C   Intravenous ganciclovir for 2–3 days followed by oral valganciclovir for 3 weeks in total
D   Oral valganciclovir for 3 weeks
E   Stop azathioprine

20. A 64-year-old woman presented to the emergency department with three episodes of haematemesis and melaena. She had a past medical history of angina and hypertension. She was taking aspirin 75 mg once daily and ramipril 2.5 mg once daily. She did not drink alcohol or smoke.

    On examination, she was pale, her pulse was 90 beats per minute and blood pressure 134/78 mmHg. She underwent a gastroscopy which showed a gastric ulcer with a non-bleeding visible vessel and altered blood in the upper gastrointestinal tract. The ulcer was injected with 10 mL of adrenaline and a clip was applied to the visible vessel. Haemostasis was achieved.

What is the most appropriate next step in management?

A   40 mg twice daily intravenous omeprazole for 3 days then convert to 40 mg twice daily oral omeprazole, and repeat endoscopy in 24 hours
B   40 mg twice daily oral omeprazole and *Helicobacter pylori* eradication and repeat endoscopy in 6–8 weeks
C   80 mg intravenous omeprazole bolus followed by a 72-hour protein pump inhibitor infusion at 8 mg/h and repeat endoscopy in 6–8 weeks
D   80 mg intravenous omeprazole bolus followed by a 72-hour protein pump inhibitor infusion at 8 mg/h, tranexamic acid and *Helicobacter pylori* eradication therapy and repeat endoscopy in 24 hours
E   80 mg twice daily intravenous omeprazole, tranexamic acid and *Helicobacter pylori* eradication and repeat endoscopy in 24 hours

21. A 54-year-old woman presented to hospital with a 3-day history of abdominal pain and nausea. She had also developed a generalised, pruritic rash. She had a history of epilepsy, atrial fibrillation and osteoarthritis, for which she was on carbamazepine, phenytoin, amiodarone, warfarin and diclofenac. She took no other medications and did not smoke or drink.

    On examination, she had a widespread urticarial rash, cervical lymphadenopathy and right upper quadrant tenderness.

Investigations:

haemoglobin 132 g/L (115–165)	eosinophils 1.5×10^9/L (0.04–0.4)
white cell count 6.4×10^9/L (4–11)	bilirubin 30 mmol/L (1–22)
platelets 189×10^9/L (150–400)	alkaline phosphatase 486 U/L (45–105)
international normalised ratio 1.2 (<1.4)	alanine transaminase 846 U/L (5–35)
neutrophils 3.6×10^9/L (1.5–7.0)	albumin 37 g/L (37–49)
lymphocytes 1.4×10^9/L (1.5–4.0)	
Paracetamol levels: normal	

What is the most likely cause?

A   Amiodarone
B   Carbamazepine
C   Diclofenac
D   Phenytoin
E   Warfarin

22. A 56-year-old woman presented with abdominal distension, which she first noticed 6 months ago. On examination, she was thin with gross abdominal distension and shifting dullness. There were no palpable masses or organomegaly.

An ascitic tap was performed:

Investigations:

white cell count 17 polymorphonuclear leukocytes (PMNs)/mm3 (<250)	
culture: no organisms seen	fluid albumin 22 g/L
fluid protein 27 g/L	serum albumin 35 g/L (37–49)

What is the most likely cause of her ascites?

A   Carcinomatosis peritonei
B   Liver cirrhosis
C   Ovarian cancer
D   Nephrotic syndrome
E   Tuberculosis peritonitis

23. A 43-year-old man presented with a history of gastro-oesophageal reflux symptoms. He underwent an upper gastrointestinal endoscopy and the following abnormalities were seen (see **Figure 4.2**).

Which one of the following is a risk factor for progression to adenocarcinoma in this disease?

A   Duration of reflux history
B   Female sex
C   Heavy alcohol use
D   Expression of p53
E   Length of Barrett's oesophagus over 3 cm

Figure 4.2 *See colour plate section.*

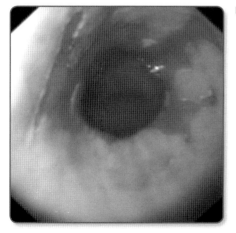

24. A 35-year-old woman presented to her general practitioner with symptoms of fatigue, for the preceding 12 months. She reported intermittent loose stools and bloating, associated with a 3-kg weight loss. She also complained of a skin rash on her arms. She had no past medical history and was on no medications.

    On examination, she looked thin and was pale. She had a blistering skin eruption covering both elbows. The rest of the examination was normal. She was referred for a skin biopsy.

    Skin biopsy – granular IgA at dermoepidermal junction

    What is the most useful diagnostic investigation?

    A   Colonoscopy and ileal biopsies
    B   Gastroscopy and duodenal biopsies
    C   Gastroscopy and small bowel biopsies with periodic acid–Schiff (pas) staining
    D   Serum acetylcholinesterase (ACE) levels
    E   Tissue transglutaminase antibodies

25. A 21-year-old male medical student presented with jaundice. 1 week ago, he returned from his elective where he had visited India, Bangladesh and Pakistan. 4 days before, he arrived back in the UK and began to feel mildly unwell with a fever. 3 days ago, he developed abdominal pain, vomiting, fever and pale stools. Today he noticed that he had yellow sclera, and came to hospital. He was not sexually active. During his elective he had not undertaken any exposure-prone procedures and had not had any transfusions, operations or needle-stick injuries. He had no previous medical problems, did not drink alcohol and was not on any medication.

    On examination, he had a soft abdomen with tender hepatomegaly. He had tender posterior cervical lymphadenopathy.

    An ultrasound of his liver was normal.

    What is the most useful diagnostic investigation?

    A   Anti-HAV IgM
    B   HBsAg
    C   Epstein–Barr virus IgM antibody
    D   HEV RNA
    E   HIV antibody

26. A 54-year-old man was reviewed in the hepatology clinic with a new diagnosis of alcohol-related cirrhosis, with no evidence of hepatic decompensation. He had no previous medical history, and had never had an upper gastrointestinal bleed.

    He underwent a gastroscopy which showed three columns of grade two oesophageal varices and portal hypertensive gastropathy in the stomach. There were no gastric varices or high-risk stigmata of bleeding.

    What is the next most appropriate management step?

    A   Combination therapy with isosorbide mononitrate and propranolol
    B   Combination therapy with propranolol and endoscopic variceal band ligation
    C   Endoscopic variceal band ligation
    D   Isosorbide mononitrate therapy
    E   Propranolol therapy

27. A 54-year-old man presented to his general practitioner with right upper quadrant pain that had been present for approximately 2 months. He was not jaundiced and had no weight loss. He had emigrated to the UK from Iran 23 years ago.
    On examination, there was tenderness in the right upper quadrant with no organomegaly or masses.

Investigations:

haemoglobin 128 g/L (130–180)	eosinophils 2.3 × 10⁹/L (0.04–0.4)
white cell count 7.8 × 10⁹/L (4–11)	bilirubin 18 mmol/L (1–22)
platelets 413 × 10⁹/L (150–400)	alkaline phosphatase 134 U/L (45–105)
neutrophils 3.2 × 10⁹/L (1.5–7.0)	alanine transaminase 28 U/L (5–35)
lymphocytes 0.5 × 10⁹/L (1.5–4.0)	albumin 36 g/L (37–49)

Liver ultrasound: 4.5×5 cm cystic lesion with an irregular cyst wall and a 3×3 cm cystic lesion with daughter cyst in right lobe of liver

What is the most likely diagnosis?

A   Amoebiasis
B   Cystadenoma
C   Echinococcal cyst
D   Polycystic liver disease
E   Simple cyst

28. A 38-year-old man presented for assessment of abnormal liver function tests. He had recently been diagnosed with emphysema and evaluation at that point indicated that he had α_1-antitrypsin deficiency.

Investigations:

bilirubin 24 mmol/L (1–22)	alanine transaminase 48 U/L (5–35)
alkaline phosphatase 189 U/L (45–105)	albumin 36 g/L (37–49)

What is the most likely genotype of his α_1-antitrypsin deficiency?

A   *PIMZ*
B   *PIMM*
C   *PISZ*
D   *PISS*
E   *PIZZ*

29. A 78-year-old man was referred for percutaneous endoscopic gastrostomy (PEG) insertion due to reduced nutritional intake secondary to a chronic disease.

In which of the following situations should PEG insertion NOT be used?

A   Cystic fibrosis
B   Motor neuron disease
C   Oesophageal carcinoma – T1N0M0
D   Peritoneal dialysis
E   Systemic sclerosis

30. A 24-year-old man presented to his general practitioner with a 2-month history of diarrhoea, bloating, tenesmus and lower abdominal pain. He had had previous episodes over the preceding 5 years, with no obvious precipitating factors. He had no weight loss and no rectal bleeding. There was no family history of inflammatory bowel disease.

On examination, he had no evidence of aphthous ulceration, and his abdomen was soft and non-tender with no masses or organomegaly. Rectal examination was normal.

Investigations:

haemoglobin 156 g/L (130–180)	C-reactive protein 9 mg/L (<10 mg/L)
white cell count 8.2 × 10⁹/L (4–11)	Tissue transglutaminase – negative
platelets 212 × 10⁹/L (150–400)	
erythrocyte sedimentation rate – 6 mm/1st h (0–20 mm/1st h)	
Faecal calprotectin – 47 μg/g	

What is the most appropriate next management step?

A   Refer for flexible sigmoidoscopy
B   Refer for endoscopy and duodenal biopsy
C   Refer for colonoscopy
D   Reassure and recommend symptomatic management
E   Send stool samples for microscopy, culture and sensitivity testing and detection of ova, cysts and parasites

31. A 19-year-old woman presented to the gastroenterology clinic with a 6-month history of 4-kg weight loss and diarrhoea associated with mouth ulcers. She had not had these symptoms prior to this episode. She opened her bowels six times per day with no blood in the stools; she had right iliac fossa abdominal pain. She had recently returned from a gap year travelling in South East Asia and Africa. She had complained of painful red eyes in the past. There was no family history of note. She had no past medical history and took no medications.

On examination, she looked thin with aphthous mouth ulcers. She was haemodynamically stable. Ophthalmological examination was normal. Abdominal examination was normal except for tenderness of the right iliac fossa. There was no genital ulceration.

Investigations:

haemoglobin 113 g/L (115–165 g/dL)	platelets 456 × 10⁹/L (150–400)
white cell count 7 × 10⁹/L (4–11)	C-reactive protein 8 mg/L (<10)

What is the most likely diagnosis?

A   Behçet's disease
B   Coeliac disease
C   Crohn's disease
D   Small bowel bacterial overgrowth
E   Tropical sprue

32. A 46-year-old woman presented with a 6-month history of difficulty swallowing foods and liquids. She reported occasional regurgitation of foods, and chest pain.

She underwent a barium swallow (see **Figure 4.3**).

What is the most likely diagnosis?

A   Achalasia
B   Diffuse oesophageal spasm

C   Hiatus hernia
D   Nutcracker oesophagus
E   Oesophageal carcinoma

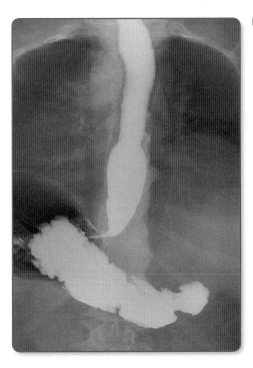

Figure 4.3

33. A 67-year-old man presented with a history of bright red rectal bleeding mixed in with his stool. He had no change in his bowel habit, and had not suffered any weight loss. He had a past medical history of atrial fibrillation and prostate cancer.

Investigations:

haemoglobin 88 g/L (130–180)   platelets 187 × 10^9/L (150–400)
white cell count 4.6 × 10^9/L (4–11)

Colonoscopy: showed the following (see **Figure 4.4**).

Figure 4.4 *See colour plate section.*

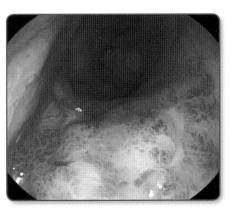

What is the most appropriate first-line treatment?

A   Argon photocoagulation
B   Prednisolone enemas
C   Sucralfate enemas
D   Topical 5-aminosalicylic acid (5ASA) treatment
E   Hyperbaric oxygen therapy

34. A 45-year-old woman presented to the clinic with abnormal liver function tests, which had been discovered on routine blood tests. She was asymptomatic.
    Investigations were performed which showed the following:

Investigations:

HBsAg: positive
HBeAg: negative
Total anti-HBc: positive
HBV DNA: 320 IU/mL
HCV IgG: positive
HCV RNA: 0 IU/mL
IgG and IgM anti-HDV: positive
HDAg: positive
HDV RNA: positive

What is the most likely diagnosis?

A   Acute hepatitis B virus (HBV), chronic hepatitis C virus (HCV), previous hepatitis D virus (HDV)
B   Acute HBV, previous HCV, acute HDV
C   Chronic HBV, chronic HCV, previous HDV
D   Chronic HBV, previous HCV, chronic HDV
E   Previous HBV, chronic HCV, previous HDV

35. A 33-year-old man with extensive ulcerative colitis was seen in the outpatient clinic. Over the last year he had required two courses of steroids for his ulcerative colitis. Recently, for a period of 2 weeks, he had experienced bloody diarrhoea five times per day with some associated abdominal pain. Two weeks ago, he had been prescribed a further reducing course of prednisolone, and after this treatment was instigated his bowel frequency had reduced to two times per day. He had no other medical problems. His current medications were 30 mg prednisolone once daily, calcium/vitamin D supplementation and mesalazine 800 mg three times daily.
    Examination was unremarkable:

Investigations:

C-reactive protein 12 (<10 mg/L)	thiopurine methyltransferase (TPMT) 50 pmol/h (26–50)
Abdominal X-ray: no toxic dilatation	
Flexible sigmoidoscopy: mild colitis	
Histology: mild colitis	
Stool culture: no ova, cysts or parasites	
Clostridium difficile: negative	

What is the most appropriate next management step?

A   Azathioprine
B   Infliximab
C   Intravenous hydrocortisone
D   6-Mercaptopurine
E   Methotrexate

36. A 45-year-old woman with a history of cirrhosis presented with worsening abdominal distension, which was causing her discomfort. She had no other past medical history and was currently taking propranolol as primary prophylaxis against variceal haemorrhage.
    On examination, she had a distended abdomen with shifting dullness indicating grade two ascites. Her abdomen was not tense. There was no evidence of encephalopathy and she was haemodynamically stable.

What is the most appropriate initial therapy?

A   Dietary salt reduction and combination therapy with spironolactone 100 mg once daily and furosemide 40 mg once daily
B   Dietary salt reduction and spironolactone 100 mg once daily
C   Dietary salt reduction and furosemide 40 mg once daily
D   Large-volume paracentesis with albumin cover
E   Large-volume paracentesis with albumin cover and spironolactone 100 mg once daily

37. A 79-year-old woman presented with symptoms of severe heartburn occurring at night, and associated with nausea but no vomiting. She had no symptoms of dysphagia or weight loss. She had never had these symptoms previously. Her past medical history consisted of hypertension, hypercholesterolaemia, depression and osteoporosis.

Which medication is the most likely cause of her symptoms?

A   Alendronate
B   Amlodipine
C   Citalopram
D   Ramipril
E   Simvastatin

38. A 28-year-old woman with colonic Crohn's disease presented with perianal pain associated with a discharge from her perineal region. She felt unwell and had a reduced appetite. She was on mesalazine 800 mg three times daily and the oral contraceptive pill.
    On examination, she had mild left-sided abdominal tenderness, and examination of her perineum revealed a perianal fistula with perianal tenderness on palpation.

What is the most appropriate next investigation?

A   Anorectal ultrasound
B   Examination under anaesthetic (EUA)
C   Fistulography
D   Pelvic MRI
E   Pelvic CT

39. An 18-year-old man was admitted with symptoms of colicky abdominal pain and vomiting. He had also been passing stools mixed with blood and mucus. He had had similar symptoms on four previous occasions, which had spontaneously resolved. He had no known medical problems.
    On examination, he was haemodynamically stable. There was a soft 'sausage-shaped' mass in the right iliac fossa but no other abnormalities.

Investigations:

haemoglobin 101 g/L (130–180)	platelets 163×10^9/L (150–400)
white cell count 4.3×10^9/L (4–11)	C-reactive protein <5 mg/L (<10)

Abdominal X-ray: intussusception
[Technetium-99m] pertechnetate scan: positive

What is the most likely diagnosis?

A   Whipple's disease
B   Henoch–Schönlein purpura
C   Meckel's diverticulum
D   Peutz–Jeghers' syndrome
E   Small bowel lymphoma

40. A 45-year-old woman presented to the emergency department with severe right upper quadrant abdominal pain. She had a 2-year history of intermittent right upper quadrant pain, which occurred approximately once a month, usually after eating, and lasted approximately 40 minutes. She had no past medical history and took no medications.

Examination was normal except for tenderness in her right upper quadrant.

Investigations:

bilirubin 16 mmol/L (1–22)	amylase 356 U/L (60–180)
alkaline phosphatase 804 U/L (45–105)	IgA 2.4 g/L (0.8–3.0)
alanine transaminase 84 U/L (5–35)	IgG 7 g/L (6.0–13.0)
albumin 38 g/L (37–49)	IgM 4 g/L (4.0–2.5)

Antinuclear antibody: negative

Ultrasound of the abdomen:
dilated common bile duct to 12 mm
no intrahepatic duct dilatation
no gallstones in the gallbladder and no filling defects in the bile ducts

Endoscopic retrograde cholangiopancreatography:
dilated 12-mm common bile duct
no filling defects seen

What is the most likely diagnosis?

A   Acute acalculous cholecystitis
B   Autoimmune cholangitis
C   Chronic pancreatitis
D   Primary sclerosing cholangitis
E   Sphincter of Oddi dysfunction (type 1)

41. A 68-year-old man presented with confusion. He had a history of short bowel syndrome after mesenteric ischaemia a year previously had led to a jejunoileal resection with jejunocolonic anastomosis. Postoperatively 120 cm of small bowel remained in situ. He was maintained on overnight enteral feeding through a percutaneous endoscopic gastrostomy tube and oral sip feeds through the day. He had diarrhoea 12–15 times per day. His current medications included thiamine 100 mg tds, omeprazole 40 mg once daily, loperamide 2 mg as required, and hydroxycobalamine injections.

On examination, he had a BMI of 20 kg/m². His Abbreviated Mental Test score was 5/10. His heart rate was 88 beats per minute, and blood pressure was 136/87 mmHg. He was warm peripherally. Cardiovascular and respiratory examination were normal. Abdominal examination revealed a midline laparotomy scar and an enterocutaneous fistula. Neurological examination was normal.

Investigations:

haemoglobin 157 g/L (130–180)	C-reactive protein 7 mg/L (<10 mg/L)
white cell count 13 × 10⁹/L (4–11)	magnesium 0.4 mmol/L (0.75–1.05 mmol/L)
platelets 386 × 10⁹/L (150–400)	pH 7.32 (7.35–7.45)
sodium 146 mmol/L (135–145 mmol/L)	P_{O_2} 13 kPa (11.3–12.6 kPa)
potassium 4.3 mmol/L (3.5–5.0 mmol/L)	P_{CO_2} 4.6 kPa (4.7-6.0 kPa)
urea 6 mmol/L (2.5–7.5 mmol/L)	BE 18 mmol/L (+/- 2 mmol/L)
creatinine 102 µmol/L (60–110 µmol/L)	HCO_3 10 mmol/L (22–30 mmol/L)
ammonia 86 µmol/L (10–20 µmol/L)	anion gap 20 mmol/L (12–16 mmol/L)

What is the most likely cause of his confusion?

A   Hypomagnaesaemia
B   Hyperammonaemia
C   Metabolic acidosis secondary to diarrhoea
D   Enterocutaneous fistula
E   D-lactic acidosis

42. A 66-year-old man presented with a 3-day history of worsening abdominal pain and distension. He felt nauseous and had been intermittently vomiting. He had not opened his bowels for 3 days, and had passed flatus only intermittently.

On examination, his pulse was 104 beats per minute and blood pressure 112/68 mmHg. Abdomen was soft, distended, with some generalised tenderness and the percussion note was tympanic.

A provisional diagnosis of small bowel obstruction was made and an abdominal CT was performed (see **Figure 4.5**).

What is the most likely cause of the obstruction?

A   Adhesions
B   Crohn's disease
C   Gallstone ileus
D   Inguinal hernia
E   Small bowel lymphoma

43. A 54-year-old man presented with vomiting, retrosternal pain and an inability to swallow his saliva. He underwent an endoscopy and was found to have a food bolus which was successfully removed. Twelve hours later, he became acutely unwell, with chest pain and shortness of breath.

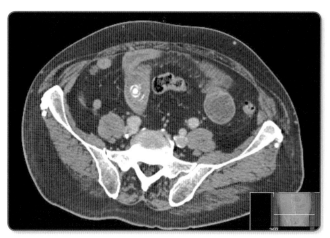

Figure 4.5

On examination, his temperature was 37.1°C, pulse 98 beats per minute, blood pressure 110/70 mmHg, respiratory rate 22 beats per minute and oxygen saturation 92% on air.

Investigations:

Chest X-ray: see **Figure 4.6**

Electrocardiogram: sinus tachycardia

What is the most appropriate next step in management?

A   Broad spectrum antibiotics
B   Furosemide

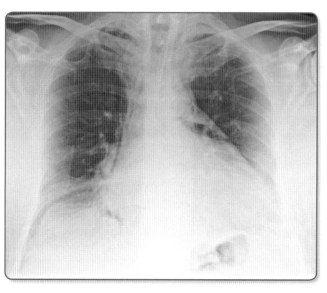

Figure 4.6

C   Low-molecular-weight heparin
D   Omeprazole
E   Salbutamol

44. A 44-year-old man presented with jaundice and abdominal pain in association with lethargy. He
had been jaundiced for 2 weeks. His abdominal pain started 3 days ago. He had no past medical
history, took no medications and there was no family history of note. He had a history of heavy
alcohol intake of over 100 units a week for the past 6 years.
    On examination, he was icteric, and had visible scratch marks on his upper body. He had
pale conjunctivae. Abdominal examination revealed a tender epigastrium and 4-cm tender,
hepatomegaly. There was no splenomegaly or ascites. Rectal examination was normal.

Investigations:

haemoglobin 88 g/L (130–180)	albumin 34 g/L (37–49)
mean corpuscular volume 108 fL (80–96)	bilirubin 167 mmol/L (1–22)
white cell count 7.4 × 10⁹/L (4–11)	alanine transaminase 56 U/L (5–35)
platelets 256 × 10⁹/L (150–400)	aspartate transaminase 64 U/L (1–31)
reticulocytes 10% (0.5–2.5)	alkaline phosphatase 168 U/L (45–105)
international normalised ratio 1.6 (<1.4)	

Antinuclear antibody – negative
Anti-smooth muscle antibody – negative
Antimitochondrial antibody – negative
HCV Ab – negative
HBsAg – negative

cholesterol 8.5 mmol/L (<5.2)   triglycerides 4.3 mmol/L (0.45–1.69)

What is the most likely diagnosis?

A   Caroli's disease
B   Crigler–Najjar syndrome
C   Gilbert's syndrome
D   Mirizzi's syndrome
E   Zieve's syndrome

45. A 72-year-old woman with a history of systemic sclerosis presented with melaena and an
associated haemoglobin drop. She underwent appropriate resuscitation with blood products and
fluids, and had an upper gastrointestinal endoscopy.

Investigations:

Upper gastrointestinal endoscopy: multiple lesions in stomach (see **Figure 4.7**).

What is the most appropriate management?

A   Adrenaline injection sclerotherapy
B   Argon photocoagulation (APC)
C   Beta-blocker
D   Corticosteroids
E   Endoscopic band ligation

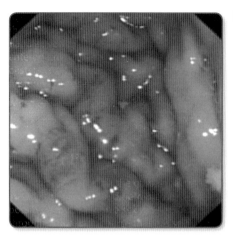

Figure 4.7 *See colour plate section.*

Answers

1. D Pancreatic pseudocyst

Pancreatic pseudocysts are a complication of chronic pancreatitis which occurs in 10–25% of patients. Pancreatic pseudocysts are localised pancreatic fluid collections which usually develop over 2–6 weeks. Raised pressure within the pancreatic ducts causes damage to the ducts, leading to leakage of pancreatic enzymes which become enclosed by a fibrotic reaction, leading to pseudocyst formation. Most will resolve spontaneously. The patient's symptoms of worsening abdominal pain, early satiety (as a consequence of the pseudocyst compressing the stomach) and nausea are classic signs of pancreatic pseudocyst formation, although pseudocysts can be asymptomatic. The incidence of adenocarcinoma of the pancreas is estimated to be 16.5 times higher in patients with chronic pancreatitis than in age-matched controls. However, in adenocarcinoma of the pancreas a longer time period of symptoms would be expected and early satiety is uncommon. The absence of jaundice makes a biliary stricture unlikely. Splenic vein thrombosis commonly presents with upper gastrointestinal bleeding from ruptured fundal varices and would not usually present with abdominal pain. Intraductal papillary mucinous neoplasms of the pancreas are not associated with chronic pancreatitis, and usually present with type 2 diabetes.

Tandon RK, et al. Chronic pancreatitis: Asia–Pacific consensus report. J Gastroenterol Hepatol 2002; 17:508–518.
Habashi S, Draganov P. Pancreatic pseudocyst. World J Gastroenterol 2009; 15(1):38–47.
Pan G, et al. Classification and management of pancreatic pseudocysts. Medicine 2015; 94(24):e960.

2. A Budd–Chiari syndrome

Budd–Chiari syndrome is characterised by hepatic venous outflow obstruction. It presents with a triad of abdominal pain, hepatomegaly and ascites. The amount of ascites present is dependent upon the extent and rapidity of the hepatic vein occlusion. Factors that predispose to the development of Budd–Chiari syndrome are acquired and inherited hypercoagulable states. Polycythaemia rubra vera (PRV) accounts for between 10% and 40% of cases. Paroxysmal nocturnal haemoglobinuria, the antiphospholipid syndrome and protein C, protein S and antithrombin III deficiency are also causes. Tumoral invasion, aspergillosis and Behçet's syndrome are rare causes.

Constrictive pericarditis manifests with tender hepatomegaly and may cause ascites, but a raised jugular venous pressure (JVP) would also be present, along with Kussmaul's sign (a raised JVP on inspiration) and a pericardial knock in 50% of cases. Hepatocellular carcinoma does not usually manifest with ascites, and is very uncommon (<2%) in those who do not have liver cirrhosis. Portal vein thrombosis does not give tender hepatomegaly as it is usually presinusoidal/prehepatic, the liver biochemistry and clotting will usually be normal and there may be splenomegaly because of portal hypertension. In tricuspid regurgitation, pulsatile hepatomegaly and a raised JVP would be present.

Menon KV, Shah V, Kamath PS. The Budd–Chiari Syndrome. N Engl J Med 2004; 350:578–585.

3. B Antibiotics and terlipressin

The patient has a suspected acute variceal haemorrhage, with evidence of significant haemodynamic instability. United Kingdom guidelines on the management of acute variceal bleed recommend antibiotics and a splanchnic vasoconstrictor such as terlipressin or somatostatin as soon as variceal haemorrhage is suspected. A meta-analysis has shown that antibiotics significantly reduce mortality in upper gastrointestinal bleeding in patients with chronic liver disease.. Terlipressin is a synthetic analogue of vasopressin and a systematic review has shown it to be effective in controlling acute variceal haemorrhage, and reducing mortality.

Beta-blockers (such as propranolol) are not recommended in acute variceal haemorrhage, as they reduce blood pressure and blunt the physiological increase in heart rate associated with bleeding. Beta-blockers are recommended as primary and secondary prophylaxis for variceal bleeding.

Tripathi D et al. UK guidelines on the management of variceal haemorrhage in cirrhotic patients. Gut 2015;0:1–25.
Garcia-Tsao, et al. AASLD practice guidelines. Prevention and Management of Gastroesophageal Varices and Variceal Hemorrhage in Cirrhosis. Hepatology 2007; 46(3):922–938.
Scottish Intercollegiate Guidelines Network. SIGN guideline 105: Management of acute upper and lower gastrointestinal bleeding, A national clinical guideline. Edinburgh: SIGN, 2008.

4.   E Thiamine administration

The patient has refeeding syndrome caused by prolonged fasting followed by rapid re-administration of a normal diet. Refeeding syndrome occurs because of the body's adaptive changes to prolonged fasting, which are designed to preserve protein and muscle. During starvation the principal adaptive changes are a reduction in the body's basal metabolic rate and a shift from carbohydrate to protein and fat use to fulfil the body's energy requirements. During prolonged starvation (in this case due to poor oral intake secondary to vomiting and alcohol dependence, followed by a hospital fast) severe depletion of intracellular phosphate, potassium and magnesium also occurs. Serum levels remain normal and so this intracellular loss is often not apparent during the fasting state. When feeding occurs after a prolonged fast, insulin levels become raised as a result of glucose absorption. Elevated insulin levels cause magnesium, glucose, phosphate and potassium to be absorbed intracellularly which can lead to a dramatic drop in serum levels of these minerals. Hyperinsulinaemia leads to the breakdown of fat, protein and glycogen, a process that requires magnesium and phosphate which further deplete serum levels. The first step in treatment consists of thiamine replacement, and then slow feeding at less than 50% of the body's requirements should be instigated if a patient has eaten little or nothing for more than 5 days. When considering enteral nutrition support, it should be started at a maximum of 10 kcal/kg/day in patients who are at high risk of developing refeeding syndrome. Electrolytes should be replaced, but thiamine administration is the first step. Without treatment refeeding syndrome can cause rhabdomyolysis and arrhythmias, and may prove fatal.

The National Institute for Health and Care Excellence (NICE). Nutrition support for adults: oral nutrition support, enteral tube feeding and parenteral nutrition. Clinical Guideline CG32. London: NICE; 2006.
Hisham M, et al. Refeeding syndrome: What is it, and how to prevent and treat it? BMJ 2008; 336:1495–1498.

5.   C Monitor LFTs and serological markers yearly

For a diagnosis of primary biliary cholangitis (PBC) to be made a combination of cholestatic liver function tests for at least 6 months and a raised anti-mitochondrial antibodies need to be present. The patient has a positive AMA but has normal cholestatic liver function tests (alkaline phosphate, bilirubin and GGT) and so does not have PBC. She has a high likelihood of developing PBC in the future and needs to be followed up with annual liver function tests, immunoglobulins and AMA titres.

PBC is a clinical diagnosis and a liver biopsy is not required to confirm the diagnosis, but it can be useful for staging activity and extent of disease and should be considered in patients who have very raised aminotransferases or a positive immunoglobulin G to rule out overlap syndromes.

Ursodeoxycholic acid and obeticholic acid are the first and second line treatments for PBC but are not appropriate management in this case as this patient does not fulfil diagnostic criteria for PBC.

Prednisolone is used as first line treatment for autoimmune hepatitis, usually in combination with azathioprine but this patient has no evidence of autoimmune hepatitis.

European Association for the Study of the Liver (EASL). Clinical practice guidelines. The diagnosis and management of patients with primary biliary cholangitis. J Hepatol 2017; 67:145–172.

6. C Lynch's syndrome

The answers are all syndromes that can cause colonic polyps.

Lynch's syndrome (hereditary non-polyposis syndrome) is a genetic disorder that is associated with a significantly increased risk of certain types of cancer (colorectal, small bowel, endometrial, renal pelvis or ureteric) and can cause colonic polyposis. It is autosomally dominantly inherited, and is due to a mismatch repair (*MMR*) gene mutation. Prior to the identification of the MMR gene diagnosis was made using the modified Amsterdam criteria.

Modified Amsterdam criteria:
- Colorectal cancer, or another Lynch's syndrome cancer, which affects three or more relatives, in at least two generations of the same family
- One affected family member has to be a first-degree relative of the other two
- One affected relative must be aged younger than 50 at diagnosis

Familial adenomatous polyposis (FAP) is an autosomally dominantly inherited syndrome. It is caused by mutations of the adenomatous polyposis coli (*APC*) gene on chromosome 5, and has a very high penetrance. It is suspected when over 100 adenomatous colonic polyps are observed at colonoscopy.

Juvenile polyposis is characterised by the presence of multiple hamartomatous colonic polyps. It is distinguished from Peutz–Jeghers syndrome, in which hamartomatous polyps are also seen, by histological differences. It typically manifests during childhood, and polyps are usually present in affected individuals before they reach the age of 20 years. MUTYH-associated polyposis is an autosomal recessive disorder which is caused by mutations in the MUTYH gene. The polyps are adenomatous or mixed adenomatous/hyperplastic.

Peutz–Jeghers syndrome is a syndrome in which pigmentation of the mucocutaneous surfaces is seen in combination with hamartomatous gastrointestinal polyps. It is inherited in an autosomal dominant fashion. There is an associated increased risk of oesophageal, gastric, pancreatic, small bowel and colorectal cancer, and a 50% lifetime risk of breast cancer.

Cairns SR, et al. Guidelines for colorectal cancer screening and surveillance in moderate and high risk groups (update from 2002). Gut 2010; 59:666–690.

7. C Mebendazole

The endoscopic image shows pinworm, or *Enterobius vermicularis*. The treatment for this is a single dose of mebendazole. It usually presents with intense pruritus ani, but can cause weight loss, irritability, diarrhoea, abdominal pain or colitis with eosinophilia. In rare cases it can colonise the female genital tract causing vaginal discharge. It is usually diagnosed via the 'Sellotape test' where the sticky side of Sellotape is placed onto the perianal skin and then examined under a microscope for ova. It has a worldwide distribution and particularly affects children.

Albendazole alone is recommended for the treatment of pinworm but steroids and albendazole together are only used where there is a suspicion of neurocysticercosis, or in the treatment of severe trichinellosis. Endoscopic removal is the treatment of choice for anisakiasis – a helminth infection. Ivermectin is used in the treatment of strongyloides infestation. Praziquantel is used to treat schistosomiasis.

Clinical Guidelines of the British Infection Society. Eosinophilia in returning travellers and migrants from the tropics: UK recommendations for investigation and management. J Infect 2010; 60:1–20.

8. B Continue clopidogrel

PY212 receptor antagonist antiplatelet agent (clopidogrel, prasugrel and ticagrelor) management for patients undergoing endoscopic procedures is based on the risk of the procedure and of the condition being treated.

PY212 receptor antagonists should be continued in low risk procedures which include diagnostic endoscopic procedures with or without biopsy (including colonoscopy), diagnostic endoscopic ultrasound, biliary or pancreatic stenting and enteroscopy without polypectomy.

In high-risk procedures such as polypectomy, endoscopic retrograde cholangiopancre-atography with sphincterotomy, ampullectomy, endoscopic mucosal resection, variceal therapy, stricture dilatation, stenting, endoscopic ultrasound with fine needle aspiration and percutaneous endoscopic gastrostomy insertion, the risk of the condition needs to be considered. In low risk conditions (ischaemic heart disease without coronary stenting, peripheral vascular disease and cerebrovascular disease) the PY212 antagonist should be stopped 5 days prior to the procedure. In high-risk conditions (patients with coronary artery stents) a cardiologist should be consulted. Stopping clopidogrel, ticragelor or prasugrel can be considered if it is over 12 months since a drug-eluting stent has been inserted, or more than 1 month following a bare metal stent insertion.

Veitch AM, Vanbiervliet G, Gershlick AH, et al. Endoscopy in patients on antiplatelet or anticoagulant therapy, including direct oral anticoagulants: British Society of Gastroenterology (BSG) and European Society of Gastrointestinal Endoscopy (ESGE) guidelines. Gut 2016; 65:374–389.

9. E Watch and wait

Chronic hepatitis B is divided into five main phases which may not always occur sequentially:

Immune-tolerance phase – Characterised by a positive HBeAg , high hepatitis B virus DNA levels, normal aminotransaminases, little or no liver necroinflammation, and virtually no or slow progression of fibrosis. Patients are highly contagious in this phase. Individuals infected as adults do not usually go through this phase.

Immune-reactive phase – patients are HBeAg positive, have elevated HBV DNA levels (but lower than the immune-tolerance phase), increased or fluctuating levels of aminotransferases, moderate or severe liver necroinflammation, and more rapid progression of fibrosis. This phase may last for several weeks to several years. During this phase there is a higher chance of spontaneous loss of HBeAg. In people who acquire the infection as adults this is the initial phase.

Immune control phase – may follow seroconversion from HBeAg to anti-HBe antibodies. During this phase HBV DNA levels can be low or even undetectable and aminotransferases are normal. Progression of fibrosis is minimal and HBsAg loss and seroconversion to anti-HBs antibodies may occur spontaneously in 1–3% of cases per year.

Immune escape phase (HBeAg-negative chronic hepatitis B) – patients are HBeAg negative and have episodic reactivation of infection with fluctuating levels of HBV DNA and aminotransferases. They can have active necroinflammation and a progression of liver fibrosis. This is due to the development of a mutation in the virus that leads to virions that fail to produce HBeAg.

HBsAg-negative phase – this occurs with loss of HBsAg. Patients are HBsAg negative, anti-HBc positive and anti-HBs may be detectable. HBV DNA is usually not detectable in the serum; however, low-level HBV replication may persist with detectable HBV DNA in the liver. Immunosuppression may lead to reactivation of HBV in these patients.

The National Institute for Health and Care Excellence (NICE) recommends patients over the age of 30 should be offered treatment when HBV DNA levels are above 2000 IU/mL, and the serum alanine aminotransferase is above the upper limit of normal on two tests which take place at least 3 months apart. Antiviral treatment should be offered to people who are younger than 30 years if the above criteria are fulfilled, and a liver biopsy shows necroinflammation and/or fibrosis, or the patient has a transient elastography score of 6 kPa or higher.

The patient is in the immune control phase and does not fulfil criteria for treatment at present but he should be monitored closely in case he progresses to the immune escape phase.

The National Institute for Health and Care Excellence (NICE). Clinical Guideline 165. Hepatitis B (chronic): diagnosis and management. London: NICE, 2013.

10. D Magnetic resonance cholangiopancreatography (MRCP)

The patient has cholestatic liver function tests with a negative antimitochondrial antibody and is likely to have primary sclerosing cholangitis (PSC). PSC is a cholestatic liver disease that is characterised by multiple intra- and extrahepatic biliary strictures. These occur as a result of chronic inflammatory changes leading to fibrosis of the bile ducts. It is diagnosed in patients with cholestatic abnormalities of their liver function tests in whom cholangiography shows segmental dilatation and multifocal strictures of the intra- and extrahepatic bile ducts, and in whom there has been exclusion of secondary causes of sclerosing cholangitis.

Cholangiography is essential for the diagnosis, and the gold standard used to be endoscopic retrograde cholangiopancreatography (ERCP); however, this procedure is complicated by pancreatitis and sepsis in 5% of cases. MRCP and ERCP have been shown to have similar diagnostic accuracy in the diagnosis of PSC, and therefore MRCP is the most appropriate next investigation in this patient. ERCP still has an important role in equivocal cases, as MRCP can miss early cases without bile duct dilatation, and for therapeutic intervention such as stent insertion.

European Association for the Study of the Liver. EASL Clinical Practice Guidelines: Management of cholestatic liver diseases. J Hepatol 2009; 51:237–267.

11. C Oesophageal candidiasis

Odynophagia (pain on swallowing) is a classic symptom of oesophageal candidiasis. Patients are often able to pinpoint the pain to a very specific retrosternal point. The main risk factor for oesophageal candidiasis is immunosuppression, one of the causes of which is diabetes. Other common causes of immunosuppression leading to oesophageal candidiasis are HIV infection (where it is an AIDS-defining illness), broad-spectrum antibiotic treatment and haematological malignancies. Cytomegalovirus can cause oesophagitis, but it is usually seen only in advanced AIDS and there is nothing in this woman's history to indicate this diagnosis. Eosinophilic oesophagitis commonly affects men in their 20s to 30s and usually presents with dysphagia and/or food impaction. Presentation with odynophagia is uncommon. Oesophageal carcinoma is usually painless and presents with dysphagia. Achalasia does not present with odynophagia but presents with dysphagia and reflux of food.

Pappas PG, Kauffman CA, Andes D, et al. Clinical practice guidelines for the management of candidiasis: 2009 update by the Infections Diseases Society of America. Clin Infect Dis 2009; 48:503.

12. A Alcohol related fatty liver disease

There are a number of causes of hepatic iron overload, the most clinically significant of which is hereditary haemochromatosis (HH). The diagnosis of HH is made in patients with evidence of clinical iron overload. The transferrin saturation is over 50% in the majority of patients, and the ferritin is usually over 1000. Confirmation of the diagnosis is achieved by HFE (human haemochromatosis gene) homozygosity for *C282Y*, or heterozygosity for *C282Y/H63*. This patient has a transferrin saturation and ferritin level that are too low for HH, and the most likely diagnosis is haemosiderosis secondary to alcohol related fatty liver disease. The appropriate management is reduction of alcohol intake. Hepatitis C virus (HCV) can cause hepatic iron overload but this patient does not have chronic HCV, having cleared the virus spontaneously. Non-alcoholic fatty liver disease (NAFLD) can cause hepatic iron deposition, but this patient's alcohol intake of 40 units per week rules out a diagnosis of NAFLD (which by definition occurs in patients who drink less than 30 g or 3.75 units of alcohol per day). Thalassaemia also causes iron overload, but this patient has a normal full blood count, ruling out this diagnosis.

AASLD practice guidelines. Diagnosis and management of haemochromatosis. Hepatology 2001; 33(5):1321–1328.

13. E Whipple's disease

Whipple's disease is the only diagnosis given that presents with malabsorption, neurological manifestations, polyarthritis and small bowel granulomas without skin or lung involvement. Although Crohn's disease can present with malabsorption and granulomas it does not manifest symptoms of neurological involvement. Sarcoidosis can rarely cause small bowel disease, and can have neurological and rheumatological involvement. Granulomas may also be present on biopsy, but the absence of skin or lung manifestations makes this diagnosis unlikely. Small bowel lymphoma is rare and can present with malabsorption. Neurological involvement can occur but it is very unlikely in the absence of lymphadenopathy, and it does not present with arthralgia. Abdominal tuberculosis can cause small bowel granulomas, malabsorption and neurological involvement, but it does not cause a migratory polyarthritis.

Whipple's disease is a rare disorder caused by the organism *Tropheryma whipplei*. It classically presents with diarrhoea and weight loss. Rheumatological manifestations occur on average 6 years prior to gastrointestinal symptoms and classically present with a migratory polyarthritis. Neurological changes are seen in up to 63% of patients, with the most common change being cognitive impairment, and cardiac involvement manifests clinically in 17–55%. The most common cardiac manifestation is pericarditis which occurs in around 50% of affected patients. Whipple's disease is diagnosed by periodic acid–Schiff (PAS) staining of small bowel biopsy specimens which on light microscopic examination show magenta-stained inclusions within macrophages of the lamina propria.

Fenollar F, Puéchal X, Raoult D. Whipple's disease. N Engl J Med 2007; 356:55–66.

14. D Prednisolone and azathioprine

This patient has classic clinical, biochemical and histological features of autoimmune hepatitis, with evidence of bridging fibrosis on liver biopsy. This is not primary biliary cholangitis (PBC) or an overlap syndrome, as antimitochondrial antibodies (AMAs) are negative and there is no evidence of the histological biliary changes seen in PBC on liver biopsy. Therefore, ursodeoxycholic acid would not be an appropriate first-line treatment for this patient.

The criteria for treatment of autoimmune hepatitis are: (a) AST /ALT (asparate transaminase/ alanine transaminase) >5 × upper limit of normal (ULN), (b) IgG >2 × ULN, and (c) features of bridging necrosis, multilobular necrosis or cirrhosis on liver biopsy. Initial treatment should be with prednisolone in combination with azathioprine as this is the regime that combines the least side effects with maximum effectiveness of treatment. Azathioprine monotherapy is not appropriate as it takes up to 12 weeks to have a therapeutic effect and thus will not treat her acute inflammation. If patients are intolerant of steroids then ciclosporin can be considered as a second line therapy. Methotrexate is not effective in treating autoimmune hepatitis.

Gleeson D, Heneghan M. British Society of Gastroenterology (BSG) guidelines for management of autoimmune hepatitis; Gut 2011; 60:1611–1629.

15. B Chronic mesenteric ischaemia

This woman has the classic features of chronic mesenteric ischaemia. This usually presents with postprandial abdominal pain that is so severe that those affected develop a fear of eating and subsequently lose weight. The classic examination finding is of abdominal tenderness which is disproportionately mild in comparison to the severity of the reported pain. Patients with chronic mesenteric ischaemia usually have evidence of previous atherosclerotic disease such as ischaemic heart disease, cerebrovascular disease or peripheral vascular disease. Biliary colic can present with postprandial pain, but is rarely associated with weight loss. Duodenal ulcer pain typically occurs 2–3 hours after eating and in 50–80% of patients pain occurs at night. Gastric ulcers present with pain that is precipitated by food, but are not associated with weight loss. Gastric carcinoma rarely presents with postprandial abdominal pain, commonly presenting with anaemia or weight loss.

White CJ. Chronic mesenteric ischaemia: Diagnosis and management. Prog Cardiovasc Dis 2011; 54:36–40.

16. C Norepinephrine

This patient has acute liver failure secondary to a paracetamol overdose with evidence of jaundice and encephalopathy. She has persistent hypotension despite adequate fluid resuscitation with colloid and requires vasopressors. The European Association for the Study of the Liver (EASL) guidelines on the management of acute liver failure recommend norepinephrine as the first line vasopressor in this situation.

Vasopressin should be added as second line therapy in patients whose requirement for norepinephrine increases to over 0.2–0.3 µg/kg/min. Inotropes such as dobutamine and milirinone are frequently required as second line therapies, but would not be used as the initial treatment of choice.

The benefit of hydrocortisone therapy in patients with acute liver failure with shock that is resistant to vasopressors is unclear. Over 50% of patients with acute liver failure have evidence of adrenal dysfunction and the use of steroids has been shown in one study to prolong time to death and reduce vasopressor requirements potentially enabling a liver to be found for transplant. However, hydrocortisone therapy has not been shown to reduce mortality in acute liver failure, and in patients with persistent hypotension while hydrocortisone might be used, vasopressor support would be the first line therapy in this situation.

European Association for the Study of the Liver. EASL Clinical Practical Guidelines on the management of acute (fulminant) liver failure. J Hepatol 2017; 66:1047–1081.

17. C Intravenous hydrocortisone 100 mg four times daily, subcutaneous heparin, calcium supplementation

The patient has acute, severe ulcerative colitis based on the Truelove and Witts criteria. These are a combination of a stool frequency of more than six per day combined with signs of systemic toxicity: (a) pulse >90 beats per minute, (b) erythrocyte sedimentation rate >30 mm/h, (c) haemoglobin <105 g/L or (d) temperature >37.8°C. Patients who fulfil these criteria should be admitted to hospital and treated with intravenous hydrocortisone 100 mg four times daily. Oral prednisolone is not appropriate management in colitis of this severity. Ciclosporin is as an effective therapy for acute, severe ulcerative colitis but it is currently recommended first line only in patients in whom steroids are best avoided. Antibiotic therapy should only be started in acute ulcerative colitis when there is a reasonable suspicion of infection, such as recent admission to hospital, a first attack of short duration or when stool cultures are positive. Subcutaneous heparin should be given to all patients with acute, severe ulcerative colitis to prevent venous thromboembolism, and calcium supplementation should be given to all patients expected to have a course of steroids of over 6 weeks – which includes all patients with acute ulcerative colitis.

Truelove SC, Witts LJ. Cortisone in ulcerative colitis; final report on a therapeutic trial. BMJ 1955; 2:1041e8.
Travis SL, et al. European evidence-based Consensus on the management of ulcerative colitis: Current management. J Crohn's Colitis 2008; 2:24–62.
National Institute for Health and Care Excellence (NICE). Clinical Guideline 166. Ulcerative cColitis: management. London: NICE, 2013.

18. D Prednisolone

The patient has alcoholic hepatitis. Alcoholic hepatitis has certain characteristic features:
- History of excessive alcohol intake
- Jaundice with bilirubin >80 mmol/L
- Hepatomegaly
- Mild fever but no infective cause found.

There are a number of scoring systems used to assess the severity of alcoholic hepatitis but the most commonly used is the Maddrey discriminant function (MDF). A score of >32 indicates a severe alcoholic hepatitis and is an indication for treatment with steroids.

MDF = (bilirubin (in µL/17) + [(PT – control PT) × 4.6]
In this case the MDF = (170/17) + [(18 – 12) × 4.6] = 38

Where PT is prothrombin time (in seconds).

Patients with a MDF of over 32 have a predicted mortality rate of 30–50%. The STOPAH trial showed that prednisolone therapy leads to a non-significant reduction in 28 day mortality in severe alcoholic hepatitis, although a reduction in longer term mortality was not shown. Prednisolone 40 mg once daily for 28 days is recommended as the first line treatment for patients with severe alcoholic hepatitis, after effectively treating any active infection, gastrointestinal bleeding and renal impairment. Pentoxyfylline does not reduce mortality and therefore is not recommended. Nutritional supplementation may improve mortality in certain subgroups of patients, and improves biochemical parameters, but has not shown an overall survival benefit and should not be used as initial monotherapy. Supportive care would be the appropriate treatment if this was a mild or moderate alcoholic hepatitis.

Thursz M, Richardson P, Allison M, Austin A, Bowers M, Day CP et al. Prednisolone or Pentoxfylline for Alcoholic Hepatitis ; N Engl J Med 2015;372:1619-28. DOI: 10.1056/NEJMoa1412278
O'Shea RS, et al. Alcoholic liver disease. Hepatology 2010; 51(1):307.
National Institute for Health and Care Excellence (NICE). Pathways:. Alcohol-related liver disease. London: NICE, 2017.

19. A Continue current treatment

Cytomegalovirus (CMV) infection has a worldwide distribution but is most common in developing countries where prevalence can be very high (almost 100% in adults). CMV infection is usually asymptomatic, and immunosuppressive therapy only rarely causes the development of severe CMV-related disease. It more usually causes latent CMV infection to undergo a subclinical reactivation. This is usually asymptomatic or mild and self-limiting and therefore screening for latent infection is not recommended for patients commencing immunosuppressant therapy with inflammatory bowel disease. In this patient's case although there is evidence of CMV infection, with CMV IgG (indicating a risk for reactivation) and CMV DNA, and inclusion bodies within the colonic mucosa, the patient is asymptomatic and has no overt clinical disease so no specific antiviral treatment is required and the azathioprine can be continued. In severe CMV colitis, treatment with intravenous ganciclovir should be commenced, with a switch to oral valganciclovir after 2–3 days if appropriate clinically.

Rahier JF, et al. Second European evidence-based consensus on the prevention, diagnosis and management of opportunistic infections in inflammatory bowel disease. J Crohn's Colitis 2014; 8:443–468

20. C 80 mg intravenous omeprazole bolus followed by a 72-hour protein pump inhibitor infusion at 8 mg/h and repeat endoscopy in 6–8 weeks

The endoscopic finding of a non-bleeding visible vessel indicates a high risk of re-bleeding, and therefore treatment with an 80 mg bolus of omeprazole (or other comparable protein pump inhibitor), followed by an 8 mg/h omeprazole infusion for 72 hours and repeat endoscopy in 6–8 weeks is the appropriate post-endoscopy management. Haemostasis is achieved by endoscopic intervention and acid suppression therapy is given to maintain intragastric pH above 6 to stabilise clots and prevent re-bleeding. A 2014 Cochrane review does not support the use of tranexamic acid in non-variceal upper gastrointestinal bleeding, despite the appearance of a beneficial effect on mortality, due to a high dropout rate in trials. If *Helicobacter pylori* is present then eradication therapy should be started; however, in this patient a result is not given and so eradication therapy should not be started until the *Helicobacter pylori* result is known. All patients with gastric ulcers should have a repeat endoscopy in 6–8 weeks to ensure ulcer healing and exclude gastric carcinoma. There is no requirement for repeat endoscopy within 24 hours if there is no further gastrointestinal bleeding.

National Institute for Health and Care Excellence (NICE). Clinical Guideline 141. Acute upper gastrointestinal bleeding in over 16s: management. London: NICE, 2012.
Scottish Intercollegiate Guidelines Network. SIGN Guidelines. Management of acute upper and lower gastrointestinal bleeding: A national clinical guideline. Edinburgh: SIGN, 2008.
Bennett C, Klingenberg SL, Langholz E, Gluud LL. Tranexamic acid for upper gastrointestinal bleeding (Review). Cochrane Database of Systematic Reviews 2014; 11: CD006640.

21. D Phenytoin

With the exception of warfarin all of the drugs listed can result in idiosyncratic drug reactions causing hepatotoxicity. The answer in this scenario is phenytoin as this is the only drug listed that causes an immunoallergic hepatotoxicity. This is characterised by fever, lymphadenopathy, rash and severe hepatocyte injury, and can cause raised eosinophils. Sulfa drugs and halothane can also cause an immunoallergic reaction. The mechanism by which this occurs is by enzyme–drug adduction on the cell surface causing IgE release. Amiodarone causes a dose-dependent hepatotoxicity and typically causes steatohepatitis. Carbamazepine causes a mixed reaction with bile duct injury. Diclofenac causes a direct hepatotoxic reaction. With all idiosyncratic drug reactions the most important management step is identifying and stopping the causative drug. With the exception of N-acetylcysteine in paracetamol overdose there are no specific antidotes for drug-induced hepatotoxicity. Liver transplantation can be required if acute liver failure occurs, defined by jaundice followed by encephalopathy within 12 weeks, and all patients who develop this should be managed in a liver transplantation centre.

Lee WE. Drug induced hepatotoxicity. N Engl J Med 2003; 349:474–485.

22. B Liver cirrhosis

The differential diagnosis of new-onset ascites includes cirrhosis of the liver (the cause in 85% of cases), carcinomatosis peritonei, massive liver metastases, tuberculosis peritonitis, and rarer causes such as nephrotic syndrome and heart failure.

The serum–ascites albumin gradient (SAAG) is the most accurate measure for determining the cause of ascites, with a 97% accuracy in diagnosing ascites secondary to portal hypertension when a SAAG of >11 g/L is present.

The SAAG is calculated by the following equation:
SAAG = serum albumin – ascitic fluid albumin

This is more accurate than the previously favoured transudate (fluid protein <25 g/L) and exudate (fluid protein >25 g/L) because in 25% of cases patients with cirrhosis can have a fluid protein >25 g/L. For causes of ascites classified by the SAAG see **Table 4.1.**

Table 4.1 Causes of ascites by SAAG	
SAAG >11	**SAAG <11**
Cirrhosis	Carcinomatosis peritonei
Nephrotic syndrome	Tuberculous peritonitis
Heart failure	Pancreatitis

The only two answers given that could cause a SAAG >11 are cirrhosis and nephrotic syndrome. The patient has a normal albumin level and no peripheral oedema, which makes nephrotic syndrome highly unlikely, and therefore liver cirrhosis is the correct answer.

Moore KP, Aithal GP. BSG Guidelines on the management of ascites in cirrhosis. Gut 2006; 55:1–12.
European Association for the Study of the Liver (EASL). Clinical Practice Guidelines on the management of ascites, spontaneous bacterial peritonitis, and hepatorenal syndrome in cirrhosis. J Hepatol 2010; 53:397–417.

23. E Length of Barrett's oesophagus over 3 cm

The picture shows Barrett's oesophagus, more accurately known as columnar lined oesophagus (CLO). This occurs when the normal oesophageal squamous lining has been replaced by a metaplastic columnar epithelium. A diagnosis of Barrett's oesophagus is made when a segment of columnar metaplasia is seen above the gastro-oesophageal junction during endoscopy, and has been confirmed histologically. The principal clinical concern in Barrett's oesophagus is the risk of progression to oesophageal adenocarcinoma.

The factors that have been associated with progression to adenocarcinoma are:
- Older age
- Male gender
- Current tobacco smoking
- Long segment Barretts Oesophagus (over 3 cm)

Molecular markers such as p53 expression are sometimes used in research as surrogate markers of adenocarcinoma risk, but their usefulness clinically has not been ascertained and so they should be used only for research purposes. Alcohol is associated with gastro-oesophageal reflux disease but does not appear to be associated with Barrett's oesophagus.

Fitzgerald RC, di Pietro M, Ragunath K, et al British Society of Gastroenterology Guidelines for the diagnosis and management of Barrett's oesophagus. Gut 2014;63:7–42.

24. B Gastroscopy and duodenal biopsies

This patient has symptoms and signs suggestive ofcoeliac disease, with fatigue, diarrhoea and bloating, and dermatitis herpetiformis. The gold standard diagnostic test is gastroscopy and duodenal biopsies while the patient is consuming a gluten containing diet. Small intestinal biopsy shows characteristic histological changes of crypt hyperplasia and villous atrophy and an inflammatory infiltrate into the lamina propria and epithelium.

Tissue transglutaminase (TTG) antibodies are a highly sensitive test for coeliac disease, being present in over 90% of patients with untreated disease, but are less specific. They are used for serological screening for coeliac disease. Immunoglobulin A levels should always be requested when TTG antibodies are tested, as false negatives can occur in IgA deficiency. Periodic acid–Schiff staining is required to diagnose Whipple's disease. Serum angiotensin-converting enzyme levels are used to diagnose sarcoidosis, which can occasionally present with small bowel involvement; however, the rash described is not typical of sarcoidosis. A colonoscopy and ileal biopsies would be appropriate if Crohn's disease was suspected. While malabsorptive symptoms could indicate Crohn's disease, dermatitis herpetiformis is not associated with Crohn's disease.

Ludvigsson JF, Bai JC, Biagi F, et al. Diagnosis and management of adult coeliac disease: guidelines from the British Society of Gastroenterology. Gut 2014;0:1–20.

25. A Anti-HAV IgM

This patient has the classic clinical features of hepatitis A virus (HAV). This is diagnosed in the acute phase by the presence of anti-HAV IgM, which is present for 14 days to 6 months after infection. Anti-HAV IgG develops approximately 5–6 weeks after the onset of acute infection, is present in serum for many years. and confers protective immunity against further infection. HAV infection consists of four stages. The first stage is an asymptomatic incubation period, lasting on average 28 days (varying from 10 to 50 days) when viral shedding takes place. The second phase is the prodromal phase, during which symptoms of fever, dark urine, pale stools, malaise, headache and gastrointestinal upset occur. This is followed within 10 days by the development of jaundice (the icteric phase). The final phase is the convalescent phase when recovery from the infection occurs. On examination jaundice, cervical lymphadenopathy and tender hepatosplenomegaly may be seen, but examination is usually normal.

Hepatitis E virus presents in a similar way to HAV, but it has a longer incubation period of 15–60 days, with an average of 40 days from exposure to symptoms, and posterior cervical lymphadenopathy has not been reported. Hepatitis B virus (HBV) can be very difficult to differentiate from acute HAV clinically. However, medical students in the UK are screened for HBV prior to medical school entry and vaccinated if not already immune. Even if this did not happen, this patient has no risk factors for contracting HBV. The classic presentation of Epstein–Barr virus (EBV) is with a triad of fever, lymphadenopathy and sore throat, which is not present in this patient. Jaundice is uncommon in EBV occurring in less than 5% of cases. HIV seroconversion can present with generalised lymphadenopathy but does not usually present with jaundice, and, this patient has no obvious risk factors for contracting HIV.

World Health Organization Department of Communicable Disease Surveillance and Response. Hepatitis A. 2000. WHO/CDS/CSR/EDC/2000.7.
Cohen JI. Epstein–Barr virus infection. N Engl J Med 2000; 343:481–492.

26. E Propranolol therapy

Non-selective beta-blockers (NSBB) are recommended as first-line therapy for primary prophylaxis of variceal haemorrhage. They reduce portal pressure (the driver for varices formation) by decreasing cardiac output and acting as a splanchnic vasoconstrictor. The risk of a first variceal bleed in patients with grade two or three (medium or large) varices is significantly reduced by beta-blocker therapy (30% in controls versus 14% in treated patients) as is mortality. Variceal band ligation (VBL) is recommended if there are contraindications to non-selective beta blocker use. A Cochrane meta-analysis has shown a reduced risk of bleeding with VBL, but no reduction in bleeding related or overall mortality when compared with NSBB for primary prophylaxis of variceal bleeding. NSBBs are associated with reduced fatal outcomes compared with VBL, due to the risk of fatal VBL-induced bleeding, and so are recommended as first line treatment.

Isosorbide mononitrate (ISMN) is not recommended as primary prophylaxis for variceal haemorrhage because studies have shown a higher mortality in patients over 50 years receiving ISMN therapy than in those taking placebo, and ISMN when compared with placebo for the prevention of variceal haemorrhage showed higher bleeding rates.

An unblinded trial has shown a significantly lower rate of haemorrhage in combination therapy with ISMN and nadolol, compared with nadolol alone; however, two more recent, large, double-blinded, controlled trials were unable to confirm this result, and significantly more side effects were noted in the combination group, so combination therapy is not recommended.

Variceal ligation alone has been compared with combination VBL and beta-blocker therapy, but no differences in the incidence of bleeding or death were seen between groups, so this is not recommended for primary prophylaxis.

Tripathu D, Stanley AJ, Hayes PC, Patch D, Millson C, Mehrzad H et al UK guidelines on the management of variceal haemorrhage in cirrhotic patients. Gut 2015;64:1680–1704.
Garcia-Tsao G, et al. AASLD Practice Guidelines. Prevention and Management of Gastroesophageal Varices and Variceal Hemorrhage in Cirrhosis. Hepatology 2007; 46(3):922–938.

27. C Echinococcal cyst

Echinococcal (hydatid) cystic disease is usually caused by *Echinococcus granulosus* in the UK. It is most frequently found in individuals returning from the Middle East, Eastern Europe, North and East Africa and Asia. It has an incubation period of months to years, and is transmitted via ingestion of eggs from canine faeces. It commonly presents with asymptomatic cysts discovered on routine abdominal imaging, but it can present with right upper quadrant pain and fever if liver cysts leak or become infected, or with hepatomegaly, cholestasis, biliary cirrhosis, portal hypertension and ascites. The cysts can rupture into the peritoneal space, leading to anaphylaxis and secondary cyst formation. An eosinophilia is present usually only when the cyst is leaking. Cyst aspiration can be complicated by anaphylaxis and cyst dissemination and so should be carried out only in specialist centres. Treatment is based on cyst size, location and stage. Treatment is albendazole ± praziquantel ± cyst aspiration with the puncture, aspiration, injection and re-aspiration technique. Of all the causes of liver cysts given, hydatid disease is the only one that will cause an eosinophilia and the only one where daughter cysts are seen. Amoebiasis may cause an eosinophilia but it causes liver abscesses not liver cysts.

Brunetti E, Kern P, Vuitton DA. Writing Panel for the WHO-IWGE. Expert consensus for the diagnosis and treatment of cystic and alveolar echinococcosis in humans. Acta Trop 2010; 114(1):1.

28. E PIZZ

$α_1$-Antitrypsin (AAT) deficiency is caused by the inheritance of two severe deficiency alleles at the locus encoding AAT. It has a prevalence of 1 case per 3000–5000 persons in the USA. AAT is a serine protease inhibitor encoded by SERPINA-1 (also known as PI). AAT deficiency classically presents with severe, early onset, panacinar emphysema with a basilar predominance. AAT deficiency presents with predominant lung or liver involvement or both dependent on the inherited allele as indicated in **Table 4.2**:

Table 4.2 α1-Antitrypsin alleles and their phenotype		
Allele	**Risk of emphysema**	**Risk of liver disease**
PIZZ	Very high	High
MZ	Possibly increased	Possibly increased
SZ	Increased	Possibly increased

Those with the *PIZZ* allele are at high risk of lung and liver involvement, and therefore this man is most likely to have this allele. Patients with the *PIMZ* allele may be at increased risk for lung and liver disease but the evidence is not robust. There is an increased risk of chronic obstructive pulmonary disease in those with the *PISZ* allele, but it is not as high as in those with the *PIZZ* allele.

Silverman EK. Alpha 1-antitrypsin deficiency. N Engl J Med 2009; 360:2749–2757.

29. C Oesophageal carcinoma – T1N0M0

Percutaneous gastrostomy (PEG) insertion is used for the maintenance of long-term enteral nutrition in those in whom oral access is reduced. The most common indication for PEG placement is acute ischaemic or haemorrhagic stroke. In certain situations PEG placement is not appropriate, and in others caution should be used.

In T1N0M0 oesophageal carcinoma PEG insertion should not be performed as there is a potential risk of seeding of malignant cells leading to PEG stoma metastases. The placement of a PEG may also mean that if an oesophagectomy is required, the stomach will not be suitable for forming a gastric tube.

In patients with cystic fibrosis nutritional status is often poor and nutritional failure common. The placement of a PEG improves nutritional status, which can help respiratory function. Progressive neuromuscular diseases such as motor neuron disease are valid indications for PEG insertion, but when ventilatory function is compromised this should occur only after an anaesthetic assessment. PEG insertion improves nutritional status in peritoneal dialysis patients, improving the likelihood of survival and of receiving a kidney transplant, but it also increases the risk of fungal peritonitis. PEG insertion can be carried out but dialysis should not occur for 3 days prior to the procedure and prophylactic antifungal therapy should be given. In systemic sclerosis, although there is no specific outcome data, the procedure is considered safe and may reduce aspiration, and so it should be performed if clinically required.

Westaby D, et al. BSG guidelines. The provision of a percutaneously placed enteral tube feeding service. Gut 2010; 59:1592–1605.

30. Reassure and recommend symptomatic management

Faecal calprotectin is recommended by the National Institute for Health and Care Excellence (NICE) to help distinguish between irritable bowel syndrome (IBS) and inflammatory bowel disease (IBD) in primary care, and it is used when patients have with lower abdominal symptoms but cancer is not suspected. During intestinal inflammatory processes faecal calprotectin is excreted into the intestinal lumen and a raised level is seen in inflammatory bowel disease and malignancy. False positives can occur in patients taking nonsteroidal anti-inflammatory drugs and in patients with coeliac disease. Values of over 50 g/g when using faecal calprotectin ELISA tests have a 93% sensitivity and 94% specificity for distinguishing IBS from IBD. A patient with no red flag symptoms and a faecal calprotectin less than 50, as in this case, can be reassured and treated symptomatically for IBS.

In patients with no red flag symptoms and who meet the IBS diagnostic criteria then the following tests should be performed to exclude other causes: full blood count, erythrocyte sedimentation rate, C-reactive protein and coeliac disease antibody testing (tissue transglutaminase or anti-endomysial antibodies). In this patient the results of these tests were all normal, or negative, making causes of his symptoms other than IBS much less likely.

The NICE guideline on irritable bowel syndrome in adults: diagnosis and management, states that IBS should be considered in people who present with abdominal discomfort or pain, which is either associated with a change in stool consistency or frequency of bowel motions, or is relieved by opening the bowels. In addition, two of the following four symptoms should be present to make a positive diagnosis: abdominal bloating; a change in the passage of stool (i.e. urgency, straining, tenesmus); passing mucus; worsening of symptoms after eating. This patient's symptoms fulfil the IBS diagnostic criteria.

National Institute for Health and Care Excellence (NICE). Diagnostics guidance. Faecal calprotectin diagnostic tests for inflammatory disease of the bowel. London: NICE, 2013.
National Institute for Health and Care Excellence (NICE). Irritable bowel syndrome in adults: diagnosis and management. Clinical guideline 61. London: NICE , 2017.

31. C Crohn's disease

This woman has presented with malabsorption (weight loss and diarrhoea), abdominal pain and scleritis, a classic spectrum of symptoms and signs associated with Crohn's disease. Small bowel bacterial overgrowth and coeliac disease do not cause abdominal pain or scleritis, although they can cause malabsorption. Tropical sprue causes malabsorption and can cause glossitis, but not aphthous ulceration.

Behçet's disease can present in a similar way, but to diagnose Behçet's disease the following criteria must be met.

Recurrent oral ulceration which occurs at least three times in a year. AND two of the following:

- Eye lesions: anterior or posterior uveitis, retinal vasculitis or cells in the vitreous humour.
- Recurrent genital ulceration
- Skin lesions: erythema nodosum, papulopustular lesions, pseudofolliculitis or acneiform nodules in non-adolescents
- A positive skin pathergy test

Gomollon F, Dignass A, Annese V, et al. 3rd European Evidence-based Consensus on the Diagnosis and Management of Crohn's Disease 2016: Part 1: Diagnosis and Medical Management. J Crohns Colitis 2017; 11:3–25.
Kontogiannis V, Powell RJ. Behçet's disease. Postgrad Med J 2000; 76:629–637.

32. A Achalasia

The barium swallow shows the classic findings of achalasia. Achalasia is an oesophageal motor disorder that is characterised by a failure of relaxation of the lower oesophageal sphincter (LOS). Pathologically inflammatory changes are seen in the oesophageal myenteric (Auerbach's) plexus. This leads to selective loss of post-ganglionic inhibitory neurons, with the postganglionic neurons of the myenteric plexus being spared, leading to unopposed cholinergic stimulation, high basal pressures and a failure of relaxation of the LOS. The classic radiological finding on barium swallow is smooth tapering of the lower oesophagus, leading to the closed LOS, which resembles a bird's beak in appearance. Oesophageal carcinoma classically presents with a long area of irregular mucosal narrowing. A hiatus hernia appears as a widening below the LOS. Nutcracker oesophagus and diffuse oesophageal spasm are diagnoses that can be made only on oesophageal manometry.

Stavropoulos SN, Friede D, Modayil R, Parkman HP. Diagnosis and management of esophageal achalasia: BMJ 2016; 353:i2785.
Vaezi MF, et al. Practice guidelines diagnosis and management of achalasia. Am J Gastroenterol 1999; 94(12):3406–3412.

33. C Sucralfate enemas

The appearances in the endoscopic picture are of radiation-induced telangiectasia. The most common cause for this is pelvic radiotherapy for prostate carcinoma. There is minimal reliable evidence for beneficial long-term outcome with any treatment.

The first-line treatment for radiation-induced rectal bleeding is sucralfate enemas in those patients for whom it is causing a reduced quality of life, or who are anaemic.

Second line treatment involves ablation of the telangiectasia with one of the following techniques, but all have significant disadvantages which limit their use:
1. Hyperbaric oxygen therapy
2. Argon plasma photocoagulation
3. Formalin therapy

The appearances are not consistent with inflammatory bowel disease for which a topical 5ASA treatment would be given. Prednisolone enemas are not recommended in radiation enteritis.

Andreyev HJN, Davidson SE, Gillespie C, Allum WH, Swarbrick E. Practice guidance on the management of acute and chronic gastrointestinal problems arising as a result of treatment for cancer. Gut 2012; 61:179–192.

34. D Chronic HBV, previous HCV, chronic HDV

With acute HBV infection, the first marker that goes up is HBV-DNA. This is followed by HBsAg, HBeAg and anti-HBc IgM. Although anti-HBc IgM is not given, it would be expected that a patient with acute HBV infection would have high HBV DNA levels and be HBeAg positive. Chronic HBV infection is characterised by the presence of HBsAg, for more than 6 months with or without symptoms and regardless of viral load.

The presence of a positive HCV IgG antibody and negative HCV RNA indicates cleared HCV infection. There is no history of HCV treatment so she has cleared the virus spontaneously.

Hepatitis delta is a defective RNA virus. It requires HBV for its own replication, and so can only occur as a co-infection. It can occur either as an acute co-infection with HBV, which is usually self-limiting with resolution of infection but can lead to a fulminant hepatitis, or as a superinfection in those already chronically infected with HBV, where it can cause a severe chronic active hepatitis with 70–80% progressing to cirrhosis.

In acute HBV–HDV co-infection the following serological markers will be positive: HBsAg, HBeAg and HBV DNA, anti-HBc IgM, HDV RNA and hepatitis D Ag (HDAg). The development of anti-HDV antibodies occurs late in the acute phase of infection, and after infection they decline to undetectable levels. As anti-HDV appears HDAg disappears. IgG and IgM anti-HD take months to years to decline after recovery from acute infection.

In contrast in HBV–HDV superinfection, persistent HDV infection occurs in up to 90% of cases. HDV viraemia (detectable HDV RNA) appears in the pre-acute phase and is associated with active liver disease. There may be high titres of IgM and IgG anti-HDV and these can persist indefinitely. HBsAg titres and HBV–DNA can decline to almost undetectable levels with HDV co-infection but there is persistence of HBsAg and HDAg. This patient has chronic HBV–HDV superinfection as shown by the positive markers of HDV replication and a positive HDAg and positive IgM and IgG anti-HD in combination with a positive HBsAg and a negative HBeAg.

WHO, Department of Communicable Disease Surveillance and Response. Hepatitis Delta. WHO, 2001. http://www.who.int/csr/disease/hepatitis/HepatitisD_whocdscsrncs2001_1.pdf

European Association for the Study of the Liver (EASL). Recommendations on treatment of hepatitis C. J Hepatol 2017; 66:153–194.
The National Institute for Health and Care Excellence (NICE). Clinical guideline 165: Hepatitis B (chronic): diagnosis and management. London: NICE, 2013.

35. A Azathioprine

This patient has steroid-refractory ulcerative colitis, having required three courses of steroids within the last year to control his symptoms. Other causes of frequent exacerbations, such as cytomegalovirus colitis, should be excluded, and once these have been ruled out and remission has been induced thiopurine therapy with azathioprine should be started to maintain remission. A full blood count should be monitored before and after treatment starts to monitor for myelotoxicity. 6-Mercaptopurine is a metabolite of azathioprine that is associated with fewer side effects. In the UK, this is used in those who cannot tolerate azathioprine therapy. The patient has responded to oral steroids and does not currently fulfil the Truelove and Witts criteria for acute severe colitis and so does not require intravenous steroids. Infliximab can be considered in this situation, but thiopurines are the usual first-line management. There is not enough evidence regarding the use of methotrexate in steroid-refractory ulcerative colitis to recommend its use in this situation.

Truelove SC, Witts LJ. Cortisone in ulcerative colitis; final report on a therapeutic trial. BMJ 1955; 2:1041e8.
Harbord M, Eliakim R, Bettenworth D, et al. Third European evidence-based consensus on diagnosis and management of ulcerative colitis. Part 2: Current management. J Crohn's Colitis. 2017; 11(7):769–784.

36. B Dietary salt reduction and spironolactone 100 mg once daily

Cirrhosis is the most common cause of ascites, and within 10 years of diagnosis 60% of patients with compensated cirrhosis will have developed ascites. Cirrhosis causes portal hypertension, by obstructing flow through the portal vasculature. Portal hypertension has a variety of consequences including the development of portosystemic shunts and intestinal disturbances causing bacterial translocation and endotoxaemia. This leads to release of prostaglandins and nitric oxide, with subsequent vasodilatation, particularly in the splanchnic beds. The result of this is decreased renal blood flow and activation of the renin–angiotensin system leading to avid sodium and water retention and ascites. In patients with a first episode of moderate, but not tense, ascites European Association for the Study of the Liver (EASL) Guidelines recommend initial dietary salt restriction to 80–120 mmol/day, in combination with an aldosterone antagonist such as spironolactone. Spironolactone is the most effective treatment as it targets the distal tubule of the kidney where most sodium retention occurs. If there is no response to spironolactone monotherapy then frusemide should be added.

Combination first line therapy with spironolactone and frusemide is recommended for patients with recurrent ascites. In a patient with tense ascites large-volume paracentesis is recommended for symptomatic relief, but this is not recommended in patients with non-tense ascites due to the potential risk of infection. Monotherapy with furosemide is less effective than spironolactone therapy and so is not recommended.

European Association for the Study of the Liver (EASL). EASL clinical practice guidelines on the management of ascites, spontaneous bacterial peritonitis, and hepatorenal syndrome in cirrhosis; J Hepatol 2010; 53:397–417.

37. A Alendronate

Bisphosphonates, and in particular alendronate, can cause oesophageal ulceration and symptoms of heart burn. All patients taking alendronate should be advised to drink plenty of water when taking their medication and to stay upright for 30–60 minutes after taking it to try to prevent this complication. Patients complaining of dyspepsia should be asked if they are taking the following medications that cause dyspeptic symptoms: bisphosphonates, calcium channel antagonists, steroids, non-steroidal anti-inflammatory drugs, nitrates and theophyllines. Calcium channel antagonists can cause dyspepsia, but do not cause symptoms of oesophagitis. Citalopram, ramipril and simvastatin do not cause oesophagitis.

National Institute for Health and Clinical Excellence (NICE). Gastro-oesophageal reflux disease and dyspepsia in adults: investigation and management. Clinical guideline CG184. London: NICE, 2014.

38. B Examination under anaesthetic (EUA)

Perianal disease complicates Crohn's disease in 20% of cases after 10 years. The incidence varies dependent on the site of Crohn's disease, with 12% of patients with ileal disease, 15% with ileocolonic disease, 41% with colonic disease and rectal sparing, and 92% of those with colonic disease and rectal involvement being affected. The first principal of management of perianal Crohn's disease is examination of the perianal area under anaesthetic with drainage of any abscesses that are present – perianal pain nearly always indicates an abscess. This should not be delayed by performing imaging investigations first. Pelvic MRI can help assess perianal disease activity after EUA and has a 76–100% accuracy for delineating the track of fistulae. Anorectal ultrasound is highly operator dependent, but can also be useful for assessing disease activity and extent after EUA. CT and fistulography are not recommended for the investigation of fistulating Crohn's disease.

Mowat C, Cole A, Windsor A, et al. Guidelines for the management of inflammatory bowel disease in adults. Gut 2011; 60:571–607.
The Second European evidence-based consensus on the diagnosis and management of Crohn's disease: Special situations. J Crohn's Colitis 2010; 4:63–101.

39. C Meckel's diverticulum

Meckel's diverticulum is the most common congenital abnormality of the gastrointestinal tract occurring in 0.6–4.0% of people. It is caused by the failure of the omphalomesenteric duct to obliterate in infancy. It occurs in the small bowel, and is lined by ileal mucosa, with ectopic gastric mucosa within the diverticulum in up to 50% of cases. It presents with obstruction due to intussusception, ulceration, diverticulitis and perforation. Bleeding from the diverticulum can cause iron deficiency anaemia. Preoperative diagnosis is difficult but a positive [99mTc] pertechnetate scan is the most accurate diagnostic test. The tracer concentrates in ectopic gastric mucosa, hence its clinical utility. Although the other diagnoses could present with intussusception they would not cause a positive [99mTc] pertechnetate scan, and therefore the diagnosis is Meckel's diverticulum.

Sagar J, et al. Meckel's diverticulum: A systematic review. J R Soc Med 2006; 99:501–505.

40. E Sphincter of Oddi dysfunction (type 1)

Sphincter of Oddi dysfunction (SOD) is characterised by symptoms of pancreatobiliary obstruction in the absence of structural causes. Diagnosis is based on typical biliary pain lasting more than half an hour severe enough to warrant presentation to a physician or to stop daily activities, which has also occurred at least twice in the previous 12 months with no evidence of structural biliary abnormalities.

The Milwaukee criteria have been used to categorise SOD:
Type I SOD: the presence of biliary pain with an alkaline phosphatase and ALT/AST more than twice normal on at least two separate occasions, and a dilated common bile duct.
Type II SOD: biliary pain and only one or two of the criteria for SOD type 1.
Type III SOD: biliary pain and no objective criteria.

Acute acalculous cholecystitis is unlikely without the presence of elevated leukocytes and a fever. Autoimmune cholangitis is characterised by an elevated IgG level, a positive antinuclear antibody and negative anti-mitochondrial antibody. Chronic pancreatitis is unlikely to cause this pattern of elevated liver enzymes, and does not cause a dilated common bile duct in isolation. Primary sclerosing cholangitis is characterised by cholestatic abnormalities of liver function tests with multifocal strictures and segmental dilatations on cholangiopathy, which this patient does not have.

Bistritz L. Sphincter of Oddi dysfunction: Managing the patient with chronic biliary pain. World J Gastroenterol 2006; 12(24):3793–3802.

41. E D-lactic acidosis

D-lactic acidosis is a cause of confusion in patients with a short bowel and preserved colon. D-lactate is produced when colonic bacteria degrade excess fermentable carbohydrate, which is subsequently absorbed, but difficult to degrade. It should be suspected in patients with a short bowel and intact colon with a raised anion gap lactic acidosis.

Lactic acidosis secondary to gastrointestinal loss (i.e. from diarrhoea) produces a normal anion gap lactic acidosis, as do enterocutaneous fistulae. Hypomagnesaemia can cause confusion in patients with a short bowel and intact colon, but only at levels of less than 0.2. Hyperammonaemia occurs in patients with short bowel as the small amount of small bowel remaining does not produce adequate amounts of citrulline to allow detoxification of ammonia through the urea cycle. It can cause confusion, but only in patients with renal failure as the additional ammonia cannot be excreted renally. In patients with normal renal function it should not cause confusion.

J Nightingale, JM Wodward. Guidelines for management of patients with a short bowel. Gut 2006; 55(suppl IV):iv1–iv12.

42. C Gallstone ileus

Gallstone ileus is responsible for around 1–4% of small bowel obstructions (SBO), but accounts for up to 25% of non-strangulated SBO in patients aged over 65 years. It classically presents with an insidious onset over a few days, with a waxing and waning of symptoms due to the 'tumbling phenomenon' of the gallstone lodging and dislodging at various levels of the bowel. It can present with chronic or intermittent episodes of SBO. This often leads to a delay in diagnosis. The CT shows a gallstone in the small bowel, and therefore gallstone ileus is the correct diagnosis.

Gallstone ileus is treated surgically, but patients with this diagnosis may be admitted to hospital under the medical team and therefore it is an important diagnosis to be aware of. It is caused by recurrent episodes of calculous cholecystitis, resulting in inflammation and adhesions between the gallbladder wall and gastrointestinal tract, and subsequent erosion of a gallstone through the gallbladder wall into the gastrointestinal tract forming a cholecystenteric fistula, and then becoming impacted. Stones less than 2.5 cm in diameter seldom become impacted.

Nuno-Guzman CM, Marin-Contreras ME, Figueroa-Sanchez M, Corona JL. Gallstone ileus, clinical presentation, diagnostic and treatment approach. World J Gastrointest Surg 2016; 8(1):65–76.

43. A Broad spectrum antibiotics

The chest X-ray shows a pneumomediastinum, the most likely cause of which is oesophageal perforation post-endoscopy. This is a recognised complication of the procedure and occurs in an estimated 0.03% of diagnostic gastroscopies. The incidence of oesophageal perforation increases when endoscopic interventions are performed, with a risk of 0.5% in oesophageal dilatation rising up to 25% for oesophageal stent placement. The initial management of oesophageal perforation is identical to that of any other perforated viscus – intravenous fluid resuscitation, broad-spectrum intravenous antibiotics and keeping the patient nil by mouth. Opiate analgesics should be used for pain control and total parenteral nutrition should be instigated. Oesophageal perforation has a high morbidity and mortality because of the oesophagus's proximity to the mediastinum and complications of mediastinitis, empyema, sepsis and multi-organ dysfunction. The mortality rate varies from 10% to 60% dependent on when treatment is instigated. Further management can involve surgical repair or expandable polymesh stent placement.

Kaman L, et al. Management of esophageal perforation in adults. Gastroenterol Res 2010; 3(6):235–244.

44. E Zieve's syndrome

This patient has the classic features of Zieve's syndrome, an acute haemolytic anaemia that manifests with jaundice, haemolysis, hyperlipidaemia and abdominal pain in patients with excess alcohol consumption. It has a good prognosis and is treated conservatively, with cessation of alcohol intake being the most important management step. There is rarely a need for blood transfusion.

The other answers given can all cause jaundice but present very differently.

Caroli's disease is a congenital malformation of the biliary tree that causes segmental saccular dilatation of the biliary tree. It causes a non-obstructive jaundice and presents with recurrent ascending cholangitis.

Crigler–Najjar syndrome and Gilbert's syndrome are congenital disorders due to a reduction in the enzyme uridine diphosphate glycosyltransferase (UGT). Crigler–Najjar syndrome is an autosomal recessive disorder, in which there is a complete absence of the UGT enzyme (type 1) or a markedly reduced level (type 2). This results in a severe unconjugated hyperbilirubinaemia. It presents soon after birth with persistent jaundice. Type 1 is always fatal before the age of 2 years due to kernicterus. Type 2 is less severe and can be treated with phenobarbital. Gilbert's syndrome is a mild illness and is much more common. It is due to reduced activity of the UGT enzyme and results in a mild unconjugated hyperbilirubinaemia which is commonly precipitated by stress, such as viral infections. It presents with normal liver function tests and no haemolysis.

Mirizzi's syndrome occurs when gallstones become impacted in the cystic duct or Hartmann's pouch and cause external compression of the common hepatic duct. This may present with abdominal pain and obstructive jaundice but the ultrasound scan classically shows a contracted gallbladder with dilated intra- and common hepatic ducts and a normal calibre common bile duct.

Shukla S, Sitrin M. Hemolyis in acute alcoholic hepatitis: Zieve's syndrome. ACG Case Rep J 2015; 2(4):250–251.
Gitlin N. Zieve syndrome and porphyrinuria in an alcoholic. BMJ 1969; 1:96–98.
Pemberton M, Wells AD. The Mirizzi syndrome. Postgrad Med J 1997; 73:487–490.

45. A Argon photocoagulation

The endoscopic appearances shown in **Figure 4.7** are of gastric angiodysplasia. This is most commonly seen in gastric antral vascular ectasia (GAVE), also referred to as watermelon stomach (due to the appearance of columns of tortuous ectatic vessels following the longitudinal gastric folds, radiating from the pylorus, which resemble the stripes on a watermelon). It is the cause of bleeding in 4% of patients presenting with upper gastrointestinal haemorrhage. The most common presentation of GAVE is chronic gastrointestinal blood loss, usually presenting with iron deficiency anaemia.

GAVE is usually associated with chronic medical conditions, with the most common being sclerodactyly (60% of patients), cirrhosis (30% of patients), autoimmune connective tissue disorders and Raynaud's disease. Other conditions in which it has been described include scleroderma, bone marrow transplantation, chronic renal failure and cardiac disease.

First-line treatment is ablation of the vascular lesions with argon photo-coagulation (APC). APC has been shown to have a 90–100% efficacy in reducing the need for further blood transfusions. Beta blockers have been investigated as a treatment due to the association of GAVE with cirrhosis, but no significant benefit has been reported. Corticosteroids were used in the treatment of GAVE based on a small case report however, systemic side effects limit their use. There is one case report showing effective treatment of GAVE with endoscopic variceal band ligation but this is not enough evidence to change practice. Antrectomy was the definitive treatment of choice prior to endoscopic therapy, but it has a high reported mortality rate of 50% in patients with cirrhosis.

Fuccio L, Mussetto A, Laterza L, Eusebi LH, Bazzoli F. Diagnosis and management of gastric antral vascular ectasia. World J Gastrointest Endos 2013; 5:6–13.
Selinger CP, Ang YS. Gastric antral vascular ectasia (GAVE): An update on clinical presentation, pathophysiology and treatment. Digestion 2008; 77:131–137.

Chapter 5

Haematology and immunology

Questions

1. A 23-year-old woman was referred by her general practitioner with a short history of easy bruising, bleeding gums and menorrhagia. She had no past medical history and was taking no medication.

   On examination, there were numerous bruises, especially over her arms and legs. The rest of the examination was normal.

   Investigations:

haemoglobin 105 g/L (115–165)	international normalised ratio 1.0 (<1.4)
mean corpuscular volume 89 fL (80–96)	activated partial thromboplastin time 28 s (30–40)
white blood cell 5 × 10⁹/L (4–11)	
platelets 35 × 10⁹/L (150–400)	

   Peripheral blood film (see **Figure 5.1**)

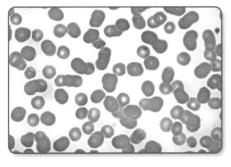

Figure 5.1 *See colour plate section.*

What is the most likely diagnosis?

A   Aplastic anaemia
B   Fanconi's anaemia
C   Paroxysmal nocturnal haemoglobinuria
D   Primary immune thrombocytopenia (idiopathic thrombocytopenic purpura)
E   Thrombotic thrombocytopenic purpura

2. A 24-year-old woman from Rwanda presented with a productive cough, weight loss and fever for the last 1 month. Other than a 6-month history of persistent diarrhoea she had no past medical history and took no regular medications.
      On examination, she had a body mass index of 17 kg/m², but was otherwise well. Examination of her chest revealed right upper zone inspiratory crackles.

Investigations:

haemoglobin 114 g/L (115–165)	IgA 2.9 g/L (0.8–3.0)
white cell count 2.1 × 10⁹/L (4–11)	IgG 8.3 g/L (6.0–13.0)
neutrophils 1.9 × 10⁹/L (1.5–7.0)	IgM 1.1 g/L (0.4–2.5)
platelets 459 × 10⁹/L (150–400)	

Chest X-ray: (see **Figure 5.2**)

Sputum: 1+ acid-fast bacilli seen

ELISpot: negative

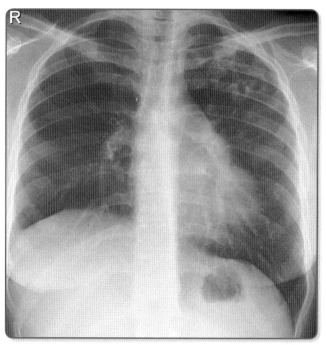

Figure 5.2

What is the most likely explanation for these results?

A   Acquired immunodeficiency
B   Common variable immunodeficiency
C   Non-tuberculous mycobacterial infection
D   Severe combined immunodeficiency
E   Surreptitious steroid use

3. A 45-year-old man presented with fever, right upper quadrant pain and deranged liver function tests (LFTs). Radiography and subsequent endoscopic retrograde cholangiopancreatography and biopsy suggested primary sclerosing cholangitis with pancreatitis. Despite steroids his LFTs continued to deteriorate and on biopsy he was found to have an autoimmune hepatitis.

   With increased immunosuppression his LFTs stabilised but he then developed renal impairment. Further imaging revealed marked retroperitoneal fibrosis.

   Investigations:

haemoglobin 98 g/L (130–180)	IgA 0.9 g/L (0.8–3.0)
white cell count 6.8 × 10⁹/L (4–11)	IgG 33.9 g/L (6.0–13.0)
neutrophils 4.6 × 10⁹/L (1.5–7.0)	IgM 2.5 g/L (0.4–2.5)
platelets 587 × 10⁹/L (150–400)	

   Antinuclear antibody negative: antineutrophil cytoplasmic antibody weakly positive perinuclear pattern

   What is the most likely diagnosis?

   A   IgA deficiency
   B   Wegener's granulomatosis
   C   Polyarteritis nodosa
   D   Hyper-IgG4 disease
   E   Sarcoidosis

4. A 22-year-old Turkish woman was admitted to hospital with pneumonia. She reported no past medical history of note and was taking no regular medications.

   Clinical examination was consistent with lobar pneumonia.

   As part of her work-up she had routine blood tests:

   Investigations:

haemoglobin 101 g/L (115–165)	red cell count 6.7 × 10¹²/µL (4.6–6.0)
mean corpuscular volume 63 fL (80–96)	HbA₂ 5.3% (1.5–3.5)
mean corpuscular haemoglobin 18.7 pg (28–32)	

   Chest X–ray: mass lesion in right mid–zone

   What is the most likely diagnosis?

   A   Alpha (α)-thalassaemia trait
   B   Beta (β)-thalassaemia trait
   C   Delta beta (dβ)-thalassaemia
   D   Thalassaemia intermedia
   E   Haemoglobin H disease

5. A 24-year-old man, originally from Ghana, developed jaundice within 48 hours of admission to hospital for treatment of pneumonia. He had no past medical history of note except for diet-controlled type 2 diabetes. He had been treated with intravenous co-amoxiclav, fluids and oxygen.

   General examination revealed conjunctival pallor and mild icterus. He was apyrexial and haemodynamically stable. Respiratory examination revealed reduced air entry and crepitations at the right lung base. There were no signs of chronic liver disease and abdominal examination was normal.

Investigations:

haemoglobin 78 g/L (130–180)	albumin 32 g/L (37–49)
mean corpuscular volume 78 fL (80–96)	protein 72 g/L (60–76)
white cell count 12 × 10⁹/L (4–11)	alkaline phosphatase 105 U/L (45–105)
platelets 236 × 10⁹/L (150–400)	alanine transaminase 36 U/L (5–35)
international normalised ratio 1.0 (<1.4)	bilirubin 54 mmol/L (1–22)

Direct agglutination test: negative

Urine: haemoglobin +
Peripheral blood film (see **Figure 5.3**)

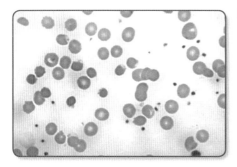

Figure 5.3 *See colour plate section.*

What is the most likely diagnosis?

A   Autoimmune haemolytic anaemia
B   Glucose-6-phosphate dehydrogenase deficiency
C   Microangiopathic haemolytic anaemia
D   Penicillin-induced haemolytic anaemia
E   Pyruvate kinase deficiency

6.   A 23-year-old man presented with a solitary cervical lymph node and progressive shortness of breath on exertion. He also described diffuse pruritus without a rash.

Investigations:

haemoglobin 104 g/L (130–180)	ESR 83 mm/h (0–16)
white cell count 11.3 x 10⁹ /L (4–11)	
neutrophils 7.1 x 10⁹/L (1.5–7.0)	
platelets 331 x 10⁹/L (150–400)	
bilirubin 20 mmol/L (1–22)	
albumin 24 g/L (37–49)	

What is the most likely diagnosis?

A   Glandular fever
B   Hodgkin's lymphoma
C   Cutaneous T cell lymphoma
D   Allergic reaction
E   Non-Hodgkin's lymphoma

7. A 16-year-old boy presented with recurrent boils, furuncles and episodes of cellulitis for many years. Several of these had been incised and drained and had grown *Staphylococcus aureus*. He had been seen by the infectious diseases team who had referred him to immunology for a further opinion.

   Investigations:

haemoglobin 144 g/L (130–180)	alanine transaminase 21 U/L (5–35)
white cell count 7.8 x 10⁹ /L (4–11)	alkaline phosphatase 79 U/L (45–105)
neutrophils 5.9 x 10⁹/L (1.5–7.0)	IgA 2.5 g/L (0.8–3.0)
platelets 241 x 10⁹/L (150–400)	IgG 9.3 g/L (6.0–13.0)
bilirubin 7 mmol/L (1–22)	IgM 2.1 g/L (0.4–2.5)
albumin 39 g/L (37–49)	

   Staphylococcus aureus toxin testing: Panton–Valentine leukocidin negative

   Neutrophil stain: fails to stain with nitroblue–tetrazolium dye

   What is the most likely cause of his immunodeficiency?

   A   Chronic granulomatous disease
   B   Familial Mediterranean fever
   C   IgA deficiency
   D   Myeloperoxidase deficiency
   E   Nephrotic syndrome

8. A 59-year-old woman presented with several months' history of increasing abdominal discomfort, indigestion, weight loss, bone pain and night sweats. She had lost 7 kg over the past 3 months. She had no previous medical history and had not travelled abroad in the past 10 years.
   On examination, she had massive hepatosplenomegaly. Respiratory, cardiovascular and neurological examinations were normal.

   Investigations:

haemoglobin 104 g/L (115–165)	platelets 408 × 10⁹/L (150–400)
white cell count 25 × 10⁹/L (4–11)	haematocrit 48.2% (38–50)

   Blood film: leukoerythroblastic with 'tear-drop' poikilocytes

   Trephine biopsy: hypercellular bone marrow

   Cytogenetic analysis: positive for *JAK2 V617F* mutation

   What is the most likely diagnosis?

   A   Chronic myeloid leukaemia
   B   Hodgkin's lymphoma
   C   Myelofibrosis
   D   Polycythaemia rubra vera
   E   Systemic mastocytosis

9. A 40-year-old woman presented to the emergency department with confusion and difficulty understanding. According to her partner she had been feeling unwell with fever for the past 2 days. She had a past medical history of systemic lupus erythematosus, and was taking hydroxychloroquine.

On examination, the patient was drowsy with a Glasgow Coma Scale score of 14/15 and a temperature of 37.7°C. She was pale and had numerous petechiae. Neurological examination revealed a receptive aphasia, but no other focal signs. The rest of her examination was normal.

Investigations:

haemoglobin 88 g/L (115–165)	bilirubin 67 mmol/L (1–22)
mean corpuscular volume 81 fL (80–96)	albumin 36 g/L (37–49)
white cell count 5 × 10⁹/L (4–11)	alkaline phosphatase 114 U/L (45–105)
platelets 37 × 10⁹/L (150–400)	alanine transaminase 29 U/L (5–35)
sodium 135 mmol/L (135–145)	international normalised ratio 1.1 (<1.4)
potassium 4.8 mmol/L (3.5–5.0)	activated partial thromboplastin time 30 s (30–40)
urea 11.2 mmol/L (2.5–7.5)	fibrinogen 2.5 g/L (1.8–5.4)
creatinine 176 µmol/L (45–90)	lactate dehydrogenase 753 U/L (10–250)
protein 73 g/L (60–70)	

Direct antiglobulin test: negative

Anticardiolipin and β2GP1 antibodies: negative

Lupus anticoagulant: negative

Peripheral blood film: indicative of microangiopathic haemolytic anaemia

What is the most likely diagnosis?

A   Catastrophic antiphospholipid syndrome (CAPS)
B   Disseminated intravascular coagulation (DIC)
C   Immune thrombocytopenia purpura (ITP)
D   Haemolytic uraemic syndrome (HUS)
E   Thrombotic thrombocytopenia purpura (TTP)

10. A 20-year-old male student was referred for investigation after failing to achieve a protective hepatitis B surface antibody after two vaccination courses and two booster vaccinations. He was known to have asthma, eczema and coeliac disease. For his asthma he took salbutamol and Seretide inhalers and had required two courses of oral prednisolone last year. He used daily topical emollients with six courses of topical steroids this year. He was not very compliant with his gluten-free diet.

Investigations:

haemoglobin 148 g/L (130–180)	IgA 1.5 g/L (0.8–3.0)
white cell count 8.9 × 10⁹/L (4–11)	IgG 7.3 g/L (6.0–13.0)
neutrophils 5.4 × 10⁹/L (1.5–7.0)	IgM 3.1 g/L (0.4–2.5)
eosinophils 0.4 × 10⁹/L (0.04–0.4)	IgE 188 kU/L (<120)
platelets 148 × 10⁹/L (150–400)	

Hepatitis BsAg – negative
Hepatitis BcAb – negative
Hepatitis BsAb <10 IU

What is the most likely explanation for vaccine non-response?

A   Atopic phenotype
B   Coeliac disease

C   Inhaled steroid use
D   Systemic steroid use
E   Topical steroid use

11. A 19-year-old man presented to the emergency department with a swollen, painful knee after a fall at work. Ultrasound of the knee raised suspicion of a haemarthrosis and on further questioning he reported nosebleeds, bleeding gums and spontaneous bruising. His mother has required blood transfusions for menorrhagia and has been told in the past that she has a type of haemophilia.

Investigations:

haemoglobin 114 g/L (130–180)	prothrombin time 12.1 s (10.9–13.2)
white blood cell 6.3 × 10⁹/L (4–11)	activated partial thromboplastin time 74.2 s (27.4–32.0)
neutrophils 3.7 × 10⁹/L (1.5–4.0)	fibrinogen 2.5 g/L (1.9–4.0)
platelets 301 × 10⁹/L (1.5–4.0)	factor VIII:C 11 iu/dL (50–150)

Hepatitis BsAg – negative
Hepatitis BcAb – negative
Hepatitis BsAb <10 IU

What is the most likely diagnosis?

A   Haemophilia A
B   Haemophilia B
C   Haemophilia C
D   Von Willebrand's disease
E   Dysfibrinogenaemia

12. A 54-year-old man attended the heart transplant clinic for routine review. He had a transplant 10 years previously. His medications include ciclosporin, azathioprine and a low dose of steroids.

Which of the following statements is correct regarding his immunosuppression medication?

A   Azathioprine acts on B cells
B   Ciclosporin acts on B cells
C   Ciclosporin can cause microangiopathy
D   Ciclosporin levels do not require to be monitored
E   Gingival hyperplasia is a common side effect of azathioprine

13. A 54-year-old man presented with a 5-month history of fatigue and abdominal discomfort. On examination, there was hepatosplenomegaly, but no significant lymphadenopathy. Numerous bruises were also noted.

Investigations:

haemoglobin 87 g/L (130–180)	neutrophils 1.0 × 10⁹/L (1.5–7.0)
white blood cell 2 × 10⁹/L (4–11)	platelets 89 × 10⁹/L (150–400)
lymphocytes 1.0 × 10⁹/L (1.5–4.0)	

Trephine bone marrow biopsy: fibrosis

Peripheral blood film (see **Figure 5.4**): the abnormal cells contain a BRAF V600E mutation on polymerase chain reaction

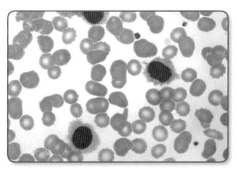

Figure 5.4 *See colour plate section.*

What is the most likely diagnosis?

A   Aplastic anaemia
B   Chronic lymphocytic leukaemia
C   Hairy cell leukaemia
D   Myelofibrosis
E   Plasma cell leukaemia

14. A 23-year-old woman was referred by her general practitioner with refractory anaemia. Her only symptom was fatigue. She had no significant past medical history and was not taking any medications, although she was previously prescribed iron sulphate tablets for 2 months without benefit. She was a personal fitness instructor, and did not smoke or drink alcohol.
     The clinical examination was normal, except for mild angular cheilitis and conjunctival pallor.

Investigations:

haemoglobin 99 g/L (115–165)	international normalised ratio 1.0 (< 1.4)
mean corpuscular volume 74 fL (80–96)	ferritin 7 g/L (15–300)
white cell count 3.5 × 10⁹/L (4–11)	vitamin B12 200 ng/L (160–760)
platelets 267 × 10⁹/L (150–400)	folate 7 ng/mL (2.0–11.0)
Peripheral blood film: see **Figure 5.5**	

What is the most likely diagnosis?

A   Anaemia of chronic disease
B   Aplastic anaemia
C   Iron-deficiency anaemia

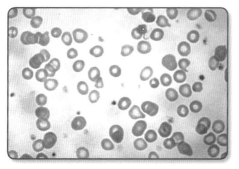

Figure 5.5 *See colour plate section.*

    D   Microangiopathic haemolytic anaemia (MAHA)
    E   Pernicious anaemia

15. A 28-year-old woman was referred to the allergy clinic complaining of a 2-year history of sneezing and itching of the nose and palate. She gained some symptomatic relief from taking chlorpheniramine at night. She reported that she had experienced similar symptoms when she visited a friend who kept cats. She did not keep pets or have regular contact with any animals. Her brother had asthma.

What is the most appropriate investigation?

    A   Cat-specific IgE serum
    B   CT of the sinuses
    C   Nasoendoscopy
    D   Peak flow diary monitoring
    E   Skin-prick testing for common aeroallergens

16. A 26-year-old woman was admitted to the emergency department with facial swelling and difficulty in breathing. She was well until 2 hours previously when she had felt some tingling in her lips and tongue. She had a similar episode a year ago for which no cause was found. She also described recurrent episodes of abdominal pain as a teenager, requiring admission but with negative investigations. She was taking no medications.
        On examination, her lips and tongue were swollen and there was some periorbital oedema.

Which one of the following is least likely regarding her diagnosis?

    A   Danazol can be given to prevent attacks
    B   Fresh frozen plasma can be given in an emergency
    C   It can be triggered by angiotensin-converting enzyme inhibitors
    D   It is highly responsive to antihistamines
    E   Oestrogen should be avoided where possible

17. An 18-year-old man presented to his general practitioner with sinusitis. He gave a history of a previous episode of sinusitis in the last year and two childhood episodes of ear infections. He was otherwise well, took no regular medication and did not require hospital treatment for any of his previous infections.

Investigations:

haemoglobin 115 g/L (130–180)	IgG 14 g/L (6.0–13.0)
white cell count 12.1 × 10⁹/L (4–11)	IgM 1.9 g/L (0.4–2.5)
IgA <0.05 g/L (0.8–3.0)	

Which one of the following is not associated with this condition?

    A   Anaphylaxis to blood products
    B   Coeliac disease
    C   Poor response to pneumococcal polysaccharide vaccines
    D   Severe life-threatening infection with encapsulated bacteria in infancy
    E   Systemic lupus erythematosus

18. A 29-year-old woman presented with several months' history of increasing fatigue and easy bruising. On examination, she appeared pale with numerous small bruises. The rest of her examination was normal.

Investigations:

haemoglobin 85 g/L (115–165)	white cell count 23 × 10⁹/L (4–11)
mean corpuscular volume 84 fL (80–96)	platelets 8 × 10⁹/L (150–400)

haemoglobin 85 g/L (115–165)

mean corpuscular volume 84 fL (80–96)

white cell count 23×10^9/L (4–11)

platelets 8×10^9/L (150–400)

Peripheral blood film: see **Figure 5.6**

What is the most likely diagnosis?

A   Acute lymphoblastic leukaemia
B   Acute myeloid leukaemia
C   Chronic lymphocytic leukaemia
D   Chronic myeloid leukaemia
E   Hairy cell leukaemia

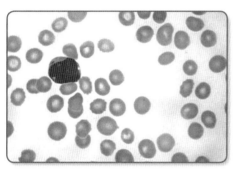

Figure 5.6 *See colour plate section.*

19. A 19-year-old dental student presented with intermittent episodes of sneezing, chest tightness and shortness of breath. On direct questioning, she reported occasional itchy rashes on her hands. The symptoms had begun after she commenced her first clinical attachment and she was worried that she would not be able to continue her studies. She had no previous history of allergies or atopy and was not taking any medications.

What is the most useful diagnostic investigation?

A   Peak flow monitoring diary
B   Sensitivity testing for common aeroallergens
C   Serum total IgE
D   Skin-prick testing for latex
E   Spirometry with bronchodilator reversibility testing

20. A 20-year-old male university student was admitted with meningitis. Prompt diagnosis and antimicrobial therapy led to a full recovery and following discharge the patient was referred to the immunology clinic.

On further questioning, he reported a history of recurrent ear, nose and throat infections throughout childhood. He confirmed that he received a meningococcal C vaccine 3 years ago prior to commencing university.

Investigations:

haemoglobin 139 g/L (130–180)	platelets 179 × 10⁹/L (150–400)
white cell count 7.8 × 10⁹/L (4–11)	IgA 0.8 g/L (0.8–3.0)
neutrophils 5.4 × 10⁹/L (1.5–7.0)	IgG 1.1 g/L (6.0–13.0)
lymphocytes 2.1 × 10⁹/L (1.5–4.0)	IgM 0.4 g/L (0.4–2.5)

HIV antibody test: negative

Reference laboratory typing of meningococcus from cerebrospinal fluid: meningococcus C

What is the most likely diagnosis?

A   Common variable immunodeficiency
B   Human immunodeficiency virus
C   Hyposplenism
D   Severe combined immunodeficiency
E   Surreptitious steroid use

21. A 23-year-old medical student presented to hospital with a 1-day history of fever and rigors. He also had headache and malaise but no neck stiffness or rash. Five days ago he returned from a 6-week elective in Thailand. He had no past medical history, and had been taking prophylactic doxycycline until a few days before his return.

On examination, the patient appeared unwell with a temperature of 38.5°C, pulse 100 beats per minute and blood pressure 90/50 mmHg.

Investigations:

haemoglobin 102 g/L (130–180)	white cell count 7 × 10⁹/L (4–11)
mean corpuscular volume 86 fL (80–96)	platelets 40 × 10⁹/L (150–400)

Peripheral blood film: see **Figure 5.7**

What is the most likely diagnosis?

A   Dengue fever
B   Dracunculiasis
C   Japanese encephalitis
D   *Plasmodium falciparum* malaria
E   Trypanosomiasis

Figure 5.7 *See colour plate section.*

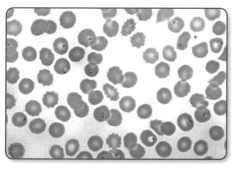

22. A 58-year-old man was admitted with purulent cough, pleuritic chest pain and a fever. A left lower lobe pneumonia was diagnosed on chest X-ray. He also had evidence of oral candida infection. He had a similar admission 4 months ago with pneumonia. There was a history of recurrent sinusitis and he had had two urinary tract infections in the last year. He was a non-smoker.

    In view of his recurrent pneumonia and abnormal chest X-ray he went on to have a chest CT which confirmed left lower lobe consolidation and also showed an anterior mediastinal mass.

    Investigations:

haemoglobin 87 g/L (130–180)	IgA 0.5 g/L (0.8–3.0)
white cell count 4.0×10^9/L (4–11)	IgG 3 g/L (6.0–13.0)
platelets 90×10^9/L (150–400)	IgM 0.2 g/L (0.4–2.5)
Human immunodeficiency virus: negative	

    What is the most likely diagnosis?

    A   Chronic granulomatous disease (CGD)
    B   Common variable immunodeficiency (CVID)
    C   Good's syndrome
    D   Wiskott–Aldrich syndrome
    E   X-linked agammaglobulinaemia (XLA)

23. A 68-year-old man with a history of severe chronic obstructive pulmonary disease (COPD) was referred to the allergy clinic by a respiratory specialist nurse. She recommended that he should receive the influenza vaccine; however, he was concerned that he may be allergic to eggs and wanted more advice. He reported that he had several episodes of lip swelling after ingesting eggs as a child. However, he admitted that he would often eat cakes containing eggs and recently ate a chocolate mousse containing raw egg white with no adverse effects.

    Investigations:

    Skin-prick testing was performed in the clinic:
    testing control 3 mm
    testing egg white 3 mm (<8 mm)

    What is the most appropriate management step?

    A   Avoid influenza vaccine
    B   Perform oral challenge test to egg white
    C   Perform specific egg-white IgE serum assay
    D   Recommend influenza vaccine
    E   Recommend *Echinacea*

24. A 30-year-old man with sickle cell disease (Hb SS) presented with shortness of breath, O_2 saturation 84% on air and a chest X-ray demonstrating diffuse pulmonary infiltrates. He was diagnosed with an acute chest syndrome.

    Which of the following is not true of the acute chest syndrome?

    A   The mortality without prompt treatment is 30%
    B   An urgent red cell exchange is required
    C   Broad spectrum antibiotics should be given
    D   High dependency monitoring is required
    E   Diuretics can improve oxygenation

25. A 43-year-old woman returned for follow-up in the rheumatology clinic. She had a diagnosis of severe rheumatoid arthritis and had been receiving methotrexate and rituximab. She was concerned because she visited a friend the day previously who had shingles. The patient could not remember if she ever had chickenpox as a child and did not think she had had shingles before.

What is the most appropriate next step in management?

A   Give oral aciclovir
B   Give intravenous ganciclovir
C   Give varicella-zoster IgG
D   Review in 1 week for signs of infection
E   Urgently test varicella-zoster IgG titre

26. A 53-year-old man was referred by his general practitioner with persistently raised white blood cell count. His only complaint was of several months' history of fatigue. There was no past medical history of note.
    On examination, he had some conjunctival pallor and moderate splenomegaly.

Investigations:

haemoglobin 107 g/L (130–180)	white cell count 63 × 10⁹/L (4–11)
mean corpuscular volume 87 fL (80–96)	platelets 512 × 10⁹/L (150–400)

Peripheral blood film: see **Figure 5.8**
Bone marrow: hypercellular with predominant granulopoiesis

Quantitative polymerase chain reaction for BCR-ABL: positive

What is the most likely diagnosis

A   Acute lymphoblastic leukaemia
B   Acute myeloid leukaemia
C   Chronic lymphocytic leukaemia
D   Chronic myeloid leukaemia
E   Hairy cell leukaemia

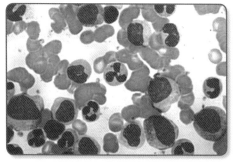

Figure 5.8 *See colour plate section.*

Answers

1.   D Primary immune thrombocytopenia

Idiopathic thrombocytopenic purpura (ITP), or immune-mediated thrombocytopenic purpura, is a common condition with incidence peaks in children and elderly patients.

In the majority of patients ITP is acute (considered chronic when >12 months) and diagnosed incidentally or after investigation of minor bleeding. Primary ITP is a diagnosis of exclusion. Malignancy and autoimmune disorders require exclusion. Major bleeding is rare, but nosebleeds and petechial haemorrhage are common. Splenomegaly, lymphadenopathy, swollen joints, or non-petechial rash suggest a secondary ITP. Blood film examination is essential but bone marrow biopsy is rarely required for diagnosis.

Management depends on the patient's age and the severity of the thrombocytopenia. In children ITP is usually managed conservatively (no treatment), even with extremely low platelet counts. In young adults, it can be managed conservatively if the platelet count is >20 x 10^9/L. If treatment is indicated, the first-line choice is glucocorticoids, intravenous immunoglobulin (IVIg) or both. Platelet transfusion should be avoided as this rarely results in a significant rise in the platelet count; if platelet transfusion is required, IVIg should be given first.

Thrombotic thrombocytopenic purpura is a microangiopathic haemolytic anaemia and is discussed in more detail in the answer to Question 9 of this chapter. Aplastic anaemia is characterised by cytopenias affecting more than one lineage, and can therefore be discounted. Fanconi's anaemia is a rare autosomal recessive disorder that presents in childhood and is a cause of aplastic anaemia. Affected individuals are often born with congenital abnormalities. Paroxysmal nocturnal haemoglobinuria is a rare haematological disorder causing intravascular haemolysis, pancytopenia and thrombosis.

2.   A Acquired immunodeficiency

This woman has the clinical, radiographic and microbiological indicators of pulmonary tuberculosis (TB) and has a likely underlying immunodeficiency. The negative interferon-γ release assay (in this example the ELISpot test) is providing a false-negative result in the immunodeficient state. An interferon-γ release assay (IGRA) allows visualisation of the secretory product of individual activated T cells (i.e. those sensitised to tuberculosis from previous exposure) in a semi-quantitative manner. It does not give rise to false-positive results in those who have received the BCG vaccine, unlike the Mantoux test (the specific epitopes used in the IGRA are present only in *Mycobacterium tuberculosis* and not in the BCG strain of *M. bovis* used in vaccination). False negative results can occur in active tuberculosis (TB), particularly in miliary TB and TB meningitis and in those with immunodeficiency due to a relative absence of circulating lymphocytes from which the IGRA can detect a response.

Severe combined immunodeficiency is rapidly fatal in childhood without intervention. The normal/mildly raised immunoglobulins and the epidemiological history point away from common variable immunodeficiency which is often characterised by hypogammaglobulinaemia. The story is not consistent with surreptitious steroid use. This patient does not have a history consistent with non-tuberculous mycobacteria.

Chin KL, Anis FZ, Sarmiento ME, et al. Role of interferons in the development of diagnostics, vaccines, and therapy for tuberculosis. J Immunol Res 2017;2017:5212910.

3.   D Hyper-IgG4 disease

This man is presenting with a multisystem disorder and a hypergammaglobulinaemia typical of hyper-IgG4 disease. This is a systemic disease characterised by multi-organ infiltration of IgG4-positive plasma cells and T lymphocytes. Elevated serum IG4 levels and immunostaining of pathological specimens with anti-IgG4 antibody are diagnostic. Serum IgG4 levels may be normal when the disease is inactive. The disease occurs predominantly in older men, and can cause inflammatory syndromes in the pancreas, biliary tree and retroperitoneum. Kidneys, lungs and prostate may be involved. Most cases of hyper-IgG4 diseases have been found to be associated with autoimmune pancreatitis. The disease usually responds well to steroid therapy, but refractory or relapsed cases can be managed with rituximab or cyclophosphamide.

There is a relatively low IgA level in this case but the clinical picture does not fit with IgA deficiency. This disease is usually asymptomatic but can have a history of increased frequency of mucous membrane infections. Polyarteritis nodosa is a medium-vessel vasculitis that can cause multi-system inflammatory change and is associated with pANCA (perinuclear anti-neutrophil cytoplasmic antibody); however, the pancreatitis, hepatitis and retroperitoneal fibrosis in this man fit more with hyper-IgG4 disease. Wegener's granulomatosis, a multisystem vasculitis is typically associated with pulmonary and renal involvement, has a cANCA (cytoplasmic ANCA) pattern. Sarcoidosis is a multi-system granulomatous condition associated with pancreatitis, hepatitis, cholangitis, retroperitoneal fibrosis and neurological symptoms which presents with mildly elevated IgG levels.

Kamisawa T, Okamoto A. IgG4-related sclerosing disease. World J Gastroenterol 2008; 14(25):3948–3955.

4. B Beta (β)-thalassaemia trait

Prior to this admission, this patient was asymptomatic. She has mild anaemia, very low mean corpuscular volume and mean corpuscular haemoglobin, and elevated red blood cell count which could be in keeping with a thalassaemia trait. The differential diagnosis is usually iron deficiency and normal iron studies are essential in diagnosing thalassaemia. Haemoglobin electrophoresis and blood film examination are required for diagnosis. Haemoglobin electrophoresis is very sensitive for detecting abnormalities of the β-chain, but not of the α-chain. Here, the haemoglobin electrophoresis reveals a moderately raised HbA_2 ($\alpha 2\delta 2$) level (>3.5%) which is sufficient to make a diagnosis of β-thalassaemia trait.

α-halassaemia traits are also associated with microcytic red cells, and low mean corpuscular haemoglobin. However, anaemia, if present, is very mild. Haemoglobin electrophoresis is normal. Genetic analysis is only indicated when the red cell indices do not suggest the diagnosis or when a female patient is pregnant and her partner is also affected.

β-Thalassaemia is divided clinically into β-thalassaemia trait where patients rarely need transfusion support, β-thalassaemia intermedia where transfusion support is needed intermittently and β-thalassaemia major where continuous transfusion support is required. As this patient has been previously well, she cannot have β-thalassaemia intermedia or major.

In β-thalassaemia intermedia and major, complications include extramedullary haemopoiesis, particularly in the liver and spleen, bony deformities, cardiac hypertrophy and iron overload from transfusions. Long-term management of these patients should be at a haemoglobinopathy centre in order to screen for these long-term conditions.

Homozygous δβ-thalassaemia is extremely rare and results in 100% fetal haemoglobin HbF ($\alpha 2\gamma 2$), due to the inability to synthesise the δ and β chains necessary for formation of HbA_2 and HbA, respectively. Anaemia is not a feature.

Haemoglobin H disease is associated with a deletion of three α-globin genes. This is associated with anaemia, microcytosis and anisopoikilocytosis on the blood film but these patients have a normal haemoglobin electrophoresis.

Hoffbrand V, Moss P, Pettit J. Genetic disorders of haemoglobin (Chapter 7). In: Essential Haematology, 7th edn. Oxford: Blackwell Publishing, 2015.
Chung SW, et al. Human embryonic zeta globin chains in adult patients with alpha thalassaemias. Proc Natl Acad Sci USA 1984; 81:6188–6191.

5. B Glucose-6-phosphate dehydrogenase deficiency

This patient, with glucose-6-phosphate dehydrogenase (G6PD) enzyme deficiency, is suffering from an acute haemolytic episode secondary to infection.

Many genetic variants of G6PD have been described, with variable levels of red cell susceptibility to oxidative stress. The two most common genetic variants have been linked to resistance to infection with *Plasmodium falciparum* and *Plasmodium vivax*.

In the absence of significant oxidant stress, patients with G6PD deficiency are usually asymptomatic. Recognised precipitants of acute haemolytic episodes include drugs (nitrofurantoin, primaquine, dapsone and others), fava beans and infection.

With G6PD deficiency, in a crisis, the patient experiences vigorous intravascular haemolysis with jaundice and haemoglobinuria. Blood tests reveal anaemia, raised bilirubin (unconjugated) and decreased levels of haptoglobin. The direct agglutination test is negative, and the coagulation profile is usually normal. Diagnosis is usually made through blood film examination with 'bite' cells and 'blister' cells. A rapid screen can be used in a well patient but this is often falsely normal in an acute crisis. Direct assays of enzyme levels are more labour intensive but can be used during an acute crisis. Treatment is supportive and by stopping precipitant medications. Transfusion may be indicated in severe anaemia.

Autoimmune haemolytic anaemias may occur in different contexts, but are associated with a positive direct antiglobulin test.

Penicillin-induced haemolytic anaemias result from the generation of antibody to a penicillin-red cell membrane complex. The anaemia resolves with cessation of treatment.

Microangiopathic haemolytic anaemia is discussed in another question. Pyruvate kinase (PK) deficiency is autosomal recessive and associated with variable levels of anaemia. Jaundice is commonplace and many patients also suffer from gallstones. Peripheral blood film tends to show poikilocytes. The diagnosis may be confirmed by enzyme assay. PK deficiency does not cause haemoglobinuria as the haemolysis is extravascular.

Hoffbrand V, Moss P, Pettit J. Haemolytic anaemias (Chapter 6) In: Essential Haematology, 7th edn. Oxford: Blackwell Publishing, 2015.
Wan GH, et al. Decreased blood activity of glucose-6-phosphate dehydrogenase associates with increased risk for diabetes mellitus. Endocrine 2002; 19:191–195.

6. B Hodgkin's lymphoma

Hodgkin's lymphoma is the most common type of malignancy diagnosed in patients aged 15–24 years. The clinical presentation is often a painless enlarged lymph node without obvious infective symptoms. Patients may suffer from pruritis, night sweats, weight loss or symptomatic anaemia but are often asymptomatic. A raised erythrocyte sedimentation rate (ESR) and low haemoglobin are strongly suggestive of Hodgkin's lymphoma.

Long-term survival from Hodgkin's lymphoma in young patients is excellent with chemo-radiotherapy. A histological diagnosis (lymph node biopsy) is essential. Bone marrow biopsy is not routinely required.

Across all groups, long-term survival for Hodgkin's lymphoma is approaching 95%, although it is becoming clear that late-stage toxicity from the chemotherapy is an emerging problem. Bleomycin is associated with a higher incidence of lung fibrosis and cardiac failure. Radiotherapy treatment increases rates of cardiovascular disease, breast and lung cancer.

This patient does not report viral symptoms, and the raised ESR and low albumin make glandular fever an unlikely diagnosis. Cutaneous T cell lymphoma and non-Hodgkin's lymphoma could account for the clinical picture but are significantly less likely than Hodgkin's lymphoma in this patient age group.

7. A Chronic granulomatous disease

This man is presenting with recurrent bacterial infections. A neutrophil functional disorder is most likely. These are a diverse group of inherited diseases in which neutrophils have a disorder of phagocytosis or deficiency in the respiratory burst. Patients with these deficiencies are vulnerable to infections with catalase-positive organisms such as *Staphylococcus aureus*. The nitroblue–tetrazolium (NBT) test is the original and most widely known test for chronic granulomatous disease – it is negative in chronic granulomatous diseases (CGD), and positive in normal individuals. In myeloperoxidase (MPO) deficiency the majority of individuals show no signs of immunodeficiency but when they present often do so with *Candida albicans* infections. Patients with MPO deficiency have a respiratory burst with a normal NBT dye test.

Treatment of CGD has historically been with long-term antimicrobial prophylaxis, but cases of CGD and MPO deficiency have undergone haematopoietic stem cell transplantation which is curative. Interferon-γ 1b has been trialled in the prevention of infection in CGD, having been shown to reduce infection frequency by 70% and to decrease its severity.

Immunoglobulin A (IgA) deficiency is usually asymptomatic but patients can have increased frequency of mucous membrane infections including urinary tract and ear, nose and throat infections. A small proportion of patients with IgA deficiency will experience anaphylaxis to blood products and caution should be exercised the first time these patients are transfused or receive intravenous immunologloglobulins.

Nephrotic syndrome can lead to a relatively immunocompromised state but the preserved immunoglobulins in this case mean that it is not the diagnosis here. Familial Mediterranean fever (FMF) is an autoinflammatory condition caused my mutations in the *MEFV* gene. Although it can cause period fevers, arthralgia, abdominal pain and serositis it does not present with recurrent staphylococcal infections. Diagnosis of FMF is through genetic testing which will diagnose approximately 97% of cases. The metaraminol provocative test, where a patient is given low dose metaraminol to provoke a painful episode is an alternative but has poor sensitivity and specificity by comparison.

Arnold DE, Heimall JR. A review of chronic granulomatous disease. Adv Ther 2017; 34:2543–2557.

8. C Myelofibrosis

The clinical case is strongly suggestive of myelofibrosis. This is a myeloproliferative disorder characterised by anaemia, a leucoerythroblastic blood appearance, tear drop poikilocytes, splenomegaly (often massive) and bone marrow fibrosis. B symptoms such as fever, night sweats and weight loss, tend to be severe. Myelofibrosis can occur *de novo* or it may develop as a complication from other myeloproliferative disorders such as polycythaemia rubra vera (PRV) or essential thrombocythaemia (ET).

Myelofibrosis is a progressive condition which often occurs in older patients where intensive therapy is unsuitable. Progression is variable, with some patients having a long indolent clinical course and others progressing rapidly. If transformation to acute myeloid leukaemia occurs, it is almost invariably fatal. Treatment of younger and fitter patients is with high-dose chemotherapy and haematopoietic stem cell transplantation. *JAK2* inhibitors such as ruxolitinib have shown promise in the COMFORT-I and COMFORT-II trials.

Polycythaemia rubra vera (PRV) is strongly linked to the *JAK2 V617F* mutation – positive in 98% of cases. In this question. However, this patient does not have polycythaemia (haematocrit >0.52 in women, >0.56 in men). Splenomegaly can be a feature of PRV but is rarely massive, and this finding would prompt investigation to rule out transformation to myelofibrosis.

Chronic myeloid leukaemia is discussed in the answer to Question 26.

Hodgkin's disease tends to present in younger patients and is rarely associated with massive splenomegaly. It is not linked to the *JAK2 mutation*.

Systemic mastocytosis is a rare myeloproliferative disorder typically characterised by haematological, gastrointestinal, cardiac and cutaneous involvement. It has a well-recognised association with recurrent anaphylaxis. The JAK2 mutation is rarely detected, whereas the c-kit mutation (A816V) is present in almost all cases.

Hoffbrand V, Moss P, Pettit J. Myeloproliferative disorders (Chapter 15) In: Essential Haematology, 7th edn. Oxford: Blackwell Publishing, 2015.

9. E Thrombotic thrombocytopenic purpura (TTP)

This patient is suffering from TTP. The condition is defined by five features: thrombocytopenia, microangiopathic haemolytic anaemia (MAHA), neurological abnormalities, renal failure and fever. All five need not be present for the diagnosis to be made, but thrombocytopenia and fever are present in almost all patients.

Laboratory findings are of thrombocytopenia, normocytic anaemia, raised levels of unconjugated bilirubin (due to intravascular haemolysis), raised lactate dehydrogenase (LDH) (both from red cell lysis and tissue infarction) and decreased haptoglobin. The peripheral blood film is the most useful diagnostic investigation and will show red cell fragmentation (schistocytes), helmet cells and confirm thrombocytopenia.

TTP diagnosis is clinical, in conjunction with blood film findings.

The mechanism underlying TTP is decreased activity of ADAMTS13 (A Disintegrin And Metalloproteinase with Thrombo Spondin motif type 13). TTP can be congenital or acquired. Congenital TTP (approximately 2–5% of cases) generally has a milder course and is caused by a defect in the gene producing ADAMTS13. Acquired TTP is the most common presentation and is clinically much more severe. This is due to an autoantibody to ADAMTS13 which inhibits its function.

Treatment with plasma exchange is initiated in any patient for whom there is a high index of suspicion. ADAMTS13 levels and autoantibody titres should be assayed at presentation but the result may take several days to be available and treatment should not be delayed. Mortality from untreated TTP approaches 90%, while with appropriate treatment the mortality is <10%.

Platelet transfusions are relatively contraindicated as they are thought to fuel the process of thrombus formation and increase the risk of myocardial infarction and stroke. Platelets should be considered only in the presence of life-threatening bleeding.

For those that present with neurological deficit, rituximab has shown some benefit in inducing remission and preventing relapse. Relapses of acquired TTP are common following the initial treatment, and are similarly managed, with the addition of further immunosuppressants.

Catastrophic antiphospholipid syndrome (CAPS) is considered a rheumatological emergency and should be suspected in any patient with multi-organ failure who has positive anticardiolipin antibodies, β-2 glyoprotein 1 antibodies or a lupus anticoagulant. Pre-existing autoimmune disease is not a prerequisite. CAPS is associated with arterial and venous thromboses, and clinical complications include stroke and renal impairment, among others. Laboratory investigations often reveal a haemolytic anaemia and thrombocytopenia. Neurological disturbance is rare, and in this patient the laboratory findings do not support CAPS.

Disseminated intravascular coagulation (DIC) occurs in response to many different underlying conditions including sepsis, malignancy and trauma. Management is treatment of the underlying cause and support with blood products. Hypofibrinogenaemia, coagulopathy and thrombocytopenia are common but do not require routine correction unless the disturbance is severe (i.e. fibrinogen <1.0 g/L, platelet count <20 x 10^9/L).

Idiopathic thrombocytopaenic purpura is discussed in the answer to Question 1.

Haemolytic–uraemic syndrome is another micro-angiopathic haemolytic anaemia and is commonly associated with *Escherichia coli* O157 septicaemia and severe diarrhoea. Severe renal impairment in conjunction with blood film findings of MAHA is characteristic.

10. B Coeliac disease

Approximately 4–10% of healthy individuals fail to elicit protective levels of hepatitis B antibodies after completing the standard HBV vaccination schedule. Human leukocyte antigen (HLA) phenotype is considered the most important genetic marker of non-response. Coeliac disease is an HLA-associated disease and non-response to hepatitis B vaccine is well documented in undiagnosed coeliac disease, particularly in those who adhere poorly to a gluten-free diet. However, in adequately treated patients re-immunisation can lead to a satisfactory HBsAb response and should be recommended.

Corticosteroids administered topically (to skin or eyes), via aerosol, or by intra-articular, bursal, or tendon injection are not contraindications to immunisation. In asthma, including those on inhaled and short-course oral corticosteroids, hepatitis B immunisation elicits good antibody response. Systemic corticosteroid therapy usually does not contraindicate immunisation when used short term (i.e. less than 2 weeks) or when being prescribed for physiological maintenance doses. Prednisolone at >20mg/day for >2 weeks is taken as a generally accepted level at which systemic immunosuppression and adverse events are more likely. Live vaccine administration should ideally not occur until 3 months after steroid discontinuation. There is currently little evidence either supporting or refuting an impact of corticosteroids in killed and sub-unit vaccinations (such as the hepatitis B vaccine). In this case the short and infrequent oral courses of steroids for the asthma cannot account for the vaccine non-response.

Ertem D, et al. The response to hepatitis B vaccine: does it differ in celiac disease? Eur J Gastroenterol Hepatol 2010; 22(7):787–793.

11. D Von Willebrand's disease

Von Willebrand's disease is the most common inherited bleeding disorder in the UK with an estimated prevalence of 1%. The majority of cases (85%) are type 1 and have few bleeding problems. Type 2 and type 3 von Willebrand's disease is much rarer and patients present with significant bleeding histories. Type 2 is further subdivided depending on the exact deficit. Most forms are autosomal dominant.

In this case the factor VIII level is low, suggesting a mild haemophilia A or von Willebrand's disease. The factor VIII level is low in von Willebrand's disease because one of the physiological roles of von Willebrand's factor is to stabilise factor VIII and prolong its half-life in serum. In this case, the patient has an affected mother. Haemophilia A is X-linked recessive and while women can be affected by being homozygotes or through extreme lyonisation in a carrier, this is extremely rare and von Willebrand's disease is the more likely disorder.

Haemophilia B is rarer than haemophilia A and is a deficiency in factor IX. It is also X-linked recessive. Haemophilia C is a deficiency of factor XI and while it is relatively common in certain ethnic populations, such as Ashkenazi Jews, it is very rare in the general population. Dysfibrinogenaemia presents with a bleeding history and normal prothrombin time/activated partial thromboplastin time. The fibrinogen level may be normal or low, but all cases are extremely rare with an incidence of approximately 1:1 million live births.

Hoffbrand V, Moss P, Pettit J. Platelets, blood coagulation and haemostasis. In: Essential Haematology, 7th edn. Oxford: Blackwell Publishing, 2015

12. C Ciclosporin can cause microangiopathy

This patient is taking a combination of commonly prescribed immunosuppressants following solid organ transplantation.

Ciclosporin and tacrolimus are calcineurin inhibitors (CNIs) and work through disruption of T-cell signalling, namely inhibiting interleukin 2. It has a narrow therapeutic window and is variably metabolised. Trough levels must be closely monitored to ensure adequate immunosuppression and to limit long-term side effects, which include nephrotoxicity. Side effects of CNIs are many and varied but the most common ones include hypertension, hyperkalaemia (type 4 renal tubular acidosis), hirsutism, gum hypertrophy (particularly with ciclosporin), tremor and thrombotic microangiopathy (TMA). Tacrolimus is also implicated in NODAT (new-onset diabetes after transplantation).

Azathioprine is an antiproliferative drug which inhibits purine synthesis, thus decreasing T-cell proliferation. Its main side effects include hepatotoxicity and myelosuppression. It is strongly associated with long-term development of skin cancers.

13. C Hairy cell leukaemia

Hairy cell leukaemia (HCL) is a malignancy of mature B cells caused by a mutation in the BRAF V600E gene. It occurs in two forms. The classical form presents with pancytopenia, bone marrow fibrosis, splenomegaly and susceptibility to atypical infections. The mechanism underlying this is poorly understood. Blood film examination often fails to yield a diagnosis as the abnormal cells are infrequent. Bone marrow aspiration and trephine, polymerase chain reaction for BRAF V600E and flow cytometry of peripheral blood can all be diagnostic. Historically, blood would have been stained for tartrate-resistant acid phosphatised (TRAP) however this is no longer routinely performed as other more sensitive techniques have become available. The variant form of HCL is a clinically more aggressive disease which presents with a high white cell count, numerous hairy cells in the peripheral blood and B symptoms.

In both forms of HCL, splenomegaly is a prominent feature and may be massive. Hepatomegaly may also arise. Abdominal discomfort may result from organomegaly or splenic infarct. Lymphadenopathy is infrequently apparent at presentation.

Aplastic anaemia may present with clinical features resulting from pancytopenia. The blood film would not be expected to reveal abnormal cells. The bone marrow biopsy typically demonstrates loss of haematopoietic cells and increased fat content. Plasma cell leukaemia may present with clinical features of acute leukaemia or myeloma; typically, an excess of plasma cells would be expected on the peripheral blood film.

Hoffbrand V, Moss P, Pettit J. Chronic lymphoid leukaemias. In: Essential Haematology, 7th edn. Oxford: Blackwell Publishing, 2015.

Cannon T, et al. Hairy cell leukaemia: current concepts. Cancer Invest 2008; 26(8):860–865.

14. C Iron-deficiency anaemia

This is a case of iron-deficiency anaemia as demonstrated by the full blood count revealing a microcytic anaemia a low serum ferritin and peripheral blood film exhibiting microcytic, hypochromic red blood cells. Pencil and target cells may also be present.

Iron studies would be expected to reveal a low serum iron, raised total iron-binding capacity and reduced transferrin saturation.

Iron-deficiency anaemia is a common condition, occuring after the reticuloendothelial iron stores are depleted. The most common causes include chronic blood loss (e.g. gastrointestinal or menstrual), increased demands (e.g. during infancy, adolescence, pregnancy, or lactation), chronic dietary insufficiency, malabsorption disorders (e.g. coeliac disease) or parasitic infiltration of the gastrointestinal tract (e.g. hookworm). Treatment is of the underlying cause as well as supplementation. Where chronic blood loss is identified, it is important to exclude an underlying bleeding diathesis and to consider urgent colonoscopy and endoscopy to rule out gastrointestinal malignancy.

Oral iron (ferrous sulphate) can be poorly tolerated, with nausea and constipation extremely common as side effects and so compliance should be evaluated. Intolerance to oral iron is an indication for intravenous iron supplementation. Historically, allergic reactions to intravenous iron led to a reluctance to recommend them but modern preparations are much safer and are suitable for routine use.

Hoffbrand V, Moss P, Pettit J. Hypochromic anaemias (Chapter 3). In: Essential Haematology, 7th edn. Oxford: Blackwell Publishing, 2015.

15. E Skin-prick testing for common aeroallergens

Her symptoms are typical of rhinitis. Patients may also report nasal discharge, blockage or congestion. Rhinitis may be allergic, non-allergic or infective. Allergic rhinitis is increasing in prevalence and affects more than a fifth of the UK population. It is more common in children with a family history of atopy. Common causes include: house-dust mite, pollen (grass, tree) and animals (cats, dogs, horses); rarer causes include: moulds, occupational (flour, animal hair).

The diagnosis is confirmed by obtaining the relevant history and examination and is supported by specific allergy testing which may include skin-prick testing for common aeroallergens and/or specific IgE testing. Given her history suggestive of cat allergy the specific IgE for cats is likely to be positive and broader testing to include all common aeroallergens including house-dust mite, grass and pollen may be more useful. Management strategies include education of allergen avoidance, nasal corticosteroids and antihistamines. Control of rhinitis may improve asthma control and immunotherapy may be highly effective in selected cases.

Peak flow monitoring may be very useful in the diagnosis and management of asthma. Nasoendoscopy and CT scanning of the sinuses may be considered if there are clinical features suggesting alternative diagnoses, such as chronic infection, nasal polyposis, malignancy or foreign bodies.

Greiner AN, et al. Allergic rhinitis. Lancet 2011; 378:2112–2122.

Scadding GK, et al. BSACI guidelines for the management of allergic and non-allergic rhinitis. Clin Exper Allergy 2017;47:856–889.

16. D It is highly responsive to antihistamines

This woman has presented with symptoms of hereditary angio-oedema, also known as C1-inhibitor (C1 esterase inhibitor) deficiency. It is a rare condition, inherited in an autosomal dominant fashion, and typically presents with a combination of cutaneous, abdominal and respiratory symptoms. Patients often describe previous episodes of angio-oedema or unexplained abdominal pain either in childhood or in early adulthood. Attacks are often associated with a prodrome around 1–2 hours before an attack, with tingling and possible mood disturbance or sensory changes.

C1 inhibitor deficiency occurs symptomatically more frequently in women, in certain variations, if treated with combined oral contraceptives or during pregnancy. It can be triggered by ACE inhibitors, although angioedema secondary to this drug occurs due to bradykinin accumulation. Antihistamines are only effective in angioedema caused by mast cell degranulation in allergic reactions. Treatment of acute attacks relies on analgesia and supportive care for mild attacks involving only limb oedema or abdominal pain, and supplementation of the C1 inhibitor or inhibition of downstream events in severe cases. Plasma derived and recombinant C1 inhibitor concentrate are available commercially but are unlikely to be available outside of specialist centres. Fresh frozen plasma can be used in an emergency but treatment usually involves large volumes with associated complications. Newer drug treatments aimed at reducing downstream activation of bradykinin include the drugs ecallantide and icatibant. These drugs have been shown to be beneficial both in acute attacks and in prophylaxis for severely affected individuals.

Danazol, a testosterone analogue, was historically used to reduce the frequency of attacks but this has been replaced by the newer drugs as danazol has numerous undesirable side effects. Tranexamic acid has been shown to be ineffective in both acute attacks and in prophylaxis and should not be routinely prescribed.

17. D Severe life-threatening infection with encapsulated bacteria in infancy

This patient has presented with selective IgA deficiency. It is the most common of the immune deficiency disorders and, depending on population, is thought to affect up to around 1 in 400 people, more frequently males. It is defined as undetectable IgA levels, with normal IgG and normal IgM levels (although a proportion of patients will also have an IgG subclass deficiency) seen persistently over the age of 4 years. Patients are often asymptomatic or not diagnosed until early adulthood and most frequently will present with recurrent upper respiratory tract infections or sinusitis. They may also present with various gastrointestinal infections and chronic diarrhoea or have a history of urinary tract infections.

Patients with selective IgA deficiency also show an increased prevalence of autoimmune conditions, such as systemic lupus erythematosus (usually without nephritis), rheumatoid arthritis and coeliac disease. They are more prone to various food allergies and atopic dermatitis. A poor response to pneumococcal polysaccharide vaccines is recognised. Because a proportion of patients with selective IgA deficiency have anti-A antibodies they have an increased risk of reactions, including anaphylaxis, to blood transfusions and intravenous immunoglobulins. Caution should be exercised if transfusing these patients for the first time, although the majority of individuals will have no adverse reaction.

Severe infection with encapsulated bacteria in infancy is associated with some of the other immune deficiencies, in particular the much rarer IgM deficiency or those with complement deficiencies, but not with selective IgA deficiency. Many patients who have isolated IgA deficiency are asymptomatic and have a very benign course; others will suffer recurrent infections with long-term sequelae such as bronchiectasis.

18. B Acute myeloid leukaemia

This patient has acute myeloid leukaemia (AML). Her peripheral blood film shows a myeloid cell containing an Auer rod in the cytoplasm, which is pathognomonic for acute myeloid leukaemia. You would not see this in chronic lymphocytic leukaemia, hairy cell leukaemia nor chronic myeloid leukaemia, hence they are not the correct choice. These topics are covered in other questions in this chapter.

Acute lymphoblastic leukaemia is the most common childhood leukaemia and may present with clinical features of bone marrow failure or organ infiltration. This is a haematological emergency and immediate specialist advice should be sought.

There are a number of immediate complications which can prove rapidly fatal. A clotting screen is an essential investigation. Some forms of AML such as acute promyelocytic leukaemia present with profound disseminated intravascular coagulation (DIC) and the mortality from intracranial haemorrhage in the first 24 hours after diagnosis has been estimated to be as high as 20%. Rapid, aggressive blood product support is often required.

Patients presenting with low neutrophil counts may have concurrent neutropenic sepsis. A raised CRP alone may be disease related, but there should be a low threshold for broad spectrum antibiotics. Patients with high white cell counts (>50) are at risk of leucostasis. This occurs when the abnormal immature cells increase plasma viscosity and frequently presents as unexplained neurological deficit or sudden collapse. These patients require urgent cytoreduction with chemotherapy or leucopheresis.

Bone marrow aspiration is essential to establish cytogenetic and molecular prognostic information for treatment, although in fragile elderly patients, the diagnosis can equally be confirmed with flow cytometry of peripheral blood.

Treatment should be started as soon as possible after diagnosis. Overall survival decreases with age at diagnosis. Patients aged 20–30 years will be expected to have approximately 60% 5-year survival, with patients >70 years old having approximately 5% 5-year survival.

19. D Skin-prick testing for latex

A dental student who develops skin rashes on her hands and respiratory symptoms soon after starting a clinical attachment is highly suggestive of latex allergy as she probably would have been wearing latex gloves. In most cases this is a type I- or IgE-mediated hypersensitivity reaction. Symptoms include a contact urticaria resulting in erythema, weals and pruritus, and occurring within minutes of skin contact. Other manifestations associated with airborne exposure of the allergens include rhinorrhoea, watery eyes and asthma. Powdered latex gloves are more likely to cause problems than powder-free gloves because of the increased amount of allergen.

The best diagnostic test is skin-prick testing which involves puncturing the skin with varying concentrations of latex extract. A positive result is when a weal develops with surrounding erythema that is equal to or greater in diameter than a histamine control (>3 mm in diameter). Skin-prick testing has a sensitivity of 65–96% and specificity of 88–94% but the results need to be correlated with clinical symptoms. Although it is a very safe test there is a possibility of developing anaphylaxis.

Peak flow monitoring and spirometry with bronchodilator testing are useful tests for the diagnosis of asthma and may be helpful in the further investigation of this patient, but the skin-prick test for latex allergy is more likely to confirm the diagnosis with the presented history. Total serum IgE may be useful in monitoring patients with chronic atopic conditions; however, it would not be diagnostic as a single investigation. Specific IgE antibody testing is a possible option and in certain countries, such as the USA, this is the preferred diagnostic test.

Royal College of Physicians. Latex allergy – Occupational aspects of management. A national guideline. London: RCP, 2008.
Cullinan P, et al. Latex allergy guideline. Clin Exp Allergy 2003; 33:1484–1499.

20. A Common variable immunodeficiency

This patient has not responded to his vaccination, with subsequent meningococcal disease. The immunoglobulin panel shows a relative pan-hypogammaglobulinaemia with markedly low IgG levels. This fits with a diagnosis of common variable immunodeficiency (CVID).

CVID is the most commonly encountered primary immunodeficiency representing a group of often heritable diseases. Presentation is varied and diagnosis is often delayed until the second or third decade of life but can be as late as the eighth. A typical history includes recurrent infections e.g ear, nose, throat, skin, and respiratory infections and often failure to develop immunity from vaccinations. The majority of CVID patients have impaired memory B cell function with a reduction in switched memory B cells. The diagnosis remains one of exclusion but new generation genetic analysis has helped identify novel mutations. Low immunoglobulin levels do point to the diagnosis but nephrotic syndrome, X-linked agammaglobulinaemia and haematological malignancies must be ruled out. Treatment is with immunoglobulin therapy either intravenously or subcutaneously.

The two most common forms of severe combined immunodeficiency (SCID) are X-linked SCID and adenosine deaminase deficiency. SCID manifests in early childhood and is rapidly fatal without bone marrow transplantation and therefore does not fit with this case. HIV could fit the history of this case but hypogammaglobulinaemia is not a feature of this disease as HIV depletes T-helper cells not B cells. Hypo- or asplenism again does not fit with the laboratory indices presented in this cases although would be consistent with the history of recurrent infections. Surreptitious steroid use does not fit with the clinical or laboratory information presented.

Park MA, et al. Common variable immunodeficiency: a new look at an old disease. Lancet 2008; 372:489–502.
Ameratunga, Ameratunga R, Brewerton M, Slade C, et al. Comparison of diagnostic criteria for common variable immunodeficiency disorder. Front Immunol 2014; 5:415.

21. D *Plasmodium falciparum*

The Giemsa-stained thin peripheral blood film reveals the distinctive ring trophozoites of *Plasmodium falciparum* malaria, as well as acanthocytosis (crenated erythrocytes). Multidrug-resistant forms of *P. falciparum* malaria are present in the rural areas of northern Thailand, especially along the Myanmar border. Furthermore, the patient appears to have discontinued his malaria prophylaxis early; it is usually recommended that it should be continued for one week after return from endemic areas.

Thrombocytopenia is a feature of falciparum malaria which is not often seen in non-falciparum infections. This can be profound and platelets should be supported to keep the platelet count >20 x 10^9/L, or for use in the event of haemorrhage. The presence (or suspected presence) of cerebral malaria or a documented parasitaemia >15% are both indications for a red cell exchange.

The most commonly used method for malaria detection is the Giemsa-stained thick and thin peripheral blood films. Differentiation between malarial species by microscopy requires considerable expertise and samples which are suspected to be positive should be referred to the local reference laboratory. A number of antigen-based tests are available. Tests for histidine rich protein-2 (HRP-2) are sensitive for falciparum malaria but not for other types. Assays for *Plasmodium* lactate dehydrogenase (pLDH) can detect and help determine the species of the parasite. Tests for *Plasmodium* aldolase are non-specific but can give rapid confirmation of a suspected positive result.

Japanese encephalitis is a mosquito-borne viral disease which is common in parts of south-east Asia and the Far East. Dengue fever is also a mosquito-borne viral disease that is endemic to many tropical and subtropical countries. Neither of these conditions is diagnosed on the peripheral blood film appearance but can be diagnosed by isolation of the virus, serological tests or reverse-transcriptase polymerase chain reaction (RT-PCR). Dracunculiasis is a parasitic disease caused by the round worm, *Dracunculus medinensis,* presenting as a painful blister that subsequently ruptures to form an ulcer, from which the adult worm emerges. It is confined to half-a-dozen African countries and is close to eradication.

Trypanosomiasis is a parasitic protozoal disease that can be diagnosed by detecting trypanosomes on the blood film. *Trypanosoma cruzi* causes American trypanosomiasis (aka Chagas' disease) and is spread by blood-sucking triatominae insects. Trypanosoma brucei gambiense and Trypanosoma brucei rhodesiense cause African trypanosomiasis (aka sleeping sickness) and these are spread by infected tsetse flies.

Basic Malaria Microscopy, Part I. Learner's Guide, 2nd edn. Geneva: World Health Organization Press, 2010.
World Health Organization Press (WHO). WHO Guidelines for the treatment of Malaria, 3rd edition. Geneva: World Health Organization Press, 2015.

22. C Good's syndrome

Good's syndrome is a rare adult-onset immunodeficiency disorder presenting around the 5th decade. It is characterised by hypogammaglobulinaemia and B-cell depletion in the presence of a thymoma. This patient has low levels of all immunoglobulin subclasses and the CT of the chest suggests a thymoma. In contrast to XLA and CVID, however, patients with Good's syndrome may also present with disorders of cell-mediated immunity, in particular to cytomegalovirus (CMV – including CMV colitis) or mucocutaneous candida infections. In addition, haematological abnormalities are common. Anaemia (including red cell aplasia and haemolytic anaemia) is seen in around 50% of cases. Many patients will also have leukopenia and some thrombocytopenia. Management of patients with Good's syndrome includes surgical removal of thymoma and immunoglobulin replacement.

Although this patient could have a CVID, the haematological disorders, the presence of *Candida* species and the findings consistent with a thymoma make the diagnosis of Good's syndrome more likely. Chronic granulomatous disease is a congenital defect of neutrophil killing and will present earlier in life, and is characterised by chronic suppurative granulomas or abscesses affecting the skin and lymph nodes, and osteomyelitis. The other two diagnoses listed are very much diseases of childhood and would not present as late as this. Wiskott–Aldrich is an X-linked condition that presents with cellular and humoral immunodeficiency, thrombocytopenia, and eczema. It typically presents after the first few months of life and survival beyond the second decade is rare. X-linked agammaglobulinaemia (Bruton's syndrome) typically manifests in childhood, particularly in boys, and also presents with recurrent bacterial infections, particularly secondary to encapsulated organisms. Treatment is with lifelong intravenous immunoglobulin.

Kelleher P, et al. What is Good's syndrome? Immunological abnormalities in patients with thymoma. J Clin Pathol 2003; 56:12–16.

23. D Recommend influenza vaccine

Influenza can be a very serious infection in certain individuals, such as those with asthma and chronic obstructive pulmonary disease. The vaccines are developed from chicken embryos and as a result patients with egg protein allergy have a theoretical risk of developing anaphylaxis when given it. Evidence suggests that in practice the risk of adverse effects is extremely rare. The current trivalent inactivated influenza vaccine has very low levels of ovalbumin and a number of international guidelines, including those of the Centers for Disease Control and Prevention, have deemed it safe to give to patients with egg allergy. Current recommendations are that skin-prick testing is no longer necessary as there is poor correlation between test result and development of adverse effects.

Egg allergy often resolves later in life and if the reaction is not too severe eggs may be cautiously re-introduced into the diet. There is interest in the use of dietary supplementation and alternative therapies to reduce the risk and duration of influenza infection. Some herbalists believe that *Echinacea* may treat common colds and other viral illnesses, but clinical trials have been inconsistent and overall do not support these claims.

Clark AT, et al. British Society for Allergy and Clinical Immunology guidelines for the management of egg allergy. Clin Exper Allergy; 40:1116–1129.
Centers for Disease Control and Prevention (CDC). Prevention and control of influenza with vaccines: recommendations of the Advisory Committee on Immunization Practices (ACIP) 2011. MMWR Morb Mortal Wkly Rep 2011; 60(33):1128.

24. E Diuretics can improve oxygenation

An acute chest syndrome in a patient with sickle cell disease is a haematological emergency. The pathophysiology underlying this is a vaso-occlusive crisis occurring within the lung alveoli. Poor flow through the alveoli results in poor oxygenation, which worsens the crystallisation of the haemoglobin S within the red blood cells. This then further reduces the flow of blood through the alveoli resulting in a cycle which ultimately, and often rapidly, results in death.

The typical presentation is with chest pain (this can be difficult to distinguish from chest wall pain without an acute chest syndrome), unexplained hypoxia and an abnormal chest X-ray. The differential diagnosis usually includes pneumonia and pulmonary embolus, as patients with sickle cell disease are predisposed to both these conditions.

Mortality without treatment is approximately 30%. Death can occur within hours, and a red cell exchange is required, in this case as soon as possible. If facilities for automated red cell exchange aren't available a manual red cell exchange is required.

As these patients can deteriorate rapidly, a high-dependency unit or ward with experience monitoring sickle cell patients is recommended. Broad spectrum antibiotics are started to cover pneumonia as the trigger for the sickle crisis, regardless of whether this is the cause of the hypoxia.

All sickle patients in crisis should be adequately oxygenated with CPAP if required, and kept well hydrated. Diuresis is sometimes incorrectly given on the suspicion that the pulmonary infiltrates represent congestive cardiac failure or fluid overload. This usually results in worsening of the underlying condition, and hence this is the incorrect statement.

Any patient who has had one acute chest syndrome is predisposed to a second and hence often started on prophylaxis in the form of hydroxycarbamide or a red cell exchange programme. The acute chest syndrome is not limited to patients who have HbSS variant disease; patients with compound variants such as SC, SDPunjab and SOarab have been found to have acute chest syndromes. The diagnosis is extremely unlikely in a patient with sickle cell trait (HbAS) although rare cases, under severe physiological stress such as cardiac bypass surgery, are reported.

25. E Urgently test varicella-zoster antibody titre

This patient is clearly immunosuppressed and has been in contact with someone with shingles, i.e. varicella-zoster virus (VZV). In patients who are at high risk of infection (e.g. transplant recipients, patients receiving chemotherapy, post-bone marrow transplantation, neonates, patients with immunodeficiencies, those taking high-dose steroids/other immunosuppressants) it is important to establish whether contact has definitely taken place and whether the contact was likely to have been infectious.

As this patient is unsure whether she has had chickenpox in the past, the most important next step is to urgently check her VZV antibody levels. If they are positive then no further action is required. If they are negative then she should be given VZV immunoglobulin. This should be given ideally within 7 days of exposure. If the result is still unknown by this point then treatment with VZV Ig should be given regardless.

There is no evidence to suggest a role for empirically treating with antivirals. As the risk of VZV infection is significant and immunosuppressed patients in particular can become very unwell with disseminated or haemorrhagic zoster, it is definitely not appropriate to do nothing or adopt a watch-and-wait policy. Ideally, even if an immunocompromised patient thinks that they have had previous exposure to VZV, their IgG levels should still be checked and the same protocol followed as above.

Department of Health. Varicella (Chapter 34). In: Immunisation against infectious disease 'The Green Book'. London: Department of Health, 2011.

26. D Chronic myeloid leukaemia

Chronic myeloid leukaemia (CML) constitutes approximately 15% of all leukaemias, and is characterised associated with an abnormal Bcr-Abl construct within the peripheral blood, usually found with PCR, as a product of the Philadelphia chromosome mutation (t9:22). CML usually presents as an incidental finding in blood tests performed for non-specific symptoms. 90% of patients present in chronic phase, where the peripheral blood shows extreme leucocytosis, often >100 x 10^9/L but with relatively preserved haemoglobin and platelet counts. The blood film shows a characteristic myelocyte peak which differentiates CML morphologically from other myeloproliferative disorders.

Of the other options, acute lymphoblastic and acute myeloid leukaemia present with bone marrow failure (typically severe anaemia and thrombocytopenia). Bone marrow showing predominant granulopoiesis makes a diagnosis of chronic lymphocytic leukaemia or hairy cell leukaemia unlikely, as does the polymerase chain reaction result.

Patients will typically have (massive) splenomegaly and on questioning will usually report symptoms of hypermetabolism such as weight loss or hyperuricaemia. The serum B12 is often extremely high although this does not add any prognostic information.

Patients presenting outside of the chronic phase are in either accelerated phase or blast crisis. This differentiation is made based upon the number of immature myeloid cells (blasts) in the peripheral blood, the presence of basophils in the blood and the platelet count. A bone marrow biopsy is usually taken at diagnosis to confirm the patient is in the chronic phase.

Hoffbrand V, Moss P, Pettit J. Chronic myeloid leukaemia. In: Essential Haematology, 7th edn. Oxford: Blackwell Publishing, 2015.

Chapter 6

Infectious diseases and genitourinary medicine

Questions

1. A 31-year-old man presented with a 3-day history of fever, a papular rash on his chest and legs, a polyarthritis affecting his right knee and right hand–third and fourth digits. He is homosexual and, 4 weeks ago, he had an episode of unprotected sexual intercourse.

   Examination revealed a warm and swollen right knee with a detectable effusion and dactylitis in the right hand. There was no palpable lymphadenopathy. His temperature was 38.3°C.

   Investigations:

haemoglobin 135 g/L (130–180)	C-reactive protein 178 mg/L (<5)
white cell count 13.2 × 10⁹/L (4–11)	erythrocyte sedimentation rate 95 mm/1st h (0–20)
neutrophils 11.2 × 10⁹/L (1.5–7)	
platelets 522 × 10⁹/L (150–400)	

   Urea and electrolytes and liver function tests: normal
   Syphilis serology: *Treponema pallidum* particle agglutination: positive
   Rapid plasma reagin: negative

   Right knee X-ray: soft tissue swelling but no periostitis

   Aspiration of the right knee effusion: 3+ white cells, no organisms seen

   Urinalysis: 1+ leukocytes, 1+ nitrites

   What is the most likely diagnosis?

   A   Disseminated gonococcal infection (DGI)
   B   HIV seroconversion
   C   Reiter's syndrome
   D   Secondary syphilis
   E   Seronegative arthropathy

2. A 43-year-old Eritrean woman who had lived in the UK for the last 6 years presented with right-sided weakness and a 3-month history of unresolving diarrhoea. She reported losing 12 kg in weight over the last year. She took no regular medications.

   Examination revealed power 2/5 in her right arm and right leg with hyperreflexia and an equivocal right plantar reflex. Cranial nerve examination detected no abnormalities. The retina could not be visualised at dilated fundoscopy. The rest of the examination was unremarkable except for obvious oral thrush.

Investigations:

haemoglobin 112 g/L (115–165)	C-reactive protein 32 mg/L (<5)
white cell count 3.3 × 10⁹/L (4–11)	erythrocyte sedimentation rate 84 mm/1st h (0–20)
neutrophils 2.9 × 10⁹/L (1.5–7)	
platelets 252 × 10⁹/L (150–400)	

Urea and electrolytes and liver function tests: normal

CT of the brain: see **Figure 6.1**

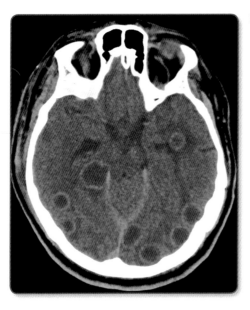

Figure 6.1

What is the most likely diagnosis?

A   Cerebral cryptococcomas
B   Cerebral lymphoma
C   Cerebral toxoplasmosis
D   Cerebral tuberculomas
E   Progressive multifocal leukoencephalopathy

3.   A 56-year-old white man presented with a 1-month history of progressive back pain and a 1-week history of night sweats and fever. He had lost 19 kg in weight over the last 6 months and had intermittent bouts of diarrhoea and constipation. On occasion he had noted fresh blood in his stool.

His pulse was 95 beats per minute, blood pressure 115/63 mmHg, respiratory rate 18 beats per minute and temperature 38.4°C. Examination revealed focal tenderness at the T8 vertebra. In the right leg, power was 4/5 and the plantar reflex was up-going. Abdominal examination was unremarkable and rectal examination revealed no masses and a normal anal tone.

Investigations:

haemoglobin 102 g/L (130–180)	platelets 622×10^9/L (150–400)
white cell count 14.2×10^9/L (4–11)	mean corpuscular volume 75.5 fL (80–96)
neutrophils 12.8×10^9/L (1.5–7.0)	albumin 30 g/L (37–49)

Urea and electrolytes and liver function tests: normal

MRI: see **Figure 6.2**

Blood cultures: Gram-positive cocci isolated from both bottles at 24 hours

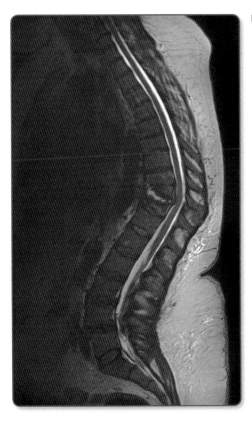

Figure 6.2

What is the most appropriate immediate management?

A   Intravenous ceftriaxone
B   Intravenous ceftriaxone and neurosurgical opinion
C   Intravenous ceftriaxone and colonoscopy with biopsies
D   Intravenous ceftriaxone and antituberculous therapy until mycobacterial smear and culture results are known
E   Intravenous vancomycin

4. A 34-year-old man, admitted with diabetic ketoacidosis, gave a 2-day history of headache, nasal congestion, periorbital swelling and a blood-stained nasal discharge.

Over the subsequent 48 hours he became drowsy and unresponsive despite correction of his hyperglycaemic state.

ENT examination revealed black, necrotic lesions on a perforated nasal septum.

Investigations:

haemoglobin 145 g/L (130–180)	platelets 553 × 10^9/L (150–400)
white cell count 9.4 × 10^9/L (4–11)	serum glucose 6.4 mmol/L (3.0–6.0)
neutrophils 8.6 × 10^9/L (1.5–7.0)	

Urea and electrolytes and liver function tests: normal

CT of the brain: no brain abnormality
marked paranasal sinus mucosal thickening
no bony destruction

Cerebrospinal fluid: white cell count 1 × 10^6/L (<5)
red cell count 4 × 10^6/L (<5)

protein 0.31 g/L (0.15–0.45)	glucose 5.2 mmol/L (3.3–4.4)

Nasal swab: *Streptococcus pneumoniae* and *Staphylococcus aureus*

What is the most likely diagnosis?

A   Dental abscess
B   Nasal diphtheria
C   Orbital cellulitis
D   Rhinocerebral mucormycosis
E   Severe maxillary sinusitis

5. A 31-year-old soldier returned from 3 weeks in the Democratic Republic of Congo and developed a fever 14 days after his return. On admission he had no localising symptoms. His observations showed temperature 39°C, pulse 115 beats per minute, blood pressure 124/70 mmHg and oxygen saturation 99% on air. There was nothing to find on examination.

Investigations:

haemoglobin 105 g/L (130–180)	platelets 15 × 10^9/L (150–400)
white cell count 2.1 × 10^9/L (4–11)	C-reactive protein 135 mg/L (<5)
neutrophils 1.1 × 10^9/L (1.5–7.0)	activated partial prothrombin time 90s (30–40s)

bilirubin 50 mmol/L (1–22)
alanine transaminase 70 U/L (5–35)
alkaline phosphatase 65 U/L (45–105)

Monospot: negative
Malaria film and rapid diagnostic test: negative

What is the most likely diagnosis?

A   Lassa fever
B   Epstein–Barr virus

C   Cytomegalovirus
D   Typhoid fever
E   Malaria

6. A 35-year-old male judo athlete presented to the emergency department with a 48-hour history
    of breathlessness, fever and a cough productive of yellow sputum with streaks of fresh blood.
    He had had recurrent attendances to his general practitioner with boils and furuncles over the
    preceding 18 months.
       His temperature was 38.7°C, pulse 120 beats per minute, blood pressure 105/55 mmHg with
    respiratory rate 24 breaths per minute and oxygen saturation 92% on air. Auscultation of his chest
    revealed coarse inspiratory crackles at the left base.

    Investigations:

haemoglobin 147 g/L (130–180)	urea 7.9 mmol/L (2.5–7.5)
white cell count 19.4 × 10⁹/L (4–11)	creatinine 89 µmol/L (60–110)
neutrophils 17.8 × 10⁹/L (1.5–7.0)	C-reactive protein 378 mg/L (<5)
platelets 769 × 10⁹/L (150–400)	

    Liver function tests: normal

    Chest X-ray: consolidation of left lower zone with an intraparenchymal abscess

    What is the most likely pathogen?

    A   Group A streptococcus
    B   *Klebsiella pneumoniae*
    C   *Streptococcus milleri*
    D   *Staphylococcus aureus*
    E   *Streptococcus pneumoniae*

7. A 29-year-old woman presented with a 12-hour history of pain, swelling and redness of her left
    leg. She reported cutting her leg shaving the previous evening but denied any travel. Throughout
    the day she had reported chills and shaking and had vomited twice since arriving in the
    emergency department.
       On examination, her left leg was red from the distal tibia to the mid-thigh, with the skin
    proximal to the erythema appearing mottled. Palpation of the mottled area exhibited surgical
    emphysema. She had a temperature of 38°C, blood pressure 95/55 mmHg, pulse 105 beats per
    minute, respiratory rate 22 breaths per minute and oxygen saturation 99% on air.

    Investigations:

haemoglobin 95 g/L (115–165)	urea 19 mmol/L (2.5–7.5)
white cell count 17.8 × 10⁹/L (4–11)	creatinine 135 µmol/L (45–90)
neutrophils 15.9 × 10⁹/L (1.5–7.0)	C-reactive protein 279 mg/L (<5)
platelets 45 × 10⁹/L (150–400)	creatine kinase 879 U/L (35–170)

    Liver function tests: normal

    What is the most likely diagnosis?

    A   Cellulitis
    B   Fournier's gangrene
    C   Meleney's gangrene
    D   Type 1 necrotising fasciitis
    E   Type 2 necrotising fasciitis

8. A 69-year-old woman presented with a 3-day history of progressive pain, erythema and swelling of the right hand, wrist and now forearm. Two days before these symptoms started she had been bitten by her cat on the thenar eminence of that hand. Over the last 24 hours she had had fevers.

    Her right hand and forearm are depicted in the clinical photo (see **Figure 6.3**). Her temperature was 38.5°C, pulse 95 beats per minute, and blood pressure 115/60 mmHg. There was lymphadenopathy in the right axillae.

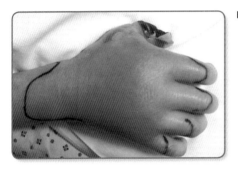

Figure 6.3 *See colour plate section.*

Investigations:

haemoglobin 11.6 g/dL (115–165)	urea 7.9 mmol/L (2.5–7.5)
white cell count 15.4 × 10⁹/L (4–11)	creatinine 82 µmol/L (45–90)
neutrophils 14.6 × 10⁹/L (1.5–7.0)	C-reactive protein 245 mg/L (<5)
platelets 210 × 10⁹/L (150–400)	creatine kinase 125 U/L (35–170)

Liver function tests: normal
Blood clotting: normal

Blood culture: Gram-negative rods in the aerobic bottle at 24 hours

What is the most likely pathogen?

A   *Capnocytophaga canimorsus*
B   *Eikenella corrodens*
C   Group A *Streptococcus*
D   *Pasteurella multocida*
E   *Staphylococcus aureus*

9. A 57-year-old man who had a metal mitral valve replacement 9 months ago presented with a 24-hour history of high fever. There were no other localising symptoms. There was no antecedent trauma, catheterisation or dental procedure. He has no known allergies.

    On examination, his temperature was 39.0°C, pulse 105 beats per minute, blood pressure 90/50 mmHg, respiratory rate 22 breaths per minute and oxygen saturation 94% on room air. There was an audible pan systolic murmur. A bedside echo in the emergency department suggested a mobile vegetation on the prosthetic mitral valve.

Investigations:

> haemoglobin 95 g/L (130–180)
> white cell count 21.5 × 10⁹/L (4–11)
> neutrophils 18.5 × 10⁹/L (1.5–7.0)
> platelets 180 × 10⁹/L (150–400)
>
> Urea and electrolytes and liver function tests: normal

What is the most appropriate empirical antimicrobial therapy?

A   Ampicillin and flucloxacillin and gentamicin
B   Vancomycin and gentamicin and rifampicin
C   Ampicillin with ceftriaxone
D   Flucloxacillin
E   Benzylpenicillin

10. A 78-year-old man presented with a 2-month history of increasing pain in his right foot and great toe. He was now unable to weight bear. He had a past medical history of hypertension, dyslipidaemia and type 2 diabetes. He was taking gliclazide, metformin, simvastatin, ramipril and amlodipine.
    On examination, there was a 3-cm ulcer over the base of his right hallux/ metatarsophalangeal joint that on probing was deep to bone. There were necrotic edges and an offensive exudate and some erythema around the ulcer. He was apyrexial and haemodynamically stable.

Investigations:

> haemoglobin 106 g/L (130–180)   creatine kinase 134 U/L (25–195)
> white cell count 10.5 × 10⁹/L (4–11)   bilirubin 6 mmol/L (1–22)
> neutrophils 6.8 × 10⁹/L (1.5–7.0)   alanine transaminase 35 U/L (5–35)
> platelets 289 × 10⁹/L (150–400)   alkaline phosphatase 456 U/L (45–105)
> urea 5.8 mmol/L (2.5–7.5)   albumin 31 g/L (37–49)
> creatinine 140 μmol/L (60–110)   HbA1c 11.8% (3.8–6.4)
> C-reactive protein 23 mg/L (<5)
>
> Foot X-ray: see **Figure 6.4**

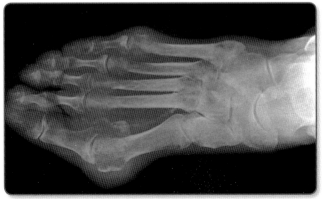

Figure 6.4

What is the most appropriate next step in management?

A Intravenous co-amoxiclav
B Intravenous flucloxacillin and benzylpenicillin
C MRI of the foot and intravenous co-amoxiclav
D MRI of the foot and intravenous flucloxacillin and benzylpenicillin
E MRI of the foot and surgical debridement with biopsy

11. A 27-year-old white woman presented to the emergency department with a 3-day history of progressive confusion, photophobia and altered sensation on the left side of her face. She worked as a business executive and frequently travelled back and forth to Europe and the USA, but had been off work for the last 8 weeks with polymyalgia rheumatica diagnosed by her general practitioner. She denied alcohol or illicit substance abuse. She denied any recent sexual relations.

On examination, there was no discernible meningism and no fever. Neurological examination showed a left trigeminal palsy. There was also a fading bruise on her upper outer thigh.

Investigations:

haemoglobin 131 g/L (115–165)	platelets 198 × 10⁹/L (150–400)
white cell count 6.1 × 10⁹/L (4–11)	C-reactive protein 45 mg/L (<5)
neutrophils 4.5 × 10⁹/L (1.5–7.0)	serum glucose 5.8 mmol/L (3.0–6.0)

Urea and electrolytes and liver function tests: normal

HIV rapid diagnostic test: negative

Cerebrospinal fluid: white cell count 18 x 10⁹ g/L (<5)
95% mononuclear
5% polymorphonuclear
red cell count <1 × 106/L (<5)
protein 0.52 g/L (0.15–0.45 g/L)
glucose 4.9 mmol/L (3.3–4.4 mmol/L)

Microscopy, culture and sensitivities: no growth

What is the most likely diagnosis?

A Herpes simplex encephalomeningitis
B *Mycobacterium tuberculosis* meningitis
C Neuroborreliosis
D Progressive multifocal leukoencephalopathy
E *Streptococcus pneumoniae* meningitis

12. A 68-year-old Indian banker presented to the outpatient department with a 4-week history of painful red nodules over the anterior aspects of both shins. His past medical history included chronic obstructive pulmonary disease for which he had previously received six courses of steroids in the last 12 months and he had lost 8 kg in weight over this period. He continued to smoke tobacco and had a 50 pack-year history.

On examination, there were, tender, smooth, shiny, 4–8 cm nodules over both anterior shins. Auscultation of his chest showed decreased breath sounds throughout but no focal abnormality. His abdomen was soft with no palpable organomegaly. There was no peripheral lymphadenopathy.

Investigations:

haemoglobin 104 g/L (130–180)	neutrophils 6.8 × 10⁹/L (1.5–7.0)
white cell count 5.9 × 10⁹/L (4–11)	platelets 364 × 10⁹/L (150–400)

Urea and electrolytes and liver function tests: normal

Antistreptolysin O titre <200 IU/mL (<200)
Hepatitis C antibody: negative
Human immunodeficiency virus antibody: negative
Epstein–Barr virus (VCA) antibody: negative
Serum angiotensin-converting enzyme 22 µg/L (<40 µg/L)

Chest X-ray: widened upper mediastinum, clear lung fields

What is the most appropriate next investigation?

A   Bronchoscopy and endobronchial ultrasound-guided biopsy
B   CT of the thorax
C   Mantoux test
D   QuantiFERON test
E   Sputum microscopy, culture and susceptibilities

13. A 21-year-old woman, who was 18 weeks' pregnant, presented with her son who had a cropping vesicular rash over his face and torso. The rash began yesterday. She was concerned over the health of her pregnancy. She was originally from Kuwait but had been in the UK for 3 years. She was asymptomatic.

On examination, she was apyrexial and examinations of her chest, abdomen and oropharynx were normal. Full dermatological examination revealed no rash.

Investigations:

haemoglobin 128 g/L (115–165)	platelets 178 × 10⁹/L (150–400)
white cell count 6.5 × 10⁹/L (4–11)	C-reactive protein <5 mg/L (<5)
neutrophils 4.8 × 10⁹/L (1.5–7.0)	

Urea and electrolytes and liver function tests: normal

Urine dipstick: normal

What is the most appropriate next step in her management?

A   Intravenous aciclovir
B   Intravenous immunoglobulin
C   Oral aciclovir
D   Send rubella and parvovirus serology from mother
E   Send varicella-zoster serology from mother

14. A 57-year-old woman presented with a 5-day history of fever dyspnoea, and a productive cough. She had recently returned from a 1-week summer holiday to Paris. She had no pets and no children.

Her temperature was 38.3°C, pulse 125 beats per minute, blood pressure 95/65 mmHg and oxygen saturation 92% on room air. Chest examination demonstrated coarse crepitations throughout both lung fields.

Investigations:

haemoglobin 123 g/L (115–165)	potassium 5.1 mmol/L (3.5–5.0)
white cell count 18.9 × 10⁹/L (4–11)	urea 13.5 mmol/L (2.5–7.5)
neutrophils 14.4 × 10⁹/L (1.5–7.0)	creatinine 87 μmol/L (45–90)
platelets 325 × 10⁹/L (150–400)	C-reactive protein 345 mg/L (<5)
sodium 132 mmol/L (135–145)	

bilirubin 20 mmol/L (1–22)
alanine transaminase 75 U/L (5–35)
alkaline phosphatase 60 U/L (45–105)

Chest X-ray: see **Figure 6.5**

What is the most likely causative organism?

A   *Legionella pneumophilia*
B   *Mycoplasma pneumoniae*
C   *Moraxella catarrhalis*
D   *Chlamydia psittaci*
E   *Streptococcus pneumoniae*

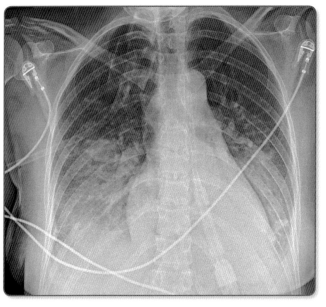

Figure 6.5

15. A 26-year-old man from Somalia presented to the emergency department after a fifth episode of haemoptysis over the preceding 24 hours. The last episode was 200 mL of fresh blood. He had lost approximately 12 kg of weight over the last 2 months and had fever and night sweats over that period.

On examination, he had a temperature of 37.8°C with a blood pressure of 105/68 mmHg and pulse 110 beats per minute. Focal crackles were heard over the upper right thorax.

Investigations:

haemoglobin 82 g/L (130–180)	potassium 3.2 mmol/L (3.5–5.0)
mean corpuscular volume 88 fL (80–96)	urea 6.4 mmol/L (2.5–7.5)
white cell count 8.6 × 10⁹/L (4–11)	creatinine 45 μmol/L (60–110)
platelets 287 × 10⁹/L (150–400)	C-reactive protein 32 mg/L (<5)
sodium 139 mmol/L (135–145)	

Chest X-ray: see **Figure 6.6**

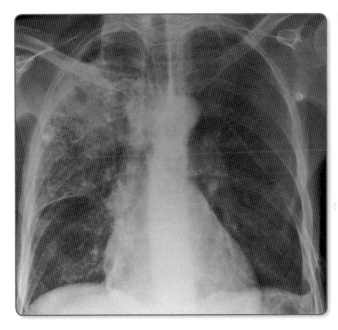

Figure 6.6

What is the next most appropriate management step?

A Bronchoalveolar lavage
B Commence intravenous co-amoxiclav and clarithromycin
C Commence oral rifampicin, isoniazid, pyrazinamide and ethambutol
D CT of the thorax
E Pulmonary angiography and embolisation

16. A 68-year-old man with bronchiectasis presented with a 7-day history of progressive dyspnoea, fever and a cough productive of foul-smelling green sputum. He had been taking azithromycin three times per week, inhaled steroids and beta-agonists.

   His temperature was 38°C, blood pressure 90/65 mmHg, pulse 80 beats per minute and respiratory rate 20 breaths per minute. Examination revealed crackles throughout both lung fields with bronchial breathing at the left base.

Investigations:

haemoglobin 135 g/L (130–180)	potassium 4.3 mmol/L (3.5–5.0)
white cell count 12.7 × 10⁹/L (4–11)	urea 9.8 mmol/L (2.5–7.5)
neutrophils 10.8 × 10⁹/L (1.5–7.0)	creatinine 90 µmol/L (60–110)
platelets 238 × 10⁹/L (150–400)	C-reactive protein 189 mg/L (<5)
sodium 145 mmol/L (135–145)	

Chest X-ray: see **Figure 6.7**

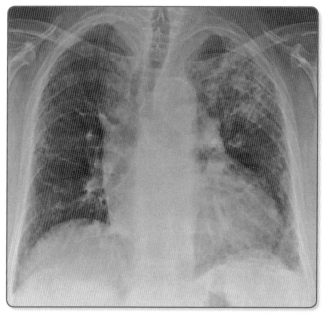

Figure 6.7

What is the most appropriate treatment?

A   Co-amoxiclav
B   Co-amoxiclav and clarithromycin
C   Doxycycline
D   Meropenem
E   Piperacillin–tazobactam

17. A 27-year-old man with acute myeloid leukaemia developed febrile neutropenia while in protective isolation 18 days after a reduced intensity allogeneic stem cell transplantation. He was started on piperacillin–tazobactam, gentamicin and vancomycin. He continued to be febrile at 48 hours and he was changed to meropenem and vancomycin. After a further 48 hours he was still febrile (38.5°C).

Examination revealed a Hickman line exiting the right anterior chest wall with a clean exit site but was otherwise unremarkable. His observations showed a blood pressure of 124/76 mmHg, pulse 90 beats per minute, respiratory rate 20 breaths per minute and oxygen saturation 98% on air.

Investigations:

haemoglobin 98 g/L (130–180)	creatinine 45 µmol/L (60–110)
white cell count 1.2 × 10⁹/L (4–11)	C-reactive protein 140 mg/L (<5)
neutrophils 0.0 × 10⁹/L (1.5–7.0)	Trough vancomycin levels 16.0 mg/dL
platelets 25 × 10⁹/L (150–400)	(in severe sepsis target range 15–20)
urea 6.7 mmol/L (2.5–7.5)	

Four sets of blood cultures showed no growth at 48 hours

What is the most appropriate next step in management?

A   Add co-trimoxazole
B   Give further dose of gentamicin
C   High-resolution CT of the thorax
D   Perform further set of blood cultures and observe
E   Remove Hickman line

18. A 24-year-old woman presented with a 24-hour history of coryza, myalgia, headache and fever. She denied breathlessness or sputum production. She was 24 weeks' pregnant but had no other past medical history.

She had a fever of 39.5°C, blood pressure 110/68 mmHg, pulse 95 beats per minute, respiratory rate 16 breaths per minute and oxygen saturation 98% on air. Examination revealed a clear chest, pink tympanic membranes and tonsillar arches with no evidence of exudate.

Investigations:

haemoglobin 114 g/L (115–165)	urea 6.7 mmol/L (2.5–7.5)
white cell count 6.8 × 10⁹/L (4–11)	creatinine 48 µmol/L (45–90)
neutrophils 1.6 × 10⁹/L (1.5–7.0)	C-reactive protein 54 mg/L (<5)
platelets 235 × 10⁹/L (150–400)	

Throat swab: normal oral flora

What is the next step in management?

A   Advice on rest and fluid rehydration
B   Amoxicillin
C   Co-amoxiclav and clarithromycin
D   Intravenous zanamivir
E   Oral oseltamivir

19. A 68-year-old man originally from Ghana presented with streaking haemoptysis in his sputum. He reported having a longstanding cough usually productive of grey sputum. This had previously been investigated and 2 years ago he was fully treated for a confirmed *Mycobacterium tuberculosis* infection. He was known to have chronic obstructive pulmonary disease and was taking Symbicort, tiotropium and salbutamol inhalers.

On examination he was well, with respiratory examination revealing only a prolonged expiratory phase but no added sounds. He was apyrexial, blood pressure 135/68 mmHg, pulse 68 beats per minute, respiratory rate 16 breaths per minute and oxygen saturation 96% on air.

Investigations:

haemoglobin 135 g/L (130–180)	urea 6.8 mmol/L (2.5–7.5)
white cell count 6.7 × 10^9/L (4–11)	creatinine 68 µmol/L (60–110)
platelets 345 × 10^9/L (150–400)	C-reactive protein 14 mg/L (<5)

Sputum microscopy, culture and sensitivities: normal oral flora

Chest X-ray (see **Figure 6.8**)

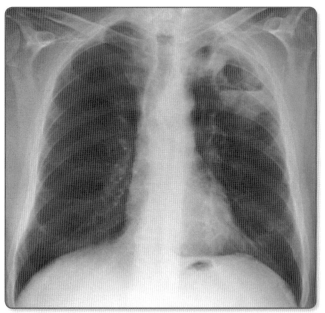

Figure 6.8

What is the next most appropriate step in management?

A   Cardiothoracic surgery opinion
B   CT of the thorax
C   Start intravenous liposomal amphotericin
D   Start oral fluconazole
E   Start rifampicin, isoniazid, pyrazinamide and ethambutol

20. A 28-year-old Somali man presented with a 2-month history of weight loss, fever, night sweats and a cough productive of grey sputum. He entered the country as an asylum seeker 6 months ago. In the past he was partially treated for tuberculosis in Somalia twice previously – at the age of 24 years and again at the age of 26 years.

Observations showed a temperature of 38°C, blood pressure 128/72 mmHg, pulse 90 beats per minute, respiratory rate 18 breaths per minute and oxygen saturation 98% on air. His weight was 51 kg and his height 173 cm. Examination of his chest revealed inspiratory crackles in the right upper zone.

Investigations:

haemoglobin 108 g/L (130–180)	urea 7.8 mmol/L (2.5–7.5)
white cell count 4.3 × 10⁹/L (4–11)	creatinine 45 μmol/L (60–110)
platelets 456 × 10⁹/L (150–400)	C-reactive protein 51 mg/L (<5)

Sputum microscopy, culture and sensitivities: normal oral flora
Sputum acid-fast bacilli: 3+

Chest X-ray: consolidation in right upper zone, calcified nodule in left upper zone

The patient was commenced on rifampicin, isoniazid, pyrazinamide, ethambutol, moxifloxacin and streptomycin.

What is next most appropriate management step?

A   Discharge home with directly observed therapy (DOT)
B   Discharge home with outpatient appointment in 2 weeks
C   Negative pressure side room admission for the first 2 weeks of therapy then DOT
D   Negative pressure side room admission until sputum culture negative
E   Side room admission for the first 2 weeks of therapy then DOT

21. A 21-year-old female student presented with a 4-day history of dysuria and a 24-hour history of fever, rigors and left loin pain. She attended the general practitioner several days ago and was prescribed oral cefuroxime but had had no relief. She reported having five to six episodes of urinary tract infections requiring antimicrobials over the last year.
     Observations showed a temperature of 38.5°C, blood pressure 95/55 mmHg, pulse 110 beats per minute, respiratory rate 16 breaths per minute and oxygen saturation 99% on air. Examination showed a clear chest and a soft abdomen but with tenderness in the left loin.

Investigations:

haemoglobin 126 g/L (115–165)	urea 5.6 mmol/L (2.5–7.5)
white cell count 15.8 × 10⁹/L (4–11)	creatinine 67 μmol/L (45–90)
neutrophils 13.1 × 10⁹/L (1.5–7.0)	C-reactive protein 308 mg/L (<5)
platelets 268 × 10⁹/L (150–400	

Urinalysis: 2+ leukocytes, 3+ nitrites, 1+ blood

Urine sputum microscopy, culture and sensitivities: E. coli (extended-spectrum β-lactamase producer)

What is the most appropriate management?

A   Intravenous cefuroxime
B   Intravenous co-amoxiclav
C   Intravenous meropenem
D   Intravenous piperacillin–tazobactam
E   Oral nitrofurantoin

22. A 34-year-old businessman who recently moved to the UK from Mumbai presented with a 7-day history of progressively worsening headache and fever and a 24-hour history of neck stiffness and photophobia. He denied any relevant past medical history.
     He had a temperature of 38°C, blood pressure 160/88 mmHg, pulse 80 beats per minute, respiratory rate 20 breaths per minute and oxygen saturation 99% on air. On examination, his Glasgow Coma Scale score was 14/15 and he appeared confused. His cranial and peripheral neurological examination detected no abnormalities.

Investigations:

haemoglobin 108 g/L (130–180)	potassium 4.1 mmol/L (3.5–5.0)
white cell count 5.6 × 10^9/L (4–11)	urea 7.6 mmol/L (2.5–7.5)
neutrophils 3.8 × 10^9/L (1.5–7.0)	creatinine 68 µmol/L (60–110)
platelets 346 × 10^9/L (150–400)	C-reactive protein 41 mg/L (<5)
sodium 131 mmol/L (135–145)	serum glucose 6.8 mmol/L (3.0–6.0)

CT of the brain: no space-occupying lesions, no acute bleed. Evidence of occipital leptomeningeal enhancement

Cerebrospinal fluid:	red cell count 10 × 10^6/L (<5)
white cell count 750 × 10^6/L (<5)	glucose 1.5 mmol/L (3.3–4.4)
lymphocytes 100 × 10^6/L	protein 1.8 g/L (0.15–0.45)

Microscopy: no organisms seen

Auramine and Ziehl–Neelsen smear: no organisms seen

What is the most appropriate next step in management?

A   Intravenous aciclovir
B   Intravenous ceftriaxone
C   Intravenous ceftriaxone and dexamethasone
D   Oral rifampicin, isoniazid, pyrazinamide and ethambutol
E   Oral rifampicin, isoniazid, pyrazinamide, ethambutol and dexamethasone

23. A 19-year-old male student presented with a 24-hour history of worsening headache, fever and photophobia. Over the last 2 hours he reported a rash appearing over his forearms. He denied any travel and was usually fit and well.

    On examination, he was febrile at 38.2°C and was lying in a darkened room. His Glasgow Coma Scale score was 15/15 and full neurological examination revealed no focal deficits. He had a purpuric non-blanching rash over his arms and shins. Fundoscopy showed clear disc margins bilaterally.

Investigations:

haemoglobin 156 g/L (130–180)	urea 5.6 mmol/L (2.5–7.5)
white cell count 18.8 × 10^9/L (4–11)	creatinine 88 µmol/L (60–110)
neutrophils 16.7 × 10^9/L (1.5–7.0)	C-reactive protein 248 mg/L (<5)
platelets 450 × 10^9/L (150–400)	

Liver function tests: normal
Blood clotting: normal

What is the most appropriate sequence of management?

A   Ceftriaxone, steroids, lumbar puncture, inform health protection unit
B   CT of the head, lumbar puncture, ceftriaxone, inform health protection unit
C   CT of the head, lumbar puncture, steroids, ceftriaxone
D   Lumbar puncture, ceftriaxone, steroids, inform health protection unit
E   Side room, lumbar puncture, steroids, ceftriaxone, inform health protection unit

24. A 27-year-old male triathlete presented with a 1-week history of fever and myalgia, and more recently a history of progressive breathlessness and cough.

On examination, he was febrile at 39°C, blood pressure 110/65 mmHg, pulse 95 beats per minute, respiratory rate 20 breaths per minute and oxygen saturation 92% on air. Auscultation of his thorax revealed focal crackles in his left lower zone. His abdomen was soft and non-tender.

Investigations:

haemoglobin 146 g/L (130–180)	creatinine 160 µmol/L (60–110)
white cell count 14.5 × 10⁹/L (4–11)	C-reactive protein 320 mg/L (<5)
neutrophils 13.9 × 10⁹/L (1.5–7.0)	creatine kinase 6729 U/L (25–195)
platelets 360 × 10⁹/L (150–400)	bilirubin 57 mmol/L (1–22)
sodium 134 mmol/L (135–145)	alanine transaminase 159 U/L (5–35)
potassium 4.4 mmol/L (3.5–5.0)	alkaline phosphatase 143 U/L (45–105)
urea 12.8 mmol/L (2.5–7.5)	albumin 23 g/L (37–49)

Urinalysis: 2+ protein, 3+ blood,

Chest X-ray: consolidation of left lower zone

What is the most likely causative organism?

A   *Haemophilus influenzae*
B   *Legionella pneumophilia*
C   *Leptospira interrogans*
D   *Mycoplasma pneumoniae*
E   *Streptococcus pneumoniae*

25. A 16-year-old boy with severe learning difficulties presented with nausea, vomiting and bloody diarrhoea. His mother reported that these symptoms had been progressing over the last 3–4 days, and he had no longer been able to go on his respite care group day trips. Other than his learning difficulties he had no medical history and took no regular medications.

On examination, he was afebrile with blood pressure 95/55 mmHg, pulse 95 beats per minute, respiratory rate 32 breaths per minute and oxygen saturation 99% on air. His chest was clear and his abdomen soft and non-tender. He had no neck stiffness or rash.

Investigations:

haemoglobin 69 g/L (130–180)	creatinine 325 µmol/L (60–110)
mean corpuscular volume 95 fL (80–96)	C-reactive protein 98 mg/L (<5)
white cell count 13.8 × 10⁹/L (4–11)	creatine kinase 105 U/L (25–195)
platelets 568 × 10⁹/L (150–400)	bilirubin 78 mmol/L (1–22)
sodium 143 mmol/L (135–145)	alanine transaminase 16 U/L (5–35)
potassium 4.3 mmol/L (3.5–5.0)	alkaline phosphatase 98 U/L (45–105)
urea 31 mmol/L (2.5–7.5)	albumin 35 g/L (37–49)

What is the most likely diagnosis?

A   *Clostridium difficile*
B   *Escherichia coli* O157
C   Leptospirosis
D   Norovirus
E   *Shigella* species

26. An 86-year-old female inpatient developed liquid diarrhoea opening her bowels 15 times in the past 24 hours. Ten days ago, she had been admitted to the orthopaedic ward for a fractured neck of femur. She had received cefuroxime and metronidazole perioperatively. Her past medical history included a previous peptic ulcer for which she was on omeprazole.

    Her temperature was 37.8°C, blood pressure 90/55 mmHg, pulse 105 beats per minute, respiratory rate 22 breaths per minute and oxygen saturation 98% on air. On examination, her abdomen was soft with tenderness in the left iliac fossa but no rebound or guarding. Her bowel sounds were hyperactive.

    Investigations:

haemoglobin 127 g/L (115–165)	creatinine 78 μmol/L (45–90)
white cell count 16.8 × 10⁹/L (4–11)	C-reactive protein 142 mg/L (<5)
neutrophils 14.9 × 10⁹/L (1.5–7)	bilirubin 6 mmol/L (1–22)
platelets 374 × 10⁹/L (150–400)	alanine transaminase 21 U/L (5–35)
sodium 149 mmol/L (135–145)	alkaline phosphatase 97 U/L (45–105)
potassium 3.8 mmol/L (3.5–5.0)	albumin 20 g/L (37–49)
urea 12.8 mmol/L (2.5–7.5)	

Stool microscopy, culture and sensitivities: no pathogens identified

What is the next step in management?

A   Intravenous immunoglobulins
B   Intravenous vancomycin
C   Oral metronidazole
D   Oral rifampicin
E   Oral vancomycin

27. A 43-year-old female travel writer presented with episodic creeping eruptions that were intensely pruritic. They could occur at any site on her body and would migrate for several centimetres over the course of several hours with an area of erythema around a track. She had no other past medical history.

    On examination her chest, abdomen and cardiovascular systems were normal. On her left calf there was a 4-cm serpiginous track with an area of 3–4 cm of erythema extending outwards. There were old excoriated areas in various locations on her body.

    Investigations:

haemoglobin 132 g/L (115-165)	platelets 213 × 10⁹/L (150–400)
white cell count 6.8 × 10⁹/L (4–11)	C-reactive protein 4 mg/L (<5)
neutrophils 4.9 × 10⁹/L (1.5–7.0)	creatine kinase 105 U/L (35–170)
eosinophils 1.2 × 10⁹/L (0.04–0.4)	

Urea and electrolytes and liver function tests: normal

What is the most likely diagnosis?

A   Cutaneous larva migrans
B   Filariasis
C   Loaiasis (*Loa loa*)
D   Schistosomiasis
E   Strongyloidiasis

28. A 35-year-old woman was referred by her primary care physician with raised transaminases, positive hepatitis B serology and a hepatitis B DNA level of 7000 IU/mL 3 months ago.

In the outpatient infectious diseases clinic nothing abnormal was detected on physical examination and vital observations were normal.

Investigations:

haemoglobin 110 g/L (115–165)	urea 6.8 mmol/L (2.5–7.5)
white cell count 5.9 × 10⁹/L (4–11)	creatinine 78 μmol/L (45–90)
platelets 190 × 10⁹/L (150–400)	C-reactive protein 5 mg/L (<5)

bilirubin 22 mmol/L (1–22)
alanine transaminase 95 U/L (5–35)
alkaline phosphatase 65 U/L (45–105)

Hepatitis B core antibody: positive
Hepatitis B surface antigen: positive
Hepatitis B e antigen: positive
Hepatitis B DNA: 24,000 IU/mL

What treatment regime is indicated?

A   Lamivudine
B   Entecavir
C   Pegylated interferon-α 2a
D   Pegylated interferon-α 2a plus ribavarin
E   None

29. A 31-year-old male doctor presented with a 4-week history of excessive flatulence, offensive belching and intermittent diarrhoea. He had returned from a 2-week trip around southern India at the same time as his symptoms had begun.

On examination, he was apyrexial and haemodynamically stable. His abdomen was soft and non-tender with no palpable organomegaly. The rest of his examination was normal.

Investigations:

haemoglobin 143 g/L (130–180)	platelets 198 × 10⁹/L (150–400)
white cell count 4.5 × 10⁹/L (4–11)	C-reactive protein 5 mg/L (<5)
neutrophils 3.9 × 10⁹/L (1.5–7.0)	

Urea and electrolytes and liver function tests: normal

Abdominal ultrasound: no abnormalities detected

What is the most appropriate next step in management?

A   Empirical metronidazole therapy
B   Entero-Test (string test)
C   Flexible sigmoidoscopy
D   Giardia serology
E   Stool ova, cyst and parasite examination

30. A 24-year-old male student from Peru presented with a self-terminating seizure during which there was urinary incontinence. The post-ictal phase was short-lived and he rapidly returned to normal. He had no past medical history and took no regular medications.

On examination, he was apyrexial and his observations were within normal parameters. Full neurological examination revealed no focal neurological deficits.

Investigations:

haemoglobin 128 g/L (130–180)	platelets 136 × 10⁹/L (150–400)
white cell count 4.6 × 10⁹/L (4–11)	C-reactive protein 5 mg/L (<5)
neutrophils 3.6 × 10⁹/L (1.5–7.0)	creatine kinase 969 U/L (25–195)

Urea and electrolytes and liver function tests: normal

Human immunodeficiency virus: negative

MRI of the brain (T2 weighted): see **Figure 6.9**

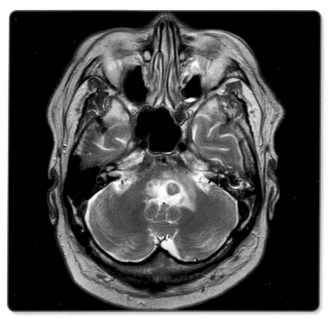

Figure 6.9

What is the most likely diagnosis?

A   Cerebral toxoplasmosis
B   Glioma
C   Neurocysticercosis
D   Progressive multifocal leukoencephalopathy
E   Racemose cyst

31. A 26-year-old male travel writer returned from a 3-month trip from Cape Town to Cairo with frank haematuria. He denied any dysuria, frequency, penile discharge or fever. He reported taking part in various outdoor activities including swimming in Lake Malawi. He reported taking over-the-counter praziquantel after this.

His observations showed a temperature of 36.8°C, blood pressure 120/65 mmHg, pulse 65 beats per minute, respiratory rate 16 breaths per minute and oxygen saturation 99% on air. Respiratory, cardiovascular, abdominal, genital and cutaneous examinations were normal.

Investigations:

haemoglobin 119 g/L (130–180)	eosinophils 1.0 × 10⁹/L (0.04–0.4)
white cell count 5.3 × 10⁹/L (4–11)	platelets 378 × 10⁹/L (150–400)
neutrophils 3.7 × 10⁹/L (1.5–7.0)	C-reactive protein 8 mg/L (<5)
Urea and electrolytes and liver function test: normal	

What is the most appropriate next step in management?

A   Flexible cystoscopy
B   Mid-stream urine for microscopy, culture and susceptibilities
C   Schistosomiasis serology
D   Stool for ova, cysts and parasites
E   Terminal stream urine for ultrafiltration and microscopy

32. A 16-year-old boy with sickle cell disease presented with bony pain in his left shin. This had been present for 1 week. He admitted to several episodes of fever over the preceding days. He had recently returned from a family trip to Nigeria.
    His observations showed a temperature of 38.3°C, blood pressure 145/75 mmHg, pulse 95 beats per minute, respiratory rate 18 breaths per minute and oxygen saturation 98% on air. On examination his chest was clear and his abdomen was soft with a 1-cm palpable spleen. His left anterior tibial plateau was hot with some overlying erythema.

Investigations:

haemoglobin 76 g/L (130–180)	potassium 4.1 mmol/L (3.5–5.0)
white cell count 17.8 × 10⁹/L (4–11)	urea 9.8 mmol/L (2.5–7.5)
neutrophils 15.9 × 10⁹/L (1.5–7.0)	creatinine 56 µmol/L (60–110)
platelets 687 × 10⁹/L (150–400)	C-reactive protein 178 mg/L (<5)
sodium 138 mmol/L (135–145)	creatine kinase 96 U/L (25–195)
Plain X-ray of the left leg: soft tissue oedema left leg with tibial periostitis	
Blood cultures: Gram-negative rod isolated at 12 hours	

What is the most likely pathogen?

A   *Brucella abortus*
B   *Pseudomonas aeruginosa*
C   *Salmonella* species
D   *Staphylococcus aureus*
E   *Streptococcus pyogenes*

33. A 17-year-old male student from the Ukraine presented with a 24-hour history of fever, odynophagia and dysphagia 3 days after returning from visiting his relatives.
    On examination, he was drooling and had a mucus discharge from his right nasal passage. Oropharyngeal examination revealed an adherent pseudomembrane on the tonsillar arch. There was cervical and submandibular lymphadenopathy. He had a temperature of 38.0°C, blood pressure 120/65 mmHg, pulse 55 beats per minute, respiratory rate 24 breaths per minute and oxygen saturation 98% on air.

Investigations:

haemoglobin 104 g/L (130–180)	platelets 647 × 10⁹/L (150–400)
white cell count 14.6 × 10⁹/L (4–11)	C-reactive protein 235 mg/L (<5)
neutrophils 12.9 × 10⁹/L (1.5–7.0)q	

Chest X-ray: normal

Electrocardiogram: first-degree heart block

What is the most appropriate next step in management?

A   Benzylpenicillin
B   Diphtheria antitoxin
C   Erythromycin
D   Metronidazole
E   Tetanus antitoxin

34. A 26-year-old male doctor presented with a needle-stick injury. He had been assisting in a laparotomy for a perforated bowel in an 86-year-old woman when a surgical needle had penetrated his glove and drew blood. He washed it profusely with soap and water immediately after the injury.
    On examination, he was anxious but otherwise well. There was a small puncture mark on his left thumb.

What is the most appropriate immediate management step for the doctor?

A   Administration of a hepatitis B booster vaccination
B   Administration of hepatitis B immunoglobulin
C   Baseline HIV, HBV and HCV testing
D   Hepatitis B sAb testing and a save serum sent from the doctor
E   The affected doctor should return to the 86-year-old woman and request permission to test her for HIV, HBV and HCV

35. A 26-year-old businessman returned from a 1-month trip to Thailand with a short history of fever, myalgia and a transient maculopapular rash. He admitted to spending the majority of his time in Bangkok frequenting brothels and only intermittently used condoms. His last sexual health screen just prior to this trip was normal.
    His observations showed a temperature of 37.8°C, blood pressure 130/65 mmHg, pulse 68 beats per minute, respiratory rate 16 breaths per minute and oxygen saturation 99% on air. On examination, he had a clear chest and soft abdomen. He had cervical lymphadenopathy and inspection of his oropharynx revealed oral candidiasis.

Investigations:

haemoglobin 126 g/L (130–180)	neutrophils 3.1 × 10⁹/L (1.5–7.0)
white cell count 3.2 × 10⁹/L (4–11)	platelets 120 × 10⁹/L (150–400)

Urea and electrolytes and liver function tests: normal

Malaria film and malarial antigen test: negative

Human immunodeficiency virus rapid diagnostic test: negative

What is the next most appropriate investigation?

A   CD4 count
B   HIV antibody testing

C HIV p24 antigen
D HIV resistance testing
E HIV viral load quantification

36. A 36-year-old man presented with a 48-hour history of fever 7 days after return from visiting his relatives in Botswana. A full systems review revealed no other symptoms.
    He had a temperature of 38.5°C, pulse 110 beats per minute, blood pressure 110/65 mmHg and oxygen saturation 99% on air. His chest was clear and his abdomen was soft with no organomegaly. He was cachectic and on inspection of the oropharynx had oral thrush. Examination of his skin revealed a large black skin lesion on his upper arm.

Investigations:

haemoglobin 145 g/L (130–180)	C-reactive protein 31 mg/L (<5)
white cell count 16.9 × 10⁹/L (4–11)	bilirubin 7 mmol/L (1–22)
neutrophils 16.1 × 10⁹/L (1.5–7.0)	alanine transaminase 30 U/L (5–35)
lymphocytes 0.1 × 10⁹/L (1.5–4.0)	alkaline phosphatase 98 U/L (45–105)
platelets 389 × 10⁹/L (150–400)	albumin 32 g/L (37–49)

Urea and electrolytes: normal

Urine dip: 1+ protein

First malaria film: no parasites seen

Blood cultures: Gram-negative bacilli in both bottles at 12 hours

What is the most likely diagnosis?

A Enteric fever
B HIV seroconversion
C Malaria
D Non-typhi salmonellosis
E Urological sepsis

37. A 31-year-old man from Australia presented with a 2-month history of an ulcer on his left calf which had been steadily growing in size. It was not painful and not pruritic. He had not had any previous similar lesions. He arrived in the UK from Victoria, Australia 3 months ago.
    On examination, there was a 3 × 4 cm deep ulcer with ragged undermined edges extending several centimetres beyond the visible wound. Probing the wound did not elicit pain. Otherwise examination was normal.

Investigations:

haemoglobin 129 g/L (130–180)	C-reactive protein 9 mg/L (<5)
white cell count 6.7 × 10⁹/L (4–11)	random glucose 5.6 mmol/L (3.0–6.0)
platelets 256 × 10⁹/L (150–400)	

Urea and electrolytes and liver function tests: normal

What is the most likely diagnosis?

A Buruli ulcer
B Diabetic ulcer
C Leishmaniasis
D Lepromatous leprosy
E *Mycobacterium marinum*

38. A 25-year-old woman presented 4 weeks after a trip to Belize with a non-healing lesion on her left forearm. She denied any fever or night sweats and had been otherwise well. She had tried topical over-the-counter emollients and had had two courses of antimicrobials from her general practitioner with no improvement.

On examination, there was a 3-cm-diameter, roughly circular lesion with rolled edges ulcerating through the dermis. There was a smaller 2 to 3-mm satellite lesion adjacent to the main ulcer. Inspection of the oropharynx was normal, as was abdominal examination.

Investigations:

haemoglobin 135 g/L (115–165)	C-reactive protein 14 mg/L (<5)
white cell count 7.1×10^9/L (4–11)	glucose 4.9 mmol/L (3.0–6.0)
platelets 281×10^9/L (150–400)	
Urea and electrolytes and liver function tests: normal	

What is the most likely diagnosis?

A   Ecthyma
B   Erysipelas
C   Impetigo
D   Leishmaniasis
E   *Mycobacterium marinum*

39. A 41-year-old woman presented with a 5-day history of myalgia, fever and headache 7 days after return from her honeymoon in Sri Lanka. She took Malarone daily and was vaccinated for hepatitis A and typhoid fever before embarking on her trip.

Her observations showed temperature 39°C, pulse 110 beats per minute, blood pressure 95/55 mmHg and oxygen saturation 99% on air. On examination, there was a fine, macular rash on her torso but otherwise chest, abdominal and neurological examination was normal.

Investigations:

haemoglobin 138 g/L (115–165)	alkaline phosphatase 87 U/L (45–105)
white cell count 3.2×10^9/L (4–11)	albumin 36 g/L (37–49)
neutrophils 1.1×10^9/L (1.5–7.0)	serum glucose 6.1 mmol/L (3.0–6.0)
platelets 100×10^9/L (150–400)	fibrinogen 2.8 g/L (1.8–5.4 g/L)
C-reactive protein 25 mg/L (<5)	prothrombin time 12 s (11.5–15.5)
bilirubin 8 mmol/L (1–22)	activated partial thromboplastin time 31 s (30–40)
alanine aminotransferase 59 U/L (5–35)	
First malaria film: negative	
Cerebrospinal fluid:	protein 0.30 g/L (0.15–0.45)
white cell count <1 x 10^6/L (<5)	glucose 5.2 mmol/L (3.3–4.4)
red cell count <1 × 10^6/L (<5)	

What is the most appropriate next step in management?

A   Fresh frozen plasma
B   Intravenous ceftriaxone
C   Intravenous fluids
D   Intravenous quinine
E   Intravenous zanamivir

40. A 38-year-old woman returned from a 2-week honeymoon in the Seychelles with a 3-day history of fever and marked arthralgia of the knees and small joints of the hand. She stated that she took regular malaria prophylaxis and received the correct vaccinations.

    On examination, she had a faint macular rash predominantly over her torso. Examination of her hands revealed a good range of movements and no palpable pannus. There was no discernible joint effusion in either knee. Otherwise examination was normal.

Investigations:

haemoglobin 125 g/L (115–165)	platelets 347 × 10⁹/L (150–400)
white cell count 4.1 × 10⁹/L (4–11)	C-reactive protein 21 mg/L (<5)
Urea and electrolytes and liver function tests: normal	

What is the most likely diagnosis?

A   Chikungunya
B   HIV seroconversion
C   Japanese encephalitis
D   O'nyong-nyong
E   Syphilis

41. A 32-year-old man originally from Brazil and recently arrived in the UK presented with a 48-hour history of a rash preceded by 4 days of myalgia, itchy eyes and fever. He described the rash as starting on his scalp before spreading to his thorax and limbs. He lived with his wife and 5-year-old son.

    He had a temperature of 38.8°C, pulse 100 beats per minute, blood pressure 130/75 mmHg and oxygen saturation 99% on air. On examination, he had a diffuse maculopapular rash extending across his face, torso and proximal limbs. Inspection of his oropharynx was normal. There was no palpable adenopathy.

Investigations:

haemoglobin 168 g/L (130–180)	platelets 378 × 10⁹/L (150–400)
white cell count 3.1 × 10⁹/L (4–11)	C-reactive protein 53 mg/L (<5)
Urea and electrolytes and liver function tests: normal	
Monospot: negative	

What is the most likely diagnosis?

A   HIV seroconversion
B   Infectious mononucleosis
C   Measles
D   Rubella
E   Syphilis

42. A 68-year-old man presented with a 24-hour history of confusion. He had no past medical history and took no regular medications.

    His temperature was 37.8°C, pulse 85 beats per minute, blood pressure 125/72 mmHg and oxygen saturation 99% on air. On examination his respiratory, cardiological and abdominal examination was normal. Neurological examination showed no cranial or peripheral signs. Abbreviated Mental Test Score was 4/10. Examination of the skin revealed healing scabs below the knee on the left lateral aspect.

Investigations:

haemoglobin 138 g/L (130–180)	platelets 265 × 10⁹/L (150–400)
white cell count 6.8 × 10⁹/L (4–11)	C-reactive protein 21 mg/L (<5)
neutrophils 3.8 × 10⁹/L (1.5–7.0)	serum glucose 6.5 mmol/L (3.0–6.0)

Urea and electrolytes and liver function tests: normal

Urine dipstick: negative

CT of the brain with contrast: no acute haemorrhage. No infarct

Cerebrospinal fluid:	red cell count 13 × 106/L (<5)
white cell count 482 x 10⁶/L (<5)	protein 0.7 g/L (0.15–0.45)
mononuclear 90%	glucose 4.5 mmol/L (3.3–4.4)

What is the most likely diagnosis?

A   Bacterial meningitis
B   Herpes simplex virus (HSV) encephalitis
C   Neuroborreliosis
D   Tuberculous meningitis
E   Varicella-zoster virus (VZV) encephalitis

43. A 56-year-old man presented with a 1-week history of fever and a 1-day history of confusion. According to his next of kin he returned from a 2-month trip to Ghana 2 weeks ago, where he was visiting relatives.

He had a temperature of 38.7°C, pulse 110 beats per minute, blood pressure 140/85 mmHg, respiratory rate 24 beats per minute and oxygen saturation 99% on air. There was neck stiffness but no focal neurological deficit. His chest and abdominal examinations were normal. There was no rash and inspection of his oropharynx was normal.

Investigations:

haemoglobin 119 g/L (130–180)	urea 10.5 mmol/L (2.5–7.5)
white cell count 5.4 × 10⁹/L (4–11)	creatinine 129 µmol/L (60–110)
platelets 56 × 10⁹/L (150–400)	C-reactive protein 13 mg/L (<5)

Liver function tests: normal

Malaria film: 3% *Plasmodium falciparum* trophozoites

What is the most appropriate next management step?

A   CT of the brain
B   Intravenous artesunate
C   Intravenous quinine
D   Lumbar puncture
E   Oral quinine

44. A National Health Service trust plans to introduce a new test for *Clostridium difficile*, which is cheaper than the test currently used. The ward is trialling this new test on samples sent from patients. There is concern about the validity of a negative result, since patients are being moved out of side rooms when they might still have *C. difficile*. This is discussed with the laboratory and data are collected comparing new and old (gold standard) tests. The data are depicted in the table below.

	Old test positive	Old test negative	
New test positive	3	1	75%
New test negative	3	15	83%
	50%	94%	

What is the calculated negative predictive value of the new test?

A   20%
B   50%
C   75%
D   83%
E   94%

45. A 58-year-old man was 7 days postoperative from a Hartmann's procedure for perforated diverticulitis. He had been on broad spectrum antimicrobials since the operation. He had had further fevers for the previous 48 hours despite escalating the antimicrobial therapy, and the surgical team has requested a medical review.

   On examination, he had a temperature of 38.5°C, pulse 115 beats per minute, blood pressure 105/65 mmHg, respiratory rate 22 beats per minute and oxygen saturation 97% on air. He had a peripherally inserted central venous catheter (PICC) in situ for total parenteral nutrition which had only been inserted 48 hours ago and looked clean. He had a urethral catheter in situ which had been replaced 3 days before, and the urine had no obvious sediment. Chest examination was normal. Abdominal examination demonstrated mild tenderness around the operative site but his abdomen was soft and there were active bowel sounds.

Investigations:

haemoglobin 97 g/L (130–180)   platelets 568 × 10⁹/L (150–400)
white cell count 13.3 × 10⁹/L (4–11)   C-reactive protein 155 mg/L (<5)

Urea and electrolytes and liver function tests: normal
Blood cultures taken 48 hours ago: no growth at 2 days
Mid-stream urine taken 48 hours ago: no growth

Chest radiograph taken today: no focal lung opacification

What is the most likely diagnosis?

A   Central venous catheter infection
B   Healthcare associated pneumoniae
C   Healthcare associated influenza
D   Urethral catheter associated urinary tract infection
E   Disseminated candidiasis

Answers

1.   A   Disseminated gonococcal infection (DGI)

This presentation most likely indicates an infective or post-infective picture and of those listed Reiter's syndrome, DGI or HIV seroconversion would fit with the 4-week timeline. DGI occurs in 1–2% of gonococcal infections and is caused by haematogenous spread of the bacteria from the initially infected mucosal membranes. DGI presents with a migratory polyarthralgia, particularly affecting the knees, elbows and often more distal joints, and can be associated with a tenosynovitis commonly affecting the wrist or Achilles flexor tendon sheaths. The cutaneous manifestations consist of painful maculopapular through to pustular lesions, and are usually peripherally located. Culture of the gonococcus is rare, particularly after administration of antimicrobial agents and polymerase chain reaction-based techniques from either mucosal/genital swabs or joint aspirates are needed. DGI necessitates a 7- to 14-day course of a third- or fourth-generation cephalosporin.

Secondary syphilis usually manifests several months after the initial painless ulcer of primary disease. Positive TPPA (*Treponema pallidum* particle agglutination) and enzyme immunoassay represent exposure of the patient to syphilis, and will remain positive for life even if the disease is treated. RPR (rapid plasma reagin) or VDRL (Venereal Disease Reference Laboratory) is a non-treponemal test that represents a measure of activity and active disease usually gives a positive RPR/VDRL titre. Reiter's syndrome includes a triad of a large joint inflammatory arthritis (commonly affecting the knee or sacroiliac joint, less likely to affect the small joints of the hand), ocular inflammation (a uveitis or conjunctivitis), and either a urethritis in men or a cervicitis in women. HIV seroconversion can present with a rash (which may be papular or maculopapular), fever and although arthropathy can be associated with HIV this usually only becomes apparent with CD4 counts less than 200 rather than as part of a seroconversion complex.

Rice PA. Gonococcal arthritis (disseminated gonococcal infection). Infect Dis Clin North Am 2005; 19(4):853–861.

2.   C   Cerebral toxoplasmosis

The patient has presented with what appears to be advanced HIV disease and is likely to have a CD4 count of well below 200. In addition to the neurological diagnosis, the history suggests opportunistic infections of the gastrointestinal system (which include *Cyclospora, Isospora, Microsporidium* and *Cryptosporidium* species in HIV-positive patients), eyes (particularly cytomegalovirus, toxoplasmosis and tuberculosis) and there is significant oral candidiasis.

In patients with advanced HIV, neurological presentations have a wide differential diagnosis and all the answers listed must be considered. The MRI appearance of multiple, thin-walled, ring-enhancing lesions with little oedema strongly suggests a diagnosis of cerebral toxoplasmosis. Definitive diagnosis can be obtained only with a neurosurgical or stereotactic biopsy, although circumstantial evidence can be gathered less invasively. In this case toxoplasmosis serology would be useful (and likely to show a strong dye test reaction), and a serum cryptococcal antigen would be negative.

This patient needs referral to an HIV centre, pyramethamine–sulfadiazine antitoxoplasmosis therapy and a reducing course of steroids for her cerebral disease with an urgent ophthalmological review. Antiretroviral therapy must be considered once the opportunistic infections are diagnosed and treatment commenced.

Contini C. Clinical and diagnostic management of toxoplasmosis in the immunocompromised patient. Parasitologia 2008; 50(1-2):45–50.

3.   B   Intravenous ceftriaxone and neurosurgical opinion

This is likely to be a pyogenic spinal/paraspinal infection that needs broad-spectrum antimicrobial therapy and an urgent neurosurgical opinion both to consider drainage of the collection and for possible stabilisation of the spine.

Streptococcus bovis and the *S. milleri* group of streptococci (*S. anginosus, S. constellatus* and *S. intermedius*) are all Gram-positive cocci and are frequently associated with abscesses. When these bacteria are isolated from sources outside the lumen of the gut, a search for a gastrointestinal malignancy should also be initiated as their movement to distal tissues usually indicates a gut mucosal disruption.

The duration of the symptomatology and marked weight loss may well point to an underlying gut cancer warranting further investigation once the spine has been stabilised and the sepsis syndrome controlled. The alternative to a malignant process would be a mycobacterial infection, possibly ileal tuberculosis (TB). However, the short duration of fever is likely to represent cytokine activation by the pyogenic collection and goes against a tuberculous diagnosis. Initiation of antituberculous therapy is a considered intervention and the indications to start this in the acute setting without suggestive microbiology are limited to TB meningitis.

Gelfand MS, Bakhtian BJ, Simmons BP. Spinal sepsis due to *Streptococcus milleri*: two cases and review. Rev Infect Dis 1991; 13(4):559–563.

4. D Rhinocerebral mucormycosis

Rhinocerebral mucormycosis is an opportunistic infection of the sinuses and brain caused by saprophytic fungi. The infection can rapidly result in death if urgent surgical debridement is not available. CT recognition of mucormycosis is facilitated by a clinical story of rapid progression of sinofacial disease with a background of immunosuppression or diabetes. Evidence of bone destruction on CT, historically a strong pointer towards *Mucor/Zygomycetes* species, is considered a late finding. Swabs sent for microscopy, culture and sensitivities usually show mixed upper respiratory tract flora and only if the clinician asks for a fungal stain and culture will laboratory results be helpful. Aggressive urgent debridement by an ENT surgeon is the mainstay of therapy, and can result in marked disfigurement of the patient. Medical care should focus on reversal of the immunocompromising state where possible – or in this case normalisation of blood sugar, in conjunction with aggressive antifungal therapy.

Nasal diphtheria produces few symptoms other than a watery or bloody discharge. There is often a small membrane visible in the nasal passages.

Orbital cellulitis is an ophthalmic emergency and often presents with erythema and oedema of the eyelids, ophthalmoplegia, fever, pain and a pink eye. Severe infections can spread to adjacent posterior ethmoidal cells which lie close to the optic canal and hence orbital cellulitis can quickly threaten sight.

Safar A, et al. Early identification of rhinocerebral mucormycosis. J Otolaryngol 2005; 34(3):166–171.

5. A Lassa fever

There are four main viral haemorrhagic fever viruses – Lassa, Ebola, Marburg and Crimean–Congo. While the first three are predominantly confined to sub-Saharan Africa, the latter has a much wider geographical area of endemicity. All four of the viral haemorrhagic fevers can present with undifferentiated fever (i.e. no other localising signs or symptoms) although pharyngitis, conjunctivitis, a faint morbilliform rash, or headache and confusion may all appear as the disease progresses. The incubation period can be up to 21 days, but more frequently less than 14 days. Lassa fever specifically is endemic in West Africa with occasional epidemics. It is transmitted by contact with infected rodent urine or droppings. As with all the viral haemorrhagic fevers, person-to-person transmission through bodily fluids is possible and care of these patients is hazardous. Thrombocytopaenia and deranged clotting (in particular the activated partial prothrombin time) is common. Definitive diagnosis is through specialist public health laboratories, and where cases are suspected close liaison with infectious diseases and public health consultants is needed prior to any blood samples being taken from a patient. Management is supportive only, but should be undertaken by specialists at a national level, and only conducted in a high-level isolation unit. Mortality is particularly high.

Epstein–Barr virus and cytomegalovirus can also both present with undifferentiated fever, but more likely is an infectious-mononucleosis-like illness with cervical adenopathy. The monospot test detects heterophile antibodies and although reasonably specific for Epstein–Barr virus has only a 70–90% sensitivity – the negative test in this case makes infective mononucleosis less likely but does not exclude it.

Malaria is common in West Africa and although often presents as undifferentiated fever, is associated with thrombocytopaenia, but on the whole no clotting abnormalities. Typhoid fever is also common in West Africa and also presents with fever and few other signs and symptoms, but thrombocytopaenia and leukopaenia is rare (indeed neutrophilia is more common) and clotting is preserved.

Moore LS, Moore M, Sriskandan S. Ebola and other viral haemorrhagic fevers: a local operational approach. Br J Hosp Med. 2014;75:515–22.

6.   D *Staphylococcus aureus*

The most common causes of intraparenchymal lung abscesses in the UK are *Klebsiella pneumoniae*, the milleri streptococci and *Staphylococcus aureus*. In south-east Asia *Burkholderia pseudomallei*, the causative organism of malleoidosis, should also be considered. This organism is the second most common cause of pneumonia after *Streptococcus pneumoniae* and requires use of broader-spectrum antimicrobials for community-acquired pneumonia in this district. The preceding history of recurrent boils and furuncles, with the now rapid progression of respiratory symptoms, makes a Panton–Valentine leukocidin-producing strain of *Staphylococcus aureus* the most likely causative organism. These strains are well documented to be transmitted by close bodily contact, particularly in close contact sports (such as judo). Identifying Panton–Valentine leukocidin-producing *S. aureus* from clinical indicators early in the course of the presentation can markedly change antimicrobial management. The Health Protection Agency has released specific guidance on this matter as outlined in the further reading below.

The lung abscesses caused by *Klebsiella pneumonia* and the milleri streptococci are usually a little more indolent. The former is the cause of Friedlander's pneumonia, whereas the latter can occur in isolation from oropharyngeal aspiration or as part of a more disseminated abscess formation, often from a source further down the gastrointestinal tract.

Streptococcus pneumoniae most frequently causes a lobar pneumonia, rarely causing intraparenchymal abscesses. Group A streptococcus is a rare cause of lower respiratory tract infections, more commonly causing upper respiratory tract pathology and also skin and skin structure infections.

Health Protection Agency. Guidance on the diagnosis and management of PVL-associated *Staphylococcus aureus* infections (PVL-SA) in England, 2nd edn. London: Health Protection Agency, 2008.

7.   E Type 2 necrotising fasciitis

The rapid soft tissue progression with systemic compromise suggests a diagnosis more severe than cellulitis. Necrotising infections can broadly be divided into three groups. Type 1 (or Meleney's) occurs following trauma or surgery and often begins as a simple periwound superficial infection before rapid subsequent systemic disturbance. Type 1 fasciitis is polymicrobial in nature with bacterial synergy propagating the disease process. This means that breadth of antimicrobial cover with urgent plastic surgical debridement is key.

Fournier's gangrene is similarly polymicrobial and is typically described as occurring in the anogenital area, arising most frequently in diabetic patients. Similar breadth of antimicrobial cover with early involvement of a urologist is necessary.

Type 2 necrotising fasciitis is typically monomicrobial and is most commonly caused by group A streptococci, although *Staphylococcus aureus* can also cause this process with toxin production causing the extensive local tissue damage. This commonly presents with rapid progression of skin erythema and disproportionate pain with or without surgical emphysema on examination. Antimicrobial therapy should be directed towards Gram-positive organisms with high-dose penicillin/flucloxacillin [unless MRSA (meticillin-resistant *S. aureus*) is suspected] with synergistic aminoglycoside use but importantly also with a toxin production-inhibiting antimicrobials such as high-dose clindamycin. Again, early plastic surgical involvement is of high importance.

Type 3 necrotising fasciitis is typically caused by Gram negative organisms from marine environments, such as *Vibrio vulnificus* or *Aeromonas hydrophilia*.

Antimicrobials, although beneficial, will not reverse the metabolic upset and should be selected based upon whether the presentation is more in keeping with a type 1, 2 or 3 necrotising fasciitis picture. The addition of clindamycin to the regimen, particularly in high doses, aids in halting toxin production from the causative pathogens at a ribosomal level. Transfer to theatre and surgical incision should not be delayed pending imaging – necrotising fasciitis is a surgical emergency and even small delays can increase the area of tissue needing to be debrided and the associated mortality rate.

Davoudian P. Necrotising fasciitis. Cont Ed Anaes Crit Care Pain 2012;12:245–250.
Wong CH, et al. The LRINEC (Laboratory Risk Indicator for Necrotizing Fasciitis) score: a tool for distinguishing necrotizing fasciitis from other soft tissue infections. Crit Care Med 2004; 32:1535–1541.

8.   D   *Pasteurella multocida*

Cat and dog bites can lead to both severe local soft tissue infections and systemic infective syndromes. This case describes a cellulitic process that is slowly developing systemic compromise and is due to a Gram-negative organism. *Pasteurella* species is the stereotypical pathogen from domesticated animal bites and is usually successfully treated with co-amoxiclav which in addition will cover a wealth of other pathogens that may also be present. On occasion *Pasteurella* species can cause a more deep-seated local infection including osteomyelitis and has been documented to cause endocarditis following animal bites.

Capnocytophaga canimorsus is also a commensal of cat and dog oropharynges but is a much rarer cause of human disease following bites. It usually causes a rapid systemic collapse, frequently complicated by disseminated intravascular coagulopathy.

Eikenella corrodens is a commensal of the human oropharynx and causes indolent infections following human bites and also in intravenous drug users who lick their needles. This pathogen is one of the HACEK group of organisms (*Haemophilus* species, *Aggregatibacter* species, *Cardiobacterium hominis*, *Eikenella corrodens* and *Kingella kingae*) and is well documented as a cause of endocarditis.

Staphylococcus aureus and group A streptococci are Gram-positive organisms and are well documented as causes of cellulitis. They most frequently enter the subcutaneous tissues though cuts, grazes, microabrasions or onychogryphotic nails. These two pathogens can cause infective processes following bites but are more commonly encountered following human rather than animal bites.

Oehler RL, et al. Bite-related and septic syndromes caused by cats and dogs. Lancet Infect Dis 2009; 9(7):439–447.

9.   B   Vancomycin and gentamicin and rifampicin

This vignette describes a case of early (ie <12 months) prosthetic valve endocarditis. The hypotension and tachycardia mean that antimicrobial therapy cannot be delayed until the causative organism is identified and empirical antimicrobial therapy must be instigated in the emergency department. A cardiothoracic opinion should be urgently explored to determine the risk/benefit of early versus late valve surgery. Formal echocardiography is needed, and in conjunction with the surgeons the degree of anticoagulation will need to be reviewed to minimise the risk of embolic phenomena from the valvular vegetation.

The most common causes of early prosthetic valve endocarditis are staphylococci (including *Staphylococcus aureus*, meticillin resistant *S. aureus* (MRSA), and coagulase-negative staphylococci), streptococci, and enterococci. The antimicrobial regime necessarily has to remain broad and include cover for resistant pathogens (such as MRSA). The regime advocated by the European Society of Cardiology is vancomycin, gentamicin and rifampicin. Care must be taken to monitor levels as nephrotoxicity may otherwise occur.

Empirical therapy for native valve endocarditis, or late (i.e. >12 months) prosthetic valve endocarditis is suggested to be ampicillin with flucloxacillin and gentamicin. Confirmed

Staphylococcus aureus (meticillin susceptible) can be treated with flucloxacillin alone, whilst enterococcal endocarditis can be treated with ampicillin with ceftriaxone and streptococcal endocarditis by benzylpenicillin. These treatment regimes should be discussed with infection specialists, and titrated according to susceptibility testing.

Habib G et al. 2015 ESC Guidelines for the management of infective endocarditis. Euro Heart J. 2015;36(44):3075–3123.

10. E MRI of the foot and surgical debridement with biopsy

The foot X-ray shows periosteal reaction at the base of the first metatarsophalangeal joint with marrow oedema. Diabetic foot ulcers should be managed by those with a specialist interest in a multidisciplinary team involving diabetologists, vascular surgeons, and infectious disease physicians or clinical microbiologists. Limb retention with local debridement and prolonged courses of antimicrobials can be attempted, but amputations are still sometimes necessary. Clarification of whether there is bone involvement is necessary and is most easily achieved through MRI. The polymicrobial nature of these wounds means that deep tissue samples (or preferably bone samples where there is an osteomyelitis) should have full culture and susceptibility performed to allow directed antimicrobial therapy. This increases both the effectiveness of the antimicrobial regimen but also reduces side effects and adverse events from unnecessary antibiotics, including development of resistant organisms and *Clostridium difficile* infections.

Where empirical antimicrobial therapy is indicated – i.e. in the case of presentation of diabetic foot with systemic compromise – the choice of antimicrobials should cover both Gram-positive and Gram-negative pathogens as well as anaerobes. Common regimens include ciprofloxacin and clindamycin or ceftriaxone and metronidazole.

Scottish Intercollegiate Guideline Network. Management of Diabetes. Guideline 116. Edinburgh: SIGN, 2010.

11. C Neuroborreliosis

Neuroborreliosis is one of the more severe presentations of Lyme disease. Lyme disease can broadly be divided into early local manifestations (such as the typical erythema migrans target-like lesions), early disseminated complications (including meningitis, facial nerve palsies and encephalitis) and late complications (including arthritis and acrodermatitis chronicum atrophicans). Meningitis typically results in a cellular cerebrospinal fluid (CSF) with mononuclear cells predominating and a raised CSF protein. CSF can be sent for western blotting to detect *Borrelia burgdorferi*-specific proteins, whereas serum may reveal an antibody response. The international epidemiological picture of infected tick prevalence and locations of documented human case changes and updates can be found on both the Public Health England and Centre for Communicable Disease Control websites. Guidelines on the treatment of Lyme disease and post-tick-bite prophylaxis have recently been published as outlined in the further reading sections.

Mycobacterium tuberculosis meningitis is a possibility but the isolated cranial nerve palsy does not quite fit and the CSF white cell count is less than that expected as is the CSF protein. CSF polymerase chain reaction for *M. tuberculosis* is available but lacks specificity and a large volume sample (6–8 mL) for mycobacterial culture is still the recommended diagnostic path.

Stanek G, et al. Lyme borreliosis: clinical case definitions for diagnosis and management in Europe. Clin Microbiol Infect 2011; 17(1):69–79.

12. A Bronchoscopy and endobronchial ultrasound-guided biopsy

The history presented suggests either malignancy – most likely to be primary lung cancer – or post-primary pulmonary tuberculosis (TB). The latter is probably more likely and may well have reactivated given the steroid use over the preceding few months. The examination indicates erythema nodosum, of which TB is a recognised cause – other causes are somewhat excluded by the other investigation results.

The key to diagnosis of TB is through biopsy, histology and microbiological culture. A bronchoscopy with endobronchial ultrasound-guided biopsy will facilitate this and provide a specimen for histopathology which will help to exclude malignancy. Bronchoalveolar lavage can be performed for mycobacterial culture.

Given that this patient is from an area of the world where TB is endemic a QuantiFERON® test will undoubtedly return a positive result and not be helpful. Similarly, a Mantoux test will be reactive and even if >15 mm would not provide enough evidence to avoid the need for bronchoscopy. A CT of the thorax in this patient is necessary but again will not provide a definitive diagnosis.

Amicosante M, Ciccozzi M, Markova R. Rational use of immunodiagnostic tools for tuberculosis infection: guidelines and cost effectiveness studies. New Microbiol 2010; 33(2):93–107.

13. E Send varicella-zoster serology from mother

The child in this case has a rash typical of varicella, a respiratory and contact-transmitted virus with a high secondary attack rate. In those born and brought up in northern Europe most will have encountered chickenpox as a child and will be immune, but in those from more equatorial regions the prevalence is lower and so adults often remain non-immune. Pregnant mothers and those with immunocompromised conditions with a significant exposure to varicella or a zoster rash must have their chickenpox history elucidated. Those who give a clear history of previous chickenpox can be considered to be immune – whether pregnant or otherwise immunocompromised. Those who do not give a clear history must have their varicella-zoster IgG sent urgently. If negative they may benefit from intravenous varicella immunoglobulin but if positive varicella-zoster IgG will not provide any additional benefit. Varicella-zoster IgG determination can be made and immunoglobulin given where necessary up to 10 days after the exposure.

Non-immune mothers who become infected and are not given immunoglobulin can develop fetal complications which are dependent upon gestation:

- Up to 20 weeks: risk of limb hypoplasia, microcephaly, cataracts, and fetal death.
- Second and third trimesters: ophthalmic complications, microcephaly, skin scaring.
- 1 week before to 1 week after gestation: neonatal varicella characterised by severe pneumonitis and hepatitis.

Oral aciclovir plays no role in pregnancy-associated varicella. Intravenous aciclovir may be indicated in neonatal varicella or if the mother develops complications of varicella disease. In non-vesicular rashes rubella and parvovirus should be considered but not in this case.

Department of Health. Immunisation against infectious disease. The Green Book. London: Department of Health, 2007.

14. A *Legionella pneumophilia*

This patient has a multi-lobar pneumonia with a hyponatraemia and a mild transaminitis, all fitting with an atypical cause of community acquired lower respiratory tract infection. This, combined with the recent travel history to an urban centre, makes *Legionella pneumophilia* the most likely causative pathogen. Legionellosis, or Legionairre's disease, is caused by a Gram-negative bacteria and can be associated with outbreaks particularly linked to aerosolised water, such as air-conditioning units or water towers. Diagnosis is typically through urinary antigens (although these only detect serotype 1) or through sputum culture, although discussion with the microbiology laboratory is warranted as non-standard culture media are needed. Treatment is with either a quinolone or a macrolide – beta lactam antimicrobials are not advocated for legionellosis. In the UK, legionellosis is a notifiable disease.

Mycoplasma pneumoniae can cause a multi-lobar community acquired pneumoniae with transaminitis and hyponatraemia, but usually occurs in 3–4 yearly cycles frequently in the winter. *Chlamydia psittaci* is another cause of atypical community acquired pneumonia, but is associated with keeping birds. *Streptococcus pneumoniae* is a cause of typical community acquired pneumonia and classically causes a lobar pneumonia without disturbed liver function tests. *Moraxella catarrhalis* can cause pneumonia, but more typically in those with structural lung disease (such as chronic obstructive pulmonary disease).

Phin N et al. Epidemiology and clinical management of Legionnaires' disease. Lancet Infect Dis. 2014;14(10):1011–1021.

15. E Pulmonary angiography and embolisation

The weight loss, fever and night sweats in a patient from sub-Saharan Africa with right apical consolidation make pulmonary tuberculosis the most likely diagnosis in this case. This patient will need sputum samples forwarding for an auramine/Ziehl–Neelsen smear and mycobacterial culture, and, if sputum cannot be provided, a bronchoscopy and bronchoalveolar lavage will be needed. The patient may also need a CT of the thorax to establish the parenchymal architecture and whether there is any mediastinal lymphadenopathy that might be amenable to endobronchial ultrasound-guided biopsy. The patient should also receive broad-spectrum antimicrobial cover for standard community-acquired pneumonia and will probably need to commence antituberculous therapy.

However, the large-volume haemoptysis, anaemia and haemodynamic compromise make pulmonary angiography and embolisation of any actively bleeding arterioles the most pressing intervention. Tranexamic acid can be given to try to ameliorate the symptoms but, with the degree of haemoptysis presented in this case, an urgent interventional radiology opinion must be obtained, from the nearest tertiary referral centre if not available locally.

Andersen PE. Imaging and interventional radiological treatment of haemoptysis. Acta Radiol 2006; 47(8):780–792.

16. E Piperacillin–tazobactam

Patients with structural lung disease – particularly cystic fibrosis and bronchiectasis – often develop infective complications from pathogens not typically encountered in community-acquired infections. In this case the patient's foul-smelling sputum, fever and focal chest signs indicated a pneumonic process and although *Streptococcus pneumoniae*, *Haemophilus influenzae* or *Mycoplasma pneumonia* may be the cause (i.e. co-amoxiclav and clarithromycin would be appropriate for this CURB65 3 pneumonia), *Pseudomonas* species must be considered and appropriately covered by the antimicrobial regimen. Of the options available this leaves piperacillin–tazobactam or meropenem. Ciprofloxacin would be an alternative antipseudomonal agent but its use is restricted in many hospitals because of concerns over *Clostridium difficile*-associated diarrhoea. Piperacillin–tazobactam has a narrower spectrum of activity over meropenem and as such would be the preferred option in this case.

Azithromycin, although having no antipseudomonal activity itself, has been recommended under specific circumstances to reduce the frequency of infective exacerbations of bronchiectasis – acting predominantly through immunomodulatory mechanisms. Use of azithromycin in this way should be instigated only by specialist physicians experienced in its use.

Amsden GW. Anti-inflammatory effects of macrolides--an underappreciated benefit in the treatment of community-acquired respiratory tract infections and chronic inflammatory pulmonary conditions? J Antimicrob Chemother 2005;55(1):10–21.

17. C High-resolution CT of the thorax

Patients with similar presentations to this are commonly encountered on the haematology wards and most hospitals have established neutropenic sepsis protocols. A neutropenic state predisposes patients to rapidly progressing infections – most commonly from gastrointestinal tract migration of native flora – but investigations to rule out common foci should be undertaken at the outset of a neutropenic fever, i.e. mid-stream urine, sputum microscopy culture and sensitivities, a plain chest X-ray and blood cultures both peripherally and from any indwelling lines that may be present. Broad-spectrum antimicrobials should be commenced and should include a β-lactam with antipseudomonal cover, an aminoglycoside and if an indwelling line is in situ it is advisable to include a glycopeptide. If there is no resolution of fever at 48 hours a reassessment should be made and the antibacterial spectrum increased. If after a further 48 hours there is still no resolution of the fever consideration of whether there is line sepsis, *Pneumocystis jiroveci* pneumonia or fungal infections must be made. Line sepsis may be indicated by positive blood cultures – even if positive for microbes considered contaminants in other circumstances (e.g. coagulase-negative staphylococci), or suggested by a red or weeping exit site. Where concerns exist about line sepsis the line should be removed. Pneumocystis pneumonia might be suggested by a marked hypoxia, or early desaturation on exercise, or by chest X-ray changes which may include bilateral parenchymal opacification with basal sparing. Treatment of pneumocystis pneumonia would include high-dose co-trimoxazole. Investigation for yeast forms of fungal disease is through blood cultures but the low sensitivity of these is well documented. High-resolution CT of the thorax allows indirect diagnosis of fungal lung disease caused both by yeasts and by filamentous fungi and where available galactomannan can be useful. Galactomannan assays detect fungal antigens – particularly from filamentous fungi – and so suggest invasive disease; however, they can produce false-positive results with piperacillin–tazobactam treatment. Fungal nodules on the CT or other changes consistent with fungal disease necessitate broad-spectrum antifungal therapy.

Tissot F, Agrawal S, Pagano L, et al. ECIL-6 Guidelines for the treatment of invasive candidiasis, aspergillosis and mucormycosis in leukemia and hematopoietic stem cell transplant patients. Haematologica 2017;102:433–444.

18. E Oral oseltamivir

This patient presents with a probable influenza in the context of pregnancy. The National Institute for Health and Clinical Excellence (NICE) guidelines outline appropriate use of antiviral agents and define groups who are at risk of complications from influenza and hence should receive antiviral therapy. For endemic or seasonal influenza these include patients with chronic heart, liver, neurological and kidney disease. Patients who are pregnant and those with diabetes mellitus should also receive the vaccine, as should those with asthma and chronic obstructive pulmonary disease.

In epidemic or pandemic influenza outbreaks these guidelines may be altered and attempts at containment may be made – usually with the goal of delaying rather than preventing spread and allowing time for vaccine production.

Antivirals are recommended for pregnant women as worse clinical outcomes (increased hospital admissions, increased need for ventilator support, increased mortality) have been noted in this cohort. Oseltamivir is indicated as a first line therapy for pregnant women with influenza, and the summary of product characteristics for Tamiflu suggests that it does not indicate direct or indirect harmful effects with respect to pregnancy, embryonal/fetal or postnatal development'.

Public Health England. PHE guidance on use of antiviral agents for the treatment and prophylaxis of seasonal influenza. Version 8. London: PHE, 2017.

19. B CT of the thorax

This patient presents with haemoptysis but is haemodynamically stable with normal haemoglobin. The clinical and laboratory findings make a bacterial pneumonic process as the cause for the haemoptysis unlikely, and the previous history of full treatment for pulmonary tuberculosis make this a less likely, but not impossible, cause for this presentation. The radiographic findings of an apical cavity with crescent sign strongly suggest a mycetoma. This should be further investigated with thoracic imaging – in the stable patient a CT would be most appropriate but angiographic studies with potential coiling of bleeding vessels would be more appropriate if there was on-going haemoptysis. Cardiothoracic review should occur in every case of massive haemoptysis, and may also be appropriate in this case but not before a diagnosis has been made. Bronchoscopic examination with washings may provide more information.

Systemic antifungals have only a limited role in management of pulmonary mycetomas, with poor penetration of the drug to the needed site of activity. Interventional instillation of antifungals into the cavity has also met with limited success. The mainstay of treatment remains angiographic or surgical. Where antifungals are started, *Aspergillus* species must be covered and the agents most frequently used are liposomal amphotericin or itraconazole. Fluconazole has no role in treatment of any filamentous fungi, its spectrum of activity being limited to *Candida albicans*.

There is no indication to start another course of antituberculous therapy in this patient. However, sputa should be submitted for mycobacterial culture and if a bronchoscopy is performed washings should similarly be cultured.

Kapur S, Louie BE. Haemoptysis and thoracic fungal infections. Surg Clin North Am 2010;90(5):985–1001.

20. D Negative pressure side room admission until sputum culture negative

The concern with this patient, who has previously been treated for tuberculosis twice and now is diagnosed for a third time, is that he may have multidrug-resistant tuberculosis (MDRTB). MDRTB is defined as tuberculosis that is resistant to both rifampicin and isoniazid. Extended drug-resistant tuberculosis (XDRTB) is defined as that which is resistant to rifampicin, isoniazid, a quinolone and a second-line injectable drug.

This patient's acid-fast bacilli smear-positive sputum could have a rifampicin polymerase chain reaction performed which could provide a rapid mode of detecting possible rifampicin resistance with approximately 95% confidence. However, true confirmation of whether this patient has true MDRTB will require the mycobacteria to grow (0–8 weeks – typically 1–3) and then have drug susceptibilities performed (2–4 weeks).

Patients with suspected or confirmed MDRTB should be managed in strict respiratory isolation. Patients may need to be transferred to a hospital with appropriate negative pressure facilities, under the care of a respiratory physician with a specialist interest in this field.

National Institute for Health and Clinical Excellence. NICE guideline NG33 Tuberculosis. London: NICE, 2016.

21. C Intravenous meropenem

This patient has a pyelonephritis caused by an extended-spectrum β-lactamase (ESBL)-producing E. coli. The most common cause of urinary tract infections is *E. coli*, accounting for around 70%. Resistance rates vary but in England and Wales community rates of ESBL-producing E. coli are generally <5%. Risk factors for community ESBL infection include:
- Genitourinary pathology
- Previous bacterial infection
- Previous intravenous antibiotic treatment
- Hospitalisation in the previous 12 months
- Previous exposure to oral second-generation cephalosporins.

ESBL-producing bacteria exhibit resistance to all cephalosporins and treatment with penicillin-inhibitor compounds is also not advised given the high risk of failure. The majority of ESBL-producing bacteria retain susceptibility to nitrofurantoin. However, it concentrates well in the urine, and is often effective for uncomplicated lower urinary tract infections; it has no discernible activity in parenchymal infections or bacteraemias. Carbapenems retain activity against ESBL-producing bacteria and are effective in treating pyelonephritis and any bacteraemia that may result.

Park SH, Choi SM, Lee DG, et al. Impact of extended-spectrum β-lactamase production on treatment outcomes of acute pyelonephritis caused by *Escherichia coli* in patients without health care-associated risk factors. Antimicrob Agents Chemother 2015;59(4):1962–68.

22. E Oral rifampicin, isoniazid, pyrazinamide, ethambutol and dexamethasone

This patient presents with an indolent meningitis and epidemiological risk factors for tuberculous disease. The finding of leptomeningeal enhancement supports a diagnosis of tuberculous meningitis but is not conclusive. The cerebrospinal fluid microscopy and biochemistry are also in keeping with this diagnosis – the lack of visualisation of acid-fast bacilli is not surprising and should not detract from the accumulated evidence that this is tuberculosis (TB).

Antituberculous therapy should be initiated as soon as possible with adjunctive corticosteroid treatment. A Cochrane meta-analysis looking at tuberculous meningitis in immunocompetent children and adults has found that corticosteroid use in this condition imbues a relative risk reduction of 0.69 (95% CI 0.52–0.92). Concerns over the potential for corticosteroids to adversely alter the pharmacokinetic properties of TB medications are unsubstantiated, and the incidence of gastrointestinal bleeding from the dexamethasone remains low.

National Institute for Health and Clinical Excellence (NICE). NICE guideline NG33 Tuberculosis. London: NICE, 2016.

23. E Side room, lumbar puncture, steroids, ceftriaxone, inform health protection unit

Bacterial meningitis is a medical emergency and management should be performed confidently and in a timely fashion. Isolation of the patient will reduce the risk of onward spread in the emergency department. In cases where there are no signs of raised intracranial pressure a lumbar puncture should not be delayed in order to perform a CT of the brain; however, in HIV-positive patients a CT should be performed as the risk of space-occupying lesions increases markedly. If the lumbar puncture is going to be delayed for more than 30 minutes ceftriaxone should be given and the lumbar puncture performed when possible. The continuing care of the patient should involve close and regular monitoring. The health protection unit should be informed by telephone to contact trace and give antibacterial prophylaxis to those considered at risk. Within the department those exposed to respiratory secretions from the patient should contact occupational health to be assessed for similar prophylaxis.

The role of steroids in bacterial meningitis is continuously under review. A recent Cochrane review found that corticosteroids significantly reduced hearing loss and neurological sequelae, but did not reduce overall mortality. Other randomised controlled trials have found that the benefit is found in those with streptococcal meningitis more than meningococcal. The steroids must be given before or with the antimicrobials, but not after.

Brouwer MC, et al. Corticosteroids for acute bacterial meningitis. Cochrane Database Syst Rev 2013; (6):CD004405.
National Institute for Health and Clinical Excellence (NICE). Clinical guideline 102. Meningitis (bacterial) and meningococcal septicaemia in under 16s: recognition, diagnosis and management. London: NICE, 2015.

24. C *Leptospira interrogans*

This patient has liver derangement, acute kidney injury and a pneumonic process. He is young and has risk factors for exposure to water sources. Leptospirosis, or Weil's disease, is acquired from coming into contact with water that has been contaminated by urine from infected animals. Clinically it can occur 4–14 days after exposure and can manifest in a range of severities from a 'flu-like illness' through to pneumonia, meningitis, myocarditis, hepatitis and renal interstitial tubular necrosis.

Streptococcus pneumoniae is the most common cause of community-acquired pneumonia and, although renal impairment can occur, liver derangement is not common. Haemophilus species is another common cause of community-acquired pneumonia, more commonly occurring in those with structural lung disease. *Mycoplasma* species typically occurs in 3- to 4-yearly cycles although sporadic cases can occur. It should be considered where there are more diffuse bilateral pneumonic changes and is often associated with hyponatraemia and a mild transaminitis.

Legionella species abides in many water sources and aerosolisation can lead to inhalation and subsequently either a transient febrile illness (Pontiac fever) or a pneumonia. It is typically acquired from air conditioning but also from residential complexes and hospitals where the water supply is poorly maintained.

Cost F, et al. Global morbidity and mortality of leptospirosis: a systematic review. Plos Neglect Trop Dis 2015; 9(9):e0003898.

25. B *E. coli* O157

This patient presents with non-specific complaints but laboratory findings that fit with haemolytic uraemic syndrome (HUS). *Escherichia coli* O157 is the commonest cause of this in the UK, usually occurring in defined outbreaks linked to breakdown in hand hygiene in those with close contact with animals – several high-profile cases recently have occurred in children on day trips to petting zoos. Diagnosis is through culture of stool samples but results can take up to 48 hours so empirical management must be based upon the clinic picture. Antibiotic therapy should be avoided if possible in HUS as death of the *E. coli* O157 can result in an increased toxaemia and worsening parameters. Management is predominantly supportive with blood products and dialysis – plasma exchange has been used in some cases with varying success.

Leptospirosis can present in a non-specific manner but would not typically manifest as acute kidney injury and blood dyscrasias without an apparent hepatitis. Norovirus can cause an acute vomiting syndrome but would be unlikely to cause the laboratory findings shown. Similarly *Clostridium difficile* can cause a colitis that typically presents as diarrhoea rather than vomiting and, although insipient renal failure can occur, the severity in this case is out of keeping with the history.

Shigella species can cause a dysenteric presentation and vomiting can be a feature. Shigella outbreaks are also not uncommon in schools and institutions and the history in this case could point to shigellosis; however, the laboratory indices are disproportionately deranged for this, in isolation, to account for the presentation.

Pennington H. *Escherichia coli* O157. Lancet 2010;376:1428–1435.

26. E Oral vancomycin

This patient presents with a picture consistent with *Clostridium difficile*-associated diarrhoea. *Clostridium difficile* is a commensal in less than 2% of the adult population, but has been noted in over 20% of the over 65-year-old population. When the luminal flora is disturbed by systemic antimicrobial therapy, *C. difficile* infection, resistant to most frequently used antimicrobials, can cause a clinical picture of diarrhoea that can develop into a fulminant colitis. Risk factors for acquisition of *C. difficile*-associated diarrhoea include:

- Increasing age
- Severity of underlying diseases
- Non-surgical gastrointestinal procedures
- Presence of a nasogastric tube
- Administration of antibiotics
- Stay on an intensive therapy unit
- Duration of antibiotic course
- Duration of hospital stay
- Antiulcer medications.

Standard therapy is oral metronidazole, but for severe disease oral vancomycin has been shown to have increased efficacy. Markers for severe disease include:

- White cell count $>15 \times 10^9$/L
- Creatinine >50% above baseline
- Temperature >38.5°C
- Severe colitis (abdominal signs, radiology or on endoscopy).

In severe *C. difficile* infection cases not responding to oral vancomycin, addition of intravenous metronidazole is recommended. The addition of oral rifampicin or intravenous immunoglobulin may also be considered although there are no firm data to support this. Even with initial resolution relapse rates are approximately 20%. Some patients require colectomy and indicators for a surgical review include megacolon (dilatation >10 cm), perforation or septic shock.

Public Heath England (PHE). Updated guidance on the management and treatment of *C. difficile* infection. London: PHE, 2013.

27. E Strongyloidiasis

Strongyloides stercoralis is a soil-transmitted helminth that initially enters humans in its larval stage through dermal penetration. It then migrates to the lungs (and can cause an eosinophilic pneumonia) before establishing an intestinal luminal infestation. Once established in the bowel the infection is usually asymptomatic but can in some cases cause a change in bowel habit, bloating, anorexia and sometimes nausea. *Strongyloides* species that escape from the gut can migrate to various anatomical areas including the skin, where they cause a cutaneous reaction termed 'cutaneous larva currens' characterised by a rapidly moving serpiginous rash with local histamine release. Hyperinfection syndrome can occur in those with Th2-oriented immunosuppression. This includes those with human T-lymphotropic virus type-I (HTLV-1) infection, as well as those who have had some forms of chemotherapy for malignancy, high-dose corticosteroids, or who are on immunosuppressant therapy following solid organ or bone marrow transplantation. Hyperinfection syndrome is not particularly seen in those with HIV infection. Investigation is typically through stool examination for ova, cysts and parasites – three specimens should be submitted for examination as faecal concentration of the larvae is variable.

Schistosomiasis can cause a cercarial dermatitis where the metacercariae enter (i.e. in the parts of the body that enter the infested waters). This typically resolves several days to 2 weeks after inoculation. Filariasis can cause lymphatic sclerosis while lymphadenitis and nocardiasis can cause chronic cutaneous scarring. Cutaneous larva migrans causes a slowly progressive serpiginous rash. *Loa loa* can cause calabar swellings over bony prominences.

Moore LSP, Chiodini PL. Tropical helminths. Medicine 2010;38(1):47–51.

28. C Pegylated interferon-α 2a

Hepatitis B is a blood-borne virus transmitted through bodily fluids (such as sexual contact, blood transfusion and needle sharing), including vertical transmission from mother to child. Prevalence varies globally, but there are particularly high levels in South East Asia and sub-Saharan Africa. It is thought there are in excess of 350 million chronic carriers of hepatitis B, with varying levels of infectivity. Infectivity can be inferred from laboratory markers, with those who have circulating hepatitis B (HBV) DNA levels of greater than 2000 IU/mL, or hepatitis e-antigen positivity the most infective.

In the UK, treatment for patients with hepatitis B is offered based upon several criteria: age, HBV DNA levels of >2000 IU/mL, ALT>30 IU/mL, or evidence of cirrhosis or necroinflammation or fibrosis on biopsy. First line treatment is pegylated interferon-α 2a for 48 weeks in the first instance. For patients whose HBV DNA level does not decrease sufficiently, or who do not convert from being e-antigen positive, or in those who relapse, long-term prescription of tenofovir disoproxil or entecavir is indicated. Lamivudine can be added to tenofovir disoproxil in resistant disease.

National Institute for Health and Clinical Excellence (NICE). Clinical guideline 165. Hepatitis B (chronic): diagnosis and management. London: NICE, 2017.

29. E Stool ova cyst and parasite examination

This patient presents with typical symptoms of giardiasis. *Giardia lamblia* is a protozoa acquired through faeco-oral transmission and is prevalent in much of the tropics but particularly the Indian subcontinent. It causes offensive and frequent belching and flatulence, and can progress to diarrhoea and abdominal cramps. Giardiasis is usually self-limiting; however, prolonged symptoms do occur in some individuals. Treatment is with metronidazole in the first instance, although for those cases in which there is clinical failure re-treatment with tinidazole has been documented to have a higher efficacy.

Diagnosis is predominantly though stool examination for ova, cysts and parasites. Three stool specimens should be submitted as sensitivity is 50–70% with a single stool rising to 90% after three specimens. If cysts cannot be identified in stool but there is still a clinical suspicion of giardiasis the Entero-test can be used as a second-line investigation and is relatively non-invasive compared with oesophagogastroduodenoscopy and biopsy for parasitological examination.

The Entero-test involves a string-containing capsule being swallowed where it sits in the upper gastrointestinal tract for several hours before being withdrawn and sent for microscopy. Serological tests are not readily available.

Empirical metronidazole therapy could be initiated in this case but a firm diagnosis should be sought in all cases and additionally parasites often coexist. Therefore in this case, where there are risk factors for acquisition of other helminths, stool examinations for ova cysts and parasites may enable identification of co-infection which may require therapy other than metronidazole.

Pawlowski SW, Warren CA, Guerrant R. Diagnosis and treatment of acute or persistent diarrhoea. Gastroenterology 2009;136(6):1874–1886.

30. C Neurocysticercosis

Neurocysticercosis is the leading cause of epilepsy in the developing world and is caused by the helminth *Taenia solium* (pork tape worm). This parasite is transmitted either through ingestion of infected raw or undercooked meat or through the faeco-oral route. When infected meat is ingested, intestinal taeniasis results. This is usually asymptomatic but on occasion results in a change of bowel habit or generalised abdominal discomfort. When transmission occurs through a human-to-human faeco-oral route cysticercosis can result. The cysticerci can disseminate to all tissues, including the central nervous system. The resulting clinical presentation depends upon the location of cysts, but focal neurological signs or seizures (focal partial or generalised tonic–clonic) can result. If the cysticerci lodge near the cerebral ventricular system, hydrocephalus can occur. Racemose cysts are particular manifestations of neurocysticercosis in which a cyst forms in the subarachnoid space which can cause marked occlusive and mass effects. Brain CT or MRI appearances in neurocysticerci can vary markedly. Younger cysticerci can appear as hypodense cysts which may or may not have associated oedema. In more established neurocysticercosis they can have the appearance of ring-enhancing lesions or become calcified. Managing neurocysticercosis should initially involve anticonvulsant therapy. Use of anthelmintic agents in neurocysticercosis should be managed with care as increased seizure activity can occur and advice on use of albendazole or praziquantel should occur only under expert guidance.

Cerebral toxoplasmosis is uncommon in immunocompetent individuals, as is progressive multifocal leukoencephalopathy caused by the John Cunningham virus. Multiple gliomas are a rare entity.

Abba K, Ramaratnam S, Ranganathan LN. Anti-helmintics for people with neurocysticercosis. Cochrane Database Syst Rev 2010;(3):CD000215.

31. E Terminal stream urine for ultrafiltration and microscopy

This patient presents with risk factors for schistosomiasis (bilharzia) and a clinical syndrome that would fit with urinary disease (*Schistosoma haematobium*) which is prevalent throughout the lakes and rivers of east Africa. Schistosomes live in water snails and enter the human through dermal penetration of water-exposed tissues – therefore, acquisition does not necessitate swimming but only wading in infested water sources. Following acquisition, the schistosomes migrate haematogenously to either the perivesicular vascular plexus (*Schistosoma haematobium* resulting in haematuria) or the mesenteric vascular system (*Schistosoma mansoni* and *Schistosoma japonicum*, presenting with abdominal pain, bloody stool or with sequelae from hepatomegaly or splenomegaly). Errant schistosomes can migrate to all areas, causing particular problems when they enter the cerebrum or paraspinal tissues.

Diagnosis is either through direct examination (terminal stream urine for *S. haematobium*; stool ova cyst and parasite examination for *S. mansoni* and *S. japonicum*) or through serology. In this case the on-going haematuria increases the probability of urine microscopy providing the diagnosis and will be considerably faster than serology. Serological tests should always be interpreted with caution as antibody positivity lasts for many years and remains positive even after treatment of the underlying disease.

Treatment is with praziquantel, but this is only active against the adult worms so when empirical treatment is used (as in this case – often self-administered by travellers) it should be taken 6 weeks after exposure to allow immature worms to become susceptible. Prolonged (years) untreated infection with *S. haematobium* can predispose to transition cell carcinoma of the bladder and urological referral for cystoscopy is indicated in these cases.

Moore LSP, Chiodini PL. Tropical helminths. Medicine 2010;38(1):47–51.

32. C *Salmonella* species

The clinical presentation here is one of osteomyelitis of a long bone with a documented Gram-negative bacteraemia. The Gram-positive organisms staphylococci and streptococci are the commonest causes of osteomyelitis. However, in patients with sickle cell disease *Salmonella* (non-*typhi*) species are a relatively common cause of osteomyelitis. Capillary occlusion secondary to intravascular sickling causes decreased gut mucosal integrity permitting salmonella invasion. Expanded bone marrow with sluggish blood flow leads to an ischaemic focus for *Salmonella* to sequester. Occasionally multiple sites which may be symmetrical are involved. Distinguishing salmonella osteomyelitis from bone infarctions in the absence of positive microbiology can be difficult and radionuclide bone studies and MRI are often needed. Treatment is with prolonged courses of antimicrobials – ceftriaxone is frequently used and the majority of *Salmonella* species remain susceptible.

  Brucella species is a Gram-negative organism acquired from ruminants – particularly goats and cows – and can cause deep-seated infections including septic arthritis and osteomyelitis. The presentation is often more indolent, however, and fever and night sweats are often predominating symptoms. It is difficult to isolate from microbiological cultures and serology is useful. Treatment again needs to be for a prolonged duration but β-lactams are ineffective and treatment usually involves rifampicin, doxycycline and gentamicin.

Battersby AJ, Knox-Macaulay HH, Carrol ED. Susceptibility to invasive bacterial infections in children with sickle cell disease. Pediatr Blood Cancer 2010;55(3):401–406.

33. B Diphtheria antitoxin

This patient presents with a severe upper respiratory tract infection with evidence of a tonsillar pseudomembrane that fits with a diagnosis of diphtheria. There is evidence of toxin-related sequelae with first-degree heart block apparent on the ECG. Diphtheria is a droplet-spread bacteria which is very infrequently seen in countries with developed immunisation programmes but is becoming prevalent once again – particularly in eastern Europe and Russia. Two to five days after exposure upper respiratory tract symptoms develop and can progress rapidly to cause both local airway issues and systemic toxic pathology – including most importantly cardiac conduction defects. Diagnosis is through throat swab for microscopy, culture and susceptibility testing, but the rapid progression and severity of cardiac sequelae when they are apparent mean that empirical treatment must often be initiated.

  Although the infection can be treated with any of the antimicrobials cited in the question, the cardiac conduction defect noted on the patient's ECG necessitates administration of diphtheria antitoxin as a matter of emergency. This patient should remain on a cardiac monitor until his rhythm returns to normal and his airway will need to be monitored in case of compromise.

  The possibility of on-going spread to non-immunised people or those in whom vaccination has waned (immune response to vaccine is thought to last approximately 10 years) necessitates immunisation or booster vaccination for contacts.

Salisbury D, Ramsay M, Noakes K. Immunisation against infectious diseases. London: The Stationery Office, 2006. http://immunisation.dh.gov.uk/gb-individual-current-chapters (last accessed October 2018).

34. D Hepatitis B sAb testing and a save serum sent from the doctor

Needle-stick injuries do occur even when all safeguards are adopted. Three main blood-borne viruses can be transmitted – hepatitis B (transmission rate is up to 30% in unvaccinated individuals), hepatitis C (transmission is approximately 3%) and HIV (transmission is approximately 0.3%). All healthcare professionals should be vaccinated against hepatitis B although some are non-responders. For that reason all those who suffer a needle-stick injury from a contaminated needle should have their HBsAb titre checked and if < 10 mLU/mL hepatitis B immunoglobulin is indicated. A review of vaccination history is also indicated and if necessary a hepatitis B booster vaccination should be administered. These two interventions should not occur without checking the HBsAb titre and obtaining a vaccine history.

There is no indication for baseline testing for HCV and HIV in the recipient of the needle-stick injury and this information may have consequences for the future if a healthcare professional. Therefore, only a save serum is indicated in the first instance.

If the donor in the needle-stick injury is known (in this case the 86-year-old patient) the donor should be consented for testing for hepatitis B, hepatitis C and HIV, but this should be undertaken by another healthcare professional – not the individual who sustained the injury, in order to avoid conflict of interest.

NHS employer's guidelines. Needlestick injury. London: NHS; 2010.

35. C HIV p24

Human immunodeficiency virus (HIV) seroconversion typically presents with fever, rash, headache, odynophagia, adenopathy, and often perioral ulcers and oropharyngeal or genital thrush. This syndrome usually occurs within 3 months of acquisition and often much sooner. In this case the haematological parameters suggest a lymphopenia (absolute lymphocyte count can be a maximum of 0.1×10^9/L given the total white cell count and the neutrophil count).

HIV rapid diagnostic tests measure antibodies and historically have a 'window' period of 3 months (12 weeks). The currently prevalent fourth-generation tests cut this 'window' period to just 4 weeks during which time they may give a false-negative result. Where early diagnosis needs to be made several different tests can be performed, but most guidelines now stipulate p24 antigen detection as being the most useful with a faster result available than requesting viral load quantification and a greater specificity than CD4 counts. Repeating HIV antibody testing is necessary but this should be done after the window period has elapsed and will not provide a timely result where one is necessary. All positive HIV test results need to be confirmed with a second test. HIV resistance testing should be performed in all newly diagnosed cases of HIV prior to commencement of highly active antiretroviral therapy.

UK National Guidelines for HIV Testing. British HIV Association British Association of Sexual Health and HIV British Infection Society, 2008.

36. D Non-*typhi* salmonellosis

This man presents with undifferentiated fever and HIV and as such the most likely diagnosis is non-*typhi* salmonellosis. In HIV-positive patients the incidence of non-typhi salmonella bacteraemia is 40–100 times that in immunocompetent individuals. It typically presents with a Gram-negative sepsis picture of fever, hypotension and a neutrophilia. Non-*typhi Salmonella* species do not cause the typical rose spots and relative bradycardia described in enteric fever, and although HIV-positive patients can get *S. typhi* or *S. paratyphi* A, B and C, the features of this presentation are more in keeping with non-typhi salmonellosis. The clinical indicators of oral candidiasis and what is likely to be Kaposi's sarcoma on this man's arm suggest that his absolute CD4 count is under 200 cells/mm^3. The presence of this advanced pathology suggests that this is not a seroconversion presentation.

Although the diagnosis of urological sepsis is possible, the lack of lower urinary symptoms and absence of nitrites or leukocytes in the urine dipstick make this diagnosis less likely. The negative malaria film makes it unlikely that there is a dual infection and the absence of a thrombocytopenia also goes against malaria. However, the patient should still have two further malaria films to make sure that there is not a low level parasitaemia contributing to his presentation.

Fernández Guerrero ML, et al. Focal infections due to non-typhi *Salmonella* in patients with AIDS: report of 10 cases and review. Clin Infect Dis 1997;25(3):690–697.

37. A Buruli ulcer

Mycobacterium ulcerans is endemic in central Africa, South and Central America, south-east Asia and Australia – particularly in areas of the coast of Victoria. It is an environmental organism most often associated with water sources but the exact mechanism of transmission is unclear. The clinical appearance usually begins with a pruritic nodule but over a period of 1–2 months the nodule ulcerates. The action of the mycolactone toxin produced by M. ulcerans causes local tissue destruction but this is usually painless. The undermined edges around the ulcer often extend far beyond the edge of the visible ulcer – up to 15 cm have been recorded. Diagnosis is through tissue biopsy and mycobacterial culture. Treatment for small lesions can be with rifampicin with streptomycin/clarithromycin but medical treatment has a low success rate. Surgical debridement is the mainstay of therapy with skin grafting often necessary given the wide margins needed.

Leprosy does cause anaesthetic areas and although there are visible dermal lesions these are not ulcerated to the extent noted in this case. Leishmaniasis causes ulcers with rolled edges, not undermined, and is often painful. Diabetic ulcers can be painless in neuropathic patients and extensive in nature. However, this diagnosis is unlikely in this young man with no past medical history with a normal random glucose.

Walsh DS, Portaels F, Meyers WM. Buruli ulcer: Advances in understanding *Mycobacterium ulcerans* infection. Dermatol Clin 2011;29(1):1–8.

38. D Leishmaniasis

This woman presents with a skin lesion unresponsive to two courses of antimicrobial treatment, to which impetigo, erysipelas and ecthyma would have responded. Leishmaniasis is caused by a parasite transmitted through sandfly bites. It is prevalent in much of Central and South America and the Middle East as well as in sub-Saharan Africa and into South Asia. There are several different species of *Leishmania* and pathophysiology depends to some extent on the species acquired:

- Cutaneous (typically *L. major*): typically appears as a lesion at the site of the bite with an ulcer forming, often with rolled edges. Secondary bacterial infection can occur.
- Mucocutaneous (including *L. viannia*): begins with skin lesions spreading to mucous membrane areas – particularly the nose and mouth.
- Visceral (including *L. donovani*): progresses from skin lesions to splenomegaly and fever and is often fatal.

Diagnosis is by biopsy for histopathological examination. Samples can also be forwarded for polymerase chain reaction in an attempt to speciate the organism but this is available only in specialist areas. Treatment is of itself potentially toxic, with amphotericin or sodium stibogluconate. Intralesional therapy can be given for cutaneous lesions; systemic therapy is needed for the other forms.

Impetigo is a pustular bacterial skin infection (staphylococci or streptococci) often characterised by thick yellow crusts forming around the ruptured pustules. Ecthyma is a similar process to impetigo (also staphylococci or streptococci) but with deeper structures becoming ulcerated. Erysipelas describes a rapidly spreading soft tissue infectious process typically caused by group A streptococci. Historically the term was used to describe facial lesions associated with *Streptococcus pharyngitis*. *Mycobacterium marinum* causes fish tank granuloma; the absence of fish contact in the history makes this diagnosis unlikely.

Moore EM, Lockwood DN. Leishmaniasis. Clin Med 2011;11(5):492–497.

39. C Intravenous fluids

This patient has dengue fever presenting with the classic history of fever, myalgia, headache and rash with a transient leukopenia and a mild transaminitis. Dengue is an arthropod-borne virus transmitted by day-biting mosquitos. There are four serotypes spread across the tropics. Initial infection with dengue typically presents with fever/arthralgia/rash although retro-orbital headaches can feature as can myalgia. Second exposure to a different serotype to that first encountered can progress to dengue haemorrhagic fever – a phenomenon of antibody-mediated enhancement. This can result in clotting derangement and haemorrhage as well as tissue oedema, including the pulmonary parenchyma. In this patient there is a tachycardic, hypotensive response that warrants rehydration but no signs of dengue haemorrhagic fever which may necessitate blood products.

The good concordance with Malarone and the negative first malaria film indicate that, although malaria should be ruled out with two further malaria films, there is no evidence to warrant initiation of empirical intravenous quinine. The typhoid vaccination, tachycardic response to infection, relative neutropenia and absence of a C-reactive protein response would go against enteric fever necessitating ceftriaxone. The normal cerebrospinal fluid would also confirm that ceftriaxone is not needed to cover for meningitis. Although the presentation could fit with influenza, dengue is more likely, and even if construed as influenza the treatment of choice, in the absence of overwhelming ventilatory failure, would be oral oseltamivir.

Teixeira MG, Barreto ML. Diagnosis and management of dengue. BMJ 2009;339:b4338.

40. A Chikungunya

This patient has a fever–arthralgia–rash presentation with a relative neutropenia and a low-level C-reactive protein after returning from an area known to have endemic chikungunya and dengue. Chikungunya is an arthropod-borne virus prevalent across the Indian ocean with spread to Italy now reported. Presentation is with fever–arthralgia–rash, arthralgia being predominant; sometimes joint pain continues for several months after the inoculation. Treatment is supportive with analgesia and non-steroidal anti-inflammatory drugs for the arthralgia.

The rash of syphilis can be macular, papular or maculopapular but classically occurs all over the body, including the palms and soles, whereas in this case the rash was over her torso. HIV seroconversion can present with fever, arthralgia and a macular rash but is less likely given the timeline and travel history. Headache or confusion which would make one concerned about encephalitis is absent; although Japanese encephalitis is arthropod borne and is in south-east and south Asia the presentation is not consistent with this diagnosis. O'nyong-nyong presents similarly to other fever–arthralgia–rash viruses but is confined to the east of sub-Saharan Africa.

Thwaites GE, Day NP. Approach to fever in the returning traveler. N Engl J Med 2017;376:548–560.

41. C Measles

This man comes from a country with a low rate of completed childhood vaccination schedules and his arrival in the UK with a child of school-age puts him at risk of what are typically considered childhood diseases. Measles is a respiratory droplet-spread virus that is highly contagious, with a 90% secondary attack rate in the non-immune. It typically presents 2 weeks after exposure with a viral prodrome followed by conjunctivitis, a descending maculopapular rash and fever. Koplik's spots are sometimes visible in the oral cavity from 24 hours prior to the rash appearing until 24–48 hours after the skin rash is visible, when they disappear. As such Koplik's spots, although pathognomonic when seen, should not detract from the diagnosis when absent. A relative lymphopenia and on occasion transient neutropenia can occur. Confirmation of the diagnosis is with a salivary swab for IgM or serology although the latter takes considerably longer. Treatment is supportive. Prognosis is good, with neurological sequelae of encephalitis or secondary bacterial pneumonia being rare in the UK. Subacute sclerosing panencephalitis can occur 5–10 years after acquisition in 1/25,000 cases and is untreatable. The mumps–measles–rubella (MMR) vaccine provides over 90% protection against measles and can be given as post-exposure prophylaxis up to 72 hours after exposure.

Secondary syphilis usually presents with a diffuse, non-pruritic, maculopapular rash that can affect the palms and soles and does not demonstrate a descending progression. HIV seroconversion can present with a diffuse, maculopapular rash and, although the patient should have a HIV test, the social history, the presence of conjunctivitis and the absence of adenopathy are not typical. Infectious mononucleosis caused by the Epstein–Barr virus and infectious mononucleosis-like syndrome caused by cytomegalovirus can present with a rash, the former classically after amoxicillin. However, adenopathy is almost universally present and a mild transaminitis is frequent. The negative monospot does not rule out Epstein–Barr virus but does decrease the likelihood of this diagnosis. Rubella can also present with a descending rash but typically causes posterior occipital and postauricular adenopathy.

Muscat M. Who gets measles in Europe? J Infect Dis 2011; 204(1):S353–365.

42. E Varicella-zoster encephalitis

This man has evidence of a resolving left L5 dermatome zoster rash and a new confusional state; there is reactive lymphocytosis (mononuclear) in the cerebrospinal fluid. The most likely cause is varicella-zoster encephalitis. During the viraemia of primary varicella and of zoster, cerebrospinal fluid (CSF) can have low numbers of lymphocytes and there may be VZV DNA detectable by polymerase chain reaction. However, the clinical manifestations of encephalitis associated with this are rare, but serious when they do occur. The encephalitis is not only due to the presence of the virus but also because of a vasculopathic process in response to this. Treatment is therefore with intravenous aciclovir but also with consideration as to whether steroids are required.

Tuberculous meningitis presents with a more subacute history than here. The CSF would show a similar mononuclear white cell picture, but would have a higher protein and a low CSF glucose. Neuroborreliosis again typically presents with a more subacute history with lethargy and focal neurological deficits although confusion can be a feature; CSF shows mononuclear white cells predominating with a high protein and a low glucose. The scabbing rash described in this case should not be confused with a Lyme disease eschar which would occur longer before the neurological presentation and would not be evident at this stage. Herpes simplex virus encephalitis presents very similarly to varicella-zoster encephalitis and would be more likely if it were not for the dermatomal rash. Bacterial meningitis typically has a much higher CSF white cell count and polymorphonuclear cells predominate.

Solomon T, et al. Management of suspected viral encephalitis in adults – Association of British Neurologists and British Infection Association National Guidelines. J Infection 2012;64:347–373.

43. C Intravenous artesunate

Malaria is caused by one of five mosquito-transmitted parasites – *Plasmodium falciparum, P. vivax, P. ovale, P. malariae* and *P. knowlesi*. Of these *P. falciparum* is the most likely to cause fatal disease. In children the most common complications are renal failure, cerebral malaria and severe anaemia. In adults renal failure and cerebral malaria also occur but instead of anaemic complications acute respiratory distress syndrome can occur. Cerebral malaria, even when treated, has a fatality of up to 20%. This patient presents with confusion and a stiff neck and a high percentage parasitaemia of *P. falciparum* malaria. A CT of the brain and lumbar puncture should be performed to look for concomitant disease processes but the most important step in the management of this patient is to treat the malaria without delay.

Historically quinine has been the antimalarial treatment of choice: oral in non-severe cases and intravenously where necessary. However, quinine is associated with QT prolongation and hence cardiac rhythm abnormalities and also with hypoglycaemia (as is malaria itself). Patients receiving intravenous quinine should be on a cardiac monitor and have regular blood sugar measurements. Artemisinin derivatives such as artesunate have a far better safety profile than quinine with fewer serious side effects. A large multi-country, randomized clinical trial on the treatment of severe malaria including cerebral malaria definitively showed decreased mortality rates with artesunate (15%) compared with quinine (22%).

Lalloo D, et al. UK malaria treatment guidelines 2016. J Infection 2016;72:635–649.

44. D 83%

Defining a diagnosis by a test outcome is dependent upon the test providing the correct result. Assigning characteristics to a test can be done in several ways but must always be in reference to the true diagnosis. In conditions where there is a pre-existing gold standard tests must be compared with that standard. Typically, four clinical aspects of a test are discussed: sensitivity, specificity, positive predictive value and negative predictive value.

Table 6.1 Comparing a new test with an existing 'gold standard' test

	Old test positive	Old test negative	
New test positive	a	b	*PPV* = a/(a + b)
New test negative	c	d	*NPV* = d/(c + d)
	Sensitivity = a/(a + c)	*Specificity* = d/(d + b)	

NPV, negative predictive value; PPV, positive predictive value.

The negative predictive value is a summary statistic describing the proportion of individuals with a negative test result who truly do not have the condition.

The positive predictive value is a summary statistic describing the proportion of individuals with a positive test result who truly do have the condition.

Sensitivity relates to the test's ability to identify positive results.

Specificity relates to the ability of the test to identify negative results.

False positives, i.e. those in box 'b' in the table above, represent a type I error and can lead to inappropriate rejection of a true null hypothesis. A type II error is the wrong decision that is made when a test fails to reject a false null hypothesis. A type II error may be compared with a so-called *false negative* in other test situations and is represented by those in box 'c' in the table above.

Harris M, Taylor G. Medical Statistics Made Easy, 2nd edn. Banbury: Scion Publishing Ltd, 2008.

45. E Disseminated candidiasis

Postoperative infections following abdominal surgery, particularly where there has been potential for spillage of gastrointestinal luminal contents, can be due to either luminal bacteria, or fungi. The majority of luminal bacteria are susceptible to standard antimicrobial regimes (such as co-amoxiclav, cefuroxime and metronidazole, or piperacillin–tazobactam). Continued fevers/raised inflammatory markers despite appropriate antibacterial therapy should raise the question of either (a) resistant bacteria, (b) a defined collection in the operative field, or (c) a fungal infection.

The clinical *Candida* score allows a risk analysis for the likelihood of a fungal infection in this patient cohort:

- 2 points for severe sepsis
- 1 point for parenteral nutrition
- 1 point for abdominal surgery
- 1 point for multi-focal *Candida* spp. colonisation

The score is out of 5, with a score of 2 or less having a 3% risk of disseminated candidiasis, a score of 3 having 8% risk, a score of 4 (such as this case) having 16% risk and a score of 5 having 24% risk. It is generally accepted that one should empirically start antifungal therapy where the clinical *Candida* score is 4 or more, and consider it where there is a score of 3.

The absence of focal chest findings on examination, and a clear chest radiograph make a healthcare associated pneumonia an unlikely diagnosis in this case. Similarly, the short duration of insertion of both the urinary catheter, and the peripherally inserted central catheter, and absence of local signs of inflammation around these devices, make these unlikely sources for the ongoing inflammatory response. While healthcare-associated influenza outbreaks do occur, they are infrequent and without epidemiological evidence to support this, and in the presence of a leucocytosis and high C-reactive protein, this is an unlikely diagnosis in this case.

Chapter 7

Neurology, ophthalmology and psychiatry

Questions

1. A 71-year-old widowed man, with a 2 month history of rapidly progressive cognitive decline and clumsiness, was admitted to hospital after concerns were raised by his neighbour. He was withdrawn, irritable, confused and unkempt.

   On examination, the patient was gaunt and inactive. He was easily startled and, despite making eye contact, was not engaging verbally. Cardiorespiratory and abdominal examinations were normal. Neurological examination was limited by poor compliance but signs of myoclonus and ataxia were apparent.

   Investigations:

MRI of the brain: symmetrical hyperintensity within the striatum	
Cerebrospinal fluid (CSF):	Serum glucose 5.3 mmol/L (CSF:blood ratio 0.6)
Opening pressure 13 cmH$_2$0	
CSF white cell count 4/mm^3 (100% lymphocytes)	
CSF protein 0.4 g/L	
CSF glucose 3.2 mmol/L	
CSF culture and Gram stain: no organisms seen	
CSF protein 14-3-3: positive	
Electroencephalogram: generalised periodic spike–wave activity	

   What is the most likely diagnosis?

   A   Corticobasal degeneration
   B   Isolated cerebral angiitis
   C   Limbic encephalitis
   D   Sporadic Creutzfeldt–Jakob disease
   E   Variant Creutzfeldt–Jakob disease

2. A 54-year-old man presented to the outpatient clinic with a 3-month history of worsening pain
    radiating from neck to the posterolateral aspect of the left arm and forearm. It was a constant
    deep ache, with superimposed shooting pains.
        On examination, there was no obvious muscle wasting of the left arm or hand. Power was
    graded 4/5 (on the Medical Research Council scale) in left elbow extension, wrist flexion and
    finger extension. The left triceps reflex was depressed. Numbness to pinprick was detected over
    the left middle finger.

    What is the most likely diagnosis?

    A   Left C6 radiculopathy
    B   Left C7 radiculopathy
    C   Left C8 radiculopathy
    D   Left Erb's palsy
    E   Left radial nerve palsy

3. A 25-year-old man was brought to the emergency department after suffering a traumatic head
    injury.
        He underwent a CT of the head (see **Figure 7.1**):

    What does the CT of the head show?

    A   Left subdural haematoma
    B   Left extradural haematoma
    C   Right subdural haematoma
    D   Right extradural haematoma
    E   Subarachnoid haemorrhage

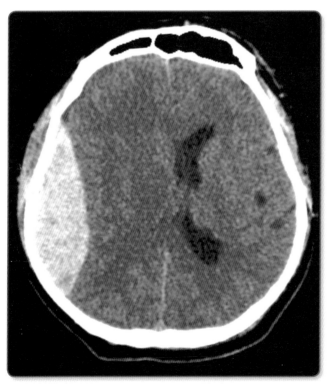

Figure 7.1

4. A 73-year-old man presented to the emergency department after awaking with loss of vision in his left eye (see **Figure 7.2**).

What is the most likely diagnosis?

A   Central retinal artery occlusion
B   Central retinal vein occlusion
C   Cytomegalovirus retinitis
D   Preretinal haemorrhage
E   Retinal detachment

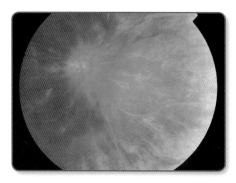

Figure 7.2 *See colour plate section.*

5. A 71-year-old man was brought to the emergency department with fever, tremor and agitation. His past medical history was of type 2 diabetes with peripheral neuropathy for which he was taking regular metformin and duloxetine. One day earlier, he had also started taking citalopram for treatment of depression.

On examination, temperature was 38.8°C, pulse 106 beats per minute and blood pressure 142/91 mmHg.

He was profusely sweaty, tremulous and confused with a Glasgow Coma Scale score of 12 (eyes 3, speech 4, motor 5). There was some neck stiffness, but no rash or photophobia. Cranial nerve examination revealed marked opsoclonus. Limb examination revealed increased tone and hyperreflexia throughout. Sustained clonus was elicited at the ankles.

Investigations:

MRI of the brain: normal

What is the most likely diagnosis?

A   Dopamine dysregulation syndrome
B   Malignant hyperthermia
C   Meningoencephalitis
D   Neuroleptic malignant syndrome
E   Serotonin syndrome

6. A 35-year-old woman presented with a 1-week history of increasingly confused behaviour and memory complaints. She had a cold with fever and headache 10 days prior to presentation but otherwise her only past medical history was a diagnosis of depression 8 months ago for which she had received cognitive behavioural therapy, although recently she had become very withdrawn and paranoid. Over the course of a week she became increasingly agitated before becoming obtunded and catatonic with abnormal orofacial movements requiring admission to intensive care.

    Her lumbar puncture results showed a mild cerebrospinal fluid pleocytosis, MRI showed non-specific changes and an EEG showed slowed delta wave activity.

    What is the most likely diagnosis?

    A   Schizophrenia
    B   Voltage-gated potassium channel antibody encephalitis
    C   Bickerstaff's encephalitis
    D   *N*-methyl-D-aspartate receptor antibody encephalitis
    E   Conversion disorder

7. A 79-year-old man presented to the emergency department with a transient ischaemic attack (TIA) that manifested as left facial droop, dysarthria and left-sided hemiparesis. Clinical signs resolved completely within 2 hours of onset. The patient was diabetic and hypertensive, with no past medical history of TIA or stroke. His current medications include metformin, ramipril and simvastatin. He was a lifelong non-smoker.

    On examination, blood pressure is 135/85 mmHg, pulse rate 70 beats per minute and rhythm regular. There are no carotid bruits and no neurological signs.

    His HbA1c was 8.1% (3.8–6.4).

    Using the $ABCD_2$ assessment tool, what does the patient score?

    A   3
    B   4
    C   5
    D   6
    E   7

8. A 38-year-old woman presented with fever, back pain, paraparesis and urinary retention.
    An MRI of the whole spine was performed (see **Figure 7.3**).

    What is the most likely diagnosis?

    A   Intervertebral disc prolapse
    B   Paraspinal abscess

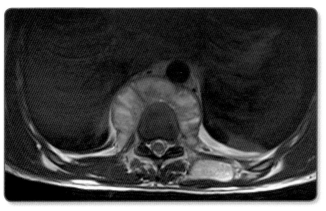

Figure 7.3

    C   Syringomyelia
    D   Transverse myelitis
    E   Vertebral metastases

9.   A 59-year-old woman presented with a 4-month history of continuous unilateral headache. She described a persistent, left, frontotemporal, throbbing pain with ocular involvement. Additionally, there were daily paroxysms of severe pain with associated excessive lacrimation, eyelid oedema and rhinorrhoea lasting anywhere from a few minutes to half an hour. They had been occurring approximately five times per day but did not wake her from sleep. She had no past medical history, and was taking paracetamol daily with little or no symptomatic relief. She worked as a supermarket cashier, did not smoke and did not drink alcohol.

      Physical examination was normal and fundoscopy was unremarkable.

Investigations:

MRI of the head: normal
MRA of the intracranial vessels: normal

What is the most likely diagnosis?

    A   Analgesic overuse headache
    B   Cluster headache
    C   Hemicrania continua
    D   Tension-type headache
    E   Migraine without aura

10. Routine fundoscopy was performed on a 71-year-old man (see **Figure 7.4**).

What is the most likely diagnosis?

    A   Cholesterol embolus
    B   Diabetic retinopathy
    C   Glaucoma
    D   Macular hole
    E   Normal

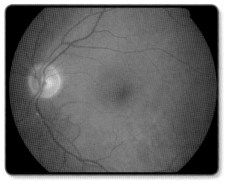

Figure 7.4 *See colour plate section.*

11. A 73-year-old man presented with a 1-year history of left hand tremor, falls and depression. He stated that he experienced a lot of difficulty using his left hand and did not feel that it was under his control. His wife also added that he is no longer able to do crossword puzzles.

On examination, speech was non-fluent but easily intelligible. His Abbreviated Mental Test score was 8/10. He had a mild resting tremor of the left hand with abnormal flexion at the wrist. There were occasional jerking movements of the limbs. Tone was increased in the left arm, with cogwheeling at the wrist. Mild weakness was present throughout. Coordination was poor, and ideomotor apraxia was evident. Reflexes and sensation were normal. Gait was slow and unsteady. Cranial nerve examination revealed limited upgaze with diplopia. Fundoscopy was also normal.

Investigations:

> MRI of the brain: moderate frontoparietal atrophy and some evidence of small vessel ischaemic disease

A trial of dopamine conferred minimal symptomatic relief.

What is the most likely diagnosis?

A   Corticobasal degeneration
B   Frontotemporal dementia
C   Parkinson's disease
D   Progressive supranuclear palsy
E   Vascular dementia

12. A 25-year-old woman with a history of idiopathic, generalised, tonic–clonic seizures attended the outpatient clinic for her annual review. She was diagnosed, aged 18 years, following two seizures in the same year.

She underwent MRI of the head and a sleep-deprived electroencephalogram (EEG), both of which were normal. Sodium valproate was commenced following the second seizure, and she had remained seizure free on a dose of 500 mg twice daily ever since.

She is now wishing to start a family and she doesn't want to take anything that may be harmful during pregnancy.

What is the most appropriate management?

A   Stop all treatment
B   Switch to carbamazepine
C   Continue valproate in view of the risk of seizure recurrence on cessation
D   Repeat a sleep-deprived EEG before making any decision
E   Switch to lamotrigine

13. A 72-year-old man was brought to hospital following a fall in which he sustained a head injury. He was taking warfarin for atrial fibrillation.

A CT of the head was performed (see **Figure 7.5**).

What is the diagnosis?

A   Bilateral acute subdural haematoma
B   Bilateral acute-on-chronic subdural haematoma
C   Bilateral chronic subdural haematoma
D   Bilateral extradural haematoma
E   Subarachnoid haemorrhage

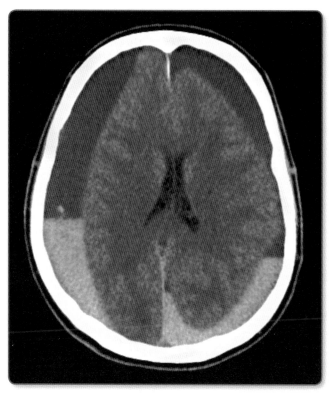

Figure 7.5

14. A 62-year-old woman was referred by her optician, following a routine eye test (see **Figure 7.6**).

What is the most likely diagnosis?

A   Branch retinal vein occlusion
B   Cholesterol emboli
C   Diabetic retinopathy
D   Hypertensive retinopathy
E   Macular degeneration

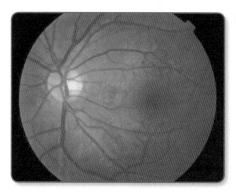

Figure 7.6 *See colour plate section.*

15. A 45-year-old Indian man was seen in the clinic with a 1-month history of bilateral wrist weakness. For the past 4 months he had been taking an Ayurvedic medicine for chronic fatigue symptoms but now he felt worse and had also developed insomnia, abdominal discomfort and constipation. He was on no other medications and did not smoke or drink alcohol.

On examination, the patient did not appear in distress. A line of bluish-black discoloration was noted along the gingival margin. Muscle bulk was normal with no wasting or fasciculations. Tone was normal throughout. There was bilateral weakness in wrist extension. Coordination and reflexes were normal. There was no sensory involvement.

What is the most likely cause?

A   Arsenic
B   Beryllium
C   Lead
D   Mercury
E   Thallium

16. A 32-year-old woman with no past medical history presented with a generalised tonic–clonic seizure after becoming acutely confused in the third trimester of her first pregnancy.

An MRI of the brain was performed (see **Figure 7.7**).

What is the most likely diagnosis?

A   Herpes encephalitis
B   Intracerebral haemorrhage
C   Multiple sclerosis

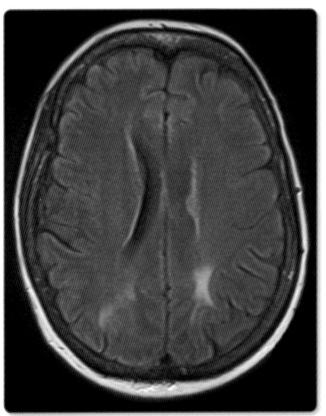

Figure 7.7

D   Posterior reversible encephalopathy syndrome
E   Progressive multifocal leukoencephalopathy

17. A 30-year-old man was brought into the emergency department unconscious (see **Figure 7.8**).

What is the most likely cause of the fundoscopic appearance?

A   Branch retinal artery occlusion
B   Choroidal haemangioma
C   Cytomegalovirus retinitis
D   Myelinated fibres
E   Traction retinal detachment

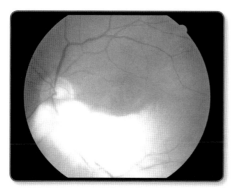

Figure 7.8 See colour plate section.

18. A 38-year-old woman presented to the emergency department after awaking with complete
blindness. There was no past medical history. Indeed, her only visits to the doctor had been
for routine women's health checks and minor ailments. None the less, she did report feeling
'very depressed' after having been recently made redundant from her high-powered job as an
executive at a city investment bank. She was single, had no financial concerns and did not use
recreational drugs.
     On examination, the patient was unable to differentiate between light and dark. Pupillary
responses to light were normal. Visual threat response was intact. Eye movements were full and
conjugate. Fundoscopy was normal. Formal assessment in the ophthalmology clinic failed to
identify any organic pathology.

Investigations:

MRI of the brain: normal

Visual-evoked potentials: normal

What is the most likely diagnosis?

A   Conversion disorder
B   Factitious disorder
C   Malingering
D   Somatisation disorder
E   Undifferentiated somatoform disorder

19. A 25-year-old woman presented with severe headache, nausea and confusion. It came on abruptly while out shopping. There was no past medical history. Her only regular medication was the combined oral contraceptive pill.

On examination, her Glasgow Coma Scale score was 14. There was a receptive aphasia. A contrast-enhanced CT was performed (see **Figure 7.9**).

What is the most likely diagnosis?

A   Dural sinus thrombosis
B   Intracerebral haemorrhage
C   Cerebral infarction
D   Subarachnoid haemorrhage with communicating hydrocephalus
E   Subarachnoid haemorrhage with non-communicating hydrocephalus

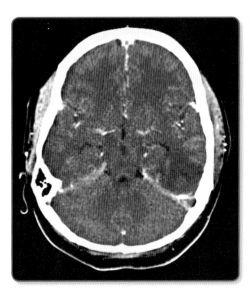

Figure 7.9

20. An 82-year-old man with a history of recently treated prostate cancer, presented with a 2-month history of swallowing difficulties and dysarthria. Examination showed him to have fluctuant weakness in eye opening, palate and tongue movement.

Investigations with formal lung function showed a forced vital capacity (FVC) of 2.6 L. His acetylcholine receptor antibody test was negative. A brain MRI scan was normal as was a CT scan of the chest, abdomen and pelvis.

What would be the most appropriate first line treatment?

A   Plasma exchange
B   High-dose steroids
C   Intravenous immunoglobulin
D   Riluzole
E   Treat the prostate cancer

21. A 61-year-old man presented to the clinic with a 5-month history of progressive weakness of his limbs, most markedly his left arm. He also reported mild difficulty in swallowing of recent onset but no cough or problems with speech. He had no significant past medical history and was on no regular medications.

    On examination, there was muscle wasting and weakness of both upper and lower limbs, with prominent 'guttering' of the dorsum of the left hand. There were numerous diffuse fasciculations. Tone and coordination were normal. Reflexes were brisk, and plantar responses were upgoing bilaterally. There was no sensory involvement. Gait was normal.

    Cranial nerve examination revealed a brisk jaw jerk, and slight wasting of the tongue with infrequent fasciculations.

    Investigations:

MRI of the head and whole spine: normal
Nerve conduction studies: normal sensory study normal motor conduction velocities with no evidence of block reduced amplitude of compound muscle action potentials
Electromyography: active denervation with partial reinnervation

    What is the most appropriate management?

    A Baclofen
    B Diazepam
    C Galantamine
    D Intravenous immunoglobulin
    E Riluzole

22. An 18-year-old woman was referred by her general practitioner, following routine fundoscopy. She reported no visual disturbance (see **Figure 7.10**).

    What is the most likely diagnosis?

    A Choroidal melanoma
    B Chorioretinitis
    C Macular degeneration
    D Macular hole
    E Photocoagulation scarring

Figure 7.10 *See colour plate section.*

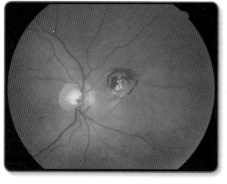

23. A 25-year-old man was referred with a 6-month history of increasing back pain and stiffness affecting his trunk and limbs. He had also been experiencing painful spasms in his arms and legs.

On examination, he was noted to have a bolt upright posture. There was increased tone and stiffness in the upper and lower limbs. Power and reflexes were normal.

Investigations:

> Electromyography: continuous motor unit activity in the paraspinal muscles

What is the most appropriate next investigation?

A   Anti-glutamic acid decarboxylase (GAD) antibody
B   Anti-myelin-associated glycoprotein antibody
C   Anti-*N*-methyl-d-aspartate receptor antibody
D   Anti-striated muscle antibody
E   Anti-Yo antibody

24. A 49-year-old man presented with severe headache, nausea and confusion. No other history was available.

On examination, his Glasgow Coma Scale score was 14 and there were no focal neurological signs.

A CT of the head was performed (see **Figure 7.11**).

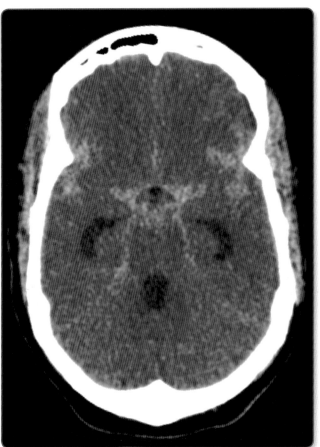

Figure 7.11

What is the most likely diagnosis?

A   Dural sinus thrombosis
B   Extradural haematoma
C   Intracerebral haemorrhage
D   Subarachnoid haemorrhage with communicating hydrocephalus
E   Subdural haematoma

25. A 22-year-old man presented with blurred central vision following blunt trauma to his left eye. He commented that straight lines appeared wavy (see **Figure 7.12**).

What is the most likely diagnosis?

A   Drusen
B   Macular hole
C   Normal appearance
D   Optic atrophy
E   Retinal detachment

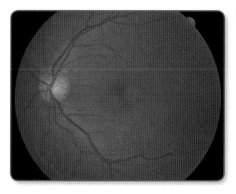

Figure 7.12 *See colour plate section.*

26. A 19-year-old man presented to the emergency department having been assaulted. He has superficial knife wounds to his thigh and hand. He describes the incident as his wounds are dressed and managed. Although he is in a cubicle, the police arrive after the incident was reported to them by a bystander. They talk to the receptionist and establish that a patient with knife wounds is in the department but the receptionist refers them to you for further information. He is medically fit to be interviewed but the patient does not wish to talk to the police. They are insisting on interviewing him.

What is the most appropriate course of action?

A   Take the police to the patient
B   Tell the police what you know of the patient and the incident but deny them access to him
C   Give the police the name and address of the patient only
D   Tell the police you cannot give them any information
E   Tell the police what you know of the incident only but do not give them the patient's details

27. A 55-year-old man was referred to the neurology clinic with a 6-month history of dizziness and falls. On direct questioning he also reported erectile dysfunction and episodes of urinary incontinence during this period.

    On examination, his pulse was 74 beats per minute, blood pressure 128/72 mmHg on lying which dropped to 104/58 mmHg on standing and was associated with symptoms of dizziness. He was generally slow with a marked torticollis and mildly increased tone throughout all limbs. Myoclonic jerks were noticed in the fingers of the outstretched hands. There was a generalised weakness throughout the limbs. Deep tendon reflexes were brisk throughout and plantars were upgoing bilaterally. Gait was mildly ataxic. Cranial nerve examination was normal except for slow pupillary responses to light.

Investigations:

serum ceruloplasmin 310 mg/L (200–350)	urinary copper 25 µg in 24 hours (<50)
MRI of the brain: atrophy of the putamen	

    The patient's symptoms do not improve with levodopa.

What is the most likely diagnosis?

A   Corticobasal degeneration
B   Multiple system atrophy
C   Parkinson's disease
D   Progressive supranuclear palsy
E   Wilson's disease

28. A 38-year-old woman presented with rapidly progressive, bilateral, central visual field loss, as well as bilateral arm and leg weakness several weeks after a flu-like illness. She also reported a short history of bladder and bowel dysfunction. There was no past medical history.

    On examination, there was a quadriparesis, with brisk deep tendon reflexes. The patient was able to stand only with assistance. Cranial nerve examination revealed bilateral central visual field loss, with fundoscopic evidence of bilateral optic neuritis.

Investigations:

MRI of the brain: normal	
MRI of the cervical spine: hyperintense cord lesion consistent with transverse myelitis (spanning C3–6)	
Visual-evoked potentials: delayed	
Cerebrospinal fluid:	
opening pressure 20 cmH$_2$O	protein 0.7 g/L (0.15–0.45)
white blood cell 100/mm^3 (<5)	glucose 4.0 mmol/L (serum 6.6 mmol/L)
Negative for oligoclonal bands	

What is the most useful diagnostic test?

A   Anti-aquaporin-4 antibody
B   Anti-GAD antibody
C   Anti-GQ1b antibody
D   Anti-*N-methyl*-d-aspartate receptor antibody
E   Anti-voltage-gated potassium channel antibody

29. A 27-year-old woman presented with several months' history of severe daily headache which was worse in the morning and associated with nausea. She also experienced episodes of pulsatile tinnitus. On a few occasions, she had experienced very brief bilateral visual loss when bending over to pick things up. Past medical history included polycystic ovarian syndrome. Her only medication was metformin.

On examination, she had some hirsutism and her body mass index was 28 kg/m². Visual acuity was 6/9 in both eyes and her visual fields were not obviously constricted. Fundoscopy revealed bilateral papilloedema. The rest of her neurological examination was normal.

Investigations:

MRI of the brain: empty sella turcica
MR venogram: normal
Lumbar puncture (cerebrospinal fluid analysis): opening pressure 30 cmH₂O (10–20) white cell count 0/mm³ (<5) protein 0.3 g/L (0.15–0.45) glucose (cerebrospinal fluid:blood ratio) 0.65 (0.5–0.8)

What is the most appropriate management?

A   Commence acetazolamide
B   Refer for insertion of a ventriculoperitoneal shunt
C   Refer for optic nerve sheath fenestration
D   Refer to a neuro-ophthalmologist for formal visual assessment
E   Serial lumbar punctures with drainage of cerebrospinal fluid to normal pressure range

30. An 82-year-old man presented with a 6-month history of progressive central visual loss (see **Figure 7.13**).

What is the most likely diagnosis?

A   Age-related macular degeneration
B   Choroidal melanoma
C   Epiretinal membrane
D   Preretinal haemorrhage
E   Retinal detachment

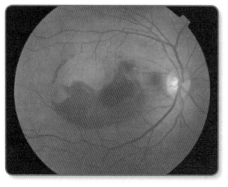

Figure 7.13 *See colour plate section.*

31. A 75-year-old man presented with hemiplegia. Diffusion-weighted MRI of the brain was performed (see **Figure 7.14**).

Which of the following is the most likely diagnosis?

A   Left anterior cerebral artery territory infarct
B   Left middle cerebral artery territory infarct
C   Left posterior cerebral artery territory infarct
D   Right middle cerebral artery territory infarct
E   Right posterior cerebral artery territory infarct

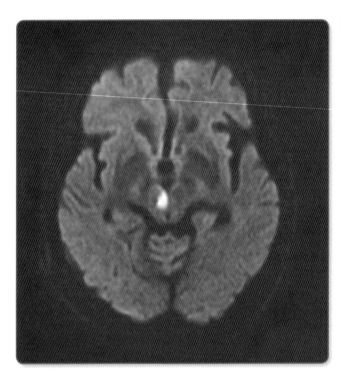

Figure 7.14

32. An 18-year-old schoolgirl presented with headache. Since adolescence, she had experienced simple headaches around the time of her periods, responsive to over-the-counter analgesia. However, these had transformed over the past 2 years. She was now suffering from unilateral throbbing headaches, associated with nausea and photophobia, lasting from several hours to a whole day at a time. There were no obvious triggers for the headache, and it did not wake her from sleep. She had not enjoyed a headache-free day for more than 2 months and was very anxious that the headaches would affect her performance in upcoming exams.

She wore reading glasses, and last had her sight checked by an optician 4 months ago. There was no past medical history of note. She was on the combined oral contraceptive pill and took analgesic medications such as co-codamol and ibuprofen in variable doses on a daily basis. She had no family history of migraine.

She lived with her parents, consumed five to six cups of coffee per day, smoked five cigarettes per day and drank 10 units of alcohol at weekends. She had a healthy diet but took no regular exercise.

Physical examination was completely normal and fundoscopy was unremarkable.

What is the most appropriate next step in this patient's management?

A   Avoid combined oral contraceptive
B   Commence propranolol prophylaxis
C   Lifestyle changes (reduce caffeine and alcohol intake, stop smoking, take regular exercise)
D   MRI of the head
E   Stop all analgesics

33. A 45-year-old man presented with deterioration of vision in his right eye (see **Figure 7.15**).

What is the most likely diagnosis?

A   Branch retinal artery occlusion
B   Branch retinal vein occlusion
C   Cholesterol embolus
D   Cytomegalovirus retinitis
E   Hypertensive retinopathy

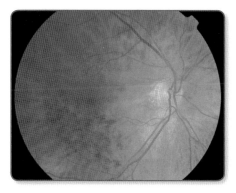

Figure 7.15 *See colour plate section.*

34. A 28-year-old man with epilepsy, who had been completely seizure free for the past 3 years on treatment with sodium valproate, wished to discontinue drug therapy.
    He had a clean driving licence and driving was not essential for his job. He knew that he was required to inform the Driver and Vehicle Licensing Authority, and would need to stop driving from commencement of withdrawal, but was unsure of how long he had to stop driving for.

For how long after cessation of treatment will the patient need to refrain from driving?

A   1 month
B   3 months
C   6 months
D   12 months
E   18 months

35. A CT of the head was performed on a 78-year-old man with clinical features of acute stroke (see **Figure 7.16**).

What is the most likely diagnosis?

A   Acute left frontal infarct and old right frontal infarct
B   Acute left parietal infarct and old left frontal infarct
C   Acute left occipital infarct
D   Acute right frontal infarct and old left frontal infarct
E   Acute right parietal infarct and old right frontal infarct

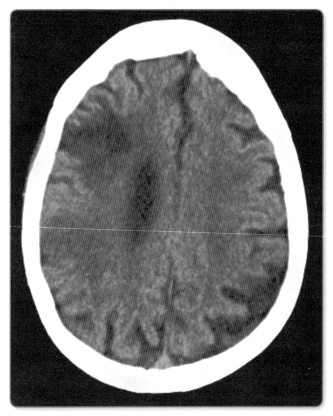

Figure 7.16

36. A 70-year-old woman presented with acute deterioration in vision in her right eye (see **Figure 7.17**).

What is the most likely underlying cause?

A   Diabetic retinopathy
B   Disseminated intravascular coagulation
C   Malignant hypertension
D   Retinal tear
E   Valsalva's retinopathy

Figure 7.17 *See colour plate section.*

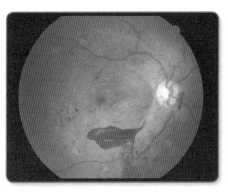

37. A 32-year-old woman presented to the emergency department after awaking with diplopia and problems with balance. She had no past medical history and was not taking any regular medications.

   On examination, she was oriented and alert. Cranial nerve examination revealed a complex ophthalmoplegia and reduced pupillary response to light. Fundoscopy was normal. Peripheral nervous system examination revealed normal tone and power. However, deep tendon reflexes were markedly depressed throughout. Plantar responses were downgoing. Moderate gait and truncal ataxia were apparent with choreoathetosis on limb examination.

   Investigations:

   MRI of the brain: normal

Cerebrospinal fluid (CSF) analysis:	protein 0.6 g/L (0.15–0.45)
white blood cell 8 cells/mm^3 (<5)	CSF culture and Gram stain: no organisms seen
glucose (CSF:blood ratio) 0.6 (0.5–0.8)	
opening pressure 18 cmH$_2$O	CSF viral polymerase chain reaction: negative
QG1b antibody: positive	

   What is the most likely diagnosis?

   A   Bickerstaff's brain-stem encephalitis
   B   Guillain–Barré syndrome
   C   Lambert–Eaton syndrome
   D   Miller Fisher syndrome
   E   Wernicke's encephalopathy

38. A 36-year-old woman presented with several years' history of headache, neck pain and restricted neck movements.
   Examination revealed a dissociated sensory loss.
   An MRI of the spine was performed (see **Figure 7.18**):

   What does the MRI show?

   A   Cervical spondylosis with syringomyelia
   B   Cervical spondylosis and Chiari I malformation with syringomyelia
   C   Cervical spondylosis and Chiari II malformation with syringomyelia
   D   Chiari I malformation with syringomyelia
   E   Chiari II malformation with syringomyelia

39. A 42-year-old man receiving monthly infusions of natalizumab for severe relapsing–remitting multiple sclerosis presented with a single generalised tonic–clonic seizure.

   Which of the following is associated with natalizumab?

   A   Acute disseminated encephalomyelitis
   B   Lathyrism
   C   Neuromyelitis optica
   D   Progressive multifocal leukoencephalopathy
   E   Transverse myelitis

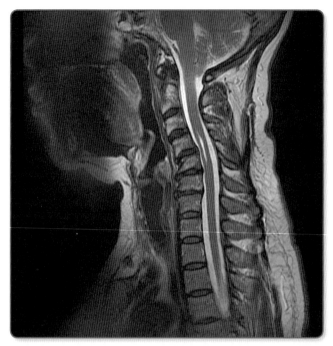

Figure 7.18

40. A 57-year-old man presented with left upper limb weakness. As part of the examination, fundoscopy was performed (see **Figure 7.19**).

What is evident on fundoscopy?

A   Central retinal artery occlusion
B   Diabetic retinopathy
C   Glaucoma
D   Hypertensive retinopathy
E   Optic atrophy

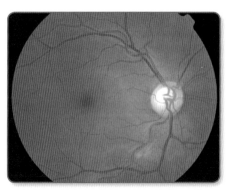

Figure 7.19 *See colour plate section.*

41. A 38-year-old man was referred with a 1-year history of progressive weakness of his arms and hands. He complained of increasing difficulty in typing and troublesome cramps affecting his left arm in particular.

On examination, there was no obvious muscle wasting. No fasciculations were observed. Tone was mildly reduced in the upper limbs. There was accompanying moderate weakness, which was most prominent in the extensors of the left arm. Lower limb tone and power were normal. Coordination was normal throughout. Reflexes were depressed. Sensory examination and gait were normal.

Investigations:

Antiganglioside antibodies: anti-GM1 positive
MRI of the cervical spine: normal
Cerebrospinal fluid (CSF) analysis: opening pressure 16 cmH$_2$O glucose (CSF: blood ratio) 0.6 protein 0.7 g/L (0.15–0.45) white blood cell count 1 cell/mm^3 (<5)

What is the most likely diagnosis?

A   Amyotrophic lateral sclerosis
B   Chronic inflammatory demyelinating polyneuropathy
C   Charcot–Marie–Tooth disease type 1
D   Mononeuritis multiplex
E   Multifocal motor neuropathy with conduction block

42. A 72-year-old woman was referred with a 3-year history of troublesome tremor which caused her to frequently spill drinks. She had noticed that her symptoms were worse with stress. There was a family history of an older half-sister who had recently been diagnosed with Parkinson's disease.

On examination, the patient appeared anxious. There was prominent titubation (head tremor) as well as staggering gait and symmetrical tremor of the outstretched hands. No resting tremor was observed. Tone, power and deep tendon reflexes were normal. Tests of coordination revealed a moderate kinetic tremor. Gait was normal.

Investigations:

MRI of the brain: normal

What is the most appropriate next step in management?

A   Apomorphine challenge
B   [123I] FP-CIT single photon emission computed tomography (SPECT) (DaT scan)
C   Levodopa challenge
D   Propranolol
E   Reassurance and discharge

43. A 28-year-old woman presented with reduced vision in her right eye with pain on eye movement. There was no previous medical history. However, on direct questioning, she reported that 5 months ago she experienced an episode of numbness of her right arm lasting several days and after a fall 10 years ago she had been left with weakness and intermittent numbness in her left leg which worsened in warm weather

On examination, there was reduced visual acuity, impaired colour vision and a relative afferent pupillary defect in the right eye. Fundoscopy revealed corresponding optic atrophy.

Investigations:

Visual-evoked potentials: delay on the right

An MRI of the brain was performed (see **Figure 7.20**).

Which management option might be considered to prevent progressive deterioration of this condition?

A   Intravenous immunoglobulin
B   Rituximab
C   Nataluzimab
D   High dose intravenous methylprednisolone
E   Plasma exchange

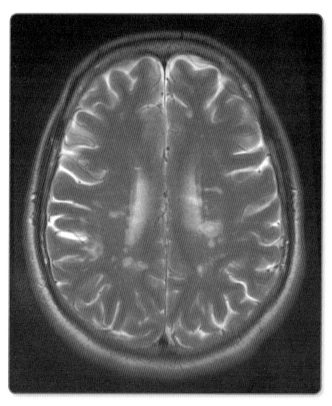

Figure 7.20

44. A 45-year-old homeless man presented with confusion and unsteadiness.

On examination, the patient was unkempt and smelled strongly of alcohol. He was apathetic and restless. His Glasgow Coma Scale score was 14 (eyes 4, speech 4, motor 6), temperature 36.1°C, pulse 73 beats per minute, blood pressure 104/64 mmHg, respiratory rate 16 breaths per minute, and oxygen saturation 96% on air. Capillary blood glucose was measured as 2.9 mmol/L. Neurological examination revealed nystagmus, truncal ataxia, broad-based gait, sensorimotor peripheral neuropathy and positive Romberg's test. The Abbreviated Mental Test score was 6/10.

What is the most appropriate next step in management?

A   Intramuscular lorazepam
B   Intravenous dextrose
C   Intravenous thiamine
D   Oral aciclovir
E   Oral olanzapine

45. A 61-year-old man presented to his optician for a routine assessment (see **Figure 7.21**).

What is the most likely diagnosis?

A   Choroidal haemangioma
B   Chorioretinitis
C   Onchocerciasis
D   Photocoagulation scarring
E   Retinitis pigmentosa

Figure 7.21 *See colour plate section.*

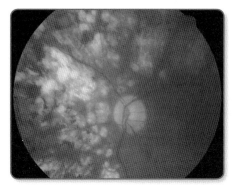

46. A 57-year-old man presented with a 6-month history of persistent burning pains in both feet. This has been particularly troubling at night, and has been affecting his sleep. There was no past medical history and he was not taking any regular medications.

Motor examination of the lower limbs was normal. Sensory examination revealed reduced sensation to pinprick, and thermal hypoaesthesia, to low-shin level bilaterally. Proprioception and vibration sense were normal. Romberg's test was normal, as was gait.

Investigations:

oral glucose tolerance test 9.9 mmol/L at 2 hours (<7.8)
Nerve conduction studies: normal

What is the most likely diagnosis?

A   Conversion disorder
B   Diabetic amyotrophy
C   Mononeuritis multiplex
D   Restless legs syndrome
E   Small fibre neuropathy

47. A 58-year-old man presented to the emergency department with sudden loss of memory. He had been found to be behaving oddly while playing tennis, repeating questions about the time of day and unable to recall what he's doing. On review he was disoriented to time and place and had difficulty following three-stage commands. He was able to recall distant events in his past but had no recollection of his recent vacation to South Africa 3 weeks ago. There were no physical neurological findings. The episode of absolute confusion lasted for 4 hours with gradual resolution over the next 6 hours. 24 hours later he had no recollection of the episode but appeared to have fully recovered his memory otherwise. He had no significant past medical history and was not a smoker.

    CT head imaging did not reveal any abnormality.

What is the most likely diagnosis?

A   Temporal lobe epilepsy
B   Hypoxic brain injury
C   Transient ischemic attack
D   Transient global amnesia
E   Encephalitis

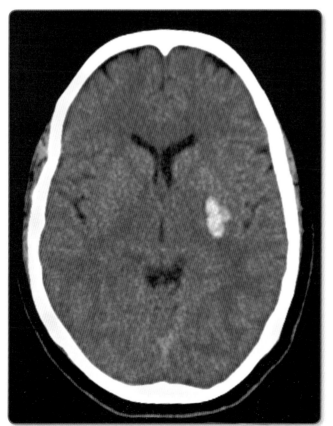

Figure 7.22

48. A 70-year-old woman presented to the emergency department. The ambulance crew reported that she has been found unconscious on the floor by her sister after not answering her phone for 2 days. On the way to the hospital she had a 30-second self-terminating generalised tonic–clonic seizure. Her past medical history included hypertension, treated with ramipril and she was taking atorvastatin for hypercholesterolaemia. She was said to enjoy a daily nightcap.

In the emergency department she scores 8 on the Glasgow Coma Scale (eyes 2, voice 2, motor 4). She is tachypnoeic, tachycardic with an irregular pulse and was hypertensive with a blood pressure of 196/105 mmHg. Her finger prick blood glucose was 3.9 mmol/L. She was noted to have a right-sided hemiparesis on examination with eyes rolled back deviating to the right and dampened reflexes with an up going plantar's reflex on the right. She has three further seizures in the emergency department without regaining consciousness between episodes. An ECG shows atrial fibrillation.

A CT of the head was performed (see **Figure 7.22**).

Which of the management options below should come next following initial benzodiazepine treatment?

A   Intravenous labetalol
B   Phenytoin infusion
C   Thiamine infusion
D   Propofol infusion
E   Neurosurgical referral

Answers

1. D Sporadic Creutzfeldt–Jakob disease

This is a prion protein disease characterised by rapid-onset dementia, myoclonus and ataxia. Extrapyramidal features are not uncommon. Akinetic mutism rapidly ensues, and the condition typically proceeds to death within 6 months of onset. Routine blood tests are often unremarkable. MRI often reveals symmetrical hyperintensity in the striatum and/or cerebral cortex. Cerebrospinal fluid is usually normal, except for elevated 14-3-3 protein (this is a useful marker of prion protein disease; however, it may sometimes be elevated in stroke or rapidly progressive dementias). An electroencephalogram (EEG) reveals generalised periodic sharp waves in the majority of patients with the sporadic variant. Brain biopsy may be necessary for definitive diagnosis. There is no effective treatment.

There are three forms of Creutzfeldt–Jakob disease (CJD): familial, sporadic and variant. The familial form is due to heritable mutation within the prion protein (PrP) gene. It accounts for 5–15% of cases. Average onset is in the sixth decade. Sporadic CJD is due to spontaneous misfolding of the prion protein, or somatic mutation within the gene. Its incidence is 1 per million per year, and it accounts for 85% of cases. Peak age of onset is the seventh decade of life and median duration of illness is 4.5 months. Variant CJD is the human form believed to be related to bovine spongiform encephalopathy (BSE) and is thought to be secondary to ingestion of contaminated meat products. Variant CJD presents at a younger age (median age of onset 28 years), with median illness duration of 14 months, with different MRI appearances of more prominent involvement of the pulvinar and medial thalamic nuclei, and the EEG is normal or non-specifically abnormal. Iatrogenic CJD results from the use of contaminated surgical equipment, pituitary products and blood transfusion.

Corticobasal degeneration typically occurs in the seventh decade. It is a cause of dementia and myoclonus. There is usually akinetic rigidity with 'alien limb' phenomenon. The latter refers to the feeling that the affected limb is not under the patient's control. Protein 14-3-3 is not typically detected.

Isolated cerebral angiitis is rare. It is a granulomatous small and medium vessel vasculitis of the brain, resulting in multiple infarcts. It can present with headache, encephalopathic features and focal neurological signs.

Limbic encephalitis is an autoimmune inflammatory process which can occur as a paraneoplastic syndrome. It presents with anterograde and retrograde amnesia. Often, there is an acute confusional state, with personality and behavioural change. MRI typically reveals symmetrical hyperintensity within the mesial temporal lobes. Cerebrospinal fluid analysis tends to reveal a mild pleocytosis with positive oligoclonal bands. Diagnosis of this condition warrants investigation for an underlying cancer if it is not overt (typically by positron emission tomography). Paraneoplastic antibodies associated with this condition include anti-voltage-gated potassium channel, anti-Hu, anti-Ta/ma2, ANNA 3 and anti-CRMP5/CV2. Limbic encephalitis is often linked to cancers of the lung (particularly small cell lung cancer), testis, breast and thymus. Initial treatment may include steroids, plasma exchange or intravenous immunoglobulin. However, definitive treatment requires identification and elimination of any underlying cancer, if possible.

Clarke C, et al. Dementia and cognitive impairment (Chapter 8). In: Neurology: A Queen Square Textbook, 2nd edn. Oxford: Blackwell Publishing, 2016.
Manji H, et al. Neurological Disorders (Chapter 4). In: Oxford Handbook of Neurology. Oxford: University Press, 2007.

2. B Left C7 radiculopathy

This causes pain, myotomal weakness and numbness in the pattern described. C7 is the principal root underlying the triceps jerk. C6 radiculopathy causes weakness of elbow flexion and wrist extension, depressed biceps and supinator jerks, and numbness in the lateral forearm extending to the thumb and index finger. C8 radiculopathy causes weakness in finger flexors and extensors, abductor digiti minimi and first dorsal interosseous; it causes numbness in the medial forearm extending to the ring and little fingers. Spurling's test is a test for vertebral foraminal compression of the cervical nerve roots. The neck is extended and rotated towards the affected side, and downward pressure is applied on the head; the test is positive if symptoms are elicited in the affected dermatomal distribution. The test is of high specificity, but low sensitivity. Muscle wasting commonly occurs in association with longstanding or severe radiculopathies.

Erb's palsy is due to C5 and C6 root injury, which is often caused by shoulder dystocia at birth. It is characterised by the 'waiter's tip' appearance (weakness being in shoulder abduction, external rotation of the arm, elbow flexion and wrist extension).

The radial nerve and its branches are responsible for extension throughout the upper limb. The only flexion that it supports is at the elbow with the wrist semi-pronated which is achieved through its innervation of brachioradialis. The radial nerve subserves triceps and supinator jerks. It innervates skin directly in the dorsum of the hand (thumb, forefinger, middle finger and lateral half of the ring finger), and indirectly in the arm and forearm through several cutaneous branches (posterior cutaneous nerve of the arm, inferolateral cutaneous nerve of the arm and posterior cutaneous nerve of the forearm). The extent of motor and sensory involvement will depend on the point at which the nerve is injured in its anatomical course.

Snell RS. Clinical Neuroanatomy, 7th edn. Philadelphia, PA: Lippincott, Williams & Wilkins, 2010.

3. D Right extradural haematoma

This is a typical appearance of an extradural haematoma. It is usually due to laceration of the middle meningeal artery following blunt trauma. The dura mater, which lines the cranium, peels away to the suture lines as blood collects in the extradural space; this gives rise to the convex appearance. Urgent neurosurgical referral for evacuation of the haematoma should be sought.

Perron AD. How to read a head CT scan (Chapter 69). In: Adams JG (ed.) Emergency Medicine. Philadelphia, PA: Saunders, 2008.

4. B Central retinal vein occlusion

This is a typical fundoscopic appearance of central retinal vein occlusion (CRVO); there are flame-shaped intraretinal haemorrhages in all four quadrants and oedema of the optic disc. The condition is more common with increasing age, and can be ischaemic or non-ischaemic in aetiology. Risk factors include hypertension, dyslipidaemia, diabetes mellitus, smoking, thrombophilia and raised intraocular pressure. Typically it presents with severe painless reduction of vision. Ischaemic CRVO is more severe, whereas non-ischaemic CRVO may present with fewer symptoms and signs.

Central retinal artery occlusion usually presents as acute onset of unilateral severe reduction of vision. The typical appearance is of a pale fundus with a cherry-red spot at the macula.

Cytomegalovirus retinitis is slowly progressive; fundoscopy usually reveals perivascular infiltration and haemorrhage (so-called 'pizza' appearance).

Preretinal haemorrhage usually presents as a boat-shaped haemorrhage, and is due to bleeding into the potential space between the retina and vitreous (e.g. from a posterior vitreous detachment/macroaneurysm/proliferative diabetic retinopathy). This is shown elsewhere.

In retinal detachment there is usually a well-defined border between attached and detached retina, with the latter typically being greyer in colour and out of focus. Normally, the detachment starts peripherally and progresses centrally. It presents with a curtain-like defect in the visual field, associated with sudden onset of floaters and flashing lights.

Wong T, et al. Retinal-vein occlusion. N Engl J Med 2010; 363:2135–2144.

5. E Serotonin syndrome

This patient is most likely to be suffering from serotonin (5HT) syndrome, a drug reaction characterised by neuromuscular excitation, autonomic stimulation and changes in mental state. Onset is usually over 24 hours of commencing the offending agent(s). Classes of drug that have been implicated include monoamine oxidase inhibitors (MAOIs), selective serotonin reuptake inhibitors (SSRIs), serotonin–noradrenaline reuptake inhibitors (SNRIs), tricyclic antidepressants, lithium, opiates and triptans.

Clinical features are variable but include hyperthermia, tachycardia, hypertension, mydriasis, profuse sweating, hyperactive bowel sounds, increased tone, hyperreflexia, tremor, opsoclonus (uncontrolled eye movements), and spontaneous or sustained clonus. The Hunter serotonin toxicity criteria can be used to make the diagnosis. Management is by withdrawal of the suspected causative agent and basic supportive measures. There is some anecdotal evidence supporting the use of the $5HT_2$ antagonist cyproheptadine. Similarly, some evidence exists to support the use of chlorpromazine in severe cases. Most cases resolve within 24 hours.

Neuroleptic malignant syndrome (NMS) is characterised by hyperthermia, severe muscular rigidity and autonomic dysfunction. The syndrome may complicate the use of neuroleptic or atypical antipsychotic medications. Clinical features may include severe lead-pipe rigidity, tremor, dystonia, fever, tachycardia, labile blood pressure, tachypnoea, profuse sweating and acute confusion. Treatment is supportive with cessation of the antipsychotic. The history of antipsychotic drug usage and clinical finding of severe rigidity can usually differentiate NMS from serotonin syndrome. Hyperreflexia and clonus are not prominent features of NMS.

Meningoencephalitis is not the most likely diagnosis in view of the history and clinical examination, which are in keeping with serotonin syndrome.

Dopamine dysregulation syndrome has been described in patients with Parkinson's disease who develop an addiction to their dopamine replacement therapy. Use of dopaminergic medications escalates beyond clinical need and is associated with the development of impulse control disorders (such as pathological gambling, excessive shopping, hypersexuality).

Malignant hyperthermia occurs in patients with an autosomal dominant mutation in the ryanodine receptor. Exposure to halogenated anaesthetic gases, such as halothane, or depolarising muscular relaxants, such as suxamethonium, may precipitate the condition. There is an extremely high mortality rate in untreated patients. Standard treatment is with dantrolene sodium and general supportive measures. Once diagnosed, future exposure to precipitants should be avoided.

Dunkley EJ, et al. The Hunter serotonin toxicity criteria: simple and accurate diagnostic decision rules for serotonin toxicity. Q J Med 2003; 96:635–642.
Boyer EW, Shannon M. The serotonin syndrome. N Eng J Med 2005; 352:1112–1120.

6. D *N*-methyl-D-aspartate receptor encephalitis

This woman is displaying signs of an autoimmune encephalitis (AE). AE is commonly a paraneoplastic phenomenon. This presentation fits with that of *N*-methyl-D-aspartate receptor encephalitis (NMDAR) which typically presents below the age of 45 and has a female:male ratio of 4:1. It is commonly associated with ovarian teratoma.

It is associated with antibodies against the GluN1 subunit of the NMDA receptor and the characteristic stages of the illness include a viral prodromal period followed by progression within 3–14 days of psychiatric symptoms. Patients often present to the mental health services prior to developing more typical neurological symptoms such as memory complaints, speech and language disintegration (including mutism) and seizures. Catatonia correlates with autonomic instability and abnormal movements, with stereotypical oro-lingual-facial dyskinesias or limb and trunk choreoathetosis.

Treatment for AE primarily consists of immunomodulation with high-dose intravenous corticosteroids, intravenous immunoglobulins or plasma exchange, with second line options including rituximab and cyclophosphamide. Status epilepticus can develop with refractory seizures requiring multiple antiepileptics or intensive care support to achieve control.

Voltage gated potassium channel (VGKC) complex antibody encephalitis presents with confusion and memory complaints. It is due to antibodies against the potassium channel complex. Antibodies to the leucine-rich, glioma-inactivated 1 (LG 1) protein are associated with faciobrachial dystonic seizures whereas anti-contactin-associated protein-like 2 (CASPr2) antibodies are more common in elderly men who have additional cerebellar signs.

Bickerstaff's brainstem encephalitis includes a triad of abnormal mental status, bilateral external ophthalmoplegia, and ataxia. IgG anti-GQ1b antibodies are highly specific for this disorder, and the related Miller–Fisher syndrome.

Schizophrenia is a chronic psychiatric diagnosis with onset most commonly in an individual's 20s and 30s. It consists of positive psychotic symptoms, negative symptoms (difficulty initiating speech, loss of emotion, lack of pleasure or enjoyment) and thought disorganisation (confused and disordered thinking and speech, trouble with logical thinking). Often impaired cognition is present due to problems with attention, concentration and memory.

Conversion disorder does not present with stereotypical abnormal movements, a pleocytosis on lumbar puncture, and is not antibody mediated. It is covered in the answer to Question 18 in more detail.

Graus F, Titulaer MJ, Balu R, et al. A clinical approach to diagnosis of autoimmune encephalitis. The Lancet. Neurol 2016; 15:391–404

7. D 6

The $ABCD_2$ score can be used to categorise patients presenting with transient ischaemic attack (TIA) into low, moderate and high risk for subsequent stroke. Patients are assigned scores from 0 to 7 using the following criteria:

Age	>60 years (1 point)
Bloodpressure	systolic >140 mmHg or diastolic >90 mmHg (1 point)
Clinical presentation	speech impairment without focal weakness (1 point)
	focal weakness (2 points)
Duration	10–59 minutes (1 point)
	>59 minutes (2 points)
Diabetes	yes (1 point)

The patient in question has an $ABCD_2$ score of 6 at presentation. Therefore, he has a high risk of stroke. Indeed, the risk is estimated to be 8% over the ensuing 2 days, as shown in **Table 7.1**.

Table 7.1 Risk stratification for stroke using the $ABCD_2$ score			
$ABCD_2$ score	Within 2 days	Within 7 days	Within 90 days
Low risk (<4)	1.0%	1.2%	3.1%
Moderate risk (4–5)	4.1%	5.9%	9.8%
High risk (>5)	8.1%	11.7%	17.8%

Johnston SC, et al. Validation and refinement of scores to predict very early stroke risk after transient ischaemic attack. Lancet 2007; 369:283–292.

8. B Paraspinal abscess

The axial MRI reveals a large paraspinal abscess. The prevertebral collection contains septations, and there appears to be extension into the left paravertebral musculature.

Mechanical intervertebral disc prolapse is not typically associated with fever. Syringomyelia is associated with dissociated sensory loss, and is identified as a fluid-filled cavity within the central cord, usually at the level of the cervical spine. Transverse myelitis has many potential causes, and may present with back pain, fever, paraparesis and sphincter dysfunction but its appearance on MRI is, of course, different. Almost always there will be central cord enhancement on T2 weighting. Vertebral metastases again have a different appearance on MRI and may cause neurological symptoms due to cord compression, possibly as a result of pathological vertebral fracture, and may rarely be associated with fever.

Hong SH, et al. Imaging assessment of the spine: Infection or an imitation. Radiographics 2009; 29:599–612.

9. C Hemicrania continua

Hemicrania continua is a rare headache characterised by persistent unilateral pain, with frequent superimposed episodes of severe pain, excessive lacrimation, conjunctival injection, mild miosis, eyelid oedema, nasal congestion and rhinorrhoea. It is expected to respond completely to treatment with indometacin.

According to the International Classification of Headache Disorders, analgesic overuse headache is present >15 days per month. It must have at least one of the following features: bilateral distribution, pressing or tightening quality, mild/moderate intensity. There should be a clear history of worsening headache during the period of analgesic use, and it should revert to the underlying type and frequency of headache within 2 months of cessation of analgesic use.

Attacks of migraine without aura may occur at variable frequency, but usually last for between 4 hours and 3 days. At least two of the following features should be present: unilateral distribution, moderate or severe intensity, aggravation by routine physical activity. In addition, nausea/vomiting and/or photophobia/phonophobia should be present.

Cluster headache is the term given to bouts of severe unilateral headache, centred on the orbital, supraorbital or temporal regions. There is usually marked parasympathetic autonomic involvement including: ipsilateral conjunctival injection, excess tearing, nasal congestion, rhinorrhoea, eyelid oedema, facial/forehead sweating, ptosis, miosis or general restlessness. The frequency of attacks is variable, ranging from one every other day up to as many as eight per day, with each lasting from 15-180 minutes. Typically, they occur in the early morning. The frequency of attacks is less frequent outside the cluster period. Cluster headaches are more common in men.

Tension-type headache is the most common primary headache. It is divided into infrequent episodic, frequent episodic and chronic forms. These, in turn, are further classified according to the presence or absence of pericranial tenderness. Two of the following need to be present: bilateral distribution, pressing/tightening quality, mild/moderate intensity, no aggravation by routine physical activity. Nausea and vomiting should not be present (mild nausea is permitted in the chronic subtype). Photophobia or phonophobia should not both be present. The frequency varies by subtype, as does the duration. Refer to the International Classification of Headache Disorders for the full diagnostic criteria.

Clarke C, et al. Headache (Chapter 12). In: Neurology: A Queen Square Textbook, 2nd edn. Oxford: Blackwell Publishing, 2016.
International Headache Society. The International Classification of Headache Disorders, 2nd edn. Oxford: Blackwell Publishing, 2003.

10. A Cholesterol embolus

This is the classic appearance of a cholesterol embolus (also known as a Hollenhorst plaque). It is present in a branch of the inferotemporal retinal artery. The blood flow in this branch distal to the embolus is surprisingly good – this is due to the presence of collateral circulation from an unoccluded branch (seen just on the right of the embolus). Studies of patients with asymptomatic retinal cholesterol emboli reveal an association with hypertension and smoking. Not surprisingly, it is a marker of reduced long-term survival.

Glaucoma typically causes pallor and cupping of the optic disc. Diabetic retinopathy and macular holes are discussed elsewhere.

Hollenhorst RW. The significance of bright plaques in the retinal arterioles. JAMA 1961; 178:23–29.
Bruno A, et al. Concomitants of asymptomatic retinal cholesterol emboli. Stroke 1992; 23:900–902.

11. A Corticobasal degeneration

Parkinsonian features may be a manifestation of Parkinson's disease or a different condition. In this case, the apraxia is the red flag.

This patient most likely suffers from corticobasal degeneration, a rare neurodegenerative disorder associated with the aggregation of tau proteins. Apraxia, 'alien limb' phenomenon, cognitive decline, extrapyramidal features of akinesia, rigidity and tremor, are highly suggestive of the disease. Progression is insidious with eventual involvement of all four limbs; a supranuclear gaze paresis may also develop. The clinical response to dopamine is often poor.

Parkinson's disease and progressive supranuclear palsy are discussed in the answers to Questions 28 and 42.

Frontotemporal lobe dementia encompasses different clinical subtypes, all of which develop insidiously. Onset is usually in middle age. Histopathologically, there is cortical neuronal loss, gliosis and inclusion body formation within the frontotemporal lobes (which may appear atrophied on MRI). A strong underlying genetic basis has been described, with there being an autosomal dominant pattern of inheritance and variable penetrance in up to 50% of affected patients. There is an association with amyotrophic lateral sclerosis with a repeat expansion mutation of the C9ORF72 gene. Personality and behavioural changes are common in the frontal variant, with blunted affect, disinhibition and perseveration being prominent findings. Episodic memory is typically unaffected. The progressive non-fluent aphasia variant presents with effortful, non-fluent speech, loss of intonation and rhythm, and word-finding difficulty. There is often difficulty in understanding full sentences. The temporal variant presents with marked impairment of semantic memory. Patients exhibit difficulty in using and understanding both spoken and written language. Vocabulary is limited, speech is impoverished, and word-finding difficulties and paraphasias (incorrect use of words, e.g. pencil instead of pen) are common. Patients often experience difficulty in identifying familiar people as well as common objects. Parkinsonian features are relatively uncommon in the frontotemporal lobe dementias.

Vascular dementia is associated with the usual risk factors for ischaemic disease (smoking, hypertension, dyslipidaemia, diabetes and positive family history). The history is of stepwise deterioration. Clinical features may include dementia, pseudobulbar palsy, parkinsonian signs, pyramidal weakness with brisk deep tendon reflexes, upgoing plantars, positive primitive reflexes and the 'marche a petit pas' gait. MRI typically reveals multiple bilateral cortical and subcortical foci of high signal on T2 weighting. Leukoaraiosis may also be evident within the periventricular white matter.

Clarke C, et al. Movement Disorders (Chapter 6). In: Neurology: A Queen Square Textbook, 2nd edn. Oxford: Blackwell Publishing, 2016.
Brooks D. Diagnosis and management of atypical parkinsonian syndromes. J Neurol Neurosurg Psychiatry 2002; 72:i10–16.

12. E Switch to lamotrigine

All antiepileptic drugs (AEDs) are associated with an increase in birth defects. Sodium valproate has the poorest record, with an unacceptably high risk of up to 40% for developmental disorders and 10% for birth defects. Since March 2018, NICE have updated their guidance, and if a woman on valproate is planning a pregnancy an appropriate revised plan for antiepileptic treatment should be put in place after discussion with the neurologist.

Treatment options depend on epilepsy severity and would usually consist of a gradual transfer onto an alternative therapy. Lamotrigine or levetiracetam would be reasonable in young patients who have had juvenile myoclonic epilepsy. This has a high risk for recurrence off treatment. Carbimazapine may worsen symptoms. In a patient who has been seizure free for a number of years on low dose therapy the risk of seizure recurrence on cessation of treatment, might be expected to be relatively low. The patient needs to be fully aware of the potential risks to herself and her future pregnancy should she have further generalised tonic–clonic attacks; these include potential hypoxic brain injury and sudden unexplained death in epilepsy (SUDEP). The incidence of SUDEP may be as high as 1 death per 100 patients per year, in severe epilepsy.

Sleep deprivation can decrease the seizure threshold; therefore, a repeat sleep deprivation EEG would not be unreasonable. If it were negative, as was the case previously, it would be reassuring but would not guarantee the absence of further seizures.

Clarke C, et al. Epilepsy and Related Disorders (Chapter 7). In: Neurology: A Queen Square Textbook. 2nd Edition Oxford: Blackwell Publishing, 2016.

13. B Bilateral acute-on-chronic subdural haematoma

This CT of the head shows bilateral acute-on-chronic subdural haematoma, as evidenced by the pooling of fresh blood (hyperdense) within the existing old subdural haematomas (hypodense).

This patient requires immediate treatment with a four-factor prothrombin complex concentrate (such as Octaplex) to reverse the effects of warfarin, if it has not already been given. Note that the British Committee for Standards in Haematology has issued guidelines that recommend that such treatment be given prior to imaging in any patient on warfarin with a clear history of head injury in whom there is a strong suspicion of an intracerebral bleed. Urgent neurosurgical referral is necessary.

Perron AD. How to read a head CT scan (Chapter 69). In: Adams JG (ed.) Emergency Medicine. Philadelphia, PA: Saunders; 2008.
Keeling et al. British Society for Haematology guidelines on oral anticoagulation with warfarin, 4th edn. Br J Haematol 2011; 154:311–324.

14. C Diabetic retinopathy

The digital retinal photograph demonstrates features of mild background diabetic retinopathy. Changes include microaneurysms (dot haemorrhages) and blot haemorrhages. Preproliferative diabetic retinopathy includes background changes plus flame haemorrhages and 'cotton-wool' spots. Features of diabetic maculopathy, such as hard exudates, may also arise. Other features of preproliferative disease include intraretinal microvascular abnormalities (IRMAs – seen as small patches of fine, flat, tortuous vessels), venous beading and venous tortuosity. This condition may progress to proliferative diabetic retinopathy, which is characterised by neovascularisation (new vessel formation) on the retina or optic disc.

Branch retinal vein occlusion is more localised. Hypertensive retinopathy usually presents with fewer hard exudates. Cholesterol emboli and macular degeneration are briefly described elsewhere.

Frank R. Diabetic type and retinopathy. N Engl J Med 2004; 350:48–58.

15. C Lead

Ayurvedic medicines have an association with heavy metal ingestion. In adults, lead poisoning typically manifests in non-specific symptoms such as fatigue, insomnia and irritability but can be associated with abdominal pain, constipation and peripheral motor neuropathies (especially wrist-drop and foot-drop). A bluish-black line of discoloration along the gingival margin is highly suspicious for lead poisoning. In children, lead toxicity has a significant effect on the brain and the level of exposure is said to correlate with intellectual impairment. Anaemia may also result from lead poisoning, with characteristic basophilic stippling evident on the blood film.

Acute arsenic poisoning may present with confusion, diarrhoea and vomiting, and hypovolaemic shock. Cardiac arrhythmias are a recognised feature. Chronic poisoning may present with painful peripheral sensory neuropathy, dermatitis, and hepatic and renal impairment. Mees' lines may be detected in the fingernails (these appear as transverse lines, which are usually white, and may be single or multiple).

Beryllium, if inhaled, may cause acute chemical pneumonitis or chronic granulomatous disease of the lungs (chronic beryllium disease). It may also cause contact dermatitis.

The effects of mercury poisoning vary depending on whether exposure is to inorganic elemental mercury or its organic form, methylmercury. The latter is more toxic and may result in a wide range of features including paraesthesia, tremors, ataxia, visual and auditory impairment, and cognitive decline. In severe poisoning, it may progress to coma and death. Chronic inorganic mercury poisoning is associated with an erythematous papular rash, proteinuria and anaemia. Neurological signs include tremor, ataxia and myopathy. Cognitive decline and behavioural change are common. Signs of encephalopathy may ensure.

Features of thallium poisoning include diarrhoea and vomiting, acute confusion, alopecia and Mees' lines. Chronic poisoning may cause a painful peripheral neuropathy.

Clarke C, et al. Toxic, metabolic and physical insults (Chapter 19). In: Neurology: A Queen Square Textbook, 2nd edn. Oxford: Blackwell Publishing, 2016.
Ernst E. Heavy metals in traditional Indian remedies. Eur J Clin Pharmacol 2002; 57(12):891–896.
Saper RB, et al. Heavy metal content of ayurvedic herbal medicine products. JAMA 2004; 292(23):2868–2873.

16. D Posterior reversible encephalopathy syndrome

The history and imaging findings are consistent with a diagnosis of posterior reversible encephalopathy syndrome. This form of encephalopathy is associated with acute hypertensive episodes (e.g. in eclampsia or renal disease), and the use of immunosuppressant medication (especially, following organ transplantation). It is thought that the condition results from dysregulation at the blood–brain barrier resulting in either a mechanical effect caused by a rise in hydrostatic pressure or by a toxic effect of circulating immunosuppressant drugs.

Clinical presentation may be with confusion, depressed conscious level, headache, cortical blindness or seizures. A timely MRI of the brain may reveal evidence of vasogenic oedema within the white matter of the occipital or parietal lobes. The condition is often completely reversible if the underlying cause is promptly addressed.

Herpes encephalitis is usually caused by HSV-1 (herpes simplex virus 1) and may present with fever, headache, depressed conscious level, personality/behavioural change, dysphasia or generalised tonic–clonic seizures with olfactory or gustatory aura. The MRI of the brain usually reveals vasogenic oedema within the inferior and medial temporal lobe which may extend into the insular cortex or frontal lobe. There may be bilateral involvement.

Intracerebral haemorrhage, multiple sclerosis and progressive multifocal leukoencephalopathy are discussed elsewhere.

Clarke C, et al. Disorders of consciousness, intensive care neurology and sleep (Chapter 20). In: Neurology: A Queen Square Textbook, 2nd edn. Oxford: Blackwell Publishing, 2016.
Hinchey J, et al. A reversible posterior leukoencephalopathy syndrome. N Engl J Med 1996; 334:494–500.

17. D Myelinated fibres

This is typical of the appearance of myelinated fibres. It is a fairly common finding resulting from anomalous myelination of nerve fibres anterior to the lamina cribrosa. It is usually asymptomatic. It usually appears feather like at its edges and can obscure the retinal vessels. It follows the path of the nerve fibre layer, which sweeps in an arch from the optic disc.

Branch retinal artery occlusion, choroidal haemangioma, cytomegalovirus retinitis and traction retinal detachment have different appearances and are described elsewhere.

Golnik K. Congenital optic nerve anomalies. Curr Opin Ophthalmol 1998; 9(6):18–26.

18. A Conversion disorder

The patient is suffering from conversion disorder. This is a condition in which there is a neurological deficit that cannot be accounted for by an underlying organic disorder. It precipitates subconsciously as a reaction to psychological stresses or conflicts and causes functional impairment. In a number of cases, the patient exhibits a lack of concern about the physical condition, although it should be noted that this is an unreliable sign. For the full diagnostic criteria, please refer to the Diagnostic and Statistical Manual of Mental Disorders (5th edn).

Factitious disorder and malingering are possibilities, but are less likely. Both are conditions in which symptoms or signs of illness are intentionally produced or feigned for the purpose of achieving some type of external gain. In factitious disorder, the primary motivation is to assume 'the sick role'. In contrast, the external gain in malingering is typically through financial compensation, work avoidance or access to narcotic drugs. Our patient does not fit the typical profile for either of these conditions.

Somatisation disorder can be discounted because it is defined by the presence of many physical complaints before the age of 30 years, which have prompted treatment-seeking behaviour or have resulted in significant functional disturbance at social, occupational or other important levels. Investigations should not reveal evidence of an underlying condition that can fully account for the patient's symptoms. The symptoms are not intentionally produced.

Undifferentiated somatoform disorder can also be excluded on the basis that symptoms must have been present for 6 months or longer. It is a condition in which there are one or more physical complaints that cannot be fully accounted for by any underlying medical condition, following adequate investigation. The condition causes distress to the patient or results in impaired functioning at social, occupational or other important levels. The symptoms are not intentionally produced, and they are not better accounted for by another mental health disorder

For full diagnostic criteria of the above listed conditions, please refer to the Diagnostic and Statistical Manual of Mental Disorders (5th edn).

American Psychiatric Association. DSM-V-TR: Diagnostic and Statistical Manual of Mental Disorders, 5th edn. Washington DC: American Psychiatric Association, 2013.
Stone J, et al. La belle indifference in conversion symptoms and hysteria. Br J Psychiatry 2006; 188:204–209.

19. A Dural sinus thrombosis

The contrast-enhanced CT reveals a filling defect in the left sigmoid sinus ('empty delta' sign), consistent with dural sinus thrombosis. Furthermore, this is complicated by venous infarction of the left temporal lobe, which would account for the receptive aphasia. Onset of headache is usually gradual, but can be of the sudden 'thunderclap' type as in this case. Subarachnoid haemorrhage is an important differential, but is clearly excluded by the CT, as is an intracerebral haemorrhage. Note that the 'empty delta' sign, which is most often found in superior sagittal sinus thrombosis, is due to contrast enhancement at the margins of a non-enhancing thrombus.

Perron AD. How to read a head CT scan (Chapter 69). In: Adams JG (ed). Emergency Medicine. Oxford: Saunders, 2008.

20. C Intravenous Immunoglobulin

This patient is suffering from myasthenia gravis (MG), an autoimmune disorder affecting the neuromuscular junction. It has two peaks of incidence, the first being in the second and third decades and the second in the sixth and seventh decades. It can occur as ocular or generalised forms. Clinical features include diplopia, blurred vision, ptosis, weakness of facial muscles, speech/swallowing difficulties, respiratory compromise and proximal limb weakness.

The diagnosis is usually suggested by the history, as in this case, and can be confirmed with serological and electromyographic (EMG) tests. Three quarters of MG patients are seropositive for anti-acetylcholine receptor antibodies. Over half of the remaining ~25% of MG patients are seropositive for anti-muscle-specific kinase (MuSK) antibodies. The Tensilon test (administration of intravenous edrophonium to observe for transient alleviation of symptoms) is rarely used to make the diagnosis; it is contraindicated in heart disease.

EMG studies are very useful in confirming the clinical diagnosis. Increased jitter (a measure of variation in the interpotential interval on a single-fibre EMG [SFEMG]) is highly sensitive for MG (93% in ocular MG, 99% in generalised MG), but not highly specific as it generally signifies problems in transmission at the neuromuscular junction. Normal SFEMG in a weak muscle practically excludes the diagnosis. Decrements in compound muscle action potentials on repetitive nerve stimulation are probably the most specific finding for MG, but not the most sensitive.

Following diagnosis, CT/MRI should be performed to exclude thymoma. Approximately 15% of MG patients have a thymoma, a small minority of which have malignant features. Thymectomy is indicated for all MG patients, from late childhood to age 60 years, who are seropositive for anti-acetylcholine receptor antibodies.

Medical treatment options include anticholinesterases, steroids, steroid-sparing immunosuppressants, intravenous immunoglobulin and plasma exchange. Patients without bulbar or respiratory symptoms can be treated with symptom control using anticholinesterase drugs (e.g. pyridostigmine). Disease control with steroids followed by steroid-sparing agents is often necessary. Steroid treatment should start at a low dose with gradual increase over a few weeks to avoid worsening symptoms that can occur with acute high dose treatment. Azathioprine or methotrexate are commonly prescribed over the long term.

Patients with respiratory or bulbar symptoms should be monitored in a hospital setting with forced vital capacity (FVC) monitoring in case ventilatory support is required. This man has an FVC at the low end of normal and with the bulbar symptoms described, more urgent treatment would be required. Due to practicalities and availability, intravenous immunoglobulin is the first line treatment over and above plasmapheresis.

Clarke C, et al. Nerve and muscle disease (Chapter 10). In: Neurology: A Queen Square Textbook. Oxford: 2Nd edn. Oxford: Blackwell Publishing, 2016.
Witoonpanich R, et al. Electrophysiological and immunological study in myasthenia gravis: diagnostic sensitivity and correlation. Clin Neurophysiol 2011; 122:1873–1877.

21. E Riluzole

This patient has characteristic features of amyotrophic lateral sclerosis (ALS), a subtype of motor neuron disease. The presence of mixed upper and lower motor neuron signs in both upper and lower limbs is strongly suggestive of motor neuron disease (MND). Unfortunately, this is an incurable condition. In the UK, the only licensed pharmacological treatment for ALS is riluzole, which is thought to act by blocking glutamate activity. It is believed that it does so by increasing glutamate uptake by spinal neurons rather than by directly antagonising glutamate receptors. Studies show that treatment with riluzole has a small but significant effect in slowing disease progression; on average, the time to tracheostomy is prolonged by 2–4 months.

All MND patients should be referred to a specialist clinic for regular monitoring and timely supportive management.

National Institute for Health and Clinical Excellence. NICE Guidelines. TA20: Motor neuron disease: riluzole–guidance. London: NICE, 2001.

22. B Chorioretinitis

This is a typical appearance of chorioretinitis, a condition that may arise secondary to infection with *Toxoplasma gondii*, cytomegalovirus or numerous other pathogens. Infective causes may be congenital or acquired. Non-infectious causes include sarcoidosis and Behçet's disease.

Choroidal melanoma is often asymptomatic and discovered incidentally. It has a fairly characteristic appearance on fundoscopy; however, the tumour can be variably pigmented or, indeed, amelanotic.

Macular degeneration, macular holes and photocoagulation scarring are described elsewhere.

Leitman M. Manual for Eye Examination and Diagnosis, 8th edn. Chichester: Wiley-Blackwell, 2012.

23. A Anti-glutamic acid decarboxylase (GAD) antibody

This patient has features of stiff-person syndrome, an autoimmune disease. It is sometimes associated with diabetes mellitus, and anti-GAD antibodies are frequently detected at high titre. Electromyography usually reveals continuous motor unit activity in affected axial and proximal limb muscles. A good response is usually achieved with high-dose baclofen or diazepam. Plasmapheresis and intravenous immunoglobulin (IVIg) have also been used successfully in these patients.

Anti-myelin-associated glycoprotein antibody is associated with demyelinating polyneuropathies. Anti-*N*-methyl-d-aspartate receptor antibody is associated with encephalitis and is found predominantly in women; a significant proportion of these cases are paraneoplastic, usually arising secondary to ovarian teratoma. Anti-striated muscle antibody is detected in a high percentage of young myasthenia gravis patients with thymoma, anti-Yo antibody is associated with paraneoplastic cerebellar degeneration. Screening for an underlying cancer should be undertaken (the antibody is linked to gynaecological and breast cancers in women).

Clarke C, et al. Movement disorders (Chapter 6). In: Neurology: A Queen Square Textbook, 2nd edn. Oxford: Blackwell Publishing, 2016.
Levy LM, et al. The stiff-person syndrome: An autoimmune disorder affecting neurotransmission of γ-aminobutyric acid. Ann Intern Med 1999; 131:522–530.

24. D Subarachnoid haemorrhage with communicating hydrocephalus

This man's CT scan reveals a subarachnoid haemorrhage with communicating hydrocephalus: there is blood in the basal cisterns and in both Sylvian fissures. The dilated 4th ventricle is suggestive of a communicating hydrocephalus.

Extradural haematoma, dural sinus thrombosis, intracerebral haemorrhage and subdural haematoma may all present similarly but would have different bleed patterns on a CT scan. Extradural haematoma has a lentiform shape haemorrhage; subdural haematoma is cresenteric; intracerebral haemorrhage would show blood deep within and/or around the cerebral tissue and dural sinus thrombosis, although it may only show a sinus thrombosis, may also show subcortical infarct.

Perron AD. How to read a head CT scan (Chapter 69). In: Adams JG (ed). Emergency Medicine, 1st edition. Saunders; 2008.

25. B Macular hole

The appearance of a yellow ring with a central defect at the fovea is characteristic of a macular hole. The diagnosis can be confirmed with optical coherence tomography. A macular hole usually presents in the elderly female spontaneously, but can develop following blunt trauma to the eye.

Drusen are deposits of lipid and protein in Bruch's membrane, and appear as small yellowish deposits. They are the cardinal sign of early age-related macular degeneration. Optic atrophy is observed as a very pale optic disc with sharply defined margins.

Leitman M. Manual for Eye Examination and diagnosis, 8th edn. Chichester: Wiley-Blackwell, 2012.

26. D Tell the police you cannot give them any information

Confidentiality is one of the cornerstones on which the doctor–patient relationship is based. Breach of confidentiality should occur only in exceptional circumstances and only when failure to disclose information may put the patient, or another, at risk of death or serious harm, or when it is likely to help in the prevention or prosecution of a serious crime. The General Medical Council (GMC) provides guidance on this in *Good Medical Practice* and their associated documents.

This guidance relating to gun and knife wounds outlines a two-stage strategy:
1. The police must be quickly informed when a person arrives with a gunshot or knife injury. This will enable the police to make a risk assessment of the situation. They have a responsibility of assessing further risk to the patient, hospital and staff, and other members of the public.
2. Patients should be asked if they wish to speak to the police. If they agree then a medical assessment of their fitness should be made and the timing of the interview dictated accordingly. If they are adamant that they do not wish to talk to the police the clinician responsible must make a professional judgement about whether disclosure of patient details is justified in the public interest. Where possible patients should be informed of the decision to disclose their details and the justification for this. This should also be documented in patients' notes.

General Medical Council. Good Medical Practice. London: GMC, 2006.

27. B Multiple system atrophy

Multiple system atrophy (MSA; previously known as Shy–Drager syndrome) is a sporadic, progressive, adult-onset neurodegenerative disease that may present with a combination of parkinsonian signs, autonomic dysfunction, cerebellar ataxia and pyramidal effects. It typically presents in the sixth decade. It is characterised by autonomic dysfunction with parkinsonism (MSA-P) or cerebellar ataxia (MSA-C). Clinical features may include orthostatic hypotension, urinary incontinence, erectile dysfunction, cold dusky peripheries, bradykinesia, rigidity, marked antecollis, action tremor, postural instability, dysarthria, dysphonia, dysphagia, cerebellar ataxia, emotional lability, daytime stridor/worsening snoring/sleep apnoea, etc. Resting tremor is uncommon. Cognitive decline is not considered to be in keeping with the diagnosis. MRI of the brain may be completely normal; however, putaminal, cerebellar or brainstem atrophy is not uncommon. Occasionally, the 'hot cross bun' sign (a radiological sign) may be detected in the pons on T2-weighted MRI. Treatment is supportive. Mean survival is 7 years.

Progressive supranuclear palsy (previously known as Steele–Richardson–Olszewski syndrome) is a sporadic neurodegenerative disease, defined by the presence of tau-positive neurofibrillary tangles in the substantia nigra, dentate nucleus, globus pallidus and subthalamic nucleus. Cortical involvement is variable. The defining clinical feature is a supranuclear gaze palsy affecting voluntary upgaze and/or downgaze; however, a full range of reflex eye movements is preserved (as can be demonstrated with the oculocephalic reflex). Other features include akinetic rigidity (predominantly axial), a propensity to fall backwards from early on in the disease, dysarthria, dysphagia, frontalis overactivity, impaired frontal executive function and personality change. MRI may reveal midbrain atrophy, with T2-weighted signal hyperintensity in the periaqueductal grey matter and globus pallidus. There may also be frontotemporal atrophy. As for MSA, response to levodopa is poor, management is supportive and mean survival is 7 years.

Corticobasal degeneration and Parkinson's disease do not explain this presentation and are described elsewhere. Similarly, Wilson's disease would not be expected to present in this way, and would be unlikely in a patient of this age; it is excluded by the normal copper studies.

Clarke C, et al. Movement disorders (Chapter 6). In: Neurology: A Queen Square Textbook. 2nd edn. Oxford: Blackwell Publishing, 2016.
Manji H, et al. Neurological disorders (Chapter 4). In: Oxford Handbook of Neurology. Oxford: Oxford University Press, 2007.

28. A Anti-aquaporin-4 antibody

This patient most likely has neuromyelitis optica (also known as Devic's disease), an antibody-mediated demyelinating disease. Typical presentation is with transverse myelitis and/or optic neuritis, following a prodromal flu-like illness. Optic neuritis is often painful and may be unilateral or bilateral, and can present with complete visual loss. It may follow a monophasic or relapsing and remitting course. Mean age of onset is 40 years, and it is more common in women than men (4:1). There is an association with connective tissue diseases and autoimmune endocrinopathies.

Neuroimaging usually reveals a hyperintense intrinsic cord lesion extending over at least three vertebral segments (with complete cross-sectional involvement of the cord, and enhancement with gadolinium). Brain imaging will usually be of normal appearance. Investigations should be performed to exclude other causes of transverse myelitis. Visual-evoked potentials would be expected to be delayed if there is optic nerve involvement. Anti-aquaporin-4 IgG is frequently detected in neuromyelitis optica, but is not associated with multiple sclerosis. Lumbar puncture usually reveals normal opening pressure, cerebrospinal fluid pleocytosis and raised protein. Oligoclonal bands are present in up to a third of patients.

Anti-GAD antibody is associated with type 1 diabetes mellitus and stiff-person syndrome; anti-GQ1b antibody is associated with Miller Fischer syndrome; anti-N-methyl-d-aspartate receptor antibody is associated with a form of encephalitis; anti-voltage-gated potassium channel antibody is associated with limbic encephalitis.

Wingerchuk DM, et al. International consensus diagnostic criteria for neuromyelitis optica spectrum disorders. Neurology 2015;85(2):177–189.

29. A Commence acetazolamide

This woman has idiopathic intracranial hypertension (also known as pseudotumour cerebri), which can be diagnosed using these criteria:

1. Symptoms and signs of generalised intracranial hypertension in an alert and oriented patient
2. No localising signs (except nerve VI palsy)
3. Normal neuroimaging (apart from signs of raised intracranial pressure)
4. Lumbar puncture with raised opening pressure
5. Normal cerebrospinal fluid analysis
6. No other cause for intracranial hypertension.

Most patients present with severe headache which may be associated with nausea and vomiting or synchronous pulsatile tinnitus. There may also be retro-orbital pain associated with eye movements, transient visual obscurations associated with posture, horizontal diplopia-associated abducens nerve palsy, reduced visual acuity, relative afferent pupillary defect, constricted visual fields and an enlarged blind spot. MRI is normal except for signs of raised intracranial pressure (including the appearance of an empty sella turcica). Intracranial mass lesions and dural sinus thrombosis must be excluded.

Patients should be reassured and advised to lose weight and restrict salt intake in the first instance. Pharmacological treatment is often commenced at diagnosis; first-line therapy is with the carbonic anhydrase inhibitor, acetazolamide. Furosemide and topiramate may also be used. A referral to a neuro-ophthalmologist should be made for visual assessment, but surgical interventions such as optic nerve sheath fenestration or ventriculoperitoneal shunts are not usually necessary. Repeat lumbar punctures with cerebrospinal fluid drainage may provide temporary symptomatic relief, but these are rarely used in isolation.

Clarke C, et al. Neuro-ophthalmology (Chapter 14). In: Neurology: A Queen Square Textbook, 2nd Edn Oxford: Blackwell Publishing, 2016.
Friedman DI, Jacobson DM. Diagnostic criteria for idiopathic intracranial hypertension. Neurology 2002; 59(10):1492.

30. A Age-related macular degeneration

Age-related macular degeneration (ARMD) is the most common cause of irreversible visual loss in the western world. It occurs as exudative (wet) and non-exudative (dry) forms. The pathophysiology of the two related conditions is not clearly understood.

This patient has exudative ARMD, as evidenced by the characteristic appearance of subretinal blood and fluid at the macula. This leakage occurs secondary to underlying choroidal neovascularisation (CNV). The condition typically presents with blurred central vision, or central visual loss (scotoma) in severe cases. Onset is usually insidious but, in some instances, may be acute.

The non-exudative form is characterised by the presence of multiple small perimacular deposits of white/yellow extracellular material within Bruch's membrane. In a significant minority, the condition may progress to the exudative form.

Fluorescein angiography and optical coherence tomography are useful in assessing the severity of the condition. Treatment of exudative ARMD is with laser photocoagulation to destroy areas of CNV or anti-vascular endothelial growth factor agents to prevent CNV (ranibizumab or aflibercept are currently available). Stem cell therapy is showing promise for the future.

Retinal detachment, choroidal melanoma and preretinal haemorrhage are addressed elsewhere. An epiretinal membrane (sometimes known as a macular pucker) is a transparent layer of scar tissue which forms over the surface of the retina, often in response to ageing and detachment of the posterior vitreous. As the scar tissue contracts it exerts traction on the retina and may cause distortion of vision. It can be treated surgically, by vitrectomy.

de Jong PT. Age-related macular degeneration. N Engl J Med 2006; 355:1474–1485.

31. E Right posterior cerebral artery territory infarct

High signal is detected within the right cerebral peduncle. This is consistent with a right posterior cerebral artery territory infarct.

Caplan, LR. Caplan's Stroke: A Clinical Approach, 4th edn. Philadelphia, PA: Saunders Elsevier, 2009.
Wardlaw J. Diagnosis of stroke on neuroimaging. BMJ 2004; 328:655.
Clarke C, et al. Stroke and cerebrovascular diseases (Chapter 5). In: Neurology: A Queen Square Textbook, 2nd edn. Oxford: Blackwell Publishing, 2016.

32. E Stop all analgesics

This young woman is suffering from chronic daily headache. In the first instance, all analgesics should be stopped. It would then be reasonable to make a fuller assessment of headache type and frequency; a headache diary is useful for this purpose. Once the analgesics have been stopped, a preventive such as propranolol or amitriptyline can be introduced. It is said that preventives are often unsuccessful where analgesics are being overused. Clearly, lifestyle changes can be beneficial for headache, but the analgesic overuse is a more pressing issue as it is likely to be significantly contributing to her daily headache. The combined oral contraceptive does not have to be stopped as this patient is not suffering from migraine with aura (in which its use is absolutely contraindicated according to the World Health Organization); however, it can be associated with worsening headache so it may be helpful for the patient to contemplate switching to an alternative form of contraceptive anyway. There is no indication for MRI of the head at present.

Clarke C, et al. Headache (Chapter 12). In: Neurology: A Queen Square Textbook, 2nd edn. Oxford: Blackwell Publishing, 2016.
World Health Organization. Medical Eligibility Criteria for Contraceptive Use, 4th edn. Geneva: WHO, 2009.

33. B Branch retinal vein occlusion

The fundoscopic appearance of a single well-confined region of intraretinal haemorrhage within one quadrant is characteristic of branch retinal vein occlusion. Most cases are thought to be due to compression of a branch retinal vein by the corresponding artery which shares the same adventitious sheath. There is a possibility that some people are anatomically predisposed to the condition, but it has been linked to hypertension, hypercholesterolaemia and thrombophilia. It presents clinically as painless deterioration in the vision of one eye, but may be asymptomatic especially if the vein occlusion is away from the macula (i.e. nasal).

  The fundoscopic appearance of an acute branch retinal artery occlusion is usually of focal retinal pallor within the affected territory. There may also be evidence of oedema, and the embolus itself may be visible within the occluded vessel. The vessel distal to the embolus may be attenuated and eventually may become thread-like in appearance.

  Cholesterol embolus, cytomegalovirus retinitis and hypertensive retinopathy are discussed elsewhere.

Wong T, et al. Retinal-vein occlusion. N Engl J Med 2010; 363:2135–2144.

34. C 6 months

This is in accordance with the current Driver and Vehicle Licensing Authority guidelines. Although these guidelines are specific to the UK, other countries most likely have similar recommendations regarding driving while on antiepileptic medication.

Drivers Medical Group. For Medical Practitioners: At a glance. Guide to the current Medical Standards of Fitness to Drive. Swansea: DVLA, 2012.

35. E Acute right parietal infarct and old right frontal infarct

The CT of the head reveals an isodense lesion within the right parietal lobe, with loss of grey–white differentiation, and sulcal effacement representing a relatively recent stroke. In addition, there is a large hypodense region in the right frontal lobe, with associated atrophy, consistent with an older established infarct.

Wardlaw J. Diagnosis of stroke on neuroimaging. BMJ 2004; 328:655.
Clarke C, et al. Stroke and cerebrovascular diseases (Chapter 5). In: Neurology: A Queen Square Textbook, 2nd edn. Oxford: Blackwell Publishing, 2016.

36. A Diabetic retinopathy

This digital retinal photograph reveals proliferative diabetic retinopathy complicated by preretinal haemorrhage. Signs of proliferative change include neovascularisation of the retina and optic disc, and retinal fibrosis. Features of background and preproliferative diabetic retinopathy such as microaneurysms, blot haemorrhages, hard exudates and 'cotton-wool' spots are also observed.

Unfortunately, neovascularisation can lead to preretinal and vitreous haemorrhage (since the new vessels are fragile and prone to bleeding), and eventually tractional retinal detachment. Panretinal laser photocoagulation is the treatment of choice, and it dramatically reduces the risk of such sight-threatening complications.

This patient should be referred urgently for ophthalmology review.

Macroaneurysm, posterior vitreous detachment, retinal tears and Valsalva's manoeuvres may all cause preretinal haemorrhage.

Frank R. Diabetic retinopathy. N Engl J Med 2004; 350:48–58.

37. D Miller Fisher syndrome

This patient is most likely to be suffering from Miller Fisher syndrome, a condition characterised by ophthalmoplegia, ataxia and areflexia. It is widely considered to be a variant of Guillain–Barré syndrome (GBS). Preceding recent infection, especially with *Campylobacter jejuni* or *Haemophilus influenzae,* predisposes to the condition. GQ1b antibody is detectable in ~95% of cases of Miller Fisher syndrome. Cerebrospinal fluid protein is elevated in ~60% of cases. The condition is usually self-limiting, the exception being when it occurs as a GBS overlap syndrome, in which it may rarely progress to generalised severe weakness, requiring close monitoring and support. In such cases, treatment may entail plasma exchange or intravenous immunoglobulin.

GBS causes acute neuromuscular weakness. It develops in the wake of a predisposing infection (*Campylobacter jejuni*, cytomegalovirus, *Mycoplasma pneumoniae*, Epstein–Barr virus, HIV, *Haemophilus influenzae*). Characteristic features include acute ascending sensorimotor neuropathy and areflexia. Cranial nerve involvement and autonomic dysfunction may also be present with arrhythmias and labile blood pressure not uncommon. Potentially sight-threatening papilloedema may sometimes arise. Diagnosis is usually clinical, but nerve conduction studies may show patchy proximal and distal demyelination. Rarely, an axonal neuropathy may be present. Denervation may be detected on electromyography later in the course of severe disease. Anti-GM1 antibody is associated with severe GBS. However, anti-GQ1b antibody is detectable in a significant proportion of cases with ophthalmoplegia. Serological tests may also yield evidence of recent seroconversion, and add further support to the diagnosis.

Bickerstaff's brain-stem encephalitis is also associated with GQ1b antibody. The clinical features may also be similar to those of Miller Fisher syndrome; however, altered consciousness, hyperreflexia and extensor plantar responses are likely to be evident. In about one-third of cases, the MRI of the brain is also abnormal.

Wernicke's encephalopathy is associated with thiamine deficiency, often in the context of chronic alcoholism with the classic clinical triad of confusion, ophthalmoplegia and ataxia, (see the answer to Question 44). In this instance, Wernicke's encephalopathy is unlikely.

Lambert–Eaton syndrome is similar to myasthenia gravis in that it is associated with impaired acetylcholine activity at the neuromuscular junction. It is an autoimmune disorder, in which anti-voltage-gated calcium channel antibodies are usually present. If diagnosed, underlying malignancy, such as small cell lung cancer, needs to be excluded. In contrast to myasthenia gravis, strength transiently improves with repetitive activity.

Clarke C, et al. Nerve and muscle disease (Chapter 10). In: Neurology: A Queen Square Textbook. 2nd Edition Oxford: Blackwell Publishing, 2016.
Overell JR, et al. Recent developments in Miller Fisher syndrome and related disorders. Curr Opin Neurol 2005; 18(5):562–566.

38. B Cervical spondylosis and Chiari I malformation with syringomyelia

This patient's T2-weighted MRI of the cervical spine shows a small syrinx within the cervical spinal cord. There is cervical spondylosis at the C5–7 level. Inspection of the cerebellum reveals mild tonsillar descent through the foramen magnum, consistent with a Chiari I malformation.

Syringomyelia is when an abnormal cerebrospinal fluid-filled cavity forms within the central spinal cord. It may arise secondary to a number of other conditions, including Chiari malformations, spinal cord tumours, trauma, arachnoiditis, spinal infection and cervical spondylosis. Clinical features include a dissociated sensory loss in the upper limbs (the so-called 'cape distribution' of impaired pain and temperature sensation, with preserved proprioception and vibration sensation). This is due to disruption of the spinothalamic tracts as they cross centrally through the cord at the level of the syrinx. The dorsal columns are normally preserved. In addition, there may be muscle wasting and lower motor neuron weakness in the upper limbs. In severe cases, there may also be a spastic paraparesis below the level of the syrinx.

The Chiari I malformation is defined by descent of the cerebellar tonsils through the foramen magnum. The condition is strongly associated with syringomyelia. This is because the descended cerebellar tonsils, combined with arachnoid adhesions, can prevent normal cerbrospinal fluid pressure transmission through the foramen magnum, causing raised intracranial pressure and increased cerbrospinal fluid flow through the spinal cord aqueduct. Presentation is usually in early to mid-adulthood. Clinical features may include headache, which is exacerbated by any action that increases intracranial pressure (coughing, Valsalva's manoeuvre, bending over, etc.), nystagmus and quadriparesis.

The Chiari II malformation is congenital and is associated with myelomeningocele and hydrocephalus. It is defined by downward displacement of the medulla and the cerebellar vermis and tonsils. The fourth ventricle sometimes partially herniates through the foramen magnum. Presentation is usually in the neonatal period. Clinical features may include hydrocephalus, dysphagia, respiratory distress and quadriparesis.

Clarke C, et al. Spinal cord disorders (Chapter 16). In: Neurology: A Queen Square Textbook. 2nd edn. Oxford: Blackwell Publishing, 2016.
Butteriss D, Birchall D. A case of syringomyelia associated with cervical spondylosis. Br J Radiol 2006; 79: e123–125.

39. D Progressive multifocal leukoencephalopathy

Nataluzimab is a monoclonal antibody that acts to prevent immune cell migration across the blood–brain barrier. It binds to α_4-integrin, and inhibits its interaction with VCAM-1 (vascular cell adhesion molecule 1). At the time of writing, in the UK it is currently licensed for the treatment of rapidly evolving severe relapsing–remitting multiple sclerosis (MS).

Clinical trials show that the drug is effective in reducing relapse frequency, delaying disease progression and reducing the number of gadolinium-enhancing lesions on MRI. One of its most serious potential side effects is the development of progressive multifocal leukoencephalopathy (PML), a potentially fatal condition that results from reactivation of John Cunningham (JC) virus. Presentation is usually with focal neurological signs, cognitive decline and sometimes seizures. MRI of the brain typically reveals single or multiple high-signal lesions on T2 weighting at the interface of the grey and white matter.

PML is usually diagnosed on account of the clinical history, characteristic appearance on MRI brain and positive cerebrospinal fluid (CSF) polymerase chain reaction result for the virus.

Lathyrism results from ingestion of *Lathyrus sativus* (grass pea). It is thought to contain a neurotoxin that damages the Betz cells of the motor cortex, causing a spastic paraparesis. Acute disseminated encephalomyelitis usually occurs in childhood following an infectious febrile illness or vaccination. It may initially present with fever, meningism, headache and focal neurological signs. The condition can progress rapidly, and seizures, coma and death may ensue. MRI reveals multifocal high-signal lesions on T2 weighting, affecting both grey and white matter, which may become confluent as the disease progresses. Transverse myelitis describes a pattern of inflammation of the spinal cord and has many potential causes, including systemic inflammatory disorders, infection, demyelination, nutrient deficiency and toxins. Neuromyelitis optica is discussed elsewhere.

Clarke C, et al. Multiple sclerosis and demyelinating diseases (Chapter 11). In: Neurology: A Queen Square Textbook, 2nd edn. Oxford: Blackwell Publishing, 2016.
Clifford D, et al. Natalizumab-associated progressive multifocal leukoencephalopathy in patients with multiple sclerosis: lessons from 28 cases. Lancet Neurol 2010; 9:438–446.

40. D Hypertensive retinopathy

The fundoscopic findings of 'silver-wiring' and arteriovenous nipping are indicative of mild hypertensive retinopathy. The full grading scale is shown in **Table 7.2**. Central retinal artery occlusion and diabetic retinopathy are discussed elsewhere. Glaucoma causes pallor and cupping of the optic disc. Optic atrophy is recognisable as a pale optic disc with sharply defined borders.

Table 7.2 Classification of hypertensive retinopathy	
Grade	**Retinal signs**
Mild	• Generalised or focal arteriolar narrowing • Arteriovenous nipping • 'Silver-wiring'
Moderate	• Haemorrhage (dot, blot or flame) • Microaneurysms • Cotton-wool spots • Hard exudates
Malignant	• Signs of moderate retinopathy AND optic disc swelling
Adapted from Wong and Mitchell (2004).	

Wong T, Mitchell P. Hypertensive retinopathy. N Engl J Med 2004; 351:2310–2317.

41. E Multifocal motor neuropathy with conduction block

This patient is most probably suffering from multifocal motor neuropathy with conduction block (MMN-CB), an autoimmune demyelinating motor neuropathy. Classically it presents lower motor neuron signs. Onset is usually in the fourth or fifth decade with asymmetrical weakness and cramping within the upper limbs. Weakness is in the distribution of specific nerves (in this case, the left radial nerve) and is disproportionate to the degree of muscle wasting, which is often mild early in the condition. Muscle wasting and fasciculations tend to be late features. Cranial nerves are rarely involved. The sensory examination is usually completely normal.

Anti-GM1 antibody is often detectable. MRI of the cervical spine should be normal but is important in excluding other potential causes, such as radiculopathy. Cerebrospinal fluid (CSF) analysis is typically normal, except for slightly elevated protein (rarely exceeding 1 g/L). Nerve conduction studies are critical in confirming the diagnosis: these show multifocal conduction block. There may also be reduced compound muscle action potentials. The sensory study should be normal. Additionally, localised denervation may be detected on electromyography.

Chronic inflammatory demyelinating polyneuropathy (CIDP) is the main differential. It is characteristically a disease of mixed motor and sensory features and has a similar age of onset with a progressive or relapsing course. Clinical features include proximal and distal weakness with areflexia and tremor. Weakness is disproportional to wasting, which is a late feature. Cramping is not as prominent as in MMN-CB. Distal sensory involvement, however, is common. In terms of investigations, the CSF reveals raised protein and the nerve conduction studies should reveal demyelination in at least two nerves. There may be evidence of enlarged or gadolinium-enhancing nerve roots on the MRI. Anti-GM1 antibodies would not classically be expected.

Amyotrophic lateral sclerosis (ALS) would be expected to present with mixed upper and lower motor neuron signs. Fasciculations and muscle wasting are characteristically prominent features. Corticobulbar involvement is also common. Anti-GM1 would not be expected to be positive. ALS is discussed elsewhere.

Charcot–Marie–Tooth disease type 1 (CMT1) is a heritable demyelinating neuropathy. It is genetically heterogeneous, with variable patterns of inheritance. Typically, it presents in the first two decades of life with predominant lower limb involvement. There is usually marked symmetrical distal wasting, weakness, depressed deep tendon reflexes and deformity of the feet. Distal sensory impairment is common.

Mononeuritis multiplex describes a pattern of disease in which at least two separate nerves have been affected. There will usually be sensory and motor impairment within the distribution of the affected nerves. It arises secondary to a large number of diseases including diabetes, vasculitis, sarcoidosis, amyloidosis and Lyme disease.

Clarke C, et al. Nerve and muscle disease (Chapter 10). In: Neurology: A Queen Square Textbook. 2nd edn. Oxford: Blackwell Publishing, 2016.
Van Schaik IN, et al. Multifocal motor neuropathy (Chapter 21). EFNS guidelines 2011. In: Gilhus NE, et al (eds), European Handbook of Neurological Management, Volume 1, 2nd edn. Oxford: Blackwell, 2011.

42. D Propranolol

Essential tremor is far more common than Parkinson's disease. Most cases have an unknown genetic basis with a positive family history. Typically, it presents with a slowly progressive, bilateral, symmetrical tremor that is predominantly kinetic or postural in nature. There may also be titubation or voice tremor. Sometimes resting tremor is also present, but it is not of the 'pill-rolling' type. Essential tremor frequently responds well to alcohol. In mild cases, reassurance may be all that is necessary. In this case, however, the patient is experiencing functional difficulty and medical treatment should be offered. Propranolol or primidone is most commonly used to treat essential tremor. Rarely, in very severe intractable cases, causing significant functional impairment, deep brain stimulation or surgical ablation of the thalamic ventral intermediate nucleus may be considered.

In contrast, Parkinson's disease is usually idiopathic. Rare genetic forms with variable modes of inheritance and drug-induced forms are also recognised. It is a progressive degenerative disease that typically presents with unilateral resting tremor (characteristically 'pill rolling'). Asymmetrical bilateral involvement, with more severe symptoms on the side of initial onset, is common. Patients exhibit rigidity ('cogwheeling' and 'clasp-knife'), bradykinesia and expressionless facies. The patient's voice may become hypophonic and monotonous. The gait is noted to be 'festinant' with increased turning time. Other features may include micrographia (small handwriting), anosmia (loss of sense of smell), drooling, constipation, depression, postural instability with falls, 'freezing', sleep disturbance, psychosis (with visual hallucinations) and dementia. Diagnosis is clinical with the aid of [123I] FP-CIT SPECT (DaT scan) imaging when necessary. Treatment should be at specialist centres and a choice of dopamine agonists, levodopa or monoamine oxidase B (MAO-B) inhibitors should be discussed. Response to levodopa is very good, and it remains the key form of treatment, but motor symptoms and the 'on–off' phenomenon of dyskinesia versus rigidity complicate long-term use. Patients on any dopaminergic therapy should be counselled on the risk of developing control disorders at any stage during the course of the disease.

The National Institute for Health and Clinical Excellence guidelines advise against the use of acute levodopa or apomorphine challenges in the diagnosis of Parkinson's disease. A DaT scan can be diagnostically valuable in cases where it is clinically impossible to differentiate between essential tremor and Parkinson's disease (it measures dopamine reuptake in the presynaptic terminals of striatonigral neurons). However, in this particular patient, the history and clinical findings are characteristic of a diagnosis of essential tremor.

Clarke C, et al. Movement disorders (Chapter 6). In: Neurology: A Queen Square Textbook. 2nd Edition Oxford: Blackwell Publishing, 2016.
NICE Clinical Guidelines. Parkinson's disease: diagnosis and management in primary and secondary care (NG71). London: NICE, 2017.

43. C Nataluzimab

This patient has multiple sclerosis (MS), an inflammatory demyelinating disease of the central nervous system. The aetiology remains unknown but there is an association with some human leukocyte antigen subtypes, suggesting a genetic susceptibility. The condition is more common in women than men, and has a peak incidence in the fourth decade.

In the vast majority of patients, the disease occurs as a relapsing–remitting form. Later, it may enter a secondary progressive phase. Approximately 10% of patients have primary progressive disease. Clinical features are highly variable, depending on the location of plaque formation, but commonly include optic neuritis, cerebellar features, transverse myelitis, hemiparesis, and focal motor or sensory deficit.

The diagnosis of MS is made on the basis of the McDonald criteria. The principle is to demonstrate evidence of central nervous system inflammatory events disseminated in time and space, with other possible causes excluded. Evidence of two clinical episodes typical of MS, such as optic neuritis and a partial transverse myelitis, is sufficient to make a clinical diagnosis. Contrast MRI is frequently used to diagnose MS with contrast-enhancing lesions indicating acute lesions, alongside older non-contrast lesions implying dissemination in time and space. T2-weighted MRI usually reveals foci of high signal within the periventricular white matter, corpus callosum, brain stem, cerebellum or spinal cord.

Visual-evoked potentials or somatosensory-evoked potentials may be delayed, supporting a process of demyelination. Additionally, in nearly all patients with MS, oligoclonal bands are found in the cerebrospinal fluid, but not in the serum. However, this finding is indicative of a local inflammatory process and, therefore, is not specific to MS. Ultimately, the diagnosis requires the demonstration of dissemination of demyelinating plaques in time and space. The MacDonald criteria, which were last revised in 2010, are frequently used to guide diagnosis.

Treatment for relapsing–remitting MS is usually initiated if there are two or more relapses in a year evidenced by clinical episodes +/- MRI changes, or new MRI changes without clinical relapse in those with established disease.

The treatment is divided into two categories. Category 1 includes moderate efficacy drugs with lesser side-effect profiles taken either orally or as an injection and include dimethyl fumarate, fingolimod, interferon-β, teriflunomide and glatiramer acetate. Category 2 are the higher effective medications given as infusions and include nataluzimab (Tysabri) andalemtuzumab (Campath). The risk profile for these treatments is higher. Progressive multifocal leukoencephalopathy is strongly associated with long-term use of nataluzimab in those with a positive serum JC virus.

- Of the medications on the list nataluzimab is the only one used as a disease-modifying agent to treat MS.
- High-dose intravenous steroids are frequently given in an acute setting as they lessen the symptom duration and severity. However, they have not been shown to modify recovery in the long term.
- The other answer options (intravenous immunoglobulin, rituximab, high dose intravenous methylprednisolone and plasma exchange) are frequently used either acutely or as a second line treatment for neurological inflammatory diseases such as Guillain–Barré, chronic inflammatory demyelinating polyneuropathy, and vasculitis.

This woman is describing Uhtoff's phenomenon where symptoms worsen after overheating with, for example, hot weather or exercise. Lhermitte's sign is the sign associated with the sensation of an electric shock running down the back due to an inflammatory spinal lesion.

Clarke C, et al. Multiple sclerosis and demyelinating diseases (Chapter 11). In: Neurology: A Queen Square Textbook, 2nd edn. Oxford: Blackwell Publishing, 2016.
Scolding N, et al. Association of British Neurologists: revised (2015) guidelines for prescribing disease-modifying treatments in multiple sclerosis. Pract Neurol 2015;15:273–279.

44. C Intravenous thiamine

This patient is exhibiting features of Wernicke's encephalopathy, a potentially fatal condition of thiamine deficiency. The triad of acute confusion, ataxia and ophthalmoplegia classically defines the condition. However, the clinical presentation is variable, e.g. eye signs may range from nystagmus to complete ophthalmoplegia.

The condition may develop acutely or subacutely and is most commonly reported in those who chronically abuse alcohol. However, it may occur in a wide range of conditions that cause malnutrition (such as gastrointestinal surgery, eating disorders, malignancy). The mainstay of immediate management is parenteral thiamine replacement. Timely treatment usually results in rapid resolution of the clinical signs, and avoids the significant mortality associated with the untreated condition. In practice, intravenous Pabrinex – a cocktail of B vitamins and vitamin C – is usually administered; this helps to prevent the complications of the broader spectrum of vitamin deficiency.

Thiamine has an important role as a coenzyme in a number of metabolic pathways (including the oxidation of glucose, the catabolism of amino acids and the biosynthesis of neurotransmitters). As such, the administration of dextrose to the thiamine-deficient patient potentially accelerates neurological damage by consuming the little remaining thiamine in the oxidation of glucose. Therefore, thiamine stores should be replaced before dextrose is administered (note that, in patients with low magnesium stores, the parental thiamine may be ineffective until magnesium has been restored to a normal level).

This patient is not violently agitated and does not warrant treatment with intramuscular lorazepam. Nor is there any evidence that he is psychotic and in need of treatment with antipsychotic medication. Aciclovir is an antiviral agent and is not indicated.

Clarke C, et al. Toxic, metabolic and physical insults (Chapter 19). In: Neurology: A Queen Square Textbook, 2nd edn. Oxford: Blackwell Publishing, 2016.

45. D Photocoagulation scarring

This patient has undergone extensive laser photocoagulation of the retina to treat proliferative diabetic retinopathy. In this case, a single large blot haemorrhage is also evident inferior to the disc. Panretinal photocoagulation (PRP) is typified by multiple, well-circumscribed, punched-out areas of retinal atrophy with some reactive hyperpigmentation. This is usually applied to the entire peripheral retina but avoiding the macula.

A choroidal haemangioma is a benign tumour which, as its name suggests, is located in the choroid and appears as a well-circumscribed orange–red region on fundoscopy. They are often asymptomatic and discovered incidentally. They can, however, present with visual disturbance and there is a risk of retinal detachment due to cystic degeneration. Management is usually conservative, but photodynamic therapy may have a role in some cases.

Chorioretinitis is addressed elsewhere.

Onchocerciasis is a filarial disease (also known as river blindness) which may cause choroiditis, glaucoma and optic atrophy. It also causes punctate keratitis and, in severe cases, may result in corneal fibrosis and opacification.

Retinitis pigmentosa is characterised by a 'bone-spicule' pattern of perivascular retinal hyperpigmentation in the mid-peripheries, associated with, retinal pigment epithelium atrophy. Typically the macula is spared. The retinal arteries eventually become attenuated and thread like, and the optic disc may become pale and waxy in appearance.

Bressler N, et al. Panretinal photocoagulation for proliferative diabetic retinopathy. N Engl J Med 2011; 365:1520–1526.

46. E Small fibre neuropathy

This patient is most likely suffering from a small fibre peripheral neuropathy, which may be secondary to impaired glucose tolerance. Typically, patients complain of burning, tingling or numbness in a glove-and-stocking distribution. Symptoms are often most problematic at night, and can have a significant impact on sleep. Clinical examination reveals normal motor function, normal proprioception and vibration sense. There is usually reduced sensation to pinprick and thermal hypoaesthesia, due to involvement of small unmyelinated C-fibres and lightly myelinated Aδ-fibres. The effect is usually length dependent, so the deficit tends to affect the feet first and progresses fairly symmetrically. Concurrent involvement of the small fibres of the autonomic nervous system is not uncommon; clinical features may include orthostatic hypotension and impotence, for example. Nerve conduction studies are almost always normal. However, if necessary, a skin biopsy may be performed to help make the diagnosis; this may demonstrate a reduced density of intraepithelial C-fibres. There are numerous causes of small fibre neuropathy, including 'prediabetic' states, but a large proportion of cases are idiopathic.

Psychosomatic disorders warrant consideration in the differential list of causes, but conversion disorder is clearly not the best explanation for this patient's condition. Conversion disorder is discussed elsewhere.

Diabetic amyotrophy describes a pattern of proximal muscle weakness that may complicate diabetes. It can be discounted based on the history and clinical findings.

Mononeuritis multiplex describes a pattern of nerve damage, in which there is discrete damage to at least two separate peripheral nerves, as a result of an underlying disease (e.g. diabetes mellitus, systemic lupus erythematosus, amyloidosis, sarcoidosis, Lyme disease and many more). This condition can be discounted as the patient exhibits a 'stocking' distribution of sensory involvement, rather than a 'nerve' distribution of motor and sensory deficit.

Restless legs syndrome may occur secondary to small fibre neuropathy. However, in this patient's case, the principal problem is neuropathic pain. The diagnostic criteria for restless legs syndrome are discussed elsewhere.

Clarke C, et al. Nerve and muscle disease (Chapter 10). In: Neurology: A Queen Square Textbook.2nd Edition Oxford: Blackwell Publishing, 2016.
Devigili G, et al. The diagnostic criteria for small fibre neuropathy: from symptoms to neuropathology. Brain 2008; 131(7):1912–1925.
Papanas YN, et al. Neuropathy in prediabetes: does the clock start ticking early? Nat Rev Endocrinol 2011; 7:682–690.

47. D Transient global amnesia

This is a diagnosis predominantly based on the history of sudden onset complete memory loss affecting all memory modalities with a predominance for inability to create anterograde memory and some retrograde amnesia. The acute episode is 2–6 hours in duration with gradual return to normal over a subsequent number of hours and usually full recovery within 24 hours. Frequently there are no MRI findings but rarely if the scan is done in the hyper acute phase imaging may show a unilateral transient hyperintensity on T2 flair imaging in the hippocampus. Cerebrospinal fluid and electroencephalogram (EEG) findings are unremarkable. Transient global amnesia is frequently an isolated incident which will not recur, with peak incidence in the 5th to 7th decades. The cause is unknown but it is thought that metabolic stress causes disturbance to the delicate CA1 neurons of the hippocampus.

These are the neurons which are also first affected with a hypoxic brain injury, such as following a cardiac arrest, however the duration of the insult is usually longer resulting in more extensive memory deficit with a much slower recovery – usually months.

Transient ischaemic or epileptic attack might be considered for this patient's clinical features but in someone with no risk factors or previous seizure history they are less likely, although they do need to be considered in the differential diagnosis. Encephalitis frequently results in memory loss but not with such abrupt recovery, and the duration of illness is weeks to months.

Spiegel DR, Smith J, Wade RR, et al. Transient global amnesia: current perspectives. Neuropsychiatr Dis Treat 2017; 13:2691–2703.

48. C Thiamine infusion

This question is testing your knowledge of management of status epilepticus.

The CT of the brain in Figure 7.22 shows a small hyperdense lesion within the left basal ganglia, consistent with an intracerebral haemorrhage (ICH). The patient is demonstrating signs which indicate a left-sided cerebral event. It may be that the fall and collapse occurred as a result of this episode. An ischaemic stroke rarely causes seizures and so haemorrhagic stroke or metabolic derangement should be considered as reasons for the long time spent on the floor and are the more likely causes of the seizure activity. Thiamine would be given on account of malnutrition, especially with the suggestion of alcohol excess.

The patient has not recovered consciousness between ictal episodes so, in the context of a haemorrhagic insult, treatment for status epilepticus should be considered.

NICE guidelines divide management of status epilepticus into four stages:
1. Airway management, oxygen, cardiorespiratory support, intravenous access. Give a benzodiazapine such as diazepam or buccal midazolam in a pre-hospital setting.
2. Emergency antiepileptic drug (AED) therapy (intravenous lorazepam/diazepam plus usual AEDs), emergency investigations (blood sampling for blood gas tests, glucose, renal and liver function, calcium and magnesium, full blood count including platelets, blood clotting, AED drug levels), treat severe acidosis, administer glucose and/or thiamine if alcoholism or malnutrition is suspected.
3. Establish aetiology, alert anaesthetist/ITU, phenytoin infusion +/- phenobarbital if already on oral phenytoin or not responding, pressor therapy when appropriate.
4. General anaesthesia and transferral to an intensive care setting. Propofol, midazolam and thiopental are the primary anaesthetic drugs used and should be titrated to stop evidence of ictal activity on EEG monitoring. Sedation should continue for 24 hours after the last seizure before a weaning trial.

Management of ICH should occur in a tertiary setting with access to neurosurgery. Referral should be made for all patients with a Glasgow Coma Scale score of less than 8 or with complications of ICH such as seizures. Urgent imaging should be completed. Antihypertensives, such as intravenous labetalol, are given to reduce the blood pressure to 140 mmHg, as long as there are no contraindications to do so. There is no guidance to give prophylactic AEDs in patients with small bleeds although they are frequently prescribed as a short course of treatment, e.g. oral/nasogastric levetiracetam.

Wardlaw J. Diagnosis of stroke on neuroimaging. BMJ 2004; 328:655.
The National Institute for Health and Care Excellence (NICE). Clinical guideline 137. Appendix F – Protocols for treating convulsive status epilepticus in adults and children. London: NICE, 2016.
Clarke C, et al. Stroke and cerebrovascular diseases (Chapter 5). In: Neurology: A Queen Square Textbook. 2nd edn. Oxford: Blackwell Publishing, 2016.

Chapter 8

Oncology and palliative medicine

Questions

1. A 66-year-old man presented with symptoms of facial swelling and a feeling of fullness in the head. This had started 2 weeks ago. He had no past medical history of note and took no medication.

    On examination, he had facial plethora and swelling, raised internal and external jugular veins, and dilated veins across his superior anterior chest wall.

    Which one of the following is the least likely underlying cause of his condition?

    A   Germ cell cancer
    B   Lymphoma
    C   Myxoma
    D   Non-small cell lung cancer
    E   Small cell lung cancer

2. A 35-year-old woman was referred to the gastroenterology clinic for consideration of colorectal cancer (CRC) screening, after her brother was diagnosed with colorectal cancer at the age of 48 years.

    What is the most appropriate CRC screening programme?

    A   Colonoscopy age 45 years and then every 5 years until age 75 years
    B   Colonoscopy age 35 years, and if normal no further colonoscopies
    C   Colonoscopy age 50 years and then 10 yearly until age 70 years
    D   Colonoscopy age 55 years, and if normal no further colonoscopies
    E   Colonoscopy age 65 years and then 5 yearly until the age of 75 years

3. A 54-year-old man underwent a chest X-ray because of shortness of breath on exertion. He was a smoker of 20 cigarettes per day (35 pack-years). This demonstrated a left upper lobe mass. Further investigations are arranged.

    Investigations:

CT: 3-cm mass lesion left upper lobe ipsilateral lymphadenopathy 1.4 cm CT staging T2aN1M0 (stage IIa)
Bronchoscopy: tumour emerging from the left upper lobe bronchus
Bronchial biopsy: squamous cell carcinoma
Spirometry: forced expiratory volume 2.4 L (83% predicted)

His case was discussed by the lung cancer multi-disciplinary team

What is the most appropriate next step in management?

A Best supportive care
B Chemotherapy
C Endobronchial ultrasound
D Lobectomy
E Position emission tomography/CT (PET/CT) scan

4. A 65-year-old woman was seen in the oncology clinic to discuss treatment of her ovarian cancer. Previously she had undergone platinum-based chemotherapy but the disease had recurred.
    Further therapy with doxorubicin chemotherapy was discussed.

Which one of the following is not a recognised side effect of anthracycline-based chemotherapy?

A Cardiotoxicity
B Colonic ulceration
C Conjunctivitis
D Peripheral neuropathy
E Thrombocytopenia

5. A 58-year-old man with Duke C rectal carcinoma was receiving XELOX (capecitabine plus oxaliplatin) chemotherapy. He has been tolerating the treatment well, with nausea relieved by antiemetics. He presented 7 days after his last treatment to the emergency department with a fever and confusion at home. He was found to be tachycardic and hypotensive.

> haemoglobin 99 g/L (130 – 180)
>
> white cell count 1.1 x 10^9/L (4 – 11)
>
> neutrophils 0.1 x 10^9/L (1.8-4)
>
> platelets 75 x 10^9/L (150-400)

Which of the following is not true?

A The patient should be treated with a broad-spectrum penicillin (e.g. piperacillin/ tazobactam)
B He should be seen by an oncologist within 24 hours
C He should not receive granulocyte colony stimulating factor (GCSF)
D He requires close monitoring
E Antibiotics should be rationalised if blood cultures are positive

6. A 74-year-old retired male builder presented with a 3-month history of dull right-sided chest discomfort, shortness of breath on exertion and sweating. He had no past medical history of note. He remained active and there was no limitation to his normal activities of daily living.
    A chest X-ray was performed (see **Figure 8.1**).
    Following this he had a CT of the chest and then he was referred to the thoracic surgeons for a video-assisted thoracoscopic surgical (VATS) biopsy to confirm the diagnosis.

What is the most appropriate management?

A Cisplatin and pemetrexed
B Insertion of indwelling chest drain
C Pneumonectomy
D Radical radiotherapy
E Radiotherapy to surgical port sites

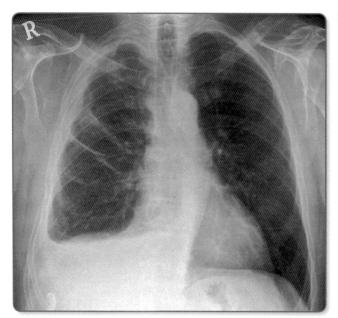

Figure 8.1

7. A 72-year-old man presented with weight loss and anaemia and was found to have a gastric carcinoma on endoscopy. He had been previously fit and well.

Investigations:

CT of the chest/abdomen/pelvis:

mass in distal gastric region

no metastases

no lymphadenopathy

Histology: gastric adenocarcinoma with HER-2-positive receptors, tumour invades the muscularis propria (T2)

What is the most appropriate management?

A   Chemoradiotherapy
B   Chemotherapy with 5-fluorouracil
C   Surgical resection and irinotecan
D   Surgical resection and radiotherapy
E   Surgical resection, chemotherapy and trastuzumab

8. A 46-year-old Chinese man was found to have a 2.5-cm liver lesion on ultrasound. He was known to have chronic hepatitis B virus cirrhosis but was not on treatment. He was fit and well and employed as a carpenter. He had no evidence of portal hypertension and had no other past medical history.
    Physical examination was normal.

Investigations:

> Triple phase CT of the liver:
> liver looked cirrhotic with irregular border but normal portal vein flow and no ascites
> single 2.5-cm nodule in segment 5 with arterial hypervascularity and delayed phase wash-out
>
> bilirubin 18 mmol/L (1–22)   albumin 34 g/L (37–49)
> alkaline phosphatase 196 U/L (45–105)   international normalised ratio 1.1 (<1.4)
> alanine transaminase 24 U/L (5–35)

What is the most appropriate management?

A   Liver resection
B   Liver transplantation
C   Radiofrequency ablation
D   Sorafenib
E   Transarterial chemoembolisation (TACE)

9. A 68-year-old man presented to the emergency department. He had no significant medical history and had been well until 3 weeks previously when he had started to experience increasingly severe back pain over his mid-spine. He had noticed over the last 2 days that he had had some difficulty in walking.

On examination of his lower limbs he had increased tone bilaterally, reduced power, 3/5 proximally and 2/5 distally, brisk reflexes and up-going plantars. He had impaired sensation to a level just below his umbilicus.

An urgent MRI of his spine confirmed a single lesion suspicious of a metastasis at T10.

Investigations:

> prostate-specific antigen 90 ng/mL (<3)

What is the most appropriate next step in management?

A   Bone biopsy
B   Chemotherapy
C   High-dose steroids and discuss with spinal surgeons
D   Non-steroidal anti-inflammatory drugs, pamidronate and discuss with spinal surgeons
E   Radiotherapy

10. A 75-year-old man presented with flank pain and macroscopic haematuria.

On examination, there was a palpable mass in the right side of his abdomen. He had a CT of the abdomen performed (see **Figure 8.2**).

Which one of the following is correct regarding the diagnosis?

A   He requires a bilateral nephrectomy
B   He requires a bone scan to assess for metastases
C   He requires a unilateral nephrectomy
D   He requires an urgent biopsy of his right kidney
E   He requires no further imaging as metastasis is rare

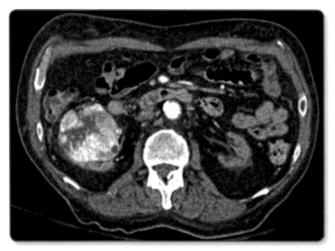

Figure 8.2

11. A 64-year-old man presented with a 2-week history of progressive shortness of breath at rest. He had advanced non-small cell lung cancer and severe chronic obstructive pulmonary disease. Six months ago, he completed four cycles of palliative chemotherapy, but his cancer had progressed and he was referred to the palliative care team. He was taking maximal inhaled bronchodilator and inhaled corticosteroids therapy and oral morphine 5 mg every 4 hours.

   On examination, he was apyrexial, respiratory rate 14 breaths per minute and oxygen saturation 95% on air. There was a small right pleural effusion.

   Investigations:

haemoglobin 107 g/L (130–180)	white cell count 6.9 × 10⁹/L (4–11)

   What is the best management step to improve the dyspnoea?

   A   Antibiotics
   B   Aspiration of effusion
   C   Blood transfusion
   D   Lorazepam
   E   Oxygen

12. An 80-year-old man with advanced refractory metastatic prostate cancer was referred to you by his general practitioner for haematuria. He had had this on and off for several years but the condition had been steadily worsening. He had recently been told that his prostate cancer has worsened and his prognosis is several months. At the time of referral he was taking apixaban for atrial fibrillation (CHA2DS2VASc score 3) and aspirin after a previous myocardial infarct 20 years ago.

   Investigations:

haemoglobin 87 g/L (130–180)	prothrombin time 14.1 s (11.5–13.2)
white cell count 2.9 × 10⁹/L (4–11)	activated partial thromboplastin time 36.3 s (26–32)
platelets 35 × 10⁹/L (150–400)	fibrinogen 1.6 g/L (1.7–4.0)

Which would be the most appropriate management of his presentation?

A   Transfuse two pool of platelets to control immediate bleeding
B   Give tranexamic acid
C   Stop aspirin and apixaban
D   Cystoscopy
E   Stop aspirin, continue apixaban

13. A 74-year-old man with a history of chronic obstructive pulmonary disease and hypertension was referred to the chest clinic with worsening shortness of breath, intermittent haemoptysis and left-sided back pain. He was an ex-smoker of 50 pack-years after quitting 5 years ago. His current medications include a combination steroid and long-acting β_2-agonist inhaler, amlodipine, aspirin and he has recently commenced co-codamol.

An urgent CT of the thorax was performed (see **Figure 8.3**).

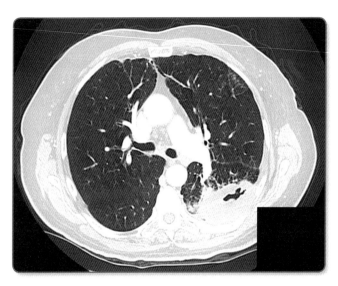

Figure 8.3

What is the most likely diagnosis?

A   Aspergilloma
B   Lung abscess
C   Small cell carcinoma
D   Squamous cell carcinoma
E   Tuberculosis

14. A 64-year-old man presented with a history of dysphagia for solids and weight loss. He had no other medical problems, and took no medication.

Investigations:

Upper gastrointestinal endoscopy: 2 × 1.5 cm neoplastic appearing lesion at 15 cm from incisor teeth

CT of the chest/abdomen/pelvis:

2-cm soft tissue mass confined to the upper oesophagus

no metastases in liver or lungs

no localised lymphadenopathy

Histology: squamous cell carcinoma

What is the most appropriate therapy?

A   Chemoradiotherapy
B   Oesophagectomy alone
C   Oesophagectomy and radiotherapy
D   Oesophagectomy with neoadjuvant chemotherapy
E   Radiotherapy

15. A 38-year-old woman presented with polydipsia and polyuria. She was found to have axillary lymphadenopathy and a breast lump which, on imaging, was suggestive of malignancy.

Investigations:

haemoglobin 121 g/L (115–165)   calcium 3.22 mmol/L (2.15 – 2.60)
white cell count 5.4 × 10⁹/L (4–11)   corrected calcium 3.43 (2.15-2.60)
platelets 235 × 10⁹/L (150-400)

She received IV pamidronate but did not respond to treatment.

Which of the following is not correct?

A   She can receive further bisphosphonates
B   This is a poor prognostic finding
C   Loop diuretics can promote calcium diuresis
D   Denosumab is the next line of treatment
E   Vitamin D supplementation is routinely indicated

16. A 56-year-old woman with a history of ischaemic heart disease was diagnosed with human epidermal growth factor receptor-2 (HER-2)-positive early invasive breast cancer. A mastectomy with adjuvant chemotherapy and trastuzumab was planned.

Which of the following is a contraindication to treatment with trastuzumab?

A   Atrial fibrillation
B   Congestive cardiac failure
C   Hypertension
D   Mitral valve prolapse
E   Previous cerebrovascular accident

17. A 57-year-old man presented with a 6-month history of intermittent abdominal pain and loose stools. He had been opening his bowel five times per day, with no associated rectal bleeding or mucus. He reported occasional episodes of facial and neck flushing. He had recently been diagnosed with asthma, for which he was taking salbutamol and beclometasone inhalers.
    On examination, he looked thin. Cardiovascular, respiratory and abdominal examinations were normal.

What is the most useful diagnostic investigation?

A   Adrenocorticotrophic hormone levels
B   C-peptide level
C   Fasting gastrin level
D   Serum 5-hydroxytryptamine levels
E   Urinary 5-hydroxyindoleacetic acid (5-HIAA) levels

18. An 84-year-old man with metastatic lung carcinoma was referred to hospital with a 3-day history of worsening shortness of breath. He was frail and largely housebound.
    On examination, his respiratory rate was 34 breaths per minute and oxygen saturations 84% on air and 92% on 10 L oxygen. Clinically he had a large right pleural effusion confirmed on chest X-ray. He had 1000 mL aspirated with a cannula and felt better. Cytology revealed malignant cells.

3 days later, the patient complained of worsening shortness of breath and a repeat chest X-ray demonstrated increased size of the pleural effusion.

What is the most appropriate next step in management?

A   Chest drain insertion and talc pleurodesis
B   Commence Oramorph
C   Commence lorazepam
D   Repeat therapeutic aspiration of 1000 mL with cannula
E   Refer for video-assisted thoracoscopic surgical (VATS) drainage and talc pleurodesis

19. A 52-year-old woman was seen in the clinic after a total thyroidectomy for medullary thyroid carcinoma. She was on levothyroxine replacement but not on any other medication. She did not have any other past medical history. She complained of episodes of sweating, flushing and palpitations associated with anxiety and headaches.

On examination, her temperature was 36.8°C, pulse 88 beats per minute, blood pressure 170/110 mmHg and respiratory rate 18 breaths per minute. There was no tremor of the outstretched hands and she was clinically euthyroid.

What is the most useful diagnostic investigation?

A   Serum corrected calcium
B   Serum parathyroid hormone level
C   Serum thyroid-stimulating hormone concentration
D   Transthoracic echocardiogram
E   Urine 24-hour metanephrines

20. A 58-year-old man presented with a single generalised tonic–clonic seizure on a background of several months' history of daily headache.

An MRI of the brain was performed (see **Figure 8.4**):

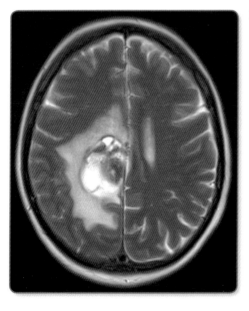

Figure 8.4

What is the most likely diagnosis?

A   Arteriovenous malformation
B   Cerebral toxoplasmosis
C   Glioma
D   Meningioma
E   Neurocysticercosis

21. A 74-year-old woman with Alzheimer's disease (Mini Mental State Examination 17/30) has been admitted with 2 days of bilious vomiting and a diagnosis of intussusception has been made. After anaesthetic review it is thought she would survive a laparotomy and surgical resolution of the intussusception. However, she is declining the operation and in two previous clinic letters over the last 3 years note is made of her wish not to have any invasive procedures or surgery to prolong her life because of her diagnosis of Alzheimer's disease. Her daughter and her son wish for her to have the operation and are arguing strongly for it to occur without further delay.

What is the most appropriate next step in management?

A   Involve the palliative care team in the decision-making process
B   Not proceed with the operation
C   Proceed with the operation
D   Talk to the family and obtain the written permission of the next of kin for the operation to proceed
E   Try to relieve the intussusception with flexible sigmoidoscopy

22. A 67-year-old woman was diagnosed with early oestrogen-positive invasive breast cancer. After surgery it was decided that she should have adjuvant chemotherapy.

What is the most appropriate management?

A   5-Fluorouracil
B   Anastrozole
C   Exemestane
D   Tamoxifen
E   Trastuzumab

23. A 62-year-old woman was referred to the chest clinic with right-sided chest pain, breathlessness, haemoptysis, weight loss and an abnormal chest X-ray. She was a lifelong heavy smoker (>80 pack-years).

Investigations:

CT of the chest and abdomen: large mass in the right lower lobe invading into the mediastinum and pericardium, extensive mediastinal lymphadenopathy and bone metastasis (T4N3M1b)

Bronchoscopic biopsies: squamous cell carcinoma

Mutation analysis: epidermal growth factor receptor negative

What is the most appropriate first-line therapy?

A   Cetuximab
B   Docetaxel
C   Gemcitabine and carboplatin
D   Pemetrexed
E   Vinorelbine

24. A 74-year-old man underwent Hartmann's procedure for a sigmoid tumour. He underwent a preoperative staging CT which showed tumour invading into the sigmoid wall and two enlarged mesenteric lymph nodes suggestive of metastasis. No distant metastases were seen.

Histology of the mass showed a 5.4-cm adenocarcinoma, with complete resection margins. The tumour had invaded the muscularis propria but no adjacent structures.

What is his TNM staging classification?

A   T1N0M1
B   T2N1M0
C   T2N0M1
D   T3N1M0
E   T4N1M0

Answers

1. C Myxoma

This man has superior vena cava obstruction (SVCO) as evidenced by his facial plethora and swelling and dilated neck and chest veins. This is an oncological emergency and requires immediate intervention.

SVCO can have malignant or non-malignant aetiology, and the latter now accounts for 35% of cases of SVCO. The most common non-malignant causes are thrombosis secondary to implanted devices such as pacemakers or catheters, fibrosing mediastinitis and aortic aneurysm. The most common malignant cause is non-small cell lung cancer accounting for 50% of malignant cases, followed by small cell lung cancer (22%), lymphoma (12%), metastatic cancer (most commonly breast – 9%), germ cell tumours (3%) and thymoma (2%). Myxomas are cardiac tumours predominantly found in the atria and are most likely to present as heart failure and not SVCO.

Management of SVCO involves urgent imaging to determine if this is luminal (e.g. thrombosis) or extraluminal (e.g. malignant). Treatment for malignant SVCO involves high dose steroids followed by chemo-radiotherapy depending on suspected tumour type. In cases where chemo-radiotherapy is inappropriate, stenting can be performed by the interventional radiologists or vascular surgeons and can be achieved via a brachiocephalic or inferior vena cava approach.

Wilson LD, Detterbeck FC, Yahalom J. Superior vena cava syndrome with malignant causes. N Engl J Med 2007; 356:1862–1869.

2. D Colonoscopy aged 55 years, and if normal no further colonoscopies

The British Society of Gastroenterology colorectal cancer (CRC) screening guidelines categorise people with a family history of CRC into high, high-moderate, low-moderate or low-risk groups, based on the presence or absence of hereditary polyposis syndromes and the age and number of affected first-degree relatives. Colorectal cancer is common, and the incidence of an affected first-degree relative (FDR) among the general population is 4–10%. In the scenario given the patient has one affected FDR aged less than 50 years which equates to a low-moderate risk, and a colonoscopy at the age of 55 years is the appropriate screening test. If this is normal then no further colonoscopies need to be done. National Institute of Health and Clinical Excellence (NICE) guidelines (issued March 2018) state that all adults aged 55 years should undergo a flexible sigmoidoscopy.

To be high risk the patient would need to have a personal or family history suggestive of, or germline mutations indicating, Lynch's syndrome, familial adenomatous polyposis, MUTYH [mutY homologue (*Escherichia coli*)]-associated polyposis (MAP), juvenile polyposis or Peutz–Jeghers syndrome. The lifetime risk of CRC in these syndromes ranges from 10% to 100%. Screening for these syndromes is covered in detail in the British Society of Gastroenterology guidelines.

The following family history would be considered high-moderate risk:

- Three affected first-degree relatives of any age. However, IF one of the three relatives is less than 50 years old then they would be considered high risk.
- If there are two affected first-degree relatives aged less than 60 OR if there are two affected relatives who have a mean age of less than 60 years AND one of them is a first-degree relative of the patient.

These patients with high-to-moderate risk should have 5-yearly colonoscopies starting at age 55 years until they are 75 years of age.

The following family history is considered to give a low-to-moderate risk:

- A single affected first-degree relative aged less than 50 years
- Two affected relatives who are aged over 60 years, of first-degree kinship.

These patients should have one colonoscopy at age 55 years and if this is normal no further colonoscopies are required.

Cairns SR, et al. Guidelines for colorectal cancer screening and surveillance in moderate and high risk groups (update from 2002). Gut 2010; 59:666–690.

3. E Position emission tomography/CT (PET/CT) scan

This patient has early disease (stages I to II) and should be considered for surgical resection. PET/CT scanning should be performed prior to attempted surgical resection because it can help determine whether there is evidence of distant metastatic disease. Malignant lesions are more likely to be 'PET avid' and demonstrate uptake of fluorodeoxyglucose (FDG). PET/CT scanning has a superior diagnostic sensitivity compared to PET scanning without a CT component. If a PET/CT scan suggests that there is lymph node involvement which would preclude surgical resection, histological confirmation needs to be performed. This approach has been shown to reduce the number of inappropriate and/or futile operations. The combination of CT and PET scanning also improves radiotherapy planning.

Techniques for nodal sampling include: endobronchial ultrasound (EBUS), which is one of the least invasive tests; endoscopic ultrasound (EUS) via the oesophagus; mediastinoscopy; mini-thoracotomy; and video-assisted thoracoscopic surgery (VATS). The last three tests necessitate general anaesthesia with its associated risks.

Patients should be considered for surgery if they are fit enough for the procedure and if predicted lung function following resection is sufficient to maintain good function. Fitness is determined by performance status, lung function [forced expiratory volume (FEV$_1$) >1.5 L for lobectomy, >2 L for pneumonectomy or more than 60% predicted] and other co-morbidities need to be considered.

Palliative chemotherapy and palliative care should be considered as primary treatments for patients presenting with more advanced disease and/or if other associated co-morbidities dictate that more radial treatments are too high risk and less likely to confer survival advantage.

The National Institute for Health and Clinical Excellence (NICE). NICE Guidelines. Lung cancer in adults. QS17. London: NICE, 2016.

4. D Peripheral neuropathy

Doxorubicin belongs to the anthracycline class of chemotherapeutic drugs. It is used in the treatment of breast, ovarian and haematological malignancies. The most important dose-related side effects are cardiotoxicity (particularly delayed cardiomyopathy in children) and myelosuppression. Cardiotoxicity with anthracyclines forces a lifetime exposure limit which is specific to each drug but cumulative across the class. Even for patients who remain under this exposure, cardiotoxicity can result in significant late morbidity and mortality.

Like most chemotherapy agents, doxorubicin also has non-specific gastrointestinal side effects such as nausea and vomiting, colonic (particularly caecal) ulceration, mucositis, and alopecia. It causes myelosuppression, including neutropenia and thrombocytopenia. Peripheral neuropathy is not associated with anthracycline administration, but is a recognised side effect of platinum based agents (e.g. cisplatin, carboplatin and oxaliplatin) and vinca alkaloids (e.g. vincristine, vinblastine).

Monseuz JJ, et al. Cardiac side effects of cancer chemotherapy. Int J Cardiol 2010; 11:3–15.

5. C He should not receive granulocyte colony stimulating factor (GCSF)

This patient has neutropenic sepsis. This is an oncological/haematological emergency associated with a high morbidity and mortality. NICE sets out the standards which should be adhered to, including prompt broad spectrum antibiotics, intensive monitoring and review within 24 hours by a clinician experienced in managing chemotherapy and its complications.

Initial antibiotic choice should be guided by local protocol, but in the absence of high risk features dual therapy with an aminoglycoside or glycopeptide is unnecessary. Antibiotic therapy should commence within 1 hour of presentation, and in centres where full blood count (FBC) test results are not expected to be available within that timeframe empirical broad spectrum antibiotic cover should be given in all patients suspected of having neutropenic sepsis. Suitable broad spectrum agents include piptazobactam or meropenem. If a positive culture is found which fits the clinical presentation, antibiotics can be de-escalated to avoid promotion of drug resistant infections.

The use of granulocyte colony stimulating factor (GCSF) is routine in patients who present with features of severe sepsis (e.g. hypotension) although use in patients without septic complications is discouraged. GCSF should be avoided in patients with myeloid malignancies such as acute myeloid leukaemia and chronic myeloid leukaemia. GCSF is indicated in septic patients post chemotherapy while the neutrophil count is <1.0 x 10^9/L and should be continued until the neutrophil count is above 1.0 on two consecutive readings.

Neutrophil and platelet counts typically nadir at between 7 and 10 days after chemotherapy and recover by day 14 to 20. Intravenous antibiotics should be continued for 48–72 hours after the last fever, depending on whether neutrophil recovery has occurred.

National Institute for Health and Care Excellence (NICE). Neutropenic sepsis: prevention and management in people with cancer [CG151]. London: NICE; 2012.

6. A Cisplatin and pemetrexed

The chest X-ray demonstrates a right-sided pleural effusion with associated pleural thickening and the history is very suggestive of mesothelioma. He was a retired builder and is likely to have had occupational exposure to asbestos. Asbestos was widely used as a building material in the 1960s and 1970s but has since been banned in the UK. Asbestos exists in several forms and these differ in their toxicity, but all are associated with asbestosis and mesothelioma. Blue asbestos (crocidolite) is the most potent carcinogen and was used for thermal insulation and cement sheeting. Brown asbestos (amosite) is also a potent carcinogen and was used for asbestos insulation boards. White asbestos (chrysotile) is the most common form found in the UK and, while still a carcinogen, is regarded as less toxic than the other forms. The mean latent interval between first exposure to asbestos and death is around 40 years. There is no significant association with smoking.

Patients may present with chest pain, which is usually dull in nature; however, pleuritic pain has also been described, and breathlessness. Profuse sweating may also be a feature. Weight loss and fatigue are rare at presentation, but are common features later in the disease. Imaging may demonstrate moderate-to-large pleural effusion, with nodular pleural thickening or pleural mass, uniform encasement of the lung with resulting small hemithorax and/or invasion of chest wall or other structures. The diagnosis should be confirmed histologically by ultrasound or CT-guided biopsy. Early use of thoracoscopy may provide diagnosis and enable management of large effusions with talc pleurodesis. The median survival is 9–12 months from diagnosis.

Patients with good performance status should be considered for palliative chemotherapy. The combination of cisplatin and pemetrexed has been demonstrated to have a response rate (tumour shrinkage >50%) of 41%.

Palliative radiotherapy may be useful, in selected patients, to help reduce chest wall pain, breathlessness and superior vena cava obstruction. Currently, there is no role for radical radiotherapy. Prophylactic radiotherapy to biopsy or surgical port sites may reduce chest wall invasion by tumour; however, a randomised study failed to demonstrate a benefit. Surgical resection remains controversial and currently there are no randomised controlled trials demonstrating survival advantage following pneumonectomy.

In patients with recurrent pleural effusion, who have failed talc pleurodesis or have trapped lung, an indwelling chest drain may be considered as a palliative option.

Van Zandwijk N, et al. Guidelines for the diagnosis and treatment of malignant pleural mesothelioma. J Thor Dis 2013; 5: E254–E307.

7.   E Surgical resection, chemotherapy and trastuzumab

Surgical resection, which may include radical gastrectomy is required for this patient. The tumour is T2 involving the muscularis propria and surgical resection alone is not recommended. Perioperative chemotherapy i.e. option C (irinotecan) in advanced gastric adenocarcinoma confers a survival benefit and is the additional treatment of choice in the UK. However, in those patients who are HER-2 receptor positive then addition of trastuzumab (Herceptin) gives an overall survival benefit and improves disease-free survival, so this should be considered in all HER-2-positive patients. Chemotherapy alone is not standard practice, and there is no role for chemoradiotherapy in gastric carcinoma.

Allum WH. BSG guidelines. Guidelines for the management of oesophageal and gastric cancer. Gut 2011; 60:1449–1472.

8.   A Liver resection

This man has hepatocellular carcinoma (HCC) on a background of hepatitis B virus cirrhosis. He has early stage cirrhosis and limited stage disease, having a single lesion which is less than 3 cm in size. He has a good performance status. The American Association for the Study of Liver Diseases (AASLD) guidelines on therapy for HCC indicate that he should have a liver resection to remove the lesion. A liver transplantation would be the treatment of choice if he had up to three nodules of less than 3 cm in diameter, and no other co-morbidities, or a single lesion less than 3 cm with evidence of a raised bilirubin or portal hypertension. Radiofrequency ablation is used for patients with three nodules of less than 3 cm who have co-morbidities that preclude liver transplantation. These are all curative treatments. Patients with multinodular HCC and a performance status of 0 should have transarterial chemoembolisation, and those with multinodular HCC or portal invasion with a performance status of 1 or 2 should be offered sorafenib. Sorafenib is a multikinase inhibitor that has been proven to give a clinically relevant improvement in time to progression and in survival.

AASLD practice guideline: Update on the management of hepatocellular carcinoma. Hepatology 2011; 53(3):1020–1022.

9.   C High-dose steroids and discuss with spinal surgeons

This patient has presented with signs and symptoms of spinal cord compression (SCC). It is a common oncological emergency, particularly affecting patients with prostate, lung, breast and haematological malignancy. Symptoms of weakness are commonly preceded by back pain. The majority of lesions (around 60%) are found in the thoracic spine but can occur at any vertebral level. As well as pain, motor and gait disturbance, patients may present with bowel and bladder disturbance. Patients presenting with such symptoms should have urgent imaging of their entire spine. MRI is the modality of choice and this should include the entire spine to look for any other evidence of metastases.

If SCC is diagnosed then high-dose steroids (dexamethasone 16 mg once daily in two divided doses with proton pump inhibitor cover) should be started immediately. This relieves the inflammation around the cord and can improve neurological symptoms and long-term neurological outcome. The case should be discussed urgently with the on-call spinal surgeons. Although radiotherapy is a treatment option if the tumour type is suspected to be radiosensitive, there is evidence that this combined with surgery rather than as an isolated treatment results in a better outcome. This is particularly true in an otherwise well patient with a good performance status, as in this case, with a single bony metastasis who would be a good surgical operative candidate. In patients who are not suitable for surgery, radiotherapy would be the best treatment after steroids are started.

Non-steroidal anti-inflammatory drugs and pamidronate are both commonly used in the treatment of bone pain caused by metastatic disease but will not improve SCC. Although bone biopsy may be of use to establish the diagnosis, it is fairly clear that this patient has metastatic prostate cancer and it is not going to alter the immediate management of his SCC. Chemotherapy is not routinely used in the treatment of SCC unless caused by a haematological malignancy as other tumour types are rarely chemosensitive.

Patchell RA, et al. Direct decompressive surgical resection in the treatment of spinal cord compression caused by metastatic cancer: a randomised trial. Lancet 2005; 366:643–648.

10. B He should have a bone scan to assess for metastases

This patient has a diagnosis of a renal cell carcinoma (RCC). RCCs constitute 80–85% of primary renal neoplasms. They are adenocarcinomas which originate from within the renal cortex. They are more common in men and there are often bilateral lesions.

RCC can present with a variety of symptoms but the classic triad is pain, haematuria and an abdominal mass. Increasingly, asymptomatic cases are being diagnosed upon finding an incidental mass on radiographic examination. They are also associated with a paraneoplastic syndrome which includes fever, weight loss, anaemia, hepatic dysfunction and hormonal effects. Hypercalcaemia is relatively common and can be as a result of parathyroid hormone-related peptide production or bone metastasis.

Often the tumours are slow growing and patients remain asymptomatic, so metastasis at the time of diagnosis is common; therefore, it is important to assess for local and metastatic spread with CT, MRI and bone scan. A renogram may help determine split function of the kidneys which may be important in planning treatment. Needle biopsy of the mass should be avoided as it is not reliable for diagnosis and there is a risk of seeding.

Surgery is curative in the majority of patients without metastases. Treatment options include radical nephrectomy or there are a variety of nephron-sparing treatments involving partial nephrectomy or radioablative techniques. Multiple monoclonal therapies are in the research phase.

Cohen HT, et al. Renal-cell carcinoma. N Engl J Med 2005; 353:2477–2490.

11. D Lorazepam

Dyspnoea can be defined as difficult, uncomfortable or laboured breathing, or when an individual feels the need for more air. Breathlessness is common and can be very distressing for patients with lung cancer and other severe respiratory disorders, and their care-givers. The mechanism of dyspnoea has been described as a mismatch between central motor activity and incoming afferent information form chemo- and mechanoreceptors. A patient's emotional state, personality and cognitive function can also alter its perception. It is important to give clear explanations of what is happening and to ensure that if possible the patient is sitting upright; opening windows and using a fan may also help. Regular doses of short-acting oral morphine every 2–4 hours may decrease the sensation of breathlessness. Panic and anxiety are frequently associated with breathlessness and a low dose of an anxiolytic such as lorazepam may be helpful.

Reversible causes should be treated where appropriate. For example, patients may benefit from antibiotics to treat superadded infections, blood transfusion in severe anaemia or from drainage of a moderate–large pleural effusion. A blood transfusion is not indicated in this situation; however, opinion varies as to the target haemoglobin level, some groups advising transfusion if haemoglobin <8. Similarly, this patient is unlikely to benefit from drainage of a small effusion that is not causing respiratory compromise – normal respiratory rate and oxygen saturation breathing air. Repeat pleural tap and/or drainage also increase the risk of further complications and potential for increasing distress. Oxygen therapy may help to resolve hypoxia but there is no evidence that supplemental oxygen will improve shortness of breath. Oxygen therapy should be prescribed to maintain target saturations of 94–98% or modified target of 88–92% if there is a history or significant risk of hypercapnic respiratory failure.

Kvale PA, Selecky PA, Prakash UB. Palliative care in lung cancer: ACCP evidence-based clinical practice guidelines. Chest 2007; 132(3):368S-403S.

12. C Stop aspirin and apixaban

This case highlights a common challenge facing medical staff with patients needing end-of-life care. Medication given as primary or secondary prevention such as antihypertensives, antiplatelet agents and the anticoagulants are generally unnecessary for patients at the end-of-life and these drugs can often cause side effects.

This patient has bone marrow failure from his metastatic prostate cancer and has suffered from haematuria intermittently. With his platelet count so low, he should not be receiving either apixaban or aspirin and these drugs are certainly exacerbating his haematuria.

Double-dose platelet infusion (giving more than one adult therapeutic dose at a time) is no longer routine practice. A single transfusion should be given, followed by an assessment of clinical response and increment before considering a further transfusion. A single pool of platelets for this patient would be appropriate.

He should not receive tranexamic acid because this is contraindicated in patients with haematuria, due to the risk of clot retention. A cystoscopy in a patient with a prognosis of only several months' survival and a well-established diagnosis is not appropriate.

Stopping aspirin but continuing apixaban might be considered if the patient was at extremely high risk of thrombosis or stroke. It is useful to consider the CHADSVASc score in this circumstance, which puts this patient at an approximately 3–4% risk of stroke from his atrial fibrillation over the next year. His risk of bleeding on anticoagulation is 100%, so the balance of risk is strongly in favour of stopping anticoagulation.

13. D Squamous cell carcinoma

The CT scan demonstrates changes in keeping with extensive emphysema and a cavitating lung mass in the left lower lobe. The most likely diagnosis in the described clinical presentation is squamous cell lung cancer. Non-small cell lung cancer (NSCLC) accounts for 75–80% of all lung cancers. Types of NSCLC include adenocarcinoma and squamous cell carcinoma.

Squamous cell lung cancer usually presents as a mass on chest X-ray, but may cavitate and look radiologically like a lung abscess. Rarely there may be multiple cavitating lesions. Squamous cell lung cancer may also be associated with hypercalcaemia (due to bony metastases or direct tumour production of parathyroid hormone-related peptide) or finger clubbing and hypertrophic pulmonary osteoarthropathy (paraneoplastic syndromes).

Aspergilloma, lung abscess and tuberculosis may also cause areas of cavitation and, although these are potential differential diagnoses, in a man of this age group with a history of chronic lung disease the likelihood of these diagnoses is lower. The patient should be referred for urgent investigations to gain a tissue diagnosis. The lesion is relatively peripheral so direct visualisation of the tumour for biopsies may be difficult at bronchoscopy. However, the presence of cavitation increases the diagnostic yield for cytology samples in bronchial washings. In patients not fit for invasive investigation, sputum should be sent for cytological testing as this may yield a diagnosis, which although it may not dictate further active treatment may help with determining prognosis and guiding further palliative approaches. The best diagnostic approach for a peripheral lesion may be via CT-guided lung biopsy. This procedure carries a risk of pneumothorax (approximately 10% risk). This patient will need to be assessed for suitability of this procedure in view of the significant emphysematous changes.

Tuberculosis (TB) more frequently appears with cavitatory change in the upper lobes; however, other appearances are well recognised and TB is recognised as a great mimic of lung cancer and should be considered as a differential diagnosis, particularly in high-risk groups. Similarly, aspergillomas typically occur in the apices: the term is used to describe a ball of fungal hyphae within a pre-existing cavity in the lung, e.g. following previous TB infection. Small cell lung cancer is not typically associated with cavitation on chest X-ray or CT.

Pentheroudakis G, et al. Cavitating squamous cell lung carcinoma-distinct entity or not? Lung Cancer 2004; 45(3): 349–355.
Soubani A, et al. The clinical spectrum of pulmonary aspergillosis. Chest 2002; 121:1988–1999.

14. A Chemoradiotherapy

The treatment of choice for proximal localised squamous cell carcinoma of the oesophagus is chemoradiotherapy. Middle and distal squamous cell carcinoma of the oesophagus can be treated with chemoradiotherapy alone or chemoradiotherapy in conjunction with surgery. Surgery alone would cause significant disability by removing the whole of the oesophagus and there is equally good survival with chemotherapy. There is no evidence to support the use of preoperative radiotherapy or adjuvant chemotherapy in squamous cell carcinoma of the oesophagus.

Allum WH. BSG guidelines. Guidelines for the management of oesophageal and gastric cancer. Gut 2011; 60:1449–1472.

15. E Vitamin D supplementation is routinely indicated

This patient is presenting with hypercalcaemia and a breast lump suggesting metastatic breast cancer. Breast cancer is the most common cancer in women and is strongly associated with hypercalcaemia. Although hypercalcaemia usually suggests metastatic disease, clinicians should be conscious of the possibility of a coincidental hyperparathyroidism. The parathyroid hormone level should be checked the first time a patient presents with hypercalcaemia, regardless of cause. In the majority of patients though, hypercalcaemia is deemed a poor prognostic finding.

Treatment is usually with hydration and bisphosphonates. Patients who are refractory to initial bisphosphonates (usually sodium pamidronate) can receive a second dose or a different bisphosphonate (such as zoledronic acid). Furosemide coupled with aggressive intravenous hydration is a useful tool as loop diuretics promote calciuria.

Denosumab is a monoclonal RANK-L inhibitor which prevents osteoclast activity. It is extremely effective in treating malignancy-associated hypercalcaemia and is the recommended second line treatment if bisphosphonates have failed.

Vitamin D levels are often normal or high in patients with malignant hypercalcaemia. While low vitamin D levels may be an indication for supplementation, this should be done in response to results, rather than as a routine intervention.

16. B Congestive cardiac failure

Trastuzumab, more commonly known as Herceptin, should be given as an adjuvant treatment in HER-2-positive breast cancer. Cardiac function should be assessed prior to treatment and women with any of the following should not be treated with trastuzumab:

- A left ventricular fraction of 55% or less
- A history of documented congestive cardiac failure
- High-risk uncontrolled arrhythmias
- Angina pectoris requiring medication
- Clinically significant valvular disease
- Evidence of transmural infarction on electrocardiograph
- Poorly controlled hypertension.

National Institute for Health and Clinical Excellence (NICE). NICE guideline 80. Early and locally advanced breast cancer: diagnosis and treatment. London: NICE, 2009.

17. E Urinary 5-HIAA (5-hydroyindoleacetic acid) levels

The patient has the classic symptoms of carcinoid syndrome. This is a syndrome that occurs when neuroendocrine tumours (NETs) metastasise to the liver, causing a direct release of serotonin, tachykinins and other vasoactive compounds into the systemic circulation. Carcinoid syndrome classically presents with flushing and diarrhoea. Seventy per cent of patients report intermittent abdominal pain, 50% report diarrhoea and 30% report flushing. Patients may also complain of rhinorrhoea, episodic palpitations and lacrimation during flushing. Pellagra, wheezing and carcinoid heart disease can occur. Urinary 5-HIAA levels are a baseline investigation for patients with symptoms suspicious of an net, and are raised in foregut and midgut carcinoid tumours. They do not confirm the diagnosis, and radiological and histological confirmation will be required. The other baseline test that should be performed in suspected NET is chromogranin A levels, which are raised in many NETs. Serum 5-hydroxytryptamine levels vary throughout the day and thus are not used clinically. Adrenocorticotrophic hormone (ACTH) levels are useful if an ectopic ACTH-producing tumour is suspected, but this patient has no symptoms to suggest Cushing's syndrome. C-peptide levels should be measured when there is a clinical suspicion of an insulinoma, but there are no symptoms of hypoglycaemia so this is unlikely. Fasting gastrin levels are raised in Zollinger–Ellison syndrome which presents with severe and recurrent duodenal ulceration.

Ramage JK, et al. BSG Guidelines for the management of gastroenteropancreatic (including carcinoid) tumours. Gut 2005; 54; 1–16.

18. A Chest drain insertion and talc pleurodesis

Malignant pleural effusions have a high risk of recurring and unless the patient has a very limited life expectancy (less than 1 month) pleurodesis should be adopted as soon as possible. Available agents include talc, bleomycin and tetracycline. Pleural aspiration should not exceed 1.5 L in a single procedure because it can be associated with the development of re-expansion pulmonary oedema.

Selected patients with malignant pleural effusions and good performance status may gain advantage from other techniques including thoracoscopy (medical or surgical video-assisted thoracoscopic surgery). Longer-term indwelling pleural catheters may also have a role in selected patients with recurrent malignant effusions, e.g. in some patients with mesothelioma.

Oramorph and lorazepam are useful agents in the palliative management of dyspnoea and may be appropriate if the patient is not a candidate for a chest drain or the effusion is not amenable to drainage.

British Thoracic Society. Pleural Disease Guideline 2010. Thorax 2010; 65(2).

19. E Urine 24-hour metanephrines

Medullary thyroid cancer (MTC) is often associated with multiple endocrine neoplasia (MEN) type 2A. The major lesion in MEN2A are medullary thyroid carcinoma, phaeochromocytoma and hyperparathyroidism.

The symptoms of episodic palpitations, anxiety and hypertension should arouse the suspicion of phaeochromocytoma in a patient with previous MTC. Hence the appropriate test in this situation would be urine 24-hour metanephrines.

Prevalence of MTC increases with age in cases of MEN2A and can reach up to 70% by the age of 70 years. After the age of 10 years the prevalence of phaeochromocytoma is up to 10–50% in this situation.

The diagnosis of clinically significant adrenal medullary disease usually follows the diagnosis of MTC. Almost all phaeochromocytomas are located in the adrenal glands. Phaeochromocytoma is almost always benign in this situation and can be bilateral in up to 50% of cases, especially after a few years.

Pacini F, et al. Medullary thyroid carcinoma. Clin Oncol (R Coll Radiol) 2010; 22(6):475–485.

20. C Glioma

All of these conditions may present with seizures. However, the appearance on the contrast-enhanced MRI of the brain is consistent with a malignant glioma. There is a large contrast-enhancing lesion in the right parietal lobe with extensive surrounding oedema. Some cystic degenerative changes are noted within the lesion.

In contrast, meningiomas are well-circumscribed extra-axial lesions. Cerebral toxoplasmosis is most common in immunocompromised individuals and usually appears as multiple ring-enhancing lesions with contrast enhancement. Arteriovenous malformations appear as an abnormal collection of entwined vessels; these may exhibit flow voids on MRI due to rapid blood flow. Cysticercosis is a parasitic disease caused by ingestion of the eggs of the pork tapeworm (*Taenia solium*). Larvae may form in the brain (neurocysticercosis). These are often very numerous and less than <1 cm diameter. They typically appear cystic and may have a visible central scolex on CT; on MRI degenerating cysts may appear as ring-enhancing lesions. Leptomeningeal enhancement is common.

Rees J, Zrinzo L. What to do with a patient who has a had a fit and the scan shows a 'glioma'? Pract Neurol 2005; 5:84–91.
Wen P, Kesari S. Malignant gliomas in adults. N Engl J Med 2008; 359:492–507.

21. B Not proceed with the operation

This patient has made repeated, sustained and documented assertions that she does not want invasive or surgical procedures to prolong her life. She now does not have capacity to make these decisions but this does not denigrate her previous statements. It is assumed that she had capacity when she made her original advance directive to refuse treatment and this must be respected. Only if there is doubt as to whether she had capacity at the time of her decision can a clinician challenge this directive, and get a court order if appropriate and there was enough time.

General Medical Council guidance gives clear advice on how to handle a situation where relatives may disagree with a patient's decision. No person may give consent for treatment to another adult. If a patient temporarily lacks capacity, their treating physician may offer to give or withhold treatment in their best interests but this does not replace the consent process. For a patient who permanently lacks capacity, treatment decisions may be made with an impartial patient advocate, through agreement at a local multidisciplinary team or by court order. The family of such a patient should be involved in any discussions, but they cannot formally give consent for treatment and they cannot supercede a previous advance directive, assuming this was put in place when the patient was of sound mind.

In an emergency situation where there is doubt and not enough time for further investigations, the clinician should do whatever he thinks best to prolong life.

General Medical Council. Treatment and care towards the end of life: good practice in decision making. London: GMC, 2010.

22. B Anastrozole

First-line adjuvant chemotherapy for postmenopausal women with oestrogen receptor-positive early invasive breast cancer is an aromatase inhibitor, either anastrozole or letrozole. Exemestane is an aromatase inhibitor but should be offered only to women who have previously been treated with tamoxifen for 2–3 years. Tamoxifen is no longer considered first-line chemotherapy and it should be offered only if an aromatase inhibitor is not tolerated or contraindicated. 5-Fluorouracil is not used in the treatment of breast cancer. Trastuzumab, more commonly known as Herceptin, is used in human epidermal growth factor receptor-2 (HER-2)-positive breast cancer not oestrogen receptor-positive breast cancer and so would not be an appropriate treatment in this case.

National Institute for Health and Clinical Excellence. NICE guideline 80. Early and locally advanced breast cancer, Diagnosis and Treatment. London: NICE, 2009.

23. C Gemcitabine and carboplatin

This patient has advanced lung cancer (stage IV disease) because he has metastatic spread and so is not a candidate for curative treatment. The management of such patients is palliative chemotherapy. Tumours should be assessed for a mutation in the epidermal growth factor receptor (EGFR) to see if they would be susceptible to EGFR tyrosine kinase inhibitors such as erlotinib and gefitinib. This is not the case here. Instead this patient would need to be given combination treatment with a platinum-based agent (such as cisplatin or carboplatin) and another agent such as etoposide, vinorelbine, paclitaxel or gemcitabine. Combination treatment first line is more efficacious than using single agent therapy.

Cetuximab is a monoclonal antibody that targets EGFR, and bevacizumab is an antibody that targets vascular epidermal growth factor. Both are second-line agents and are used in combination with chemotherapy agents.

Lal R, Enting D, Kristeleit H. Systemic treatment of non-small-cell lung cancer. Eur J Cancer 2011; 47 (3):S375–377.
Goldstraw P, et al. The IASLC Lung Cancer Staging Project: Proposals for the revision of the TNM stage groups in the forthcoming (seventh) edition of the TNM classification of malignant tumours. J Thorac Oncol 2007; 2:706.

24. B T2N1M0

The tumour/node/metastasis staging (TNM) system is overtaking the Duke's staging classification for colorectal carcinoma. The T describes how locally advanced the malignancy is, with N representing the presence and number of local lymph nodes and M representing the presence or absence of distant metastasis.

This is a useful classification as it gives a clearer idea of an individual patient's risk of response to treatment and recurrence and therefore allows evidence-based individualisation of treatment.

The classification is as follows (see **Table 8.1**):

Table 8.1 TNM staging criteria

TNM system for hypopharyngeal carcinoma

Primary tumour		Nodes		Metastasis	
TX	Not assessable	NX	Regional nodes not assessable	MX	Distant metastasis not assessable
T0	No evidence of tumour	N0	No regional node metastasis	M0	No distant metastasis
Tis	Carcinoma in situ	N1	Metastasis in single ipsilateral node (≤3 cm)	M1	Distant metastasis
T1	Tumour invades submucosa	N2	Metastasis in one to three regional lymph nodes		
T2	Tumour invades muscularis propria	N3	Metastasis in four or more regional lymph nodes		
T3	Tumour invades through the muscularis propria into the subserosa, or into the non-peritonealised pericolic or perirectal tissues.				
T4	Tumour directly invades other organs or structures, and/ or perforates visceral peritoneum				

Adapted from: Sobin LH, Gospodarowicz MK, Wittekind C (eds). TNM Classification of Malignant Tumours, 7th edn. Oxford: Wiley-Blackwell, 2009.

Chapter 9

Renal medicine

Questions

1. A 56-year-old woman with type 2 diabetes and contrast-induced acute kidney injury was admitted for a coronary angiogram. She regularly took lisinopril and metformin, both of which were withheld for the procedure.

   Her pulse was 80 beats per minute, blood pressure 130/75 mmHg, jugular venous pressure visible at 3 cm and there was no peripheral oedema. Cardiovascular and respiratory examinations were unremarkable.

   What is the most appropriate next management step to reduce the risk of contrast-induced nephropathy?

   A   0.9% NaCl 1 mL/kg per hour for 12 hours pre- and post-procedure
   B   1.26% sodium bicarbonate 3 mL/kg per hour for 1 hour pre-procedure and 1 mL/kg per hour during and post-procedure
   C   Haemofiltration immediately before and after procedure
   D   *N*-Acetylcysteine 600 mg twice daily before and after procedure
   E   No additional measure required

2. A 69-year-old man was admitted with a 7-day history of diarrhoea and vomiting. He had ischaemic heart disease, type 2 diabetes mellitus and gout. His current medications were amlodipine, metformin, gliclazide, diclofenac and bisoprolol.

   On admission, his blood pressure was 120/70 mmHg, falling to 100/53 mmHg on standing; jugular venous pressure was not visible and mucous membranes were dry.

   Investigations:

   > creatinine 420 μmol/L (90 μmol/L 3 months ago, normal range males 60–110)
   > lactate 2.4 mmol/L (0.6–1.8)

   Which one of the followings drug is most likely to be the cause of his acute kidney injury?

   A   Amlodipine
   B   Bisoprolol
   C   Diclofenac
   D   Gliclazide
   E   Metformin

3. A 68-year-old woman presented with worsening peripheral oedema over the past few weeks.

   On examination, she had pitting oedema to her thighs, and her blood pressure was 150/85 mmHg.

Investigations:

creatinine 180 µmol/L (females 45–90)	albumin 24 g/L (37–49)
Urinary protein:creatinine ratio 612 mg/mmol (<45)	
Renal biopsy (silver stain): see **Figure 9.1**	

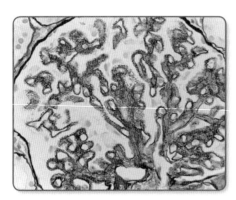

Figure 9.1 *See colour plate section.*

Which one of the following is least likely to be associated with this condition?

A   Antiglomerular basement membrane disease (Goodpasture's disease)
B   Breast cancer
C   Hepatitis B
D   Hepatitis C
E   Systemic lupus erythematosus (SLE)

4.   A 41-year-old man returned to the nephrology clinic. He had type 2 diabetes with proliferative retinopathy, treated with insulin.
      Blood pressure was 150/90 mmHg and there was no peripheral oedema. Creatinine when checked 6 months ago was 158 µmol/L.

Current investigations:

creatinine 225 µmol/L (60–110)	albumin 38 g/L (37–49)
potassium 4.9 mmol/L (3.5–5.0)	HbA1c 60 mmol/mol (<48)
Antinuclear antibody: negative	
Antineutrophil cytoplasmic antibody: negative	
Urine dipstick: protein +++, blood –	
Urinary protein:creatinine ratio 248 mg/mmol (<45)	

What is the most appropriate next step in management?

A   Amlodipine
B   Increase insulin
C   Low-potassium diet
D   Ramipril
E   Renal biopsy

5. A 54-year-old, 75-kg Afro–Caribbean man attended the renal clinic. He was known to have progressive chronic kidney disease secondary to diabetic nephropathy. He felt well and reported no specific symptoms. He had previously been seen by the dietician who advised dietary restrictions of salt, potassium and phosphate.

On examination, his blood pressure was 130/80 mmHg and he was clinically euvolaemic.

Investigations:

creatinine 420 µmol/L (350 4 months ago, 60–110)	iron 3 mmol/L (12–30)
urea 26.0 mmol/L (2.5–7.5)	corrected calcium 2.1 mmol/L (2.2–2.6)
potassium 5.5 mmol/L (3.5–5.0)	phosphate 1.84 mmol/L (0.87–1.49)
haemoglobin 94 g/L (130–180)	parathyroid hormone 18 pmol/L (7.7–12.1)
Urinary protein:creatinine ratio 339 mg/mmol (<45)	

What is the most appropriate next step in management?

A   Add ramipril to reduce proteinuria
B   Admit and start haemodialysis
C   Erythropoietin-stimulating agent (ESA)
D   Renal ultrasound to exclude obstruction
E   Start a phosphate binder

6. A 64-year-old Afro–Caribbean man presented with fatigue and increasing dyspnoea. He had type 2 diabetes mellitus and a previous myocardial infarction. He was taking gliclazide, ramipril and furosemide. Prior to this presentation he had seen his general practitioner with the same complaints; the furosemide dose was increased and he was started on a 5-day course of cephalexin for a presumed chest infection.

On examination, his blood pressure was 125/82 mmHg sitting, 115/78 mmHg standing; jugular venous pressure was not elevated and there was no peripheral oedema.

Investigations:

haemoglobin 82 g/L (130–180)	corrected calcium 2.85 mmol/L (2.2–2.6)
white cell count 8.3 × 10⁹/L (4–11)	HbA1c 8.9% (3.8–6.4)
creatinine 220 µmol/L (80 3 months ago, males 60–110)	
Urine dipstick: trace protein	

What is the most likely diagnosis?

A   Acute tubular necrosis secondary to increased furosemide
B   Acute tubulo-interstitial nephritis secondary to antibiotics
C   Diabetic nephropathy
D   IgA nephropathy
E   Multiple myeloma

7. A 70-year-old man with a history of mitral valve replacement presented with a 4-month history of general malaise and weight loss of 9 kg.

On examination, his temperature was 37.5°C, there was splenomegaly and a soft pan-systolic murmur.

Investigations:

Urine dipstick: protein ++++, blood +++	
haemoglobin 80 g/L (130–180) white cell count 3×10^9/L (4–11) platelets 45×10^9/L (150–400) creatinine 350 µmol/L (80 4 months ago, 150 2 months ago, males 60–110)	C-reactive protein 60 mg/L (<10) C3 0.42 g/L (0.65–1.9) C4 0.08 g/L (0.15–0.5)
Antineutrophil cytoplasmic antibody: positive myeloperoxidase <5 IU/mL (<5) proteinase-3 8 IU/mL (<5)	

What is the most appropriate next step in management?

A   0.5 g methylprednisolone intravenously
B   Bone marrow biopsy
C   Broad-spectrum antibiotics
D   Renal biopsy
E   Serial blood cultures

8.   A 35-year-old man presented for routine clinic review. He had received a cadaveric renal transplant 6 months previously. He was taking ciclosporin, mycophenolate mofetil and prednisolone. His baseline creatinine postoperatively had settled to around 130 µmol/L. He was well with no specific symptoms.
      On examination blood pressure was 145/85 mmHg, jugular venous pressure was not elevated, and cardiovascular and respiratory examinations were unremarkable. Abdominal examination revealed slight tenderness over his transplanted kidney.

Investigations:

creatinine 190 µmol/L
Urine dipstick: protein ++
Ultrasound: normal size renal transplant kidney with no hydronephrosis seen

On repeat testing three days later, his creatinine had risen further to 205 µmol/L.

What is the most appropriate next step in management?

A   Cytomegalovirus polymerase chain reaction
B   Renal transplant biopsy
C   Renal transplant artery angiogram
D   Transplant renogram with furosemide
E   Urine culture and empirical antibiotics

9.   A 78-year-old white woman presented with a 4-month history of weight loss, general malaise and occasional fevers. She was a smoker with a cough and at the time of admission had had two episodes of fresh haemoptysis. She had no significant past medical history and, other than a salbutamol inhaler, took no regular medication.
      Examination revealed a blood pressure of 130/75 mmHg, jugular venous pressure +2 cm, no peripheral oedema and nothing else of note.

Investigations:

creatinine 214 µmol/L (45–90)	albumin 33 g/L (37–49)
Antinuclear antibody: negative C3 normal C4 normal	Antineutrophil cytoplasmic antibody: positive (myeloperoxide <5 AU/mL, proteinase 3 <5 AU/mL)
Urine dipstick: protein +++, blood +++	
Chest X-ray: bilateral diffuse alveolar shadowing	

What is the most likely diagnosis?

A   Acute interstitial nephritis secondary to tuberculosis
B   Antiglomerular basement membrane disease
C   Membranous nephropathy associated with lung malignancy
D   Microscopic polyangiitis
E   Sepsis from a pneumonia causing acute tubular necrosis

10. A 30-year-old woman presented with a 2-month history of general malaise and intermittent fevers.
    She was found to have acute kidney injury with blood and protein on urine dipstick testing.

Investigations:

creatinine 175 µmol/L (previously 85 µmol/L, 45–90) haemoglobin 90 g/L (115–165) white cell count 11 × 10⁹/L (4–11)	platelets 90 × 10⁹/L (150–400) C3 0.5 g/L (0.65–1.9) C4 0.1 g/L (0.15–0.5)

Which one of the following is the least likely diagnosis?

A   Infective endocarditis
B   Lupus nephritis
C   Mixed cryoglobulinaemia
D   Post-streptococcal glomerulonephritis
E   Granulomatosis with polyangiitis (Wegener's granulomatosis)

11. A 72-year-old man presented to the emergency department after being found on the floor 24 hours after a fall at home.
    On examination, his blood pressure was 110/60 mmHg and his right calf was tense and swollen. Urine output was documented as 45 mL over the past 2 hours.

Investigations:

potassium 7.9 mmol/L (3.5–5.0) urea 28.5 mmol/L (2.5–7.5)	creatinine 480 µmol/L (60–110) creatine kinase 10,000 U/L (25–195)
Electrocardiogram: 98 beats per minute, sinus rhythm tented T waves broad QRS complexes	

What is the most appropriate next step in his immediate management?

A   10 mL of 10% calcium gluconate given intravenously over 5 minutes
B   10 units of short-acting insulin in 50 mL of 50% dextrose given intravenously over 20 minutes
C   5 mg nebulised salbutamol followed by 15 g calcium polystyrene sulphate (Calcium Resonium) orally four times daily
D   Emergency fasciotomy
E   Haemodialysis

12. A 71-year-old woman was admitted for a semi-elective coronary artery bypass graft. She was known to have type 2 diabetes mellitus, hypertension and stage 3 chronic kidney disease with a creatinine of 135 µmol/L. She regularly took ramipril, atenolol and insulin. She was given intravenous co-amoxiclav peri-operatively. During the operation, her mean arterial pressure was 60 mmHg for two hours.
    On the second postoperative day, there was some slight erythema around her wound site. She was apyrexial, her pulse was 84 beats per minute and blood pressure 130/75 mmHg. Her urine output was 350 mL over the previous 24 hours.

Investigations:

creatinine 380 µmol/L (45–90)	C-reactive protein 18 mg/L (<10)
white cell count 9.4 × 10⁹/L (4–11)	
Urine dipstick: protein +	
Ultrasound:	
right kidney 9.4 cm	
left kidney 10.5 cm	

What is the most likely cause of her acute kidney injury?

A   Acute tubular necrosis secondary to hypotension
B   Acute tubular necrosis secondary to sepsis
C   Acute tubulo-interstitial nephritis secondary to antibiotics
D   Contrast nephropathy
E   Renal artery occlusion

13. A 77-year-old Caucasian man underwent an elective coronary angiogram. He had a history of type 2 diabetes, hypertension, peripheral vascular disease and osteoarthritis. He smoked 20 cigarettes per day.
    Ten days following the procedure, he developed intermittent abdominal pain, for which he was given analgesia, and had a painful mottled right foot.

Investigations:

creatinine 463 µmol/L (pre-procedure 105, males 60–110)	eosinophils 1.1 × 10⁹/L (0.04–0.4)
	C3 0.14 g/L (0.65–1.90)
white cell count 7.8 × 10⁹/L (4–11)	
Urine dipstick: protein +	
Ultrasound:	
right kidney 9.1 cm	
left kidney 9.9 cm	

What is the most likely cause of his acute kidney injury?

A   Analgesic nephropathy
B   Cholesterol emboli
C   Contrast-induced nephropathy
D   Lupus nephritis
E   Renal artery stenosis

14. A 24-year-old woman presented with a 1-week history of diarrhoea and malaise. She had seen some blood in her stool and had noticed that she was bruising easily. Her bilirubin was found to be elevated and she was referred to the gastroenterologists for investigation. She had no significant past medical history and was taking no medications.
    On examination, she had icteric sclerae and bruising on her skin. Urine output was 40 mL/h.

Investigations:

haemoglobin 61 g/L (115–165)	creatinine 196 µmol/L (45–90)
white cell count 12 × 10⁹/L (4–11)	bilirubin 70 mmol/L (1–22)
platelets 40 × 10⁹/L (150–400)	lactate dehydrogenase 1900 U/L (10–250)
urea 13 mmol/L (2.5–7.5)	
Blood film: some fragmented red blood cells	

What is the most appropriate next step in her management?

A   Flexible sigmoidoscopy
B   Haemofiltration
C   Stool microscopy and culture
D   Intravenous antibiotics
E   Platelet transfusion

15. A 45-year-old peritoneal dialysis (PD) patient presented with diffuse abdominal pain and vomiting. Cloudy fluid was drained from his PD catheter. A diagnosis of PD peritonitis was made, and intraperitoneal ceftriaxone and gentamycin were commenced. After 3 days of treatment, he was feeling no better.

Peritoneal dialysis fluid:
white cell count 350/mm³, 60% neutrophils
culture: multiple gram negative organisms

What is the most appropriate next step in his management?

A   Admit for intravenous antibiotics in addition to intraperitoneal antibiotics
B   Broaden intraperitoneal antibiotics for increased gram negative cover
C   Continue current intraperitoneal antibiotics
D   Remove PD catheter under local anaesthetic, convert to haemodialysis
E   Perform CT scan of abdomen and pelvis

16. A 46-year-old woman came for review having recently been diagnosed with adult polycystic kidney disease. She had a strong family history of renal failure and intracranial haemorrhage. She was well with no symptoms of note.
    On examination, her blood pressure was 150/80 mmHg and there were bilateral masses palpable in her abdomen.

Investigations:

> Urine dipstick: protein +, blood +

Which one of the following would be the next most appropriate step in her management?

A   She should be advised to arrange for her 15-year-old son to have an ultrasound screening test
B   She should be advised that she will definitely require renal replacement therapy in the future
C   She should be counselled that there is a 25% chance that her daughter will inherit the disease
D   She should have her blood pressure repeated in 6 months to assess need for treatment
E   She should have a magnetic resonance cerebral angiogram

17. A 48-year-old man from Ghana was referred by his general practitioner with unexplained renal impairment. He had no known past medical history and took no regular medication.
    His blood pressure was 135/95 mmHg and he had mild peripheral oedema.

Investigations:

creatinine 210 µmol/L (60–110)	albumin 21 g/L (37–49)
Anti-neutrophil cytoplasmic antibody: negative	Anti-nuclear antibody: negative
C3 0.7 g/L (0.65–1.9)	C4 25 g/L (0.15–0.5)
Hepatitis B and C screen: negative	IgG 18.4 g/L (6.0–13.0)
CD4 100 × 10⁶/L (500–1200)	IgM 1.0 g/L (0.4–2.5)
HIV viral load 3500 copes/mL	IgA 1.5 g/L (0.8–3.0)
Serum electrophoresis: diffuse increase in gamma-globulins	
Urine dipstick: protein ++++, blood ++	

What is most likely to be found on renal biopsy?

A   Cast nephropathy
B   Collapsing focal segmental glomerulosclerosis (FSGS)
C   Hyaline arteriosclerosis
D   Kimmelstiel–Wilson nodules
E   Minimal change in disease

18. A 67-year-old patient presented to the transplant review clinic. He had received a cadaveric renal transplant 10 years previously. His early course had been complicated by rejection and he had been heavily immunosuppressed. At presentation he had good graft function with a baseline creatinine of 105 µmol/L and negligible proteinuria. He described symptoms of weight loss over the last 2 months and general malaise. There was no history of abdominal symptoms or fever.
    On examination, he had a large inguinal lymph node and a palpable mass in his left iliac fossa.

Investigations:

> haemoglobin 89 g/L (130–180)

Which one of the following is the most useful virological test?

A   BK virus
B   Cytomegalovirus

C   Epstein–Barr virus
D   Hepatitis B
E   HIV

19. A 40-year-old man underwent renal biopsy. He had been seen in the renal clinic when his general practitioner referred him having found a raised creatinine at his first attendance there. He had no results for comparison and had never seen a general practitioner before. He took no regular medications.

Investigations:

creatinine 315 µmol/L (60–110)

Renal biopsy (see **Figure 9.2**):

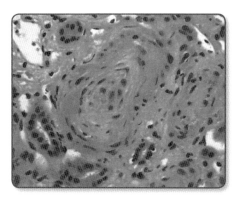

Figure 9.2 *See colour plate section.*

Which one of the following statements regarding his condition is most likely?

A   He has high blood pressure
B   He needs to start renal replacement therapy (RRT) immediately
C   He should be started on prednisolone and cyclophosphamide
D   He will definitely have nephrotic range proteinuria
E   His serum IgA will be high

20. A 50-year-old man presented with a short history of lethargy, nausea and intermittent lower back pain. He had seen his general practitioner for the back pain and was taking diclofenac as required. He had no past medical history of note. He had noticed a reduction in urine output over the past 2 days.
    His blood pressure at presentation was 190/100 mmHg and urine dipstick testing was unremarkable.

Investigations:

haemoglobin 110 g/L (130 –180)	potassium 6.3 mmol/L (3.5–5.0)
white cell count 9 × 10⁹/L (4–11)	urea 42.7 mmol/L (2.5–7.5)
erythrocyte sedimentation rate 90 mm/1st h (males 0–20)	creatinine 1024 µmol/L (60–110)
	corrected calcium 2.7 mmol/L (2.2–2.6)

He was admitted urgently to hospital and a CT was performed.

CT (see **Figure 9.3**):

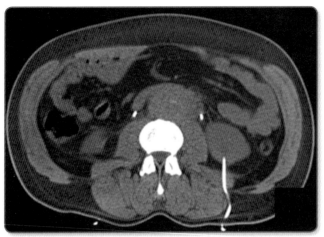

Figure 9.3

Which one of the following is not a recognised cause of his condition?

A   Beta-blockers
B   Lymphoma
C   Prostate carcinoma
D   Radiotherapy
E   Tuberculosis

21.   A 25-year-old man presented with tiredness. He had previously been found to be hypertensive, but had not attended clinic for follow-up. On further questioning, he reported persistent nausea, reduced appetite, severe muscle aches and itch for the preceding 6 weeks.
       On examination, he was fully alert, his blood pressure was 180/100 mmHg, oxygen saturation was 98% on air. He had bilateral pedal oedema.

Investigations:

haemoglobin 62 g/L (130–180)	urea 41.6 mmol/l (2.5–7.5)
mean corpuscular volume 80 fL (80–96)	creatinine 1740 µmol/L (60–110)
potassium 5.8 mmol/l (3.5–5.0)	bicarbonate 15 mmol/L (22–30)

ECG: normal sinus rhythm

Urine dipstick: blood ++, protein ++

What is the most appropriate next step in his management?

A   Give 1 L of 1.4% sodium bicarbonate intravenously
B   Create arteriovenous fistula and start haemodialysis
C   Insert dialysis catheter and start haemodialysis
D   Intravenous methylprednisolone
E   Transfuse three units of packed red cells

22.   A 37-year-old African man was referred because his blood pressure was found to be 230/150 mmHg. He had been diagnosed with hypertension by his general practitioner several years ago but had been non-compliant with antihypertensive medications. He was asymptomatic.
       On examination, there were no focal neurological signs. Blood pressure in the left arm was 235/152 mmHg and in the right arm 245/155 mmHg. His peripheral pulses were present and there were no audible bruits; there was no papilloedema.

Investigations:

Electrocardiogram:

voltage criteria for left ventricular hypertrophy (LVH)

creatinine 190 µmol/L (males 60–110)

Urine dipstick: blood +++, protein +++

What is the most appropriate next step in management?

A   Admit for intravenous antihypertensives as this is a hypertensive emergency
B   Blood pressure and creatinine – re-check next week before initiating treatment
C   Start on a single oral antihypertensive agent
D   Urgent CT of the chest and abdomen to exclude dissection
E   Urgent renal biopsy to investigate renal impairment

23. A 44-year-old female haemodialysis patient presented with increased tiredness and lethargy. The cause of her end-stage renal failure was reflux nephropathy and she had been established on thrice weekly haemodialysis for 5 years. Her haemoglobin was noted to have dropped recently and the dose of her erythropoietin (Epo), given on dialysis, had been increased accordingly.

Investigations:

---

haemoglobin 59 g/L (target 100–120)	haematocrit 30% (36–48)
white cell count 9.2 × 10⁹/L (4–11)	reticulocytes 0% (0.5–2.5)
platelets 194 × 10⁹/L (150–400)	ferritin 620 g/L (15–300)
mean corpuscular volume 82 fL (80–96)	transferrin saturation 50%*

*Transferrin saturation = serum iron ÷ total iron-binding capacity × 100 (12–45% in females)

What is the most likely diagnosis?

A   Anaemia of chronic disease
B   Chronic lymphocytic leukaemia (CLL)
C   Myelodysplasia
D   Pure red cell aplasia (PRCA)
E   Occult gastrointestinal blood loss

24. A 56-year-old man presented with confusion and weight gain. His past medical included type 2 diabetes mellitus and chronic hepatitis C infection. His medications, which had not changed recently, comprised metformin, lansoprazole and spironolactone.

On examination, he was jaundiced and had spider naevi. Blood pressure was 100/50 mmHg, jugular venous pressure was elevated at 5 cm, and he had pedal oedema. His urine output was 100 mL over 6 hours.

---

creatinine 260 µmol/L (75 one month ago, 60–110)	albumin 22 g/L (37–49)
urea 10.4 mmol/L (2.5–7.5)	bilirubin 124 mmol/L (1–22)

Urine dipstick: negative for blood and protein
Urine sodium: 5mmol/L

Ultrasound: Normal sized, unobstructed kidneys, cirrhotic liver, ascites

---

What is the most likely renal diagnosis?

A   Hepatitis C-related mesangiocapillary glomerulonephritis
B   Drug-induced interstitial nephritis
C   Acute tubular necrosis
D   Hepato-renal syndrome
E   Diabetic nephropathy

25. A 69-year-old man presented with a severe community-acquired pneumonia. He was known to have ischaemic heart disease and impaired left ventricular function. His blood pressure was 80/40 mmHg on admission.

   He received intravenous antibiotics and fluid resuscitation. Although his blood pressure rose to 100/70 mmHg, he remained oliguric with a urine output of 10 mL over 4 hours. His jugular venous pressure was elevated to the angle of his jaw, and fine bi-basal crackles were heard on auscultation of his chest. His respiratory rate was 30 breaths per minute and oxygen saturation was 92% on 0.28 FiO_2 (fraction of inspired oxygen).

Investigations:

haemoglobin 76 g/L (130–180)	potassium 6.5 mmol/L (3.5–5)
white cell count 15.6 × 10^9/L (4–11)	creatinine 250 µmol/L (baseline 100, 60–110)

What is the most appropriate next step in management?

A   Transfuse 2 units of packed red cells
B   Continuous veno-venous haemofiltration (CVVHF)
C   Further fluid challenge (1000 mL) and monitor urine output
D   Haemodialysis
E   Dopamine and furosemide infusion

26. A 36-year-old man with end-stage renal failure secondary to hypertensive nephrosclerosis presented with facial pain and deformity. He had been on renal replacement via intermittent haemodialysis three times a week for 10 years. He was non-compliant with his medications, which included 1-alfacalcidol (1-hydroxylated vitamin D), ramipril, lansoprazole and sevelamer hydrochloride (a non-calcium containing phosphate binder).

Investigations:

corrected calcium 2.8 mmol/L (target 2.1–2.37 on dialysis)	alkaline phosphatase 370 IU/L (44-147)
phosphate 2.1 mmol/L (target 1.1–1.7 on dialysis)	parathyroid hormone 223 pmol/L (target 14–63 on dialysis)
CT of the head: see **Figure 9.4**	

What is the most appropriate next step in management?

A   Start cinacalcet
B   Change phosphate binder from sevelamer to aluminium hydroxide
C   CT scan of the chest, abdomen and pelvis to exclude malignancy
D   Increase alfacalcidol dose
E   Parathyroidectomy

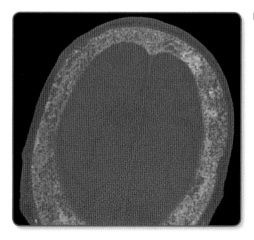

Figure 9.4

27. A 73-year-old Caucasian man was referred via his general practitioner with acute kidney injury. He had a purpuric rash over his lower limbs. He complained of generalised lethargy and weight loss. He had no significant past medical history, took no regular medication and denied using any herbal remedies.

Investigations:

creatinine 450 µmol/L (previously 100, 60–110)	C3 0.8 g/L (0.65–1.9)
	C4 0.04 g/L (0.15–0.5)
rheumatoid factor 390 IU/mL (<20)	
Urine: blood ++, protein +++	

Which test would be most helpful in making the diagnosis?

A   Antineutrophil cytoplasmic antibody
B   Cryoglobulins
C   Anti-double-stranded DNA antibodies
D   Extractable nuclear antigens (ENA)
E   Erythrocyte sedimentation rate

28. A 60-year-old woman presented with acute kidney injury. She was oliguric despite fluid resuscitation.
    Initial blood results revealed:

Investigations:

white cell count 9.6 × 10⁹/L (4–11)	urea 52 mmol/L (2.5–7.5)
C-reactive protein 18 mg/L (<10)	creatinine 920 µmol/L (45–90)
potassium 6.0 mmol/L (3.5–5.0)	

It was decided that she should start renal replacement therapy. A dialysis catheter was inserted and she commenced heparin-free haemodialysis. After 3 hours of dialysis she complained of headache and nausea. After a further 30 minutes she became confused and then had a generalised seizure.
On examination, she had no focal neurological signs and plantar reflexes were equivocal.

Investigations:

potassium 4.0 mmol/L (3.5–5.0)	creatinine 680 µmol/L (45–90)
urea 21 mmol/L (2.5–7.5)	

What is the most likely cause of her symptoms?

A   Cardiac arrhythmia
B   Dialyser reaction
C   Disequilibrium syndrome
D   Intracranial bleed
E   Sepsis

29. A 42-year-old man with acute lymphoblastic leukaemia was started on chemotherapy. Over the next 48 hours his urine output was noted to decrease.

Investigations:

potassium 6.9 mmol/L (3.5–5.0)	uric acid 840 µmol/L (110–420)
creatinine 300 µmol/L (60–110)	lactate dehydrogenase 600 U/L (10–250)
phosphate 3.1 mmol/L (0.8–1.4)	

Which one of the following is the least useful treatment for this condition?

A   Allopurinol
B   Calcium gluconate
C   Mesna
D   Rasburicase
E   Intravenous sodium bicarbonate

30. A 42-year-old woman presented with lethargy, fatigue and intermittent fevers. She had a history of asthma and had recurrent chest infections requiring several courses of oral antibiotics over the previous 6 months. She had had to increase her inhaler use. She had also had intermittent abdominal pain and diarrhoea over the previous month.
      On examination, her blood pressure was 140/80 mmHg and she had an isolated wheeze on the right side of her chest. Her abdomen was soft and minimally tender.

Investigations:

haemoglobin 95 g/L (115–165)	urea 23 mmol/L (2.5–7.5)
white cell count 11.5×10^9/L (4–11)	creatinine 351 µmol/L (45–90)
platelets 505×10^9/L (150–400)	C3 1.0 g/L (0.65–1.9)
eosinophils 1.4×10^9/L (0.04–0.4)	C4 0.4 g/L (0.15–0.5)

Antineutrophil cytoplasmic antibody: positive
myeloperoxidase (MPO) 80 AU/mL (<5)
proteinase-3 4 AU/mL (<5)

Urine dipstick: blood +++, protein +++

Blood tests repeated the following day showed that her creatinine had increased to 443 µmol/L.
      Renal biopsy: focal and necrotising crescentic glomerulonephritis with one granuloma seen in the interstitium.

What is the most likely cause of her symptoms?

A   Allergic granulomatosis and angiitis (Churg–Strauss syndrome)
B   Granulomatosis and polyangiitis (Wegener's granulomatosis)
C   Post-infectious glomerulonephritis
D   Strongyloides infection
E   Tubulo-interstitial nephritis secondary to antibiotics

31. A 36-year-old male haemodialysis patient was admitted for a live-related renal transplant. Tissue typing for major antibody incompatibility was negative and blood groups were matched. He received standard immunosuppression at induction and was prescribed standard maintenance doses.

    Initially he produced good volumes of urine (>200 mL/h), but after 24 hours his urine output suddenly decreased to 10 mL/h despite adequate fluid administration, and he became acutely tender over the graft.

    What is the most likely cause for these symptoms?

    A   Acute tubular necrosis
    B   Pyelonephritis
    C   Hyper-acute rejection
    D   Ureteric obstruction
    E   Renal vein thrombosis

32. A 48-year-old man was found to have progressive chronic kidney disease on routine blood tests. He had a long history of Crohn's disease, requiring multiple bowel resections of the previous 15 years. His estimated glomerular filtration rate had reduced from 66 to 39 mL/min/1.73 m^2 over the space of 3 years.

    Aside from longstanding loose bowel motions, he reported no new symptoms or any change to his medications for several years. He took azathioprine and lansoprazole.

    Aside from surgical scars and a thin build, clinical examination was unremarkable.

    Investigations:

    creatinine 173 µmol/L (60–110)   Ultrasound: bilateral cortical and
    Urine microscopy: positively birefringent crystals   medullary calcification
    under polarised light

    What is the most likely diagnosis?

    A   Drug-induced crystalluria
    B   Oxalate nephropathy
    C   Cystinuria
    D   Urate nephropathy
    E   Ethylene glycol toxicity

33. A 35-year-old woman underwent renal biopsy to investigate progressive renal impairment with proteinuria.

    Renal biopsy (Congo red staining): see **Figure 9.5:**

    Regarding this patient's diagnosis, which one of the following is incorrect?

    A   If renal biopsy is insufficient rectal biopsy can aid diagnosis
    B   It is associated with familial Mediterranean fever
    C   It is associated with rheumatoid arthritis
    D   The prognosis is good with steroids
    E   The patient should be screened for a plasma cell dyscrasia

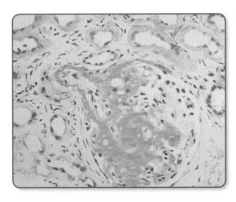

Figure 9.5 *See colour plate section.*

34. A 74-year-old woman presented with lethargy and back pain, and was found to have abnormal kidney function. She had no significant past medical history and took no regular medications.

Investigations:

haemoglobin 88 g/L (115–165)	creatinine 407 μmol/L (45–90)
white cell count 9.6 × 10⁹/L (4–11)	total protein 96 g/L (60–76)
urea 26.4 mmol/L (2.5–7.5)	albumin 34 g/L (37–49)

Renal biopsy: see **Figure 9.6**

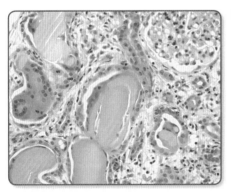

Figure 9.6 *See colour plate section.*

What is the most likely diagnosis?

A   AA amyloidosis
B   Cast nephropathy
C   Cryoglobulinaemia
D   Sarcoidosis
E   Tubulo-interstitial nephritis

35. A 75-year-old woman presented feeling weak. She had had diarrhoea and vomiting for 3 days. She was initially taking bendroflumethiazide but had stopped this 1 day previously.

On examination, she was alert and oriented. Her pulse was 100 beats per minute. Her blood pressure 100/60 mmHg when standing and 80/51 mmHg when supine.

Investigations:

sodium 120 mmol/L (135–145)	thyroid-stimulating hormone 2.0 mU/L (0.4–5.0)
urea 12.2 mmol/L (2.5–7.5)	free thyroxine 20 pmol/L (10–25)
creatinine 94 µmol/L (females 45–90)	urine osmolality 410 mosmol/kg (500–800)

What is the most appropriate management?

A 0.9% NaCl intravenously
B 2.7% NaCl intravenously
C Demeclocycline
D Fluid restriction <1 L/24 h
E Tolvaptan

36. A 45-year-old woman with a history of renal transplantation 15 years previously presented with shingles and commenced treatment with oral aciclovir. She had previously been heavily immunosuppressed for rejection. She had also had a recent admission for *Pneumocystis jiroveci* pneumonia and was treated with co-trimoxazole, which she was still taking at a prophylactic dose. Her other medications included ciclosporin, mycophenolate mofetil and prednisolone. In addition, she had recently been started on allopurinol following an attack of gout.
    She returned to the clinic 2 weeks later for routine blood tests.

Investigations:

haemoglobin 115 g/L (115–165)	urate 500 mmol/L (females 110–360)
white cell count 7.4 × 10^9 (4–11)	corrected calcium 2.5 mmol/L (2.2–2.6)
platelets 320 × 10^9 (150–400)	phosphate 1.1 mmol/L (0.8–1.4)
creatinine 500 µmol/L (baseline 130)	

Urine microscopy: birefringent needle-shaped crystals

Which drug is the most likely cause of her acute kidney injury?

A Aciclovir
B Allopurinol
C Ciclosporin
D Co-trimoxazole
E Mycophenolate mofetil

37. A 42-year-old woman presented with headaches and grade 3 hypertensive retinopathy. She had no significant past medical history and was otherwise well.
    Her blood pressure was 190/105 mmHg in both arms, heart sounds and peripheral pulses were normal, with no radio-femoral or radio-radial delay. She had bilateral ankle oedema.

Investigations:

sodium 140 mmol/L (135–145)	fasting glucose 4.2 mmol/L (3–6)
potassium 3.1 mmol/L (3.5–5.0)	

Urine dipstick: negative for blood and protein

Chest X-ray: normal

What is the most likely cause of her hypertension?

A   Acute glomerulonephritis
B   Bartter's syndrome
C   Coarctation of the aorta
D   Cushing's syndrome
E   Renal artery stenosis

38. A 51-year-old man was referred to the renal clinic for investigation of abnormal blood results. He had a history of autoimmune thrombocytopenia, treated with ciclosporin and low dose prednisolone. He had no other significant past medical history and took no other medications.

Investigations:

sodium 136 mmol/L (135–145)	bicarbonate 17 mmol/L (22–30)
potassium 5.7 mmol/L (3.5–5.0)	chloride 115 mmol/L (95–107)
creatinine 89 µmol/L (males 60–110)	urine pH 5.1
Urinary anion gap: positive	

What is the most likely diagnosis?

A   Fanconi's syndrome
B   Type 1 renal tubular acidosis
C   Type 2 renal tubular acidosis
D   Type 3 renal tubular acidosis
E   Type 4 renal tubular acidosis

39. A 45-year-old woman was referred to the emergency department with breathlessness and severe hypertension. She had a long history of Raynaud's syndrome, and more recently had developed swallowing difficulties.
      On examination, her blood pressure was 190/110 mmHg and she had fine crepitations at the lung bases.

Investigations:

haemoglobin 83 g/L (115–165)	anti-nuclear antibodies: positive
platelets 95 × 10^9/L (150–400)	anti-centromere antibody: negative
creatinine 436 µmol/L (45 – 90)	anti-Scl70 antibody: positive
	anti-RNA polymerase antibody: positive
Urine dip: negative for blood and protein	

What is the most appropriate next step in her management?

A   Renal biopsy
B   Intravenous methylprednisolone
C   Oral captopril
D   Intravenous labetalol
E   Plasma exchange

40. A 32-year-old man with a history of bipolar disorder was admitted felling generally unwell. He took regular lithium. He complained of increased thirst and generalised weakness. His urine output was 4 L per day.

Investigations:

sodium 152 mmol/L (135–145)
potassium 3.9 mmol/L (3.5–5.0)
corrected calcium 2.46 mmol/L (2.2–2.6)

glucose 7.1 mmol/L (3–6)
urine osmolality 250 mosmol/kg (500–800)

What is the most appropriate treatment?

A   5% dextrose
B   0.45% saline
C   Desmopressin (DDAVP)
D   Fluid restriction
E   Thiazide diuretic

41. A 28-year-old pregnant woman at 20 weeks' gestation was referred to the joint renal-obstetric clinic by the antenatal team as she was found to have persistent proteinuria (1+ protein on dipstick testing). She was sent for further investigations.

When interpreting these further tests, which one of the following is definitely abnormal in pregnancy?

A   Creatinine changing from 73 µmol/L in the 1st trimester to 47 µmol/L in the 3rd trimester
B   Creatinine clearance changing from 125 mL/min in the 1st trimester to 90 mL/min in the 2nd trimester
C   Glycosuria on urine dipstick
D   Sodium 132 mmol/L
E   Proteinuria 100 mg/24 hours

42. A 48-year-old woman presented to the renal transplant clinic. She received a deceased donor transplant 2 years previously and had good graft function with a baseline creatinine around 100 µmol/L. Recently, however, this had increased to 155 µmol/L over 6 months, with proteinuria (3+ protein on dipstick testing).

She was admitted for a transplant biopsy, which showed no rejection but did show some features consistent with her original renal disease.

Which one of the following conditions is not recognised as recurring in a renal transplant?

A   Diabetic nephropathy
B   IgA nephropathy
C   Mesangiocapillary glomerulonephritis type II
D   Primary focal segmental glomerulosclerosis
E   Tubulo-interstitial nephritis

43. A 32-year-old man presented with a short history of feeling generally unwell and weak. He had been found collapsed a home.

On examination, he was confused, with a Glasgow Coma Scale score of 14/15. His blood pressure was 170/90 mmHg and jugular venous pressure was visible at 4 cm. There were bi-basal crepitations on respiratory examination and heart sounds revealed a gallop rhythm. Neurological examination revealed an ataxic gait and bilateral cranial nerve VII palsies.

Investigations:

sodium 139 mmol/L (135–145)	creatinine 460 µmol/L (males 60–110)
potassium 6 mmol/L (3.5–5.0)	chloride 104 mmol/L (95–107)
urea 32 mmol/L	bicarbonate 15 mmol/L (22–30)

Urine dipstick: protein +++, blood ++

Urine microscopy: positively birefringent crystals under polarized light

What is the most likely diagnosis?

A   Ethylene glycol ingestion
B   Rhabdomyolysis
C   Severe community-acquired pneumonia
D   Salicylate overdose
E   Vasculitis with a rapidly progressive glomerulonephritis

Answers

1. A 0.9% NaCl 1 mL/kg per h for 12 hours pre- and post-procedure

Contrast-induced acute kidney injury (CI-AKI) is defined as a rise in serum creatinine by >26 µmol/L within 48 hours or by >50% from baseline, or urine output of <0.5 mL/kg/h for >6 consecutive hours, following the use of iodinated radiocontrast. It usually occurs within 72 hours of contrast exposure, and recovers over the following week; peak serum creatinine is usually around 5 days following exposure. Although generally accepted as a reversible cause of renal dysfunction, CI-AKI is an important iatrogenic cause of morbidity and mortality. It is uncommon in the general population (incidence 1–2%), but some patients are particularly vulnerable. Risk factors include chronic kidney disease (eGFR <60 mL/min/1.73 m^2), older age, cardiac failure, diabetes, nephrotoxic medications, hypovolaemia and sepsis.

Nephrotoxins should be withheld for 48 hours before and after the angiography. There is also evidence that intravenous volume expansion will reduce the risk of CI-AKI. Intravenous fluid mitigates against the afferent arteriolar vasoconstriction and osmotic diuresis caused by the contrast agent, and has been shown to reduce the incidence of CI-AKI. Various types of fluid have been compared in clinical trials: there is no evidence to support the use of hypotonic saline, and meta-analyses have found conflicting results in trials comparing 0.9% saline with isotonic (1.26%) sodium bicarbonate. Therefore, current guidelines recommend intravenous volume expansion with either 0.9% sodium chloride or isotonic (1.26%) sodium bicarbonate. It is important to examine the patient first, however: patients who are volume deplete often require a larger volume of fluid than suggested here; likewise, in patients who are fluid overloaded, intravenous fluid would be contraindicated and could be harmful. This patient appears clinically euvolaemic, so 1 mL/kg per hour for 12 hours pre- and post-procedure would suffice.

Large meta-analyses suggest that N-acetylcysteine confers no significant benefit. Continuous veno-venous haemofiltration does remove circulating contrast but there have been no large-scale trials to prove its benefit and it is clearly invasive, expensive, time-consuming and not without risk.

UK Renal Association, British Cardiovascular Intervention Society and Royal College of Radiologists. Joint Clinical Practice Guideline: Prevention of contrast induced acute kidney injury (CI-AKI) in adult patients (2013). (last accessed May 2017)
Solomon R, Dauerman HL. Contrast-induced acute kidney injury. Circulation 2010; 122(23):2451–2455.

2. C Diclofenac

Amlodipine and bisoprolol both lower blood pressure and thus can contribute to the progression to acute tubular necrosis, but they are not directly toxic to the kidneys. Gliclazide is a sulfonamide that has no association with acute kidney injury (AKI). Metformin is exclusively excreted via the kidneys, so may accumulate and cause lactic acidosis in the presence of significant renal dysfunction (it should be discontinued in patients with AKI, and avoided in patients with eGFR <30 mL/min/1.73 m^2); however, it does not cause AKI.

Non-steroidal anti-inflammatory drugs (NSAIDs; such as diclofenac) and cyclo-oxygenase (COX) inhibitors are inhibitors of prostaglandin synthesis. In situations of normal renal blood flow, prostaglandins (namely prostacyclin and prostaglandin E2) have little haemodynamic effect on the kidney. In states of reduced renal blood flow (e.g. in hypovolaemia, as present here, any type of shock, congestive cardiac failure or cirrhosis) prostaglandins maintain the glomerular filtration rate via compensatory afferent arteriolar dilatation. Attenuation of this by NSAIDs/COX inhibitors results in unopposed vasoconstriction mediated by vasopressin and catecholamines, which can cause AKI.

Murray MD, Brater DC. Renal toxicity of the nonsteroidal anti-inflammatory drugs. Annu Rev Pharmacol Toxicol 1993; 33:435.

3.　A　Antiglomerular basement membrane disease (Goodpasture's disease)

This patient has presented with nephrotic syndrome with the triad of proteinuria (6 g in 24 hours), hypoalbuminaemia and peripheral oedema. The biopsy is classic for membranous nephropathy with numerous small 'spikes' seen on the glomerular basement membrane (seen best on silver stain). Light microscopy may be normal or there may be glomerular basement membrane (GBM) thickening. On electron microscopy there will be subepithelial immune deposits. Membranous nephropathy has many associations – most importantly infections and malignancy. Detection of malignancies may be preceded by membranous nephropathy by several years.

Associations include:

Infections
Hepatitis B and C
Malaria
Streptococcal infection
Syphilis
Schistosomiasis

Neoplasms
Solid tumours – carcinoma of breast, lung, kidney, gastrointestinal tract
Haematological malignancy – Hodgkin's disease, non-Hodgkin's disease

Systemic disease
Systemic lupus erythematosus
Sarcoidosis
Autoimmune thyroiditis

Toxins
Captopril
Non-steroidal anti-inflammatory drugs
D-penicillamine
Gold

Anti-GBM disease is a rare pulmonary–renal syndrome which presents as a rapidly progressive glomerulonephritis with focal and segmental necrotising crescentic glomerulonephritis on renal biopsy; it does not cause nephrotic syndrome.

Urine protein:creatinine ratio (PCR) is a more reproducible and generally more useful measure than 24-hour urine collection. A PCR of 100 mg/mmol is approximately equal to 1 g protein per 24 hours, and a PCR of >300 mg/mmol suggests 'nephrotic range' proteinuria.

4.　D　Ramipril

Diabetic nephropathy is the most common cause of end-stage renal failure in Europe and the USA with an increased incidence in males. Renal biopsy is seldom required to establish the diagnosis, particularly in the context of established retinopathy, negative immunology testing and absence of microscopic haematuria (as seen in this case).

Good blood pressure control has been shown to slow down progression of all renal disease, particularly diabetic nephropathy which typically progresses quickly with glomerular filtration rate (GFR) declining by up to 12 mL/min per 1.73 m^2 each year. This can be reduced to 5 mL/min per 1.73 m^2 each year with tight blood pressure control. Amlodipine is a reasonable choice of antihypertensive; however, use of a long-acting, tissue-bound, angiotensin-converting enzyme (ACE) inhibitor (such as ramipril) or an angiotensin receptor blocker (ARB) may slow decline further to as little as a loss of 0.3 mL/min per 1.73 m^2 each year and should be tried as first-line antihypertensive therapy (the RENAAL trial – see below). Tight diabetic control is also important but with hypertension and heavy proteinuria the most appropriate first step is to control blood pressure. A low-salt diet would be indicated but in the absence of hyperkalaemia a low-potassium diet is less important. Potassium should be monitored closely after the addition of an ACE inhibitor. Renal artery stenosis is common, particularly in type 2 diabetes, and should be considered if the serum creatinine increases by >30% after initiation of an ACE inhibitor or if fluid retention becomes problematic.

National Institute for Health and Care Excellence. (NICE). Clinical Guideline 182. Chronic kidney disease in adults: assessment and management. London: NICE, 2014.
Brenner BM. Effects of losartan on renal and cardiovascular outcomes in patients with type 2 diabetes and nephropathy. N Engl J Med 2001; 345(12):861–869.

5. E Start a phosphate binder

This patient has blood results consistent with progressive chronic kidney disease (CKD) stage 4. Although he has a declining glomerular filtration rate (GFR) corrected for race (16 mL/min per 1.73 m^2 by the MDRD equation*) he is well and has no uraemic symptoms. He should be counselled that the need for renal replacement therapy is inevitable in the near future, and ideally he should be assessed for either elective formation of arteriovenous fistula for haemodialysis or insertion of a Moncrieff or Tenckhoff catheter for peritoneal dialysis. Younger patients should also be assessed for their suitability for transplantation, have any appropriate cardiac investigations, explore potential live donors or, failing that, be placed on the deceased donor transplantation list. The gold standard is that all of this should be done before the need to start dialysis.

Here the patient is anaemic but needs adequate iron replacement before starting erythropoietin. An angiotensin-converting enzyme (ACE) inhibitor to reduce proteinuria would be appropriate in a less advanced state of CKD; hyperkalaemia is a contraindication.

Although his creatinine has risen by 70 μmol/L this actually corresponds only to a drop in GFR of 3 mL/min per 1.73 m^2 and is very unlikely to be caused by renal tract obstruction.

The serum calcium is low and phosphate is high, with evidence of secondary hyperparathyroidism from a raised parathyroid hormone (PTH). Starting a phosphate binder would be appropriate here, to keep serum phosphate in the recommended range (see below). Hyperphosphataemia is known to exert a direct calcifying effect on coronary arteries, cardiac valves and pulmonary tissues, which are associated with increased cardiovascular morbidity and mortality. Release of parathyroid hormone (PTH) is also stimulated, leading to increased bone turnover (renal osteodystrophy).

The UK Renal Association recommends that serum phosphate should be maintained between 0.9 and 1.5 mmol/L in patients with CKD stages 3b to 5, (as in this case), and between 1.1 and 1.7 mmol/L in patients on dialysis. They also publish guidelines for PTH, as well as the recommended frequency of measurement for PTH, calcium and phosphate.

*The Modification of Diet in Renal Disease (MDRD) equation has been widely accepted as a formula to calculate estimated GFR (eGFR). It takes into account serum creatinine, age, race and gender.
The Renal Association. Clinical Practice Guideline: CKD-mineral and bone disorders. Bristol: The Renal Association, 2015.

6. E Multiple myeloma

Acute tubulo-intersitial nephritis does occur with antibiotic use but is relatively rare; associated findings are eosinophilia, moderate proteinuria (<1g/day, uPCR<100mg/mmol) or white cell casts (which may manifest as leucosuria on dipstick testing). Diabetic nephropathy is a possibility but it would be unusual for renal impairment to progress this quickly, particularly in the absence of significant albuminuria. There is no suggestion that the patient is hypovolaemic, making acute tubular necrosis less likely. The rate of decline of renal function, relatively bland urine and normal blood pressure also go against IgA nephropathy.

Acute kidney injury with anaemia and hypercalcaemia should always raise the suspicion of multiple myeloma. Serum electrophoresis, immunoglobulins, Bence Jones proteins, a bone marrow biopsy and a renal biopsy are all indicated here. Note that standard urine dipsticks detect albuminuria; therefore Bence Jones proteins (urinary light chains) will not be detectable by dipstick testing (urine protein:creatinine ratio will be raised, however).

Heher EC, et al. Kidney disease and multiple myeloma. Clin J Am Soc Nephrol 2013; 8(11):2007-17.

7. E Serial blood cultures

The two broad differential diagnoses here are a small vessel vasculitis (SVV) with a rapidly progressive glomerulonephritis (RPGN) or infective endocarditis (IE). There are features that would suggest either diagnosis. The patient clearly has rapidly progressing renal impairment with blood and protein on dipstick testing, and the positive antineutrophil cytoplasmic antibody (ANCA) suggests the diagnosis of an SVV. The complements are, however, consumed which is not in keeping with a vasculitis but rather IE, supported by the pancytopenia, splenomegaly and history of valve replacement. A renal biopsy would be helpful (showing a focal and segmental necrotising crescentic glomerulonephritis with vasculitis and a proliferative glomerulonephritis with infection) but is unsafe here because of thrombocytopenia. Pulsed methylprednisolone can be given empirically if the suspicion of RPGN is high (particularly in the context of a strongly positive ANCA), but there are too many factors pointing towards infection in this case. Broad-spectrum antibiotics would be important but not until serial blood cultures have been taken. Echocardiogram (transthoracic or transoesophageal) should be performed urgently. Bone marrow biopsy is unlikely to aid in distinguishing between SVV and IE.

It is well recognised that ANCA can be positive in conditions other than vasculitis. Infection, particularly endocarditis, and occult malignancy should be looked for where the diagnosis is not clear.

Csernok E, et al. Clinical and immunological features of drug-induced and infection-induced proteinase 3-antineutrophil cytoplasmic antibodies and myeloperoxidase–antineutrophil cytoplasmic antibodies and vasculitis. Curr Opin Rheumatol 2010; 22(1):43–48.

8. B Renal transplant biopsy

The key thing to exclude here is rejection. The patient has received a fairly recent cadaveric transplant and had good initial graft function, which is now deteriorating rapidly. An ultrasound scan has already been performed and is normal with no suggestion of hydronephrosis, thus there is little value in doing a renogram at this point to look for obstruction. His blood pressure is on the high side but there is no suggestion of salt and water retention, making transplant renal artery stenosis unlikely. There is nothing to suggest urinary tract or systemic infection; although urine should be sent for culture, there is no indication to commence empirical antibiotics. Although cytomegalovirus polymerase chain reaction should be monitored regularly post-transplantation, it is not indicated urgently here. Renal biopsy is the definitive way to diagnose rejection and should therefore be performed urgently to allow prompt treatment, if it is confirmed. UK renal Association guidelines suggest that renal allograft biopsy should be performed before treating acute rejection, unless facilitating the biopsy will substantially delay potential treatment. They also recommend that kidney biopsy be performed when there is a persistent, unexplained increase in serum creatinine, or if sustained new onset proteinuria develops (uPCR >50 mg/mmol).

The Renal Association. Clinical practice guideline. Post-operative care of the kidney transplant recipient. Bristol: The Renal Association, 2017.

9. B Antiglomerular basement membrane disease

This patient presents with acute kidney injury and evidence of pulmonary haemorrhage. Antiglomerular basement membrane (anti-GBM) disease (Goodpasture's disease) is a rare pulmonary–renal syndrome. It may present acutely with fulminant pulmonary haemorrhage and renal failure or more gradually, as in this case, with generalised symptoms of fatigue and weight loss, and subclinical pulmonary haemorrhage. Pulmonary haemorrhage is more common and severe in smokers and cigarette smoking has been proposed as a possible trigger, exposing antigenic epitopes on the basement membrane that are normally 'hidden'. Granulomatosis with polyangiitis (GPA, formerly known as Wegener's granulomatosis) is another cause of pulmonary–renal syndrome that may present in a similar way, however this is characterised by antineutrophil cytoplasmic antibodies (ANCA) directed against the neutrophil enzyme proteinase 3 (PR3), which makes this a less likely diagnosis. Microscopic polyangiitis (MPA) is another a small vessel vasculitis characterised by ANCA directed against myeloperoxidase (MPO). The patient's age and race make tuberculosis less likely, and with an acute nephritis there might be leukocytes in urine. There is nothing to suggest a membranous nephropathy (she is not nephrotic) and the chest x-ray description is more suggestive of pulmonary haemorrhage than malignancy. She is not haemodynamically compromised or obviously septic so acute tubular necrosis (ATN) is less likely and, again, the chest X-ray is more suggestive of pulmonary haemorrhage (with bilateral changes) than pneumonia.

Anti-GBM disease is caused by IgG anti-GBM antibodies against the a_3 chain of type IV collagen (found in glomerular and alveolar basement membranes), which bind and fix complement, causing local injury. Renal biopsy will show a focal and segmental, necrotising glomerulonephritis, with rupture of the basement membrane and proliferation of inflammatory cells in Bowman's space (a crescent, so-called because of its appearance on microscopy). Immunofluorescence shows linear capillary wall staining for anti-GBM (IgG) and C3 deposition.

Treatment is immunosuppression with methylprednisolone and cyclophosphamide, haemodialysis if oligoanuric (often with a low chance of renal recovery) and plasma exchange to remove circulating antibodies. Patients can be dual ANCA and anti-GBM positive and this group tends to have a better outcome.

10. E Granulomatosis with polyangiitis (Wegener's granulomatosis)

In a patient presenting with acute kidney injury in the context of systemic symptoms there are several important differential diagnoses. Often a renal biopsy is required in order to confirm the diagnosis but it is vital to first undertake a full nephritic screen. Here, the main pointer is the serum complement components, C3 and C4, which are low and indicate activation of the 'classic' complement system (see **Table 9.1**). Complement may be low in all of the options except granulomatosis with polyangiitis (GPA), an antineutrophil cytoplasmic antibodies (ANCA)-associated small vessel vasculitis in which serum complement is normal. Lupus nephritis, cryoglobulinaemic vasculitis, and infection-associated glomerulonephritis are characterised by immune deposits in the glomerulus, and activation of the complement system, and low serum complement.

Table 9.1 Hypocomplementaemia		
Disease	**C3**	**C4**
Infective endocarditis	↓	↓
Postinfectious glomerulonephritis	↓	↓/↔
Systemic lupus erythematosus	↓	↓
Essential mixed cryoglobulinaemia	↔	↓
Mesangiocapillary glomerulonephritis (MCGN) type II	↓	↔
Cholesterol emboli	↓	↔

11. A 10 mL of 10% calcium gluconate given intravenously over 5 minutes

This patient presents with acute kidney injury in the context of rhabdomyolysis. Because of widespread cell death there is accumulation of intracellular elements, particularly creatine kinase (CK), myoglobin and potassium.

In this case there is evidence of myocardial irritation on his ECG caused by hyperkalaemia, and the first and most important step is to stabilise this using intravenous calcium gluconate. If there is no improvement in ECG changes, this can be repeated after 5 minutes, up to a total of 40 mL calcium gluconate. It is important to remember that calcium gluconate (or chloride) is cardioprotective only and does not actually lower serum potassium. In addition, its protective effects will last for under an hour, so other measures must be taken.

The first measure to lower serum potassium would be an insulin/dextrose infusion (10 units of fast-acting insulin in 50 mL of 50% dextrose over 10–20 minutes through a large-bore peripheral cannula). Insulin lowers serum potassium by 0.5–1.5 µmol/L within 30 minutes by increasing Na^+/K^+/ATPase activity, which moves potassium into cells; dextrose is co-administered to prevent hypoglycaemia. It is important to remember that this does not remove any potassium from the body, which should be the goal of treatment. The effects of insulin last 2–4 hours, following which serum potassium will rise again unless steps are taken to lower total body potassium.

The only way to remove potassium from the body is by excretion in the urine or by using extra-corporeal removal (haemodialysis or haemofiltration). This patient is oliguric so is very likely developing acute tubular necrosis (ATN) secondary to myoglobinuria. Therefore, renal replacement therapy (RRT) is the definitive treatment. Haemodialysis/haemofiltration will bring serum potassium down within 30 minutes, but requires time to set up (vascular access, ward/ITU transfer and specialist nursing are needed), so calcium gluconate and insulin/dextrose are necessary as bridging measures. When using insulin/dextrose, beware of causing hypoglycaemia, especially in non-diabetic patients.

Compartment syndrome occurs either if there is compromise to the blood supply of a limb because of immobility, or from generalised muscle injury in the case of toxic or virally induced rhabdomyolysis. An urgent fasciotomy is indicated to treat the cause of the hyperkalaemia and save the limb. First, however, the patient must be stabilised with the measures described above. Nebulised salbutamol will lower serum potassium by around 1 µmol/L but also acts on the Na^+/K^+-ATPase pump, so it confers no additional benefit. In acutely unwell patients with underlying cardiac disease it may also precipitate tachyarrhythmias. Calcium Resonium is a cation exchange resin, which exchanges sodium for potassium in the gastrointestinal tract. It can be given orally or rectally (more effective) and its effect will be maximal at 24–48 hours. Clearly, this patient will require more rapid correction.

Steddon S, et al. Oxford Handbook of Nephrology and Hypertension. Oxford: Oxford University Press, 2006.

12. A Acute tubular necrosis secondary to hypotension

The causes of postoperative acute kidney injury (AKI) are many and should always be considered, particularly looking for sepsis. The prolonged period of low blood pressure here makes acute tubular injury secondary to hypotension the most likely cause of her rising creatinine, especially in the context of her risk factors and pre-existing kidney disease. When mean arterial pressure falls below 70 mmHg, auto-regulation of intra-glomerular pressure is impaired and glomerular filtration rate falls. Sepsis is another common cause of postoperative AKI, but is unlikely here, given the clinical picture. Acute tubulo-interstitial nephritis is unlikely; the onset is too quick, and it is rarely caused by co-amoxiclav. Contrast is not used in coronary bypass grafting. Renal artery occlusion is also unlikely because there has been no instrumentation or manipulation of the abdominal aorta. Features of acute renal artery occlusion are loin pain, hypertension (secondary to renin release), vomiting and fever.

13. B Cholesterol emboli

Cholesterol emboli are the most likely diagnosis in view of the patient's age, risk factors and atherosclerotic history. Caucasian men over the age of 50 are the most susceptible group. It most frequently occurs after vascular instrumentation or surgery, most commonly angiography. It can also occur in the context of thrombolysis or anticoagulation. Showers of cholesterol crystals from destabilised plaques cause partial occlusion of small arteries, which results in infarction of endarterial territories, typically the digits and the gut. Damage in the kidneys can either be acute (1–4 weeks post-procedure) from similar downstream ischaemia in the small renal vessels, or more chronic (it can occur months after the initial insult) and progressive from a secondary fibrotic response. Urine is often bland, although patients can present with heavy proteinuria. A blood eosinophilia is common and hypocomplementaemia is often seen. Treatment is largely supportive, mortality and morbidity from cardiovascular causes are high, and renal function often fails to recover.

Contrast-induced nephropathy would also be a possible cause of acute kidney injury here, but the systemic signs and the patient's symptoms point more towards cholesterol emboli. Also, the timing of the presentation is a little late for contrast-induced nephropathy, which typically occurs within 48 hours of exposure.

Although this patient has risk factors for renal artery stenosis, the acute presentation, signs and ultrasound findings go against this. Lupus nephritis is associated with hypocomplementaemia but it would be a very unlikely presentation in an elderly white man. Analgesic nephropathy would not present in such an acute way, although pain killers can be associated with acute tubulo-interstitial nephritis.

Dupont PJ, et al. Lesson of the week: Cholesterol emboli syndrome. BMJ 2000; 321:1065–1067.

14. C Stool microscopy and culture

This patient has haemolytic uraemic syndrome (HUS) associated with a diarrhoeal illness. HUS is the triad of microangiopathic haemolytic anaemia, thrombocytopaenia and acute kidney injury. 'Typical' HUS is associated with diarrhoea (D+) and caused by infection with a shiga-toxin producing bacteria, most commonly *Escherichia coli* O157:H7, hence the need to send stool microscopy urgently. Other organisms include *Shigella*, *Campylobacter* or *Salmonella*. 'Atypical' (D-) HUS can be caused by drugs (e.g. cancineurin inhibitors, quinine, the contraceptive pill), pregnancy, infection (e.g. pneumococcus), or inherited deficiencies of complement regulatory proteins (e.g. factor H).

In D+ HUS, bacterial toxins translocate across inflamed bowel mucosa into the blood, causing widespread endothelial damage, platelet activation, increased pro-thrombotic factors and release of ultra-large von Willebrand's factor. There is resultant thrombocytopenia, haemolytic anaemia and tissue ischaemia due to microcirculatory occlusion. Intra-renal vessels are affected, resulting in acute kidney injury, oliguria and hypertension.

Treatment is supportive, and confirmation of the suspected cause should be sought. Although many patients require renal replacement therapy, there is no indication for haemofiltration here. Flexible sigmoidoscopy is not indicated and would be unsafe with this degree of anaemia and thrombocytopenia. Antibiotics may increase shiga-toxin release, and should be avoided if HUS is suspected, unless there is systemic bacteraemia. There is no indication for haemofiltration in this case.

HUS and thrombotic thrombocytopenic purpura (TTP) are part of the same clinical spectrum, known collectively as the thrombotic microangiopathies. Although TTP classically causes less renal and more neurological damage, both conditions may quickly progress to multi-organ failure, and it can be difficult to differentiate between them at initial presentation. Plasma exchange is the mainstay of treatment for TTP, and is often started if there is any doubt as to the diagnosis, while waiting for confirmatory tests. Platelet transfusion can worsen the outcome by propagating small vessel occlusions, so should be avoided unless there is life-threatening bleeding.

Clark WF. HUS/TTP update. Kidney Int 2008; 75:S1–S3.

15. E Perform CT scan of abdomen and pelvis

The most likely diagnosis here is bowel perforation, which has initially been incorrectly diagnosed as peritoneal dialysis (PD) peritonitis.

PD peritonitis is a common problem, which typically presents with abdominal pain and cloudy PD effluent. The diagnosis is confirmed by microscopy and culture of the PD fluid, with >100 WBC/mm^3 being diagnostic. It is most commonly caused by gram positive cocci, which are introduced by touch contamination or skin colonisation. Gram negative organisms are responsible for around 25% of infections, but if mixed gram negative organisms are cultured (as in this case) bowel perforation should be suspected. This patient is likely to have another cause of peritonitis (e.g. appendicitis or diverticulitis). A CT scan is necessary to establish the cause before surgical intervention. At surgery, the PD catheter will have to be removed and he will be converted to haemodialysis. Each episode of peritonitis damages the peritoneal membrane and can cause adhesions, so it may not be possible to continue PD in the long term.

Intravenous antibiotics will be needed once the PD catheter has been removed, but surgical intervention is necessary as well. Continuing intraperitoneal antibiotics would not be appropriate as he is not improving on this treatment.

16. E She should have a magnetic resonance cerebral angiogram

Adult polycystic kidney disease (APKD) is a common inherited disease. It is inherited as an autosomal dominant disease, so there is a 50% chance of any offspring being affected. There are two mutations, found on chromosome 16 and chromosome 4, which are responsible for the phenotype seen. These mutations code for polycystin-1 (PKD-1) and polycystin-2 (PKD-2) respectively. PKD-1 is more common than PKD-2. Both polycystin-1 and polycystin-2 are involved in the regulation of cell proliferation and differentiation in the tubular epithelium and in the maturation of these cells. When this mechanism fails in APKD there is dysregulated cell turnover and uncontrolled growth, which results in the formation of multiple cysts. These cysts enlarge over time and there is ongoing ischaemic and fibrotic damage, resulting in progressive renal impairment.

Patients often present with a positive family history, flank or loin pain, haematuria, nocturia or hypertension. Ultrasound is the imaging of choice for diagnosis. For the best negative predictive value this should be done only after the age of 20 years.

The diagnostic criteria depend on the familial genotype and age of the patient being screened. The criteria for patients with an unknown familial genotype are summarised in **Table 9.2**.

A finding of fewer than two cysts in a patient aged over 40 years with a family history is sufficient to exclude the disease (100% negative predictive value). There are no agreed criteria for diagnosing patients without a family history. Ultrasound is less sensitive in patients below the age of 18. Screening in children is controversial, but referral for genetic counselling is suggested.

Table 9.2 Adult polycystic kidney disease diagnostic criteria for at-risk patients with an unknown genotype

Age	Criteria for diagnosis
15–39 years	≥3 cysts (unilateral or bilateral)
40–59 years	≥2 cysts in each kidney
≥60 years	≥4 cysts in each kidney

PKD-2 often presents later than PKD-1. Hypertension is often the first sign of APKD and may be present even when renal function is normal. Not all patients with APKD will progress to renal failure. A worse renal prognosis is associated with patients who are diagnosed earlier or have early hypertension, and those with PKD-1 mutations.

APKD is associated with both extrarenal cysts (particularly polycystic livers) and an increased risk of intracranial aneurysms. Around 5–10% of patients with APKD will have an intracranial aneurysm. Patients with a family history of intracerebral bleeds should have screening with an MR angiogram. Most commonly the aneurysms rupture in younger patients with poor blood pressure control and confer high mortality and morbidity.

Her blood pressure at present is too high and she should be promptly started on antihypertensives to help preserve renal function.

17. B Collapsing focal segmental glomerulosclerosis (FSGS)

This patient has significant renal impairment with a negative nephritic screen except for positive HIV virology. A low CD4 count and a high viral load indicate untreated, or undertreated, disease. HIV infection is associated with many different types of renal lesion but the most common is HIV-associated nephropathy (HIVAN). In HIVAN, which is predominantly seen in patients of African descent, there is typically a collapsing variant of focal segmental glomerulosclerosis (FSGS) caused by HIV infection of the renal proximal tubular cells and podocytes. HIVAN is characterised by heavy proteinuria (often nephrotic range, i.e. >3 g/24 h), microscopic haematuria, hypoalbuminaemia, but relatively little peripheral oedema. There is a high rate of progression to end-stage renal disease. It occurs when HIV infection is advanced (CD4 count <200) and often in the context of an AIDS-defining illness.

Hyaline arteriosclerosis is caused by uncontrolled hypertension; this patient's blood pressure is only marginally elevated and he is not on antihypertensive agents. Kimmelstiel–Wilson nodules are found in diabetic nephropathy. Minimal change, although a common cause of nephrotic syndrome, is not as a rule associated with abnormal creatinine or dipstick haematuria. Cast nephropathy is caused by multiple myeloma, which is excluded here by the serum electrophoresis result (hypergammaglobulinaemia is typical of untreated HIV infection; a paraprotein would be found in myeloma). It does not present with nephrotic syndrome.

Kaufman L, et al. The pathogenesis of HIV-associated nephropathy. Adv Chronic Kidney Dis 2010; 17(1):36–43.

18. C Epstein–Barr virus

This patient has a 10-year history of immunosuppression with a history of rejection earlier in his transplant history, which would have necessitated intense immunosuppression. All the viruses listed are important and can cause problems throughout the post-transplantation course. The key here is in interpreting the clinical picture and the time frame.

The weight loss, anaemia, lymphadenopathy and a palpable abdominal mass are clear pointers towards malignancy. Patients who have received long-term immunosuppression are at increased risk of malignancy. In particular, transplant recipients can develop post-transplantation lymphoproliferative disease (PTLD). This is most commonly a lymphoma-type condition, and is usually associated with Epstein–Barr virus (EBV). EBV infection, particularly in patients who have not previously encountered the virus, can cause uncontrolled B cell proliferation. It occurs in 1–5% of renal transplant recipients, and is more common in patients who have been most heavily immunosuppressed. Patients often respond to a reduction in their immunosuppression, but may also require chemotherapy.

Cytomegalovirus (CMV) is important to remember as a major complication of transplantation. wCMV polymerase chain reaction should be performed regularly post-transplantation. Patients can be asymptomatic but can present with systemic symptoms or involvement of many organs: colitis, pneumonitis, bone marrow suppression, transplant dysfunction, retinitis and encephalitis are all seen. CMV infection is most commonly seen in the first 6–12 months following transplantation, and it would be unusual to present at such a late stage. Although it should be checked, in this case CMV infection would not account for all the features.

BK virus (named after the initials of the first renal transplant recipient in whom the virus was isolated) is a polyoma virus that can cause graft dysfunction and ureteric stenosis, but there is nothing to suggest BK nephropathy here. Equally there is nothing to suggest hepatitis B virus infection in this case. HIV should be considered but again it is less likely, given the history.

Steddon S, et al. Oxford Handbook of Nephrology and Hypertension. Oxford: Oxford University Press, 2006.

19. A He has high blood pressure

The biopsy picture is consistent with malignant hypertension. The picture shows hyaline arteriosclerosis, and the vessel seen in the centre of the biopsy has a typical 'onion skin' appearance of the tunica media, with complete occlusion of the lumen. Vascular changes in the renal vessels from uncontrolled hypertension are a result of endothelial injury and intimal thickening. There are sub-endothelial lipid deposits and hyaline thrombi. Fibrinoid necrosis is seen in the small renal arteries.

Although this section of the biopsy looks to be severely damaged by hypertensive changes, it is impossible to comment on his prognosis based on one small segment. So, despite the fact that his renal function is already significantly impaired, it would be impossible to say that he needs immediate dialysis, although it is highly likely that renal function will continue to deteriorate over time, particularly if his blood pressure remains poorly controlled.

There is no evidence of an inflammatory or autoimmune condition in the history or on the biopsy, so starting immunosuppression is not appropriate.

It is possible that this patient could have IgA nephropathy as well as malignant hypertension, but again a larger biopsy sample including glomeruli is required to consider this diagnosis, as well as specific staining for IgA deposition. Serum IgA level is not used to make the diagnosis of IgA nephropathy.

Finally, it is not possible to comment on the extent of proteinuria just by looking at vessels on a renal biopsy. Hypertension can cause a degree of proteinuria, but nephrotic-range proteinuria indicates a glomerular lesion; there is insufficient biopsy material here to determine this.

20. C Prostate carcinoma

This patient has a diagnosis of retroperitoneal fibrosis (RPF) as seen by the inflammatory mass on the CT surrounding the aorta. He has presented with acute kidney injury secondary to obstruction from ureteric involvement (which may be as a result of reduced contractility as opposed to simply mechanical obstruction), causing hydronephrosis as seen on the imaging. There is also evidence on the CT of a nephrostomy tube in the left kidney to decompress the system.

RPF is a relatively uncommon condition and typically presents in men aged 40–60 years. It is characterised by extensive fibrosis throughout the retroperitoneum, and causes obstruction of the mid- to lower-third of the ureters. Renal impairment develops as a result of obstructive nephropathy. The exact pathogenesis of the condition is unknown, but it is believed to develop as an immunological response to antigens from atherosclerotic plaques on the aorta. It is frequently associated with aortic aneurysms.

RPF can also occur secondary to a variety of causes including drugs (classically beta-blockers, methysergide and methyldopa), lymphoma or other lymphoproliferative disorders, tuberculosis and metastatic malignancy. The patient should have a full CT to look for evidence of malignancy or lymphadenopathy, and the inflammatory mass should be biopsied to aid diagnosis. Immediate treatment is decompression of the renal tract with nephrostomy or ureteric stenting. Immunosuppression in the form of corticosteroids may reduce the inflammation and thus improve renal function, but there is an absence of evidence for long-term immunosuppression. Definitive surgery would include ureterolysis and omental wrapping.

Prostatic malignancy and hypertrophy can also present with bilateral hydronephrosis, but the level of obstruction would be lower (bladder outflow obstruction) and it would not be expected to cause the inflammatory para-aortic mass seen on the CT scan. Treatment of prostate cancer with radiotherapy could, however, cause RPF.

21. C Insert dialysis catheter and start haemodialysis

This patient has presented with end-stage renal failure and symptoms of uraemia. It is likely that he has had chronic kidney disease (CKD) for some time, which was not detected. He needs to start renal replacement therapy.

Sodium bicarbonate can be used to correct acidosis and control serum potassium. However, a large volume (2–3 L) would be needed to normalise the serum bicarbonate and this patient is already fluid overloaded. Although a blood transfusion would improve his symptoms, this should only be done on dialysis, because there is a risk of worsening fluid overload and hyperkalaemia. Aside from hyperkalaemia or severe/refractory acidosis, there are no absolute biochemical thresholds above which dialysis must be started. If serum urea increases gradually, it is often well tolerated until very high. The potassium in this case is not affecting the myocardium, and he is not in overt pulmonary oedema. His uraemic symptoms mean that dialysis is indicated.

The optimal 'access' for haemodialysis is an arterio-venous fistula (AVF), because of the reduced risk of thrombosis and infection in comparison to tunnelled dialysis catheters. However, an AVF takes around 6 weeks to mature, and this patient cannot wait that long to start dialysis.

There is nothing in the history to suggest a rapidly progressive glomerulonephritis; dipstick haematuria and proteinuria are often seen in advanced CKD, due to parenchymal scarring and hyperfiltration of the remaining nephrons. There is no indication for an urgent OGD because there is no evidence of active bleeding.

22. C Start on a single oral antihypertensive agent

Hypertensive crises can be defined as urgencies or emergencies. Features of a hypertensive emergency are encephalopathy, stroke, acute left ventricular failure and cardiac ischaemia. This patient presents as a hypertensive urgency, not an emergency. He does have evidence of target organ damage (left ventricular hypertrophy, renal impairment) but this is probably not acute as he has long-standing hypertension and no symptoms. There is nothing to suggest a dissection, but chest or back pain, or a discrepancy in blood pressure measured on each arm, would require urgent investigation.

He does have evidence of renal impairment, and blood and protein in his urine; this should be monitored. A renal biopsy is probably warranted, but this cannot be performed safely until his blood pressure is lowered. His renal function and urinary abnormalities may in fact improve with control of his blood pressure.

A hypertensive emergency should be treated with an intravenous infusion of antihypertensives, aiming for a blood pressure of 160/100 mmHg in the first day, and even lower if there is aortic dissection. Labetalol or glyceryl trinitrate are commonly used.

In this case a single oral agent can be used, for example, amlodipine 5 mg daily. Aim to bring the blood pressure down relatively slowly; a diastolic pressure of 100 mmHg is a reasonable initial target. Re-assess the patient every 2 days. It would not be reasonable to simply re-check the patient a week later; the presence of target organ damage means this is not 'white-coat hypertension' and needs immediate treatment.

Untreated, the 1-year mortality in severe hypertension is >90%; with treatment it is <10%.

Cherney D, et al. Management of patients with hypertensive urgencies and emergencies: A systematic review of the literature. J Gen Intern Med 2002; 17(12):937–945.
Steddon S, et al. Oxford Handbook of Nephrology and Hypertension. Oxford: Oxford University Press, 2006.

23. D Pure red cell aplasia (PRCA)

This patient has worsening anaemia despite adequate iron stores and erythropoietin treatment. It is not sufficient to attribute this to 'anaemia of chronic disease' as she should be able to maintain her haemoglobin with iron and erythropoietin therapy. The normal white cell count makes chronic lymphocytic leukaemia unlikely. Gastrointestinal blood loss would result in an iron deficiency anaemia: the normal mean corpuscular volume and elevated ferritin and transferrin go against this; elevated reticulocytes (indicating increased red cell production) may also been seen. Myelodysplasia is also unlikely with a normal white cell and platelet count.

The key abnormality here is the very low reticulocyte count, indicating reduced red cell production. Acquired pure red cell aplasia is a rare condition. It can be idiopathic, associated with underlying haematological/autoimmune disorders and viral infections, or secondary to neutralising autoantibodies against erythropoietin. The latter is the most likely cause in this case. Typically patients have been on erythropoietin for 6–18 months. PRCA is characterised by profound anaemia, very low/absent reticulocytes, and a virtual absence of erythroblasts in the bone marrow. Serum transferrin saturations and ferritin rise, as iron cannot be incorporated into new erythrocytes. Bone marrow aspirate should be performed and anti-erythropoietin antibodies measured. Treatment includes withdrawal of erythropoietin and transfusions for symptoms. Immunosuppressive treatment can be considered.

Casadeval N, et al. Epoetin-induced autoimmune pure red cell aplasia. J Am Soc Nephrol 2005; 16:S67–S69.

24. D Hepato-renal syndrome

This patient has presented with severe acute kidney injury (AKI) in the context of advanced liver disease with portal hypertension. Hepato-renal syndrome (HRS) should be considered a diagnosis of exclusion, as there are many other potential causes of AKI in such patients. There are two types of HRS: type 1 is characterised by a rapid onset of AKI with progressive oliguria, whereas type 2 is more chronic, with refractory ascites as the dominant feature. The pathophysiological mechanism is profound splanchnic vasodilatation, leading to effective systemic arterial blood volume depletion; this stimulates release of antidiuretic hormone (ADH) and aldosterone, leading to salt and water overload. The response of the renal vascular bed is physiological, with vasoconstriction and avid sodium retention. A urine sodium concentration of less than 10 mmol/L is traditionally seen as a cardinal feature of HRS, but this does not actually discriminate it from other forms of pre-renal AKI, so it is now thought to be less important.

This patient has signs of volume expansion and a low blood pressure, indicating a reduction in effective circulating volume and systemic vascular resistance. There is nothing to suggest hypovolaemia, but it is important to consider this: gastrointestinal haemorrhage is a far more common cause of AKI and should not be missed. Diuretic-induced hypovolaemia would manifest as progressive weight loss and elevated urinary sodium. Acute tubular necrosis typically results in elevated urinary sodium, as the tubules lose their concentrating ability. There would also be a history of infection or volume loss. Although lansoprazole can cause an interstitial nephritis, this is unlikely because it was not started recently. The bland urine dipstick result rules out mesangiocapillary glomerulonephritis (MCGN); similarly, diabetic nephropathy would be associated with proteinuria, and would not present so acutely.

The prognosis of HRS is very poor. Renal replacement therapy, if indicated, should only be considered as a bridge to liver transplantation, which is the only effective treatment.

Steddon S, et al. Oxford Handbook of Nephrology and Hypertension. Oxford: Oxford University Press, 2006.

25. B Continuous veno-venous haemofiltration (CVVHF)

This patient has presented with severe sepsis and acute kidney injury, most likely due to acute tubular necrosis (ATN). The associated mortality is high.

Although he is anaemic and would benefit from a blood transfusion, this is not safe at present – he is volume expanded, hyperkalaemic and oliguric. Equally, further fluid challenges will worsen fluid overload and pulmonary oedema once a patient is in established ATN. He is likely to require vasopressor support, but there is little evidence to support the use of 'renal dose' (i.e. low dose) dopamine or furosemide in the context of ATN.

Table 9.3 Intermittent haemodialysis versus continuous veno-venous haemofiltration		
	Intermittent haemodialysis	**Continuous veno-venous haemofiltration**
Location	Outpatient, inpatient, home	Mainly high-dependency/intensive care unit setting
Patients	Haemodynamically stable	Haemodynamically compromised
Principles	Intermittent	Slow and continuous
	No fluid replacement required	Fluid replacement required
	Dialysate required	No dialysate required
	Solute clearance by diffusion	Solute clearance by convection
Benefits	Independence for the well patient	Slower more controlled fluid shifts
	Form of long-term treatment	
Disadvantages	Large fluid shifts	High intensity care required
	Rapid correction of electrolytes	Temporary treatment

The combination of oliguria, volume overload and hyperkalaemia mean that renal replacement therapy (RRT) is required. The choice is between intermittent haemodialysis (IHD) or haemofiltration (CVVHF) – see **Table 9.3**. Haemofiltration is the appropriate treatment in this situation because it causes less haemodynamic instability. The patient has left ventricular impairment and a borderline blood pressure, so would be unlikely to tolerate haemodialysis, which involves faster blood flow through the extra-corporeal circuit. Haemofiltration is the most common method of renal replacement therapy in the intensive care unit, which is where this patient should be managed.

Ronco C, Bellomo R. Dialysis in intensive care unit patients with acute kidney injury: Continuous therapy is superior. Clin J Am Soc Nephrol 2007; 2(3):597–600.

26. E Parathyroidectomy

This patient has biochemical evidence of tertiary hyperparathyroidism. Secondary hyperparathyroidism develops in renal failure secondary to hypocalcaemia, hyperphosphataemia and low levels of activated vitamin D (hypocalcaemia is the prime stimulus). If this continues in an uncontrolled fashion (more often seen in patients who are non-compliant with vitamin D replacement and phosphate binders), hyperplasia of one or more of the four parathyroid glands can ensue, causing autonomous secretion of parathyroid hormone (tertiary hyperparathyroidism). This results in a very high parathyroid hormone level, hypercalcaemia, hyperphosphataemia and a raised alkaline phosphatase (indicating high bone turnover). Brown tumours (osteitis fibrosa cystica, the osteolytic lesions seen on the CT image) can develop as a result of excess osteoclast activity, causing bone deformity and pain.

Parathyroidectomy is the first line treatment for tertiary hyperparathyroidism. Cinacalcet is a calcimimetic agent that acts by lowering the threshold at which parathyroid hormone release is suppressed in the overactive parathyroid gland (essentially 'switching off' the hyperplastic tissue). It is used for treatment of refractory hyperparathyroidism in patients who are unfit for parathyoidectomy – there is no indication in the information given that this patient is unfit for surgery.

Calcium-based phosphate binders should be discontinued, but there no benefit in switching from sevelamer to aluminium hydroxide (another non-calcium-containing phosphate binder). The picture is not suggestive of metastatic cancer, so a full body CT is not justified. Increasing the alfacalcidol dose would further raise his serum calcium and phosphate, so this is not indicated.

The Renal Association. Clinical Practice Guideline: CKD-mineral and bone disorders. Bristol: The Renal Association, 2015.
National Institute for Health and Care Excellence (NICE). Technology Appraisal: Cinacalcet for the treatment of secondary hyperparathyroidism in patients with end-stage renal disease on maintenance dialysis therapy. London: NICE, 2007.

27. B Cryoglobulins

This man has acute kidney injury with an active urinary sediment and a rash. This makes some form of vasculitis likely. The low complement level narrows the differential diagnosis down. ANCA-associated vasculitis is not associated with hypocomplementaemia. Systemic lupus erythematosus (SLE) would be a possibility, but is unlikely in view of this patient's age, race and gender; therefore dsDNA antibodies are unlikely to help. Extractable nuclear antigens (ENA) are useful to distinguish between various connective tissue/autoimmune disorders if there is a positive antinuclear antibody (ANA); in this case we are not told that ANA is positive, thus ENA is not indicated. Erythrocyte sedimentation ratio is a non-specific marker of chronic inflammation, and will not help to establish a diagnosis.

The strongly positive rheumatoid factor, low complement (C4>C3), rash and acute kidney injury (AKI) all point towards cryoglobulinaemia. Cryoglobulins are a heterogeneous group of immunoglobulins which precipitate from plasma/serum at low temperatures (<37°C). There are many causes of cryoglobulinaemia and different ways to classify the condition, but essentially there are three categories. Type I (simple, monoclonal), which accounts for around 10% of cryoglobulinaemias, is associated with lymphoproliferative disorders; type II (mixed, monoclonal–polyclonal immune complex) and type III (mixed polyclonal–polyclonal immune complex), which account for 90% of cases, involve rheumatoid factor (an 'antibody to an antibody', typically IgM, forming complexes with the Fc portion of polyclonal IgG) and are almost always associated with hepatitis C infection.

Other important investigations would include hepatitis C (and B) serology, immunoglobulins, serum electrophoresis (warm), and a renal biopsy.

Ramos-Casals M, et al. The cryoglobulinaemias. Lancet 2012; 379:348–60.

28. C Disequilibrium syndrome

This patient has typical signs of disequilibrium syndrome. This is a central nervous system disorder that can develop during or immediately after haemodialysis. Early symptoms include headache, nausea, restlessness and blurred vision; this can progress to confusion, seizures and coma. The condition develops following rapid reduction of serum urea during haemodialysis; with insufficient time for urea equilibration across the blood-brain barrier, the resultant movement of water into the brain causes cerebral oedema. New dialysis patients are at highest risk, particularly those who are elderly with a high serum urea (>60 mmol/L). The first few dialysis sessions are therefore usually limited to a maximum of 2 hours, with slow blood flow rates and minimal fluid removal; this is usually adequate to reduce serum urea and potassium to safe levels, and avoid disequilibrium syndrome. If disequilibrium does develop, dialysis should be stopped and seizures should be treated along standard lines.

There is no indication here that the patient has had an arrhythmia, and her potassium has been lowered effectively. There are no features of sepsis in the vignette. A dialyser reaction would typically occur shortly after starting dialysis (usually within 30 minutes), and presents as an anaphylactoid reaction. An intracranial bleed is a possibility, but she has had heparin-free dialysis and the lack of focal neurological signs goes against this. She should, however, have a CT to formally exclude this diagnosis.

Levy J, et al. The Oxford Handbook of Dialysis, 3rd edn. Oxford: Oxford University Press, 2009.

29. C Mesna

This patient has tumour lysis syndrome (TLS). TLS occurs at initiation of treatment of malignancies, most commonly haematological. It may also occur spontaneously if the tumour burden is large. Hyperuricaemia, resulting from necrosis of large numbers of malignant cells, is the main cause of renal injury. Other sequelae of cell lysis are hyperkalaemia (which can rise rapidly as lysed cells release their contents), hyperphosphataemia, and elevated lactate dehydrogenase.

Ideally, at-risk patients should be identified, pre-hydrated with 0.9% sodium chloride, and given prophylactic allopurinol.

In established TLS, treatment includes aggressive fluid resuscitation to maintain a high urine output, and allopurinol to prevent the metabolism of xanthine to uric acid. Sodium bicarbonate can be used to alkalinise the urine and reduce precipitation of uric acid crystals, although maintaining a diuresis with sodium chloride is usually sufficient. Rasburicase is a recombinant version of the enzyme urate oxidase, which metabolises uric acid to allantoin. Treatment of hyperkalaemia, which would include calcium gluconate to stabilise the myocardium, may be required; haemodialysis is often also required.

Mesna is used to prevent haemorrhagic cystitis in patients treated with ifosfamide or cyclophosphamide.

Howard SC, et al. The tumour lysis syndrome. N Engl J Med 2011; 364:1844–1854.

30. A Allergic granulomatosis and angiitis (Churg–Strauss syndrome)

This patient presents with classic features of all granulomatosis and angiitis, also termed Churg–Strauss syndrome (CSS). CSS is a small and medium vessel vasculitis that typically presents with allergic rhinitis, asthma and eosinophilia, usually in the third to fifth decades. There are three stages of the disease: initially the allergic phase in which asthma begins, then the eosinophilic stage characterised by eosinophilic infiltration of various organs, and finally the vasculitic phase in which patients present with symptoms of a systemic vasculitis. Around 30% of patients have renal involvement, many of whom will have a rapidly progressive glomerulonephritis (RPGN). Antineutrophil cytoplasmic antibody (ANCA) is usually positive, and it is most commonly associated with myeloperoxidase (MPO) antibodies. The patient displays the classic picture of worsening asthma, eosinophilia, abdominal pain and diarrhoea (which usually indicates mesenteric vasculitis).

Granulomatosis and polyangiitis (Wegener's granulomatosis) is a possibility, but this is not associated with asthma or eosinophilia. Proteinase 3 (PR 3) ANCA are usually raised.

A post-infectious glomerulonephritis (GN) can also cause a necrotising GN on biopsy, but this is usually accompanied by hypocomplementaemia. Tubulo-interstitial nephritis does not cause a necrotising GN, and is not associated with ANCA.

Although strongyloides could be responsible for some of the gastrointestinal and even respiratory symptoms, with an eosinophilia, it would not be associated with an ANCA, or a rapidly progressive glomerulonephritis.

Jennette J et al. Pathogenesis of antineutrophil cytoplasmic autoantibody associated small vessel vasculitis. Ann Rev Pathol 2013; 8:139–160.
Katzenstein AL. Diagnostic features and differential diagnosis of Churg–Strauss syndrome in the lung. Am J Clin Pathol 2000; 114:767–772.

31. E Renal vein thrombosis

There are many causes for renal transplant dysfunction in the early postoperative period. Distinguishing between them relies on the clinical history and the timing of the deterioration, as well as findings on renal biopsy.

Acute tubular necrosis (ATN) is a common cause of delayed graft function and is usually seen in cadaveric organs with a long 'cold ischaemic time' (the time between removal from the donor and implantation into the recipient). Living donor transplants usually have a very short cold ischaemic time as the two operations (removal and implantation) are started at the same time. Deceased donor transplants frequently have to travel long distances between donor and recipient, so ATN is expected in the first few postoperative days. In this case the urine output is initially good, followed by a sudden reduction; in the absence of any other insult (such as hypotension), this is typical of ATN.

Graft pyelonephritis within 24 hours of implantation would be unusual. Hyperacute rejection occurs within minutes of implantation and manifests as a mottling of the transplant soon after it is perfused, and is very rare in the modern era, thanks to more sophisticated cross-matching techniques. Ureteric obstruction would also be uncommon at this early stage as it is standard practice to place a ureteric stent and urethral catheter during the operation. Extrinsic compression from a postoperative collection can cause a degree of obstruction, but this is unlikely to cause such a sudden reduction in urine output.

The abrupt onset of this problem points towards a vascular complication. Renal vein thrombosis is a relatively rare complication (incidence of up to 3%), but it usually results in graft loss. It can be caused by technical problems or a pro-thrombotic state (e.g. anti-phospholipid syndrome, seen in some patients with lupus nephritis), but often no cause is found. If suspected, an urgent ultrasound should be performed, with Doppler assessment of the renal vein and artery. Thrombectomy can be attempted but nephrectomy is common.

32. B Oxalate nephropathy

Microscopic examination of the urine is an essential part of the work-up for patients with renal impairment. All of the options given are causes of crystalluria.

Oxalate nephropathy is characterised by progressive, irreversible kidney damage due to hyperoxaluria. Hyperoxaluria can be primary (due to an inherited liver enzyme deficiency), dietary (due to intake of oxalate-rich foods, such as spinach and rhubarb), or enteric. Oxalate nephropathy should be suspected in any patient with chronic kidney disease and a history of fat malabsorption. Other causes include chronic pancreatitis, bariatric surgery and long-term use of orlistat. Binding of calcium with unabsorbed fatty acids reduces the amount of calcium available to bind with oxalate (which is present in most plant-derived foods), causing excess oxalate absorption. Urinary excretion leads to precipitation of calcium oxalate as crystals or calculi, and eventually nephrocalcinosis. Diagnosis is confirmed by 24-hour urine collection for oxalate level.

Azathioprine and lansoprazole are not known to cause crystalluria. Cystinuria is a rare autosomal recessive disorder that causes cystine stones due to excessive urinary excretion. Urate crystals are negatively birefringent under polarised light. Ethylene glycol poisoning is another cause of calcium oxalate crystals, but this would be associated with acute kidney injury.

33. D Prognosis is good with steroids

The diagnosis is renal amyloid, as shown by the dense deposition of amorphous hyaline material in the glomerulus, with positive Congo red staining (this gives 'apple green' birefringence under polarised light, to complicate matters further). There are two main forms of amyloid that affect the kidney. AA amyloid is a reactive amyloid associated with chronic inflammatory conditions, such as rheumatoid arthritis, bronchiectasis, chronic abscesses and inflammatory bowel disease. It is also associated with familial Mediterranean fever, an autosomal recessive disorder that usually occurs in people of Mediterranean origin. AL amyloid, also known as primary amyloid, is caused by monoclonal light chains produced by a plasma cell dyscrasia.

Renal involvement typically presents with heavy proteinuria ± nephrotic syndrome and progressive renal impairment. Deposits of pale hyaline material are seen in the mesangium and the capillary loops on renal biopsy and electron microscopy will show amyloid fibrils.

If the diagnosis of amyloidosis is suspected, biopsy is the definitive investigation. In the absence of renal involvement or if renal biopsy is not possible, fine-needle fat-pad or rectal biopsy can be used, which are diagnostic in 80–90% of cases.

The prognosis depends on the type of amyloid (AL worse than AA) and the extent of organ involvement. Steroids alone will not suffice as a treatment. Treatment includes removing the cause, i.e. treating the plasma cell dyscrasia in AL and the underlying inflammation in AA. Chemotherapy with melphalan and steroids is used in AL, as is haematopoietic cell transplantation. Prognosis is very poor. In AA amyloid there may be a role for cytotoxic, immunosuppressive or anti-cytokine drugs. Newer agents that interfere with amyloid fibril development are under investigation.

Dember M. Amyloidosis-associated kidney disease. J Am Soc Nephrol 2006; 17:3458–3471.

34. B Cast nephropathy

The patient has presented with multiple myeloma. The clues here are lethargy, back pain, anaemia and otherwise unexplained renal impairment. In addition there is a high total protein count with a low normal albumin, suggesting an elevated globulin (this is the paraprotein). The biopsy shows cast nephropathy with large fractured casts within dilated and atrophied tubules; some inflammatory cells are also seen.

Myeloma may cause renal impairment in several ways. Cast nephropathy ('myeloma kidney') is the most common: light chains, or fractures of them, precipitate in the tubules, causing obstruction and toxicity. Other renal manifestations of myeloma include AA amyloidosis, light chain deposition disease, or hypercalcaemia-associated AKI,.

Renal involvement develops in 50% of patients with myeloma, and is associated with increased mortality. Cast nephropathy is a medical emergency and chemotherapy (bortezomib or thalidomide with dexamethasone) should be started as soon as possible, in order to switch off paraprotein production; dialysis is often required, but renal recovery is possible.

Cryoglobulinaemia causes glomerular abnormalities (typically membranoproliferative glomerulonephritis), and there is nothing in the history to suggest this as the diagnosis. With both a tubulo-interstitial nephritis (TIN) and sarcoidosis (which causes a TIN) you would expect a much denser inflammatory cell infiltrate in the interstitium than seen here, with granulomas in the case of sarcoid. Neither of these conditions would cause large casts in the tubules.

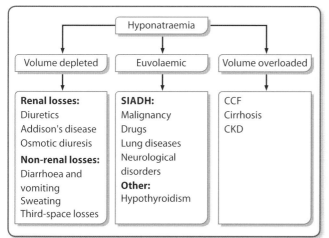

Figure 9.7 Approach to diagnosing hyponatraemia. CCF, congestive cardiac failure; CKD, chronic kidney disease; SIADH, syndrome of inappropriate antidiuretic hormone secretion

35. A 0.9% NaCl intravenously

When approaching hyponatraemia and its treatment it is vital to consider the underlying cause and, in particular, identify the patient's volume status (see **Figure 9.7**). Hyponatraemia can occur in the context of volume depletion, volume overload or euvolaemia; the causes and – importantly – treatments are very different.

Symptomatic hyponatraemia occurs when serum sodium concentration drops rapidly or to a level below around 125 mmol/L. In this case the patient is clearly volume deplete: she has orthostatic hypotension, a resting tachycardia, and a history consistent with volume loss (diarrhoea, as well as taking a thiazide diuretic). The urinary osmolality is difficult to interpret in the context of diuretic use, but in general a high urine osmolality is associated with diuretic use, adrenal insufficiency, cerebral salt wasting, salt-wasting nephropathy and the syndrome of inappropriate antidiuretic hormone secretion (SIADH).

In this case, the appropriate treatment is to restore euvolaemia and address the underlying causes. 0.9% saline is the appropriate fluid to use. Hypertonic saline should only be used if the patient has signs of cerebral oedema (confusion, impaired consciousness, papilloedema, seizure) – whatever the cause of the hyponatraemia – and is generally administered in a high-dependency setting with access to frequent blood sampling, aiming to quickly raise the serum sodium by around 5 mmol/L.

Unless there is clear evidence of acute (onset <48 hours) hyponatraemia, correction of the serum sodium should not exceed 10 mmol/L per day, in order to avoid central pontine myelinolysis (a catastrophic complication). Patients with hyponatraemia in the context of fluid overload or euvolaemia should be fluid restricted to <1 L/24 hours. If SIADH is diagnosed (hyponatraemia not on diuretics, euvolaemic, normal renal/adrenal/thyroid function, urine sodium, urine osmolality) demeclocycline or tolvaptan, which block the effects of antidiuretic hormone, may be used.

Sterns RH, et al. The treatment of hyponatraemia. Semin Nephrol 2009; 29(3):282–299.
Schrier RW, et al. Tolvaptan, a selective oral vasopressin V2-receptor antagonist, for hyponatraemia. N Engl J Med 2006; 355:2099–2112.

36. A Aciclovir

This patient has an acute kidney injury and is on many potentially toxic drugs. The distinguishing finding is crystalluria. Drugs that can precipitate as crystals include antivirals (aciclovir and indinavir), methotrexate and some antibiotics (sulfadiazine, amoxicillin). Needle-shaped birefringent needles are typical of aciclovir toxicity, and directly damage renal tubules.

Allopurinol itself is not nephrotoxic, but the dose should be adjusted in renal impairment. It should not be given with azathioprine as this can cause severe bone marrow suppression.

Ciclosporin is a commonly used immunosuppressant in renal transplantation, which must be monitored closely using trough levels because it can also be nephrotoxic at higher levels. Nephrotoxicity can result from acute tubular necrosis, arteriolar vasoconstriction, fibrosis and a thrombotic microangiopathy.

Co-trimoxazole is not nephrotoxic but must be dose-adjusted in renal impairment. It can cause leucopenia.

Mycophenolate mofetil typically causes gastrointestinal side effects; it can also cause leucopenia.

37. E Renal artery stenosis

This woman presents with uncontrolled hypertension, which is not acute – she has evidence of target organ damage with established retinopathy. This is not likely to be due to an acute glomerulonephritis as she is otherwise well and urinalysis is unremarkable. Patients with Bartter's syndrome have hypokalaemia, but they are usually normotensive (or hypotensive). Hypertension is common in Cushing's syndrome, affecting over 80% of patients, and this is associated with hypokalaemia; however, the normal serum glucose makes this unlikely. Coarctation of the aorta causes hypertension in children and young adults, more commonly in men. Clinically there would be higher blood pressure in the upper limbs, radio-femoral delay and a mid-systolic murmur. A chest X-ray may show rib notching and a 'figure-3' sign in the upper mediastinum from pre- and post-stenotic dilatation of the aorta.

Renal artery stenosis (RAS) refers to atherosclerotic narrowing of the larger renal vessels. It typically presents with hypertension which is difficult to control, and evidence of salt and water overload. Renal function is often impaired and potassium is characteristically low, due to activation of the renin-aldosterone system. It does not cause abnormalities on urine dipstick testing. A difference in kidney size of more than 1.5 cm on ultrasound suggests the diagnosis, which is confirmed with an isotope test (captopril MAG-3), CT or MR angiography. A large-scale trial found no significant benefit from angioplasty, over medical therapy alone.

The ASTRAL investigators. Revascularization versus medical therapy for renal-artery stenosis. N Engl J Med 2009; 361:1953–1962.

38. E Type 4 renal tubular acidosis

This patient has evidence of a renal tubular acidosis shown by low serum bicarbonate and a low urinary pH. Broadly speaking, the renal tubular acidoses (RTAs) are divided into proximal and distal, and differentiating between them involves interpreting the clinical context as well as the results of serum and urine biochemistry. They all cause a normal anion gap (hyperchloraemic) acidosis, as in this case.

Type 1 (distal) RTA is characterised by impaired secretion of H^+ in the collecting duct. It manifests as a hyperchloraemic hypokalaemic metabolic acidosis, and is associated with renal stones and hypophosphataemic metabolic bone disease. It can occur secondary to Sjögren's syndrome, systemic lupus erythematosus, rheumatoid arthritis, amyloidosis, analgesic nephropathy and lithium toxicity. Typically, serum potassium is low, serum bicarbonate is very low (<10 mmol/L) and the urine pH is >5.3. The urinary anion gap (u-AG = u-$[Na^+ + K^+]$ – u-$[Cl^-]$) is positive.

In type 2 (proximal) RTA, impaired reabsorption of bicarbonate in the proximal tubule causes bicarbonate wasting and systemic acidosis; it also presents as a hyperchloraemic hypokalaemic metabolic acidosis. It is caused by myeloma, amyloidosis, Wilson's disease, heavy metal toxicity and drugs (aminoglycosides, acetazolamide and antiretrovirals). Typically serum potassium is low, serum bicarbonate is low (12–20 mmol/L) and the u-AG is positive. Patients often present with other features of proximal tubular dysfunction, known as Fanconi's syndrome. Fanconi's syndrome is marked by failure to absorb many substances by the proximal tubules, including amino acids and phosphate, and often presents with bone pain and osteomalacia. Serum phosphate is low and there is glucosuria and proteinuria (tubular proteins, rather than albumin).

Type 4 RTA is much more common than types 1 or 2. It is caused by hypoaldosteronism, which results in a hyperkalaemic metabolic acidosis. It is most commonly seen in elderly diabetics, but can also be caused by drugs (particularly ciclosporin and non-steroidal anti-inflammatory drugs), obstructive uropathy and Addison's disease. Typically, the acidosis is mild (bicarbonate above16 mmol/L), and urinary pH is <5.3. The u-AG is positive.

Confusingly, there is no type 3 RTA.

Steddon S, et al. Oxford Handbook of Nephrology and Hypertension. Oxford: Oxford University Press, 2006.

39. C Oral captopril

This patient has presented with a scleroderma renal crisis (SRC). This is a rare complication of systemic sclerosis, characterised by severe hypertension and acute kidney injury.

The clues to the diagnosis here are the symptoms of scleroderma (Raynaud's and oesophageal dysmotility), pulmonary fibrosis, and the pattern of autoantibodies. Limited cutaneous systemic sclerosis (lcSSc) is usually associated with anti-centromere antibodies, whereas diffuse cutaneous systemic sclerosis (dcSSc), which more often affects other organs, is associated with anti-scl-70 and anti-RNP antibodies. Antinuclear antibodies are frequently positive in both types of SSc.

SRC is far more common in dcSSc. The hallmark is a rapidly progressive, obliterative arteriolar vasculopathy, leading to organ ischaemia and haemolytic anaemia. In the kidney, collapsed (ischaemic) glomeruli are seen, and blood vessels show typical 'onion skin' changes from hypertensive damage. A rapid decline in the glomerular filtration rate (GFR) ensues, associated with oliguria and bland urinalysis. Untreated, SRC can be rapidly fatal.

Treatment of SRC is prompt blood pressure control using angiotensin-converting enzyme inhibitors (ACEIs); captopril is the preferred agent as it has a rapid onset and short duration of action, so can be titrated easily. Unless there are signs of left ventricular failure or hypertensive encephalopathy, the aim is to gradually reduce the systolic blood pressure by 10% per day. Up to 40% of patients require renal replacement therapy.

A renal biopsy is not safe with such high blood pressure, nor is it essential to make the diagnosis. Intravenous labetalol can be used, but it is not the first line antihypertensive agent. Plasma exchange and steroids have no role in the management of SRC (high-dose steroids can in fact provoke a crisis).

UK Scleroderma Study Group. Consensus best practice recommendations: management of scleroderma renal crisis. London: UK Scleroderma Study Group, 2013.
Steddon S, et al. Oxford Handbook of Nephrology and Hypertension. Oxford: Oxford University Press, 2006.

40. E Thiazide diuretic

Hypernatraemia is relatively rare and should not generally be seen where there is free access to water. Groups of patients who are more susceptible are very young and elderly people and those who are otherwise unwell.

Broadly speaking, hypernatraemia is caused by an excess of hypertonic fluids (intravenous infusions, enteral or parenteral nutrition), excess water loss and decreased thirst (in the risk groups mentioned above). Water loss may be renal (diabetes insipidus, diuretics, osmotic diuresis), gastrointestinal (diarrhoea and vomiting, nasogastric losses) or from the skin (sweating, burns).

Treatment involves identifying and treating the underlying cause and aiming to restore normal sodium values. If the hypernatraemia is acute then it may be reversed quickly. If chronic (>24 hours), it should be corrected slowly at a rate of no more than 0.5 mmol/L per hour. The most appropriate fluid resuscitation is water by mouth or via nasgastric tube. If it must be given intravenously then either 0.45% saline or 5% dextrose can be used.

The diagnosis of diabetes insipidus (DI) can be made here partly based on clinical information – he is polyuric, suggesting an increased renal loss, there is no history of diuretic use and he does not have diabetes mellitus, making an osmotic diuresis unlikely. The diagnosis is supported by lab results, which show inappropriately dilute urine. DI can be either cranial or nephrogenic. Cranial causes include infections, vasculitis, tumours, tuberculosis or trauma, and the treatment is desmopressin (DDAVP). Nephrogenic DI, on the other hand, is often drug-induced (particularly lithium, which renders the distal tubules resistant to the actions of vasopressin) but may also be congenital, secondary to hypercalcaemia or medullary cystic disease. The treatment is with a thiazide diuretic, which causes reduced water delivery to the collecting duct. Non-steroidal anti-inflammatory drugs, which antagonise the effect of antidiuretic hormone, can also be used.

Waise A, Fisken RA. Unsuspected Nephrogenic Diabetes Insipidus. BMJ 2001; 323:96–97.

41. B Creatinine clearance changing from 125 mL/min in the 1st trimester to 90 mL/min in the 3rd trimester

There are many physiological changes that affect the kidneys during pregnancy, reflecting increased renal blood flow and glomerular filtration rate (GFR). These begin as early as 6 weeks' gestation. Effective renal blood flow increases from around 480 mL/min pre-pregnancy to a peak of around 890 mL/min in the 2nd trimester. With this, the GFR and creatinine clearance rise, peaking in the 2nd trimester, and thus it would definitely be abnormal for creatinine clearance to fall from the 1st to 2nd trimester. A fall in creatinine, conversely, simply reflects the increased GFR.

A degree of proteinuria is often seen, secondary to changes in renal haemodynamics and tubular function. This is usually no more than 260 mg/24 h. Changes in tubular function can also cause glycosuria, which does not necessarily indicate impaired glucose tolerance. If glycosuria is persistent or heavy, a glucose tolerance test is warranted.

Finally, changes in fluid status, including an increase in total body water of up to 8 L, can cause mild hyponatraemia. The normal sodium concentration is around 132–140 µmol/L.

Williams D, Davison J. Chronic kidney disease in pregnancy. BMJ 2008; 336:211–215.

42. E Tubulo-interstitial nephritis

Disease recurrence in a renal transplant affects up to 10–20% of patients and accounts for around 5% of graft failures at 10 years.

Primary focal segmental glomerulosclerosis has a recurrence rate of around 20–30%, and can occur within days of transplantation. It is thought to lead to graft loss in around 50% of cases. IgA nephropathy also commonly recurs with rates quoted between 20% and 60%. Progression of disease is usually slow but can result in graft loss in the long term.

Mesangiocapillary glomerulonephritis (MCGN), particularly type II, has also been seen to recur in allografts. Rates of between 50% and 100% are quoted for MCGN type II.

Other primary diseases that may recur include membranous nephropathy and atypical haemolytic uraemic syndrome.

Various systemic diseases also recur in the transplanted kidney, the most common of which are lupus nephritis and diabetic nephropathy.

Tubulo-interstitial nephritis is commonly secondary to drugs, or less commonly tuberculosis and sarcoid, and is not reported to recur in renal transplants.

Golgert WA, et al. Recurrent glomerulonephritis after renal transplantation: An unsolved problem. Clin J Am Soc Nephrol 2008; 3(3):800–807.

43. A Ethylene glycol ingestion

Oxalate crystals can be ovoid or pyramidal in shape and are present in hyperoxaluria or hypercalciuria. They are also a diagnostic clue in ethylene glycol poisoning. Another clue in his investigations is the raised anion gap (AG) acidosis (AG = 26 here, normal 8–16, calculate by $[Na^+ + K^+] - [Cl^- + HCO^{-3}]$).

Ethylene glycol itself causes inebriation but, more harmfully, is metabolised in the liver by successive oxidations to toxic metabolites responsible for the symptoms seen. One of these is glycolic acid; this is metabolised to oxalic acid, which can precipitate as calcium oxalate crystals in the urine. Classically, there are three clinical stages of presentation. Stage 1 is the central nervous system stage where patients display depression, ataxia, speech slurring, hallucination, convulsions, coma and vomiting. Stage 2 is the cardiorespiratory stage with tachycardia, tachypnoea, hypertension, pulmonary oedema, pneumonitis and shock. Finally, stage 3 is the renal stage with proteinuria, haematuria, flank pain, crystalluria and acute kidney injury. Renal biopsy shows acute tubular necrosis, and calcium oxalate crystals in the tubules.

Although rhabdomyolysis can cause a raised AG acidosis, there are no other clues pointing to rhabdomyolysis in the history, apart from the collapse, and it would not explain the patient's cardiovascular, respiratory or neurological symptoms, or crystalluria.

Severe sepsis, often with a raised lactate, can cause a raised AG acidosis, but again pneumonia would not account for all of the other symptoms in this patient.

Salicylate poisoning causes neurological signs and pulmonary oedema, as well as an increased AG acidosis, but does not cause acute kidney injury. Haemodialysis can be used to effectively remove salicylate.

Although a small vessel vasculitis might account for some of the patient's constitutional and neurological symptoms (vasculitis is most commonly associated with mononeuritis multiplex or peripheral neuropathy), this would not cause crystalluria.

Chapter 10

Respiratory medicine

Questions

1. A 74-year-old man was referred to the chest clinic from the emergency department. He presented following a fall on ice and was treated with simple analgesia for a minor soft tissue injury. No other injuries were sustained. He was otherwise fit and well with no history of cough, shortness of breath, chest pain or weight loss. He stopped smoking 20 years ago. He was a retired dock-yard ship-builder.

   Clinical examination was normal.

   Chest X-ray: see **Figure 10.1.**

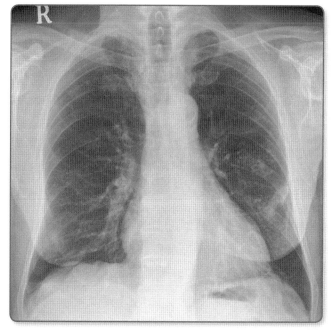

Figure 10.1

Which one of the following statements is least likely regarding the diagnosis?

A   Benign asbestos-related pleural effusions usually occur within 10 years of exposure
B   Diffuse pleural thickening may be seen in patients with a history of heavy asbestos exposure
C   High-resolution CT is more sensitive than chest X-ray in detecting pleural plaques
D   Pleural plaques are a premalignant finding
E   Pleural plaques are usually asymptomatic

2. A 21-year-old female student nurse was referred to the chest clinic for further advice following pre-employment screening. She was asymptomatic and had been previously well with no past medical history of note. She was born in London; her parents emigrated to the UK from Bangladesh 40 years ago. She lived with her parents and her three siblings and had had frequent holidays to visit relatives in Bangladesh. She received a BCG vaccine at school aged 13 years as confirmed by a scar on her left deltoid.

   Physical examination was normal.

   Investigations:

Mantoux test: 18 mm (<5 mm negative, 5–14 mm positive, >15 mm strongly positive)
Chest X-ray: lungs are clear normal mediastinal contours
Interferon release assay: positive

   What is the most appropriate next step in management?

   A Bronchoscopy
   B Chest physiotherapy for induced sputum sampling with hypertonic saline
   C CT of the chest
   D Start quadruple therapy with rifampicin, isoniazid, pyrazinamide and ethambutol
   E Treat with rifampicin and isoniazid

3. An 84-year-old man, presented to the emergency department with a 5-day history of increased breathlessness and a cough productive of green sputum. He felt tired and lethargic and had lost his appetite. His exercise tolerance had decreased such that he was short of breath on minimal exertion (baseline exercise tolerance 10 metres). He had a history of severe chronic obstructive pulmonary disease (COPD), diabetes and osteoarthritis.

   On examination, he was alert, but appeared tired. He had a low-grade fever 37.8°C and was haemodynamically stable. He was able to speak in short sentences with a respiratory rate of 34 breaths per minute. He was centrally cyanosed. Pulse oximetry showed oxygen saturation of 87% on air and 91% on 2 L/min O_2 via nasal cannulae. On auscultation, there was widespread mild wheeze.

   Investigations:

white cell count 14.3 × 10⁹/L (4–11) neutrophils 10.8 × 10⁹/L (1.5–7.0)	C-reactive protein 76 mg/L (<10)
Chest X-ray: emphysematous change in keeping with COPD no focal consolidation or mass lesion seen	
Arterial blood gases on arrival (on 2 L/min O_2 via nasal cannulae): pH 7.35 (7.35–7.45) $PaCO_2$ 7.6 kPa (4.7–6.0)	PaO_2 7.3 kPa (11.3–12.6) base excess 4 mmol/L (± 2)

   He was commenced on antibiotics, steroids, and nebulised salbutamol and ipratropium.

   What is the most appropriate next step in management?

   A Aminophylline infusion
   B Continue present treatment and re-assess within 1 hour
   C Doxapram infusion

D   Non-invasive ventilation
E   Reduce oxygen to 1 L/min via nasal cannulae and re-assess within 1 hour

4.   A 68-year-old woman presented with a 12-hour history of left-sided pleuritic chest pain and shortness of breath. She had a past medical history of hypertension and a right mastectomy for breast cancer 5 months ago. Her current medications included amlodipine and tamoxifen.

On examination, she appeared to be in moderate discomfort, but was alert and oriented and with good peripheral perfusion. Her pulse was 118 beats per minute, blood pressure 130/80 mmHg, respiratory rate 22 breaths per minute and oxygen saturation 91% on room air. Heart sounds were normal and chest was clear on auscultation. There was some swelling and tenderness of the left calf.

Investigations:

> Chest X-ray: blunting of the left costophrenic angle

What is the most useful diagnostic investigation?

A   CT pulmonary angiogram (CTPA)
B   D-dimer
C   Echocardiogram
D   Isotope lung scan
E   Doppler ultrasound of the left leg

5.   A 23-year-old female nursing student attended the chest clinic for routine review. She had had asthma since the age of 5 years and had needed multiple hospital admissions, including one admission to an intensive therapy unit for mechanical ventilation and four admissions over the past 12 months with severe exacerbations of asthma. She was a non-smoker. She had good compliance with her medications, which included: budesonide 200 µg/formoterol fumarate 6 µg two inhalations twice daily, salbutamol 100 µg two inhalations as required – used about 8 times per day, montelukast 10 mg daily and, for the last year, a maintenance dose of prednisolone 20 mg daily. She was intolerant of oral theophyllines.

Investigations:

> Skin-prick tests:
> strong positive reaction to house-dust mite
> negative for other common aeroallergens
>
> total IgE 308 IU/mL (<30)

What is the most appropriate next step in management?

A   Adrenaline by intramuscular injection for self-administration in case of emergencies
B   Aminophylline modified-release tablets
C   Home nebuliser with salbutamol and ipratropium nebulised solutions
D   Maintenance dose of prednisolone should be increased to 40 mg daily
E   Trial of omalizumab

6.   A 74-year-old woman presented with a 2-year history of increasing shortness of breath on exertion and a cough productive of white sputum. Her symptoms had not responded to three courses of antibiotics. There was no history of any fevers, night sweats or weight loss. She was born in Bangladesh and came to live in the UK 10 years ago. Her exercise tolerance was limited to 50 metres at a gentle pace. She had type 2 diabetes mellitus and hypertension. She had no previous history of respiratory illness and had never smoked. She had no known tuberculosis

contacts. She was a housewife and lived with her extended family. Her current medications included gliclazide, amlodipine, aspirin and salbutamol.

On examination, her oxygen saturation was 93% breathing room air and respiratory rate 24 breaths per minute. Chest auscultation revealed mild scattered wheeze. She also had mild ankle swelling. There was no BCG scar.

Investigations:

Spirometry:

FEV$_1$ 0.60 L (normal range 1.18–1.26)   FVC 1.20 L (normal range 1.60–1.72)

FEV$_1$ post-BD 0.62 L   FVC post-BD 1.18 L

(FEV$_1$, forced expiratory volume in 1 second; FVC, forced vital capacity; BD, bronchodilator)

What is the most likely diagnosis?

A   Adult onset asthma
B α_1-Antitrypsin deficiency
C   Congestive cardiac failure
D   Chronic obstructive pulmonary disease (COPD) secondary to biomass fuel exposure
E   Tuberculosis

7. A 46 year old woman presented to the respiratory clinic with progressive shortness of breath and a rash. Her shortness of breath had progressed over the preceding 10 years, and she had been prescribed a salbutamol inhaler by her GP which had not really improved her symptoms. She had no other past medical history. She was a current smoker, with a 4-pack per year history.

On examination she was comfortable at rest with erythematous plaques and tender nodules on her abdomen and the proximal aspect of her arms. One of the nodules had ulcerated and an oily discharge was noted. Respiratory examination revealed hyperinflation and a mild expiratory wheeze.

What is the most likely diagnosis?

A   PiZZ α_1-antitrypsin deficiency
B   PiMS α_1-antitrypsin deficiency
C   PiSS α_1-antitrypsin deficiency
D   PiMZ α_1-antitrypsin deficiency
E   PiSZ α_1-antitrypsin deficiency

8. A 28-year-old woman was referred to the medical admissions unit after consulting her obstetrician. She was 26 weeks' pregnant with her first child. 6 hours ago, she had sudden-onset, left-sided pleuritic chest pain and shortness of breath. The obstetrician examined her and reassured her that there were no concerns with the progression of the pregnancy, but requested a medical review. She had no past medical history of note.

On examination, she appeared anxious, but was comfortable at rest. Her pulse was 102 beats per minute and regular, blood pressure 110/84 mmHg, respiratory rate 24 breaths per minute and oxygen saturation 95% on air. Auscultation of the chest revealed a pleural rub at the left base. She had mild swelling of the ankles bilaterally.

Investigations:

Chest X-ray: small left pleural effusion and peripheral dome shaped pleural based opacity left base

---

Electrocardiogram: rate 102 beats per minute, sinus rhythm

What is the most appropriate next investigation?

A CT pulmonary angiogram
B D-dimer
C Doppler ultrasound of the legs
D Echocardiogram
E Ventilation/perfusion scan

9. A 23-year-old man presented to the emergency department complaining of sudden-onset, right-sided chest pain and shortness of breath. He had no past medical history of note.
    On examination, he appeared distressed with pain, respiratory rate was 24 breaths per minute, oxygen saturation 97% breathing FiO_2 (inspired oxygen fraction) 0.6 via a facemask, blood pressure 110/74 mmHg and heart rate 98 beats per minute. There were reduced breath sounds on the right.
    An urgent chest X-ray was performed: see **Figure 10.2**.

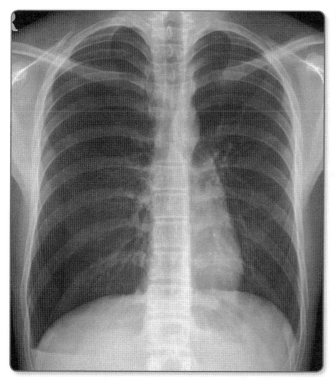

Figure 10.2

What is the most appropriate next step in management?

A Continue high-flow oxygen and observe
B Needle aspiration in right second intercostal space in the mid-clavicular line
C Insertion of large-bore surgical chest drain
D Ultrasound-guided chest drain insertion using small-bore tube in right mid-axillary line in fifth intercostal space
E Ultrasound-guided needle aspiration anterior to right mid-axillary line in fifth intercostal space

10. A 23-year-old woman presented to her general practitioner complaining of a cough, night sweats, shortness of breath and weight loss. She was born in China and had lived in the UK for 5 years.

Investigations:

haemoglobin 102 g/L (115–165)	lymphocytes 2.5×10^9/L (1.5–4.0)
white cell count 24.6×10^9/L (4–11)	neutrophils 20.8×10^9/L (1.5–7.0)
platelets 463×10^9/L (150–400)	monocytes 1.2×10^9/L (0–0.8)

Chest X-ray: see **Figure 10.3**

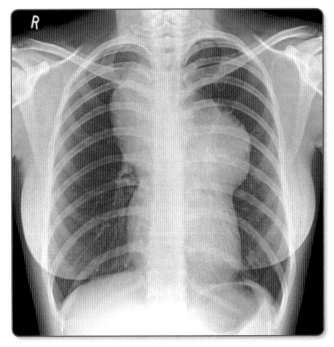

Figure 10.3

What is the most likely diagnosis?

A   Bronchogenic cyst
B   Germ cell tumour
C   Lymphoma
D   Retrosternal goitre
E   Thymoma

11. A 74-year-old woman was referred by her general practitioner to the chest clinic with a 3-year history of cough and progressive shortness of breath. Her general practitioner had prescribed her four courses of antibiotics and two short courses of steroids with little benefit. She was a non-smoker and was not taking any regular medication. She described a persistent cough productive of purulent sputum and had noticed a few episodes of blood streaking in the sputum. There was no weight loss or night sweats, but she did complain of lethargy. She had no known tuberculosis contact, but she had been admitted to hospital with a pneumonic illness in childhood.

What is the most appropriate diagnostic test?

A   Bronchoscopy
B   Chest X-ray
C   High-resolution CT of the chest
D   Serum α_1-antitrypsin level
E   Tuberculin skin test

12. A 24-year-old man with a history of asthma presented to the emergency department with a 2-day history of worsening wheeze and shortness of breath. His regular medication included budesonide/formoterol combination inhaler one puff twice daily and as required, plus montelukast. He was under outpatient follow-up with the respiratory clinic and a clinic letter stated that his best peak flow was 620 L/min.

On arrival he was alert but appeared tired and was unable to complete sentences, his oxygen saturation was 95% breathing 40% oxygen, respiratory rate 30 breaths per minute, pulse 130 beats per minute and on auscultation there was widespread wheeze. His peak flow was 180 L/min.

He was commenced on prednisolone, salbutamol nebulisers and continuous oxygen therapy (40%).

Investigations:

Chest X-ray: hyperexpanded lungs no acute lung pathology detected	
Electrocardiogram: 102 beats per minute, sinus rhythm	
Arterial blood gases on 40% oxygen: pH 7.37 (7.35–7.45)	$PaCO_2$ 4.2 kPa (4.7–6.0) PaO_2 14.3 kPa (11.3–12.6)

What is the most appropriate next step in management?

A   Increase oxygen therapy to 60%
B   Intravenous ketamine
C   Intravenous magnesium
D   Intravenous salbutamol
E   Intubation and mechanical ventilation

13. A 34-year-old man presented to the chest clinic with a 6-month history of increasing shortness of breath and a non-productive cough. He smoked 10 cigarettes per day. He had no past medical history of note and did not take any regular medication. He worked in an office with no exposure to dust or fumes. He did not keep any pets and had not recently travelled abroad.

On examination, he had finger clubbing and coarse crackles on auscultation of the lower zones. Oxygen saturation was 93% on air.

Investigations:

Chest X-ray: bilateral consolidation with thickened interlobular septa
CT of the chest: 'crazy paving pattern' of patchy airspace shadowing, with areas of normal lung
Bronchoalveolar lavage (BAL): profuse milky washings
BAL microscopy culture and sensitivity (MC&S): no organisms seen, culture negative
BAL acid-fast bacilli (AFB) / tuberculosis (TB) culture: AFB not seen, TB cultures negative
BAL cytology: granular, acellular, eosinophilic, PAS (periodic acid–Schiff)-positive deposits and foamy macrophages

What is the most appropriate treatment?

A   Antituberculous therapy
B   Co-trimoxazole
C   High-dose oral prednisolone
D   Pulsed intravenous methylprednisolone
E   Whole lung lavage

14. A 32-year-old woman was referred to the chest clinic following a third spontaneous left-sided pneumothorax. She reported shortness of breath on exertion and had previously suffered an episode of self-limiting haemoptysis. She also complained of abdominal bloating.
      Physical examination was normal.

Investigations:

Pulmonary function tests: no abnormality detected

Chest X-ray:
hyperinflated lungs with reticular shadowing
no mass lesion or pneumothorax seen

CT of the thorax:
multiple small (<1 cm) thin-walled cysts
small left-sided effusion

What is the most likely diagnosis?

A α_1-Antitrypsin deficiency
B   Catamenial pneumothorax
C   Cystic fibrosis
D   Lymphangioleiomyomatosis
E   Pulmonary Langerhans' cell histiocytosis

15. A 72-year-old man was referred to the medical admissions unit by his general practitioner. He had a 5-day history of cough with green sputum and left-sided chest pain. He was feverish and confused and had lost his appetite. He had type 2 diabetes mellitus, hypertension and hypercholesterolaemia. His medications included metformin, ramipril, simvastatin and aspirin. He was a non-smoker and lived with his wife.
      On examination, he was mildly confused, but oriented in time, place and person. He appeared flushed and was pyrexial at 38.4°C, but had cool peripheries with a systemic blood pressure of 108/58 mmHg. He had a respiratory rate of 24 breaths per minutes and oxygen saturation on air of 95%. There were coarse crackles audible in the left lower zone with dullness to percussion.

Investigations:

haemoglobin 154 g/L (130–180)	potassium 5.8 mmol/L (3.5–5.0)
white cell count 18.4 × 10⁹/L (4–11)	urea 13.4 mmol/L (2.5–7.5)
neutrophils 14.7 × 10⁹/L (1.5–7.0)	creatinine 178 µmol/L (60–110)
sodium 124 mmol/L (135–145)	

What is the most appropriate next step in management?

A   Admission to the high dependency unit for intensive monitoring
B   High-flow oxygen

C   Intravenous co-amoxiclav and clarithromycin
D   Intravenous hydrocortisone
E   Stop current medications, prescribe intravenous fluids, and oral amoxicillin and clarithromycin

16. A 16-year-old girl presented to the emergency department with a 3-day history of increasing shortness of breath, lethargy, fevers and right-sided neck discomfort. She had consulted her general practitioner 10 days previously complaining of a sore throat and was prescribed a 5-day course of erythromycin. She had no past medical history of note and did not take any regular medications. She was allergic to penicillin.

    On examination, she appeared unwell with a temperature of 38.6°C and pulse 110 beats per minute. There was tenderness of the right side of the neck. Examination of the oropharynx revealed mild erythema and bilateral tonsillar enlargement; no exudate seen. Examination of respiratory, abdominal and nervous systems was normal.

    Investigations:

Chest X-ray: thin-walled cavitating lesions in left mid-zone and right lower zone
HIV negative

    What is the most likely causative pathogen?

    A   *Cryptococcus neoformans*
    B   *Fusobacterium necrophorum*
    C   *Mycobacterium tuberculosis*
    D   *Pneumocystis jirovecii*
    E   *Staphylococcus aureus*

17. A 22-year-old male student attended a routine asthma clinic follow-up appointment. He was planning a trip to the Everest Base Camp. He suffered from mild asthma in early childhood, but had not needed to take any regular or reliever medications for more than 10 years. He had never smoked and was athletic, regularly competing in running events for his university.

    He was concerned about the potential risk of developing high-altitude pulmonary oedema.

    What is the most appropriate advice?

    A   Keep ascent to ≤300 m/day and rest every third day
    B   Keep ascent to ≤800 m/day and rest every fifth day
    C   Prophylactic dexamethasone
    D   Prophylactic nifedipine
    E   The trip should not be contemplated in view of his past medical history of asthma

18. A 36-year-old man was referred to the chest clinic following a routine medical examination as part of the visa application process for a 2-year secondment to America. He worked for a bank and had never smoked tobacco or other substances. He had no past medical history of note other than mild viral illnesses during early childhood, for which he did not require any specific treatment, and there was no family history of respiratory disease. He was fit and well.

    Investigations:

Chest X-ray: right lung appeared hyperlucent with reduced vascular marking and small pulmonary artery

    What is the most likely diagnosis?

    A a_1-Antitrypsin deficiency
    B   Congenital lobar emphysema

    C   Swyer–James–MacLeod syndrome
    D   Pneumothorax
    E   Pulmonary sequestration

19. A 29-year-old woman presented to the emergency department with a 3-day history of increased shortness of breath and wheeze. She had a history of minor coryzal symptoms and was coughing up yellow sputum. There was no history of chest pain, haemoptysis or leg swelling. She had a history of asthma, but had stopped her regular inhalers 6 weeks ago, after she discovered that she was pregnant and was concerned about the risk of steroid inhalers to the baby. Her prescribed medication consisted of a combination inhaled corticosteroid and long-acting b_2-agonist two puffs taken twice daily and as required. At presentation she was taking folic acid only and no other medication.

    On examination, she appeared stable and was able to speak in full sentences. She was afebrile. Respiratory rate was 14 breaths per minute and oxygen saturation 98% on air. There was mild wheeze throughout both lungs but no other added sounds. Peak flow rate (PEFR) was 520 L/min (patient's best previous PEFR was 540 L/min). Pulse was 80 beats per minute and blood pressure 110/76 mmHg.

    She was keen to go home. She lived with her husband and 2-year-old child. She agreed to return if her symptoms deteriorated and she was referred to the asthma clinic for further follow-up.

What is the most appropriate next step in management?

    A   Admit for regular nebulisers and observation
    B   Advise chest physiotherapy and relaxation techniques
    C   Amoxicillin and prednisolone
    D   Montelukast
    E   Restart regular inhaler corticosteroid and long-acting b_2-agonist

20. An 84-year-old man presented with haemoptysis of approximately three teaspoonfuls over the previous 24 hours. He had a 5-day history of cough productive of yellow sputum. There was no preceding history of weight loss, but he gave a 6-month history of general malaise which he had attributed to 'old age'. He had suffered from pulmonary tuberculosis in his teens and recalled that he was in hospital for 12 months. He had not had any operations. There was no other past medical history and he did not take any regular medication. He was a retired school teacher and there was no history of foreign travel or contact with industrial dusts or fumes. He was active and independent.

    One hour after arrival in the emergency department he suffered an episode of massive haemoptysis – approximately 1.5 L of fresh red blood. His pulse was 120 beats per minute and blood pressure 80/40 mmHg. He was able to maintain his own airway and his oxygen saturation was found to be 95% breathing high-flow oxygen.

    Large-bore venous access was gained and the intensive care teams were assisting in the resuscitation.

What is the most appropriate management?

    A   Arterial embolisation
    B   Fresh frozen plasma
    C   Itraconazole
    D   Surgical resection
    E   Tranexamic acid

21. A 28-year-old woman with cystic fibrosis attended for a routine follow-up appointment. She discussed with the specialist nurse that she was planning to start a family. Her genotype was ΔF508 /ΔF508. She had been well recently and had not suffered from any pulmonary exacerbations of the disease for 4 years. She did not take any regular antibiotics, performed twice daily chest physiotherapy and took regular mucolytic nebulisers. She had pancreatic insufficiency for which she took Creon 10,000 units as directed and vitamins A, D, E and K, folic acid and calcium supplements. Her husband was not a carrier of the common cystic fibrosis genes.

On examination, her chest was clear, her oxygen saturation was 97% on breathing room air and her body mass index was 17 kg/m^2.

Investigations:

> Spirometry:
> FEV$_1$ 91% predicted
> FVC 93% predicted

What is the most appropriate advice with regard to pregnancy?

A   Ciprofloxacin is the preferred antibiotic for a pulmonary exacerbation during pregnancy
B   Colomycin is the preferred antibiotic for a pulmonary exacerbation during pregnancy
C   Pregnancy should be avoided as there is a significant risk of lung function decline
D   She is unlikely to conceive without assisted conception
E   She should commence dietary supplements

22. A 54-year-old man attended the chest clinic accompanied by his wife, who complained that he was a heavy snorer and she slept in another bedroom as the snoring was so loud. The patient said he felt tired and lethargic during the day and needed to urinate at least three times during the night. His wife said that she had observed some episodes where he seemed to stop breathing and then woke up coughing and choking, but the patient did not recall these events. He often woke with a dry mouth and had occasional morning headaches.

    He had gained weight recently and wore a 46 cm (18") collar shirt. He smoked 20 cigarettes per day and drank 40 units of alcohol per week. He had hypertension and type 2 diabetes mellitus and his regular medications included metformin, ramipril and bendroflumethiazide. On examination, his weight was 110 kg and height 1.75 m giving a body mass index of 35 kg/m^2. He had no obvious craniofacial abnormality. His chest was clear.

Investigations:

> Epworth Sleepiness Score: 6/24 (<9)
>
> Sleep study: apnoea–hypopnea index 11.4/h (<5)

What is the most appropriate management?

A   Bariatric surgery
B   Continuous positive airway pressure
C   Dietary and lifestyle advice
D   Domiciliary non-invasive ventilation
E   Mandibular advancement device

23. A 76-year-old woman presented to the chest clinic complaining of a 4-month history of progressive shortness of breath, right-sided chest discomfort and a dry cough. She had weight loss of 2 kg and poor appetite. She had ischaemic heart disease, type 2 diabetes mellitus and hypertension. Two years ago, she had triple-vessel coronary artery bypass grafting (CABG) and had not experienced any further angina. She had stopped smoking 4 years ago. Her current medications included aspirin, bisoprolol, metformin, ramipril and simvastatin.

    Examination of the chest revealed reduced chest expansion on the right with dull percussion note and absent breath sounds.

    Thoracic ultrasound confirmed a large right pleural effusion and a diagnostic pleural tap was performed.

    Blood-stained fluid 20 mL was aspirated and sent for analysis together with matched venous samples:

Investigations:

Pleural fluid microbiology: Gram stain negative, no organisms seen, no growth after 5 days
Pleural fluid cytology: atypical, reactive mesothelial cells, no malignant cells seen
Pleural fluid biochemistry: protein 31 g/L lactate dehydrogenase 568 U/L glucose 4.9 mmol/L (>3.3) pH 7.4 (>7.4)
Venous biochemistry: total protein 54 g/L (60–76) lactate dehydrogenase 674 U/L (10–250) glucose 8.4 mmol/L (fasting 3.0–6.0)

What is the most likely cause of the pleural effusion?

A   Dressler's syndrome
B   Malignancy
C   Meigs' syndrome
D   Liver cirrhosis
E   Rheumatoid arthritis

24. A 38-year-old woman presented with a 6-week history of shortness of breath and cough. She had no significant past medical history and did not take any regular medication. She smoked 20 cigarettes per day. There was no history of recent foreign travel and she did not keep any birds or pets. She worked in an office and there was no history of exposure to industrial dusts or fumes.
    On examination, there was finger clubbing and fine inspiratory crackles in the lower zones on auscultation.

Investigations:

Chest X-ray: no abnormality
High-resolution CT of the thorax: ground-glass opacity in lower zones and peripheries

What is the most likely diagnosis?

A   Acute interstitial pneumonitis
B   Cryptogenic organising pneumonia
C   Desquamative interstitial pneumonia
D   Respiratory bronchiolitis-associated lung disease
E   Usual interstitial pneumonia

25. A 23-year-old female university student presented with a 2-week history of a dry cough and left-sided chest discomfort on coughing. She had no previous history of respiratory illness and did not take any regular medication. She was a non-smoker and had recently moved into a shared rented house. She appeared tired but physical examination was normal.

What is the most likely diagnosis?

A   Adult-onset asthma
B   Allergic rhinitis
C   Gastro-oesophageal reflux

D Inhaled foreign body
E Self-limiting viral illness

26. A 24-year-old man was admitted to the acute medical ward with right lower lobar pneumonia. He had no past medical history and was not taking any regular medication. There was no history of recent travel, he was a non-smoker and he worked in an office.

On admission his temperature was 38.8°C, pulse 120 beats per minute, blood pressure 124/68 mmHg, respiratory rate 34 breaths per minute and oxygen saturation 92% on air. He was not confused.

Chest X-ray showed consolidation in the right lower zone and loss of the right hemi-diaphragm. He was commenced on high-flow oxygen therapy, intravenous co-amoxiclav and clarithromycin, and intravenous fluids. The next day as he had improved clinically he was switched to oral antibiotics. Forty-eight hours after admission his condition deteriorated and he had spiking fevers, complaining of worsening shortness of breath, and respiratory rate was 28 breaths per minute with oxygen saturations of 94% on 40% oxygen.

What is the most likely cause of the deterioration in the clinical condition?

A Acute respiratory distress syndrome
B Complication of different underlying lung pathology
C Lung abscess
D Inappropriate antibiotic prescribing
E Parapneumonic effusion

27. A 46-year-old male lorry driver was referred to the sleep clinic by an occupational health physician working for the haulage company. He had recently been involved in a road traffic accident and it was suggested that he may have been at fault because of lack of due care and attention when driving.

He had no past medical history of note. He rarely drank any alcohol and smoked 20 cigarettes per day. He did not have a partner and so there was no collateral history; however, he had previously been told that he was a snorer and he reported that he frequently woke gasping for breath. He confirmed that he had excessive daytime somnolence (Epworth Sleepiness Score 16/24), poor concentration and early morning headaches.

An urgent sleep study was performed (**Figure 10.4**):

What is the most appropriate advice?

A Commence domiciliary non-invasive ventilation
B Commence modafinil
C Inform the Driver and Vehicle Licensing Authority (DVLA) and stop driving until he has received adequate treatment
D Lifestyle and dietary advice
E Surrender his licence and do not drive again

28. A 34-year-old female Zimbabwean office worker presented with progressive shortness of breath on exertion. She was diagnosed with HIV 4 years ago and was receiving antiretroviral therapy.

Pulse oximetry demonstrated desaturation on exercise. She had a loud second heart sound but no audible murmurs. Chest was clear to auscultation.

Investigations:

Chest X-ray:
no focal consolidation
prominent pulmonary arteries

CD4 count: 348 cells/mm³ (400–1600)

Viral load: undetectable

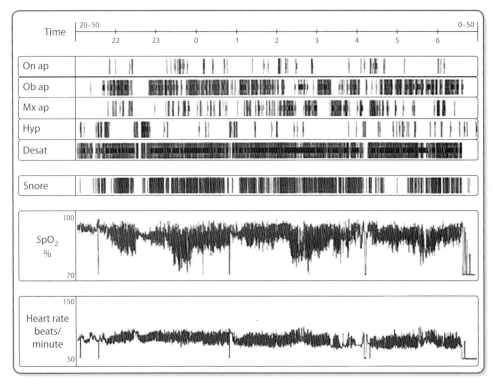

Figure 10.4

What is the most likely diagnosis?

A　Chronic thromboembolic disease
B　Intracardiac shunt across an atrial septal defect (ASD)
C　Physical deconditioning secondary to sedentary lifestyle
D　*Pneumocystis jirovecii* pneumonia
E　Pulmonary arterial hypertension

29. A 34-year-old Norwegian man was referred to the chest clinic because the chest X-ray that his general practitioner had ordered was reported as abnormal. He had a 6-week history of lethargy, fevers, painful wrists and ankles, and tender erythematous nodules on his shins. He had no recent infective illnesses. He had no past medical history of note and was not taking any regular medication.

Investigations:

Chest X-ray: see **Figure 10.5**, opposite

What is the most likely prognosis?

A　30% chance of central nervous system involvement
B　30% chance of progressive pulmonary infiltration
C　50% chance of progressive renal dysfunction
D　50% chance of symptomatic hypercalcaemia
E　90% chance of resolution of disease within 2 years

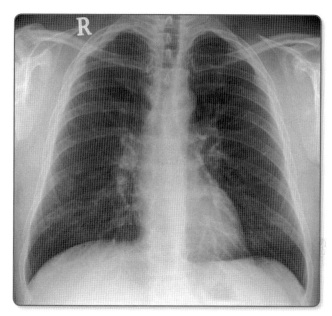

Figure 10.5

30. An influenza pandemic was declared, and a 54-year-old woman presented to the emergency department with a 24-hour history of fevers, myalgia, a sore throat and a cough productive of green sputum.

On examination observations revealed a heart rate of 90 beats per minute, blood pressure of 124/70 mmHg, respiratory rate of 24 breaths per minute, oxygen saturation of 94% on air, and a temperature of 38.6°C. Respiratory examination revealed bibasal coarse crepitations.

Investigations:

haemoglobin 134 g/L (115–165)	potassium 4.3 mmol/L (3.5–5.0)
white cell count 17.2 × 10⁹/L (4–11)	urea 6.4 mmol/L (2.5–7.5)
neutrophils 14.7 × 10⁹/L (1.5–7.0)	creatinine 110 μmol/L (60–110)
sodium 135 mmol/L (135–145)	

Chest X-ray: bilateral pulmonary infiltrates

What is the most appropriate management?

A   Oral co-amoxiclav and oral clarithromycin
B   Intravenous co-amoxiclav, oral clarithromycin and oseltamivir 75 mg twice daily for 5 days
C   Intravenous co-amoxiclav and oral clarithromycin
D   Oseltamivir 75 mg bd for 5 days
E   Oral co-amoxiclav, oral clarithromycin and oseltamivir 75 mg twice daily for 5 days

31. A 72-year-old woman presented to the chest clinic with a 9-month history of progressive shortness of breath and dry cough. Her exercise tolerance was limited to 10 metres. She did not notice any diurnal variation in her symptoms, but she was unable to lie flat and slept with three pillows. She had hypertension and hypercholesterolaemia. She was a non-smoker. Her current medications included ramipril, bendroflumethiazide, aspirin and simvastatin.

On examination, there was ankle oedema and fine end-inspiratory crackles. Oxygen saturation was 92% on air.

A CT of the chest was performed (see **Figure 10.6**).

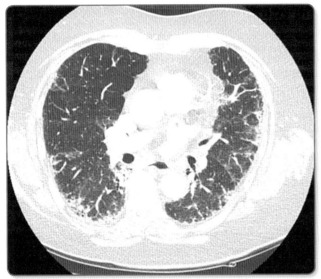

Figure 10.6

What is the most likely diagnosis?

A   Bronchiectasis
B   Cough secondary to angiotensin-converting enzyme inhibitor
C   Congestive cardiac failure
D   Desquamative interstitial pneumonia
E   Usual interstitial pneumonitis

32. A 56-year-old man was referred by the stroke team for an opinion regarding an abnormal chest X-ray. He presented with sudden-onset, left-sided weakness and was making a steady recovery with rehabilitation. The physiotherapists were concerned that he showed desaturation on standing and mobilising. He had no previous history of respiratory symptoms and no past medical history of note. He was a non-smoker.

On examination, there was telangiectasia and finger clubbing. Oxygen saturations were 93% on air. His chest was clear to auscultation.

Investigations:

Chest X-ray: 3-cm, smooth, round, intrapulmonary mass in right lower zone

What is the most likely diagnosis?

A   Asbestos-related pleural plaque
B   Lung abscess
C   Previous tuberculosis infection
D   Pulmonary arteriovenous malformation
E   Pulmonary embolism

33. A 38-year-old white businessman presented to the chest clinic with a persistent cough, wheeze and shortness of breath on exertion. He also had ongoing lethargy, fevers and minor weight loss. He suffered a flu-like illness 6 weeks ago, when on a business trip to Malaysia. He had a past medical history of mild asthma and occasionally used a salbutamol inhaler. The inhaler had not been effective recently. He did not smoke but kept a dog.

Investigations:

haemoglobin 135 g/L (130–180)	lymphocytes 3.3×10^9/L (1.5–4.0)
white cell count 21.0×10^9/L (4–11)	eosinophils 4.2×10^9/L (0.04–0.4)
neutrophils 12.3×10^9/L (1.5–7.0)	erythrocyte sedimentation rate 46 mm/1st h (0–20)

Mantoux test: 11 mm (<5 mm negative, 5–14 mm positive, >15 mm strongly positive)

Chest X-ray: bilateral reticular nodular infiltrates

What is the most likely diagnosis?

A   Churg–Strauss syndrome
B   Löffler's syndrome
C   Miliary tuberculosis
D   *Pneumocystis jirovecii* pneumonia
E   Tropical pulmonary eosinophilia

34. A 64-year-old man with bullous emphysema presented to the emergency department with sudden onset of shortness of breath and left-sided chest pain. A chest X-ray confirmed a large left-sided pneumothorax. The emergency department team inserted small bore (12 Fr) intercostal chest tube with underwater seal, and the X-ray was repeated which demonstrated that the chest tube was in a satisfactory position near the left apex and there was partial re-expansion of the left lung.

    He was prescribed regular simple analgesia and oxygen therapy to maintain oxygen saturation 94–98% and was referred to the medical team for on-going care. Forty-eight hours after admission the chest drain was still bubbling profusely. A third chest X-ray again confirmed that the chest tube remained in a satisfactory position and the lung had further expanded; however, a large left pneumothorax persisted (>2 cm rim).

    What is the most appropriate next step in management?

    A   Apply low-volume high-pressure suction to chest drain
    B   Clamp chest tube
    C   Flush chest drain with 10 mL 5% saline solution using aseptic technique
    D   Insert large-bore chest drain
    E   Refer to cardiothoracic surgeons

35. A 28-year-old man presented to the emergency department with a 4-week history of cough with purulent sputum, fever, night sweats and weight loss of 3 kg. He had no past medical history. He was a smoker of 20 cigarettes per day and drank excessive alcohol (>70 units per week). He was unemployed and of no fixed abode but was living in a charity-run shelter.

    On examination, he was unkempt and malnourished. His temperature was 37.2°C, pulse 94 beats per minute, blood pressure 110/68 mmHg, respiratory rate 18 breaths per minute and oxygen saturation 94% on air. There was no palpable lymphadenopathy. He had reduced breath sounds in the right upper zone. Cardiovascular, abdominal and nervous system examinations were normal.

    Investigations:

haemoglobin 118 g/dL (130–180)	lymphocytes 0.7×10^9/L (1.5–4.0)
mean corpuscular volume 110 fL (80–96)	sodium 134 mmol/L (135–145)
white cell count 7.8×10^9/L (4–11)	urea 4.5 mmol/L (2.5–7.5)
neutrophils 6.4×10^9/L (1.5–7.0)	creatinine 54 µmol/L (60–110)

Chest X-ray: see **Figure 10.7**

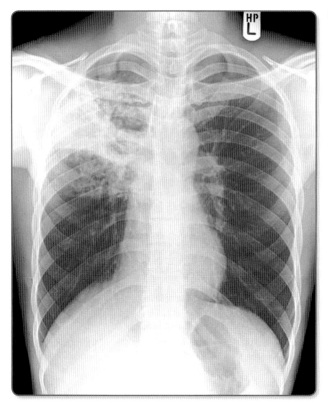

Figure 10.7

What is the most appropriate next step in management?

A   Admit to general respiratory ward for intravenous amoxicillin and clarithromycin
B   Admit to negative pressure room and send sputum samples for acid-fast bacilli and tuberculosis (TB) culture
C   Discharge with ethambutol, isoniazid, pyrazinamide and rifampicin
D   Discharge with oral amoxicillin and clarithromycin
E   Discharge with urgent follow-up in chest clinic for CT of thorax and bronchoscopy

36. A 54-year-old woman was referred by her general practitioner to the chest clinic with a 6-month history of persistent dry cough. Her symptoms occurred throughout the day but were particularly troublesome at night and when speaking on the telephone. There was no history of rhinitis or postnasal drip. She had a history of hypertension. There was no previous history of respiratory illness or atopy. Her general practitioner reviewed her medications and had stopped perindopril 8 weeks ago. Her current medications included bendroflumethiazide and candesartan; she also took over-the-counter remedies for occasional dyspepsia. She was a non-smoker and worked as a telephone receptionist. She was distressed that the cough was interfering with her work.

On examination, she appeared well but had a dry cough. Body mass index was 34 kg/m², oxygen saturation 94% on room air, heart sounds normal and chest clear to auscultation.

Investigations:

Chest X-ray: no abnormality detected

Spirometry:
FEV_1 2.23 L (80% predicted)
FEV_1 postbronchodilator 2.28 L (82% predicted)
FVC 2.76 L (85% predicted)
FVC postbronchodilator 2.73 L (83% predicted)
DLCO 78% predicted
corrected DLCO 96% predicted

(FEV_1 = forced expiratory volume 1 second; FVC = forced vital capacity; DLCO = diffusion capacity of lung to carbon monoxide)

What is the most appropriate next step in management?

A   Gastric emptying studies
B   High-resolution CT of the chest
C   Oesophageal pH manometry
D   Omeprazole
E   Prednisolone

37. A 64-year-old man presented with a persistent cough for 2 months and haemoptysis. He was referred as a 2-week wait to the respiratory physicians. He was an ex-smoker with a 20-pack per year history. He had no other medical problems. His performance status was zero.
      Investigations were undertaken which showed T2N0M0 adenocarcinoma of the lung.

Investigations:

Chest X-ray: 4 cm left upper lobe lesion

CT thorax, abdomen and pelvis: left upper lobe 4 cm lesion, with no metastatic disease and no bronchial invasion

CT PET: avid uptake in left upper lobe corresponding with lesion on CT thorax

Bronchoscopy and EBUS: left bronchial infiltrating lesion over 2 cm distal to the carina

Histology: adenocarcinoma

What is the most appropriate next step in the management of his tumour?

A   Radical radiotherapy
B   Radical chemotherapy and radiotherapy
C   Wedge resection
D   Lobectomy
E   Wedge resection followed by radical radiotherapy

38. A 72-year-old man, with type 2 diabetes mellitus, was admitted with a 4-day history of cough, drenching sweats, chest pain and loss of diabetic control.

Investigations:

> Chest X-ray: large right-sided pleural effusion
>
> Ultrasound-guided diagnostic pleural tap: purulent thick green fluid

What is the most likely infecting organism?

A   *Bacteroides* species
B   Enterobacteriaceae
C   *Staphylococcus aureus*
D   *Streptococcus milleri*
E   *Streptococcus pneumoniae*

39. A 34-year-old man presented to the chest clinic with a chronic productive cough and several episodes of haemoptysis. He gave a history of recurrent chest infections since childhood. He and his partner had recently been referred for fertility treatment.

On examination, he had finger clubbing and scattered crackles throughout both lung fields.

What is the most likely diagnosis?

A   Bronchiectasis
B   Cystic fibrosis
C   Primary ciliary dyskinesia
D   Pulmonary fibrosis
E   Pulmonary tuberculosis

40. A 56-year-old man presented with a 6-month history of a dry cough and progressive shortness of breath on exertion. The symptoms first occurred following a flu-like illness. There was no history of weight loss or on-going fevers. He had a history of rheumatoid arthritis, for which he was taking methotrexate weekly. He had never smoked.

On examination, a left-sided effusion was detected. The aspirated fluid was turbid looking. Following simple bench centrifugation, the pleural fluid remained turbid and a clear supernatant did not appear.

What is the most likely nature of the effusion?

A   Chylothorax
B   Empyema
C   Malignant effusion
D   Pseudochylothorax
E   Rheumatoid effusion

41. A 75-year-old man was referred to the chest clinic by his general practitioner. Eight weeks ago he presented with a 2-week history of cough productive of yellow sputum and his general practitioner requested a chest X-ray which was found to be abnormal. By the time of outpatient consultation, he had recovered completely; the cough had resolved and he was feeling well. He had no loss of appetite or weight. He had previously worked at a granite quarry. He had never smoked.

On examination, there was no finger clubbing, his chest was clear and oxygen saturation was 94% on air.

Investigations:

> Chest X-ray: multiple, small, dense nodules bilaterally, mainly in the upper zones

What is the most likely diagnosis?

A   Asbestosis
B   Kaolinosis
C   Progressive massive fibrosis
D   Silicosis
E   Stannosis

42. A 68-year-old woman was referred to the chest clinic following an infective exacerbation of chronic obstructive pulmonary disease (COPD). She had made a good recovery and her exercise tolerance was back to her baseline of 250 metres on flat ground. She planned to travel to Spain on a 3-hour flight in 6 weeks' time and her general practitioner requested an in-flight oxygen assessment.

Investigations:

> Oxygen saturation at rest breathing air: 93%
>
> PaO_2 after hypoxic challenge test using 15% FiO_2 for 20 min: 7.8 kPa
>
> Forced expiratory volume in 1 second (FEV$_1$): 1.48 (48% predicted)

What is the most appropriate advice?

A   Reassess in 3 weeks
B   She can fly with in-flight oxygen at a flow rate of 2 L/min
C   She can fly with in-flight oxygen at a flow rate of 4 L/min
D   She can fly without the need for in-flight oxygen
E   She should undergo exercising testing as a prelude to flying

43. A 76-year-old man with severe chronic obstructive pulmonary disease (COPD) with progressive shortness of breath was prescribed long term oxygen therapy (LTOT) by his respiratory physician.

Investigations:

Arterial blood gases on 40% oxygen:	haemoglobin 160 g/L (130–180)
pH 7.37 (7.35–7.45)	HCT 57% (40–54)
PO_2 7.24	MCV 100 fL (80–96)
PCO_2 6.8 kPa	

LTOT in patients with COPD improves which of the following?

A   Pulmonary haemodynamics
B   Health-related quality of life
C   Hospital admission rates
D   Hypercapnia
E   All of the above

44. A 74-year-old man was admitted to hospital with severe shortness of breath. He had a history of emphysema.
    On examination, he had diminished breath sounds over the left side of the chest; the trachea was central.

Investigations:

Chest X-ray: large left pneumothorax

What is the most appropriate next step in management?

A   Insert 14 Fr drain immediately above a rib margin in the scalene triangle
B   Insert 14 Fr drain immediately below a lower rib margin in the scalene triangle
C   Insert 14 Fr drain in the second intercostal space in the mid-clavicular line
D   Insert 28 Fr drain immediately above a rib margin in the scalene triangle
E   Insert 28 Fr drain immediately below a lower rib margin in the scalene triangle

45. A 53-year-old woman presented with a 2-year history of increasing wheeze and shortness of breath on exertion. She was a current smoker (30 pack-years) and had started working at a local bakery as a cleaner 3 years previously. Her wheeze improved on holiday and was better on her days off.
    On examination, she had nasal congestion and marked expiratory wheeze.

What is the most likely diagnosis?

A   Atopic asthma
B   Chronic bronchitis
C   Emphysema
D   Hypersensitivity pneumonitis
E   Occupational asthma

46. A 56-year-old woman was referred by her GP as a 2-week wait referral to the respiratory clinic after a chest X-ray performed to investigate a chronic cough showed a pulmonary nodule.
    She was an ex-smoker and had a history of hypothroidism. Her current medications were thyroxine125 µg once daily. Her father had a history of lung cancer.
    A CT was performed to further investigate.

Investigations:

CT Thorax: 10 mm solid pulmonary nodule in right upper lobe

What is the most appropriate next management step?

A   CT-PET
B   CT-guided biopsy of nodule
C   Follow-up CT in 3 months
D   Assess risk using the Brock model
E   Assess risk using the Herder model

Answers

1. D Pleural plaques are a premalignant finding

Pleural plaques are the most common manifestation of asbestos exposure and may be found in up to 50% of asbestos-exposed people. Plaques develop 20–40 years after initial exposure and the incidence increases with prolonged exposure. Pleural plaques are usually asymptomatic and present as an incidental finding. There is no evidence that plaques are premalignant. Patients with isolated pleural plaques do not necessarily need further investigations or regular follow-up; Pleural plaques can usually be diagnosed on chest X-ray however, high-resolution CT scanning is a more sensitive test to detect pleural plaques. Other forms of benign asbestos-related pleural disease include benign asbestos-related pleural effusion, diffuse pleural thickening and rounded atelectasis. Benign pleural effusions occur relatively early within 10 years of exposure and may be asymptomatic or present with pleuritic chest pain, dyspnoea and fever, and tend to resolve spontaneously. They may recur and progress to diffuse pleural thickening. There is no clear association with mesothelioma. On chest X-ray, diffuse pleural thickening may be defined as a smooth pleural opacity extending over at least a quarter of the chest wall. Symptoms are relatively common and include dyspnoea and chest pain. Pleural biopsy may be required to differentiate diffuse pleural thickening from mesothelioma. Rounded atelectasis consists of a fibrotic, invaginated pleura with fibrotic, thickened interlobular septa. It is classically seen as a 'comet's tail' on CT or chest X-ray where a thickened pleura is seen to be connected to a peripheral lung lesion by a fibrous band.

British Thoracic Society. Pleural plaques: information for health care professionals. London: British Thoracic Society, 2011.
King C, Mayes D, Dorsey DA. Benign asbestos-related pleural disease. Dis Mon 2011; 57:27–39.

2. E Treat with rifampicin and isoniazid

As in the case above, screening may identify cases of latent tuberculosis (TB). Active TB infection should be excluded by medical history, physical examination and chest X-ray and samples for TB microscopy and culture. If there is no evidence of active TB infection and the chest X-ray is normal then further investigation including bronchoscopy, induced sputa and CT scanning is not necessary and may have potential risks and side effects including significant discomfort and radiation exposure. Mantoux (with appropriate interpretation and knowledge of prior BCG vaccination) and/or interferon-γ screening tests may identify cases of latent TB infection. Certain groups with latent TB, including patients with HIV and health-care workers should be offered TB chemoprophylaxis. The most frequently offered treatment is 3 months of isoniazid and rifampicin, but isoniazid for 6 months can be used if there are concerns regarding interactions with rifampicin (i.e in those who have undergone transplantation or who have HIV). Patients who do not have TB chemoprophylaxis should be counselled to seek medical advice if they develop any symptoms suggestive of active disease and the chest X-ray should be repeated at 3 and 12 months.

National Institute for Health and Clinical Excellence (NICE). NICE guideline NG33. Tuberculosis. London: NICE, 2016.

3. B Continue present treatment and re-assess within 1 hour

Non-invasive ventilation (NIV) should be considered for all patients presenting with respiratory acidosis (pH <7.35 and Paco$_2$ >6.5 kPa) secondary to an exacerbation of chronic obstructive pulmonary disease (COPD), if standard medical treatment (controlled oxygen therapy, nebulised salbutamol and ipratropium, prednisolone ± antibiotic therapy if indicated) has not improved the situation within 1 hour. A clearly documented treatment plan for NIV, with ceilings of treatment and/or suitability for escalation to invasive ventilatory support, should be discussed and documented at the outset of treatment. It would be inappropriate to reduce the oxygen flow rate to 1 L/min as this would lead to worsening hypoxia; however, it would be appropriate to use a controlled delivery system such as a Venturi device delivering 24–28% oxygen. Nebulised treatment should continue and be delivered using air rather than high-flow oxygen to avoid over-oxygenation and possible loss of hypoxic drive.

Aminophylline may be used in reversible airway obstruction and acute severe asthma; however, there is little evidence of benefit in acute exacerbations of COPD and it may cause arrhythmias, convulsions and hypotension.

With widespread availability of NIV, respiratory stimulants, e.g. doxapram, have little role in the management of respiratory failure and are associated with a number of side effects including arrhythmias, chest pain, agitation, hallucinations and seizures.

Davidson AC, Banham E, Elliott M, et al. BTS/ICS guideline for the ventilatory management of acute hypercapnic respiratory failure in adults. Thorax 2016; 71:ii1–ii35.

4. A CT pulmonary angiogram (CPTA)

The history is suggestive of venous thromboembolic (VTE) disease with an acute pulmonary embolism (PE). The diagnosis of a PE can be difficult and involves a clinical assessment of probability. Risk factors, clinical presentation and clinical signs are taken into account and tests are performed to add weight to the clinical decision. The 2012 NICE guidelines recommend use of the two-level Wells score to estimate the pre-test probability of a PE (see **Table 10.1**).

Interpretation of two-level Wells score for PE:

Table 10.1 Two-level Wells score for PE	
Clinical feature	**Points**
Clinical symptoms of deep vein thrombosis (DVT)	3
Other diagnosis less likely than pulmonary embolism (PE)	3
Heart rate greater than 100 beats per minute	1.5
Immobilisation or surgery within past 4 weeks	1.5
Previous deep vein thrombosis or pulmonary embolism	1.5
Haemoptysis	1
Malignancy (palliative, currently being treated or treated within the last 6 months)	1
Adapted from: Wells PS, et al. Derivation of a simple clinical model to categorize patient's probability of pulmonary embolism: increasing the models utility with the SimpliRED D-dimer. Thromb Haemost 2000; 83(3):416–420.	

- Over 4 points – PE likely
- Less than 4 points – PE unlikely

In the clinical scenario described in the question there are clinical features of a DVT, PE is more likely than another diagnosis, the heart rate is greater than 100 beats per minute and there is active malignancy (total score 8.5 so PE is likely).

D-dimer testing has an important role in diagnosing and excluding PE and should be used only after a pre-test probability assessment. D-dimers are a sensitive test for VTE but not specific. D-dimers are generated as a result of fibrinolysis, which occurs in many clinical situations, including VTE, sepsis, pregnancy and neoplasia.

A low or intermediate pre-test probability score, combined with a negative D-dimer has a 92% probability for excluding PE. If there is a high clinical suspicion of PE (i.e. Wells score >4) a D-dimer should not be performed and patients should be referred for appropriate imaging. CTPA is the recommended initial lung imaging modality for non-massive PE. Urgent bedside echocardiography may be useful for diagnosing massive PE in haemodynamically compromised patients.

Ventilation–perfusion (nuclear medicine) scans may be considered if the chest radiograph is normal and if facilities are readily available, and the criteria used for reporting are standardised and significant cardiopulmonary disease is not present. If the patient presents with signs of a deep vein thrombosis, Doppler ultrasound may be sufficient to confirm the diagnosis, but should not be used as a sole test to exclude the diagnosis.

National Institute for Health and Care Excellence (NICE). Clinical guideline 144. Venous thromboembolic diseases: diagnosis. Management and thrombophilia testing. London: NICE, 2012.
The British Thoracic Society Standards of Care Committee, Pulmonary Embolism Guideline Development Group. British Thoracic Society guidelines for the management of suspected acute pulmonary embolism. Thorax 2003; 58:470–484.

5. E Trial of omalizumab

This patient with severe asthma remains poorly controlled and dependent on regular oral steroids. She may be a candidate for a trial of omalizumab. This is a humanised monoclonal antibody which binds to circulating serum IgE. It is administered by subcutaneous injection and should be initiated only in specialist centres managing patients with severe and difficult asthma. If the trial of omalizumab is successful, as indicated by improvement of symptom control, lung function and reduction in serum IgE, oral steroids may be tapered and stopped.

Patients with severe and difficult asthma should have self-management plans. With good inhaler technique and compliance with medications home nebulisers are not normally required. This patient has been intolerant of theophyllines and therefore commencing aminophylline modified-release tablets would not be appropriate. Patients may require additional oral corticosteroids to treat acute exacerbations. However, long-term high-dose steroids have a number of deleterious side effects, including osteopenia, immunosuppression, weight gain and impairment of glucose tolerance, so dose should be minimised where possible. Increasing the regular dose would not be a satisfactory long-term strategy.

It would not be appropriate to recommend adrenaline by intramuscular injection for self-administration in case of emergencies unless there was a history of anaphylaxis.

British Thoracic Society and Scottish Intercollegiate Guidelines Network. SIGN 153: British Guideline on the Management of Asthma – a national clinical guideline. London: BTS and SIGN, 2016.

6. D Chronic obstruction pulmonary disease (COPD) secondary to biomass fuel exposure

The history and spirometry findings are suggestive of COPD. Tobacco smoking is the leading cause of COPD; however, exposure to biomass fuels is an increasingly recognised cause of respiratory disease. Wood and charcoal are used by a third of the world's population for cooking and heating, and burning of these fuels indoors results in the generation of large amounts of noxious gases including carbon monoxide, hydrocarbons, oxygenated and chlorinated organics, and free radicals which have been found to increase the incidence of respiratory disease, cardiovascular disease and all-cause mortality.

α_1-antitrypsin (α1AT) deficiency is an autosomal recessive disorder that is associated with early development of emphysema. The glycoprotein protease inhibitor α1AT is produced by the liver and acts in the lungs to oppose neutrophil elastase, which destroys alveolar wall connective tissue. Insults such as tobacco smoke and infection stimulate pulmonary neutrophils and macrophages to produce increased levels of the elastase. If α1AT is deficient, the elastase cannot be opposed and the lungs are subject to proteolytic attack leading to emphysema.

Adult-onset asthma is also increasing in prevalence and congestive cardiac failure may also be a differential diagnosis; however, the fixed obstructive defect seen in the spirometry would not support either of these diagnoses.

The history is not particularly suggestive of tuberculosis (TB); however, this patient may be considered at high risk of reactivation of latent disease especially considering her ethnic background and co-morbidities, including diabetes mellitus. Patients with diabetes are at increased risk of re-activation of latent TB. Patients presenting with a chronic cough – a cough of more than 8 weeks' duration – should have a chest X-ray and patients considered to be at high risk of TB should be screened by sending three early morning sputum samples for alcohol acid-fast bacilli testing and TB culture.

Salvi SS, Barnes PJ. Chronic obstructive pulmonary disease in non-smokers. Lancet 2009; 374:733–743.

7. A PiZZ α_1-antitrypsin deficiency

The patient has evidence of emphysema and panniculitis making PiZZ α_1-antitrypsin (AAT) deficiency the most likely diagnosis. α_1-Antitrypsin deficiency associated panniculitis is a very rare disease and less than 50 cases have been described. While it can occur in any genotype of α_1 antitrypsin deficiency the majority of cases (70%) occur in women with the PiZZ genotype. The genotype of α_1-antitrypsin deficiency (i.e PiZZ, PiSZ, etc) refers to the genetic variant of the SERPINA1 gene that the individual has inherited. SERPINA1 is the gene that encodes the protease inhibitor α_1-antitrypsin. The SERPINA1 gene has over 100 genetic variants, the designation of these is alphabetical and based on their migration speed, with M (medium mobility) being the most common, and Pi Z and Pi S being the most common deficiency alleles. Severe deficiency is seen most commonly in those who are homozygous for the Z allele (PiZZ), and homozygosity for the MM allele is the most common genotype, which produces normal serum α_1-antitrypsin. The pathogenesis is not clearly defined but a decrease in α_1-antitrypsin appears to lead to neutrophil protease over activity in subcutaneous fat. Some case reports have described a dramatic response of the panniculitis to α_1-antitrypsin augmentation. Dapsone has been recommended as the first line treatment. There is no evidence that corticosteroids, nonsteroidal anti-inflammatory drugs or antibiotics have any clinical effectiveness in treatment of AAT panniculitis.

Blanco A, Lipsker D, Lara B, Janciauskiene S. Neutrophilic panniculitis associated with alpha-1-antitrypsin deficiency: an update. Br J Dermatol 2016; 174:753–762.

8. A CT pulmonary angiogram

Pulmonary embolism (PE) is one of the main causes of maternal death. The diagnosis of PE in the general population is sometimes difficult and this may be more complicated in pregnancy and the postpartum period as some of the symptoms of PE may be some of the normal symptoms of pregnancy. Accurate diagnosis is essential to reduce the risks of the side effects of inappropriate treatments, and morbidity and mortality risks of undetected PE for both the mother and the fetus. Serum levels of D-dimer increase in pregnancy, and therefore this test is not clinically useful in pregnancy and is not recommended. There is a high prevalence (70%) of deep vein thrombosis (DVT) in patients with proven PE in pregnancy and therefore compression duplex ultrasound of the leg veins may be a useful test to confirm the diagnosis without the risks associated with ionising radiation. In patients with clinical signs or symptoms of DVT and suspected PE then Doppler ultrasonography is recommended as the first line investigation, and if this is positive no further investigation is required. However, physiological changes associated with hormonal effects and the compressive effects of the gravid uterus increase leg swelling in pregnant women in the absence of a DVT and a negative Doppler should not be used to rule out PE.

When a PE is suspected and there are no symptoms or signs of a DVT then either a CT pulmonary angiogram or a ventilation/perfusion lung scan should be carried out, however in patients with an abnormal chest X-ray (as in this case) a CT pulmonary angiogram should be performed. CT pulmonary angiogram (CTPA) has a high sensitivity and specificity.

Advice to pregnant women with suspected PE regarding choice of investigation should include the fact that while the absolute risk of both is small, ventilation perfusion scanning when compared with CTPA carries a lower risk of breast cancer to the mother but a slightly increased childhood cancer risk.

Royal College of Obstetricians and Gynaecologists (RCOG). Thromboembolic disease in pregnancy and the puerperium: acute management. Green-top Guideline No 37b. London, RCOG, 2015.
British Thoracic Society Standards of Care Committee Pulmonary Embolism Guideline Development Group. British Thoracic Society guidelines for the management of suspected acute pulmonary embolism. Thorax 2003; 58:470–484.
Matthews S. Imaging pulmonary embolism in pregnancy: what is the most appropriate imaging protocol? Br J Radiol 2006; 79:441–444.

9. B Needle aspiration in right second intercostal space in the mid-clavicular line

This patient has presented with a classic history of a primary spontaneous pneumothorax (PSP) as confirmed by the chest X-ray. He has a large pneumothorax (complete collapse of right lung) and, although distressed and in pain, is still haemodynamically stable.

The clinical situation guides the management of PSP. If a patient presenting with PSP is asymptomatic and clinically stable, then a conservative approach may be appropriate. The administration of high-flow oxygen may treat associated hypoxia, but has also been demonstrated to increase the rate of resolution of the pneumothorax.

If the patient is distressed, tachypnoeic and/or hypoxic, the intial management of choice is attempted needle aspiration of up to 2.5 L of air followed by repeat chest X-ray to ensure that the lung has re-expanded. If this is successful, then no further immediate treatment may be necessary, and if the lung has partially re-expanded and the overall clinical picture has improved, then the patient may be observed. Needle aspiration may be as effective as insertion of a large-bore chest drain and may reduce the length of stay. If however, needle aspiration is unsuccessful, a small-bore chest drain may be the next best step.

Thoracic ultrasound will identify specific diagnostic features of a pneumothorax, but this practice is not necessary for routine management. Thoracic ultrasound should, however, be used for other pleural procedures including diagnostic pleural taps and chest drain insertion for pleural effusion.

MacDuff A, et al. Management of spontaneous pneumothorax: British Thoracic Society pleural disease guideline 2010. Thorax 2010; 65(2):ii18–eii31.

10. C Lymphoma

The chest X-ray demonstrates a large anterior mediastinal mass. The most likely cause of the mediastinal mass in a woman of this age group and with the blood test presented is lymphoma. The mediastinum is commonly involved in patients with Hodgkin's lymphoma. To establish the histological diagnosis of lymphoma, an adequate tissue sample is required; this should be in the form of a biopsy which may be either CT guided, via endobronchial ultrasound (EBUS), or surgical.

Common symptoms of mediastinal disease include cough, chest pain and dyspnoea, as well as symptoms relating to structural compression, e.g. dysphagia, stridor or superior vena cava obstruction. Mediastinal disorders may also be asymptomatic and found incidentally on chest X-ray. The likely nature of a mediastinal mass may be determined according to anatomical site.

Anterior mediastinal mass:
- thymoma (superior)
- thyroid (superior)
- germ cell tumour
- lymphoma
- ascending aortic aneurysm
- pleuropericardial cyst
- pericardial fat pad
- anterior diaphragmatic hernia

Superior mediastinal mass:
- bronchogenic cyst

Posterior mediastinal mass:
- neural tumour
- foregut duplication cyst
- lipoma
- descending aortic aneurysm
- posterior diaphragmatic hernia

Germ cell tumours arise from immature germ cells during development. Mature cystic teratomas represent 80% of germ cell tumours. These are benign and occur in young adults (prevalence male = female) and appear on a chest X-ray or as a well-defined mass which may contain flecks of calcification. Seminomas occur in men aged 20–40 years and are malignant.

Retrosternal goitre is usually asymptomatic unless there is tracheal compression leading to dyspnoea. Surgical resection is recommended if there is airway compromise.

Thymomas are tumours arising from the thymus and may contain functioning thymic tissue. Myasthaenia gravis (MG) occurs in 30–40% patients with thymomas; frequently this does not respond to thymectomy and may even occur after resection. Twenty per cent of patients with MG are found to have thymoma.

Duwe BV, Sterman DH, Musani AI. Tumors of the mediastinum. Chest 2005; 128(4):2893–2909.

11. C High-resolution CT of the chest

The history is suggestive of bronchiectasis which may present as recurrent lower respiratory tract infections and the expectoration of purulent sputum. Symptoms may also include chest pain, dyspnoea and haemoptysis, and the condition may progress to respiratory failure.

A chest X-ray should be performed in all suspected cases and is recommended for all patients presenting with a chronic cough (>8 weeks). However, the imaging modality of choice for diagnosing bronchiectasis is high-resolution CT (HRCT), which will demonstrate the pathognomonic features of bronchial wall thickening and dilatation. HRCT may demonstrate certain features suggesting a cause for the condition, e.g. allergic bronchopulmonary aspergillosis (ABPA) or cystic fibrosis (CF). Some routine blood tests should be performed in the work-up of all patients presenting with bronchiectasis, including serum immunoglobulins and protein electrophoresis, plus total IgE and skin-prick testing or serum IgE testing to *Aspergillus* species. Bronchoscopy is not routinely performed, unless there is a suspected endobronchial lesion, or foreign body, with associated distal bronchiectasis. Bronchoalveolar lavage may be useful to gain a microbiological diagnosis if mycobacterial infection is suspected.

α_1-Antitrypsin levels should not be routinely requested in these patients, but may be useful if HRCT demonstrates basal emphysema. A tuberculin skin test is unlikely to be helpful in a patient of this age group and is not the test of choice. Tuberculin skin tests are useful to identify cases of latent tuberculosis infection but need to be interpreted with knowledge of previous BCG vaccination history.

M C Pasteur, D Bilton, A T Hill. British Thoracic Society guideline for non-CF bronchiectasis. Thorax 2010; 65:i1–i58.

12. C Intravenous magnesium

This patient has features of life-threatening asthma as suggested by peak expiratory flow rate (PEFR) <33% of best or predicted PEFR. Other features of life-threatening asthma include the presence of: (1) a silent chest, feeble respiratory effort or cyanosis; (2) hypotension or arrhythmia; (3) altered conscious level or exhaustion. .

Following the administration of oxygen-driven nebulised salbutamol or terbutaline and ipratropium bromide and steroids, intravenous magnesium sulphate 1.2–2.0 g infusion over 20 minute should be considered. Intravenous magnesium has bronchodilator effects; however, the exact mechanism of action is unclear.

As the patient has features of life-threatening asthma, a senior physician should be called to review the patient and the patient should be referred to the intensive care team to consider transfer to the intensive care unit. If the patient is not improving the senior clinician may consider use of intravenous β_2-agonist (salbutamol) or intravenous aminophylline, or progression to mechanical ventilation.

Oxygen therapy should be given to maintain oxygen saturation between 94 and 98%; there is no benefit in maintaining saturation >98% with increased oxygen therapy. In cases of life-threatening asthma requiring intubation and mechanical ventilation, intravenous ketamine may sometimes be used to relieve intractable bronchospasm but requires expert anaesthetic supervision.

Scottish Intercollegiate Guidelines Network. SIGN Guidelines. Guideline 153: British Guideline on the Management of Asthma. Edinburgh: SIGN, 2016.
Scottish Intercollegiate Guidelines Network. SIGN Guidelines. Management of acute severe asthma in adults in hospital, 2008.

13. E Whole lung lavage

The history, radiological findings and bronchoalveolar lavage (BAL) results are suggestive of pulmonary alveolar proteinosis (PAP). PAP is a rare alveolar defect due to failure of alveolar macrophages to remove surfactant, leading to the accumulation of proteinaceous material within the alveoli. The condition presents between 30 and 50 years age and male smokers are at higher risk. Patients may present with breathlessness and a dry cough and/or with superadded infection, causing acute onset of symptoms in association with fever. Opportunistic infection is the major complication (*Nocardia* species, fungi and mycobacteria) due to the impaired host defence secondary to surfactant accumulation.

Diagnosis is suggested by typical CT appearances – 'crazy paving pattern' of patchy airspace shadowing, with areas of normal lung and confirmed by bronchoalveolar lavage showing foamy, large macrophages with eosinophilic granules and PAS positive extracellular globular hyaline material. The treatment of choice is repeated therapeutic whole lung lavage. This is performed at specialist centres under general anaesthetic using single lung ventilation via a double-lumen endotracheal tube. Repeated warm saline lavage is used to wash the bronchial tree and characteristic milky lavage fluid is obtained. The prognosis with whole lung lavage is generally good.

Atypical infections are common and specific antibiotics should be administered if cultures are positive. There is no role for empirical antituberculous therapy or co-trimoxazole. There is no benefit from treatment with steroids which may increase the risk of opportunistic infections.

Borie R, et al. Pulmonary alveolar proteinosis. Eur Respir Rev 2011; 20(120):98–107.

14. D Lymphangioleiomyomatosis

Lymphangioleiomyomatosis (LAM) is a disorder characterised by the abnormal proliferation of smooth muscle and perivascular cells throughout the lungs, airways, blood vessels and lymph system. Progressive nodular infiltration of the lymphatics and airways leads to the formation of cysts throughout the lungs one of the characteristic lesions in LAM. The disease affects women of child-bearing age (and postmenopausal women taking hormone replacement therapy). It is a rare disorder, affecting 1 in 1.1 million, and is of unknown cause. Of adult women with tuberous sclerosis 40% develop the pulmonary changes seen in LAM.

Clinical features include pneumothorax (often recurrent), dyspnoea, chest pain, cough, haemoptysis, and pulmonary haemorrhage, chylothorax and pleural effusion. Other organs may be affected by the condition. Angiomyolipoma, a benign renal tumour, occurs in 50% of LAM patients and patients should be screened for these lesions with abdominal CT. Within the pelvis, cystic masses (lymphangioleiomyomas) may occur that enlarge during the day, leading to fullness and bloating. There is also an increased chance of developing meningioma.

Diagnosis is confirmed by a lung biopsy fulfilling characteristic pathological criteria plus a compatible or characteristic lung high resolution CT (HRCT) or a characteristic lung HRCT and one or more of the following features: lymphangioleiomyoma, renal angiomyolipoma, thoracic or abdominal chylous effusion, tuberous sclerosis or lymph node involvement by lymphangioleiomyomatosis.

Patients should be referred to a specialist centre for further management. The course and prognosis of LAM are very variable. Hormonal manipulation with progesterone has been tried, but there are no randomised placebo controlled studies. If airflow obstruction is present inhaled bronchodilators should be trialled as a quarter of patients will have some response. Oestrogens should be avoided. Patients should be advised that pregnancy may accelerate the disease process. Lung transplantation may be necessary; however, LAM can recur in the transplanted lung.

α₁-Antitrypsin deficiency, catamenial pneumothorax (pneumothorax occurring during menstruation probably secondary to thoracic endometriosis), cystic fibrosis and pulmonary Langerhans' cell histiocytosis (rare condition of pulmonary infiltration with histiocytes) may also present or be complicated by recurrent pneumothoraces; however, the CT appearance described is not typical of these conditions (**Table 10.2**).

Johnson SR, Cordier JF, Lazor R, et al. European Respiratory Society guidelines for the diagnosis and management of lymphangioleiomyomatosis. Eur Resp J 2010; 35:14–26.
Harari S, Torre O, Moss J. Lymphangioleiomyomatosis: what do we know and what are we looking for? Eur Respir Rev 2011; 20(119):34–44.

Table 10.2 Typical CT finding of conditions associated with recurrent pneumothorax	
Diagnosis	**Typical CT findings/notes**
α₁-Antitrypsin deficiency	Bullous emphysema
Catamenial pneumothorax	Often normal CT – diagnosis confirmed by video-assisted thoracoscopic surgery (VATS)
Cystic fibrosis	Bronchiectasis – predominantly in upper zones
Lymphangioleiomyomatosis	Multiple, small (<1 cm), thin-walled cysts
Pulmonary Langerhans' cell histiocytosis	Multiple nodules, thin and thick walled, varying sizes (reflecting different ages of nodules), may cavitate

15. C Intravenous co-amoxiclav and clarithromycin

This patient has the history, signs and investigation findings suggesting severe community-acquired pneumonia (CAP). Patients with severe pneumonia should be treated as soon as possible with intravenous antibiotics, e.g. co-amoxiclav and clarithromycin.

The severity of pneumonia may be graded according to the CURB65 score and the score should be interpreted in conjunction with clinical judgement. One point is scored for each positive finding to provide a score out of 5.

C – confusion [Abbreviated Mental test (AMT) score <8/10]
U – urea >7.0 mmol/L (normal range 2.5–7.5 mmol/L)
R – respiratory rate >30 breaths per minute (normal range 12–18 breaths per minute)
B – blood pressure <90 mmHg systolic or <60 mmHg diastolic
65 – age >65 years

Patients with a CURB65 score >3 are at higher risk of morbidity and mortality. Patients with CURB65 scores of 4 and 5 should be considered for transfer to the critical care unit. These patients should have early senior review.

Patients with a low CURB65 score (0 or 1) are at low risk and may be treated with oral antibiotics at home if there are no concerning features and the patient has sufficient support in the community.

Oxygen saturations should be monitored and patients should be prescribed and administered appropriate oxygen therapy to maintain an oxygen saturation of 94–98% (unless there is a history or significant risk of hypercapnic respiratory failure). There is no evidence for the routine use of steroids in the management of severe pneumonia.

British Thoracic Society Standards of Care Committee. The British Thoracic Society Guidelines for the management of community acquired pneumonia in adults. Update 2009. Thorax 64 (suppl III).

16. B *Fusobacterium necrophorum*

The history of an infective illness in a previously well young person with pharyngitis, 'angina' (neck pain) and lung cavitation is suggestive of Lemierre's syndrome. This rare illness is usually, but not exclusively, caused by the anaerobe *Fusobacterium necrophorum*, an organism that can colonise the oral cavity, but may occasionally lead to bacteraemia. The history described is typical of the syndrome which, although still rare, appears to be increasing in incidence with recent efforts to reduce inappropriate antibiotic prescribing for pharyngitis-type illnesses.

In addition to the above findings the syndrome includes thrombosis of the internal jugular vein (suppurative thrombophlebitis) as a result of spread of infection to the neck and carotid sheath. Septic embolisation to the lung may occur with subsequent cavitation and/or abscess formation. Other complications may also include empyema, and abscesses in bones, joints and other organs. Treatment of the condition requires a prolonged course of metronidazole (6 weeks) and a penicillin (or appropriate alternative if penicillin allergic). The role of anticoagulation is controversial.

Cryptococcus neoformans, Pneumocystis jirovecii, Rhodococcus species and fungi are causes of lung cavitation in HIV infection and other immunocompromised patients. Lung cavitation may occur secondary to community-acquired pneumonia and may complicate approximately 16% of *Staphylococcus aureus* pneumonias. *Staphylococcus aureus* is also the most common causative organism of lung abscesses secondary to septic embolisation in right heart endocarditis in intravenous drug abusers. Tuberculosis may cause lung cavitation; however, the typical presentation would be more prolonged than the case described above.

Riordan T. Human infection with *Fusobacterium necrophorum* (necrobacillosis), with a focus on Lemierre's syndrome. Clin Microbiol Rev 2007;20:622–659.

17. A Keep ascent to ≤300 m/day and rest every third day

Minor effects of altitude sickness may be due to hyperventilation provoked by hypoxia at altitude and may include light-headedness, fatigue, peripheral paraesthesia, nausea and anorexia, headaches and sleep disturbance. The major concerns of altitude sickness are high-altitude pulmonary oedema (HAPE) and high-altitude cerebral oedema (HACE). These conditions are caused by hypoxia itself, may develop rapidly and are potentially fatal.

The risk of altitude sickness increases with the rate at which altitude is attained. The risk may be reduced by keeping the ascent to ≤300 m/day and resting every third day. Minor symptoms resolve with rest, analgesia and adequate hydration but descent may be necessary to control the symptoms. Acetazolamide may be useful as prophylaxis and to treat minor symptoms, by provoking a mild metabolic acidosis and allowing greater hyperventilation in response to hypoxia without the usual alkalosis. It is recommended when rapid ascent is unavoidable.

Such a trip should be planned and expert medical advice may be needed, but many patients who suffer from mild asthma in childhood are not affected later in adult life and so this should not be an absolute contraindication to the trip.

Nifedipine may be used in the treatment of HAPE to reduce pulmonary artery pressure although its use for prophylaxis is controversial. Dexamethasone is used in the management of HACE to reduce cerebral oedema.

Imray C, et al. Acute altitude illnesses. BMJ 2011; 343:d4943.

18. C Swyer–James–MacLeod syndrome

Swyer–James–MacLeod's syndrome is due to parenchymal and vascular maldevelopment, following childhood bronchiolitis obliterans. The condition may be asymptomatic but can present with recurrent chest infections and bronchiectasis. The disease usually presents in childhood with recurrent pulmonary infections, but patients who are asymptomatic or have minimal symptoms may be diagnosed in adulthood. It can be diagnosed on routine chest X-rays, which may demonstrate a hyperlucent lung, with reduced vascular markings and a small pulmonary artery. Pulmonary function tests usually show an obstructive pattern.

α_1-Antitrypsin deficiency is an autosomal recessive condition associated with early onset emphysema. Emphysematous change is accelerated in smokers and causes bilateral disease.

Congenital lobar emphysema is a congenital abnormality that causes the overinflation of a lobe due to localised bronchomalacia or bronchial obstruction. It may cause wheeze and/or chest wall deformity. The condition may resolve spontaneously during development through childhood.

In cases of pneumothorax there would be absent rather than reduced pulmonary markings if complete or a visible lung edge in partial collapse; there is more likely to be a typical history of either trauma or sudden-onset pleuritic pain and shortness of breath.

Pulmonary sequestration is a congenital abnormality resulting from a segment of lung without a bronchial connection and therefore reduced ventilation. The segment of lung may be supplied by an aberrant artery. Most are left sided (most common in left lower lobe). This condition is often associated with other congenital abnormalities, but may be detected on routine chest X-rays. Surgical resection may be necessary if there is repeated infection.

Sen HS, Taylan M, Abakay O, Sezgi C, Cetincakmak MG. Adult diagnosis of Swyer–James–Macleod syndrome: retrospective analysis of four cases. Respir Care 2014; 59:e51–e54.

19. E Restart regular inhaler corticosteroid and long-acting β_2-agonist

The presentation suggests a mild exacerbation of asthma which may be as a result of a viral illness and is probably exacerbated by stopping the regular prescribed medications. The patient is well and lives with her husband and so may be safely discharged home with advice.

Pregnancy can affect asthma and asthma can affect the outcome of pregnancy. Generally, a third will improve during pregnancy, a third will notice no change in their symptoms and a third will deteriorate. The course of asthma is likely to be similar in successive pregnancies.

Pregnant women with asthma should be counselled to continue their normal asthma medications and should be monitored closely throughout pregnancy and provided with a written asthma management plan. Smoking cessation advice should be given if indicated.

The risk to the fetus of uncontrolled asthma outweighs any small risk of asthma medication and steroid should be continued. With this history provided above there is no clear indication for admission for nebuliser or for oral antibiotics or steroids. Relaxation techniques may be of use but only in addition to the recommended medication.

There are limited data for the safety of leukotriene receptor antagonists, e.g. montelukast, and manufacturers recommend that these drugs are not commenced in pregnancy but should be continued if this is already an established medication as the risk of deterioration of symptoms outweighs the potential for side effects.

Scottish Intercollegiate Guidelines Network (SIGN). SIGN Guideline 153. British guideline on the management of asthma. Edinburgh: SIGN, 2016.

20. A Arterial embolisation

Massive haemoptysis (>500 mL in 24 hours) is a life-threatening emergency, with a mortality of up to 80%. Priorities need to include: airway protection and ventilation, cardiovascular support with large-bore ± central access, fluid resuscitation with blood and clotting factors ± inotropes. A chest X-ray should be performed in all cases and cross-sectional imaging with multidetector CT should be performed after the chest X-ray. The initial management of choice, if available locally, is arterial endovascular embolisation. Tranexamic acid may be useful, but the principal management is arterial embolisation. Surgical resection is the first line treatment if there is iatrogenic pulmonary artery rupture or chest trauma and may be required if other measures fail. In some cases, active treatment may be inappropriate and palliative treatment with oxygen and opiates may be necessary.

The history suggests that an aspergilloma may be the cause of the haemoptysis. An aspergilloma is a ball of fungal hyphae occurring within a cavity in the lung. Aspergillomas are often asymptomatic; however, up to 75% will present with haemoptysis. Superadded infections may provoke exacerbations. Sometimes there are systemic symptoms such as malaise and fever, and treatment with itraconazole may be considered. Itraconazole will not eradicate the fungus, but may reduce the cavity size and reduce the chance of haemoptysis.

Larici AR, Franchi P, Occhipinti M, et al. Diagnosis and management of hemoptysis. Diagn Interv Radiol. 2014; 20:299–309.

21. E She should commence dietary supplements

Women with cystic fibrosis (CF) are often subfertile; however, some patients may conceive naturally and if possible pregnancy should be planned to optimise the mother's physical and nutritional status. The outcome of a pregnancy is improved by optimising and maintaining pulmonary function and weight gain throughout the pregnancy. She has a body mass index (BMI) of 17 and should be advised to optimise her nutritional status before becoming pregnant. It is likely that dietary supplementation will be necessary. A pre-pregnancy target BMI of 22 is recommended. Close monitoring with regular dietician, chest physiotherapy and support from the other members of the multi-disciplinary CF team is essential throughout pregnancy. Pregnancy does not affect survival when compared with the entire female CF population, but impaired pulmonary function with forced expiratory volume$_1$ <60% predicted is the main predictor of worse maternal and fetal outcome.

Most antibiotics used to treat pulmonary exacerbations of CF are safe in pregnancy; however, ciprofloxacin, chloramphenicol, metronidazole and intravenous colimycin should be avoided. Aminoglycosides should be used with caution and close level monitoring carried out as there is a risk of fetal ototoxicity.

Genetic counselling and screening should be offered to CF patients and their partners. CF is an autosomal recessive disorder. The *CFTR* gene is located on the long arm of chromosome 7. Carrier frequency in the white population is 1:25. ΔF508 is the most common mutation. More than 1000 different mutations of the *CFTR* gene are recognised and the 30 most common abnormalities (>99.5% of the abnormalities) are screened for by a screening blood test, so if the partner is not a carrier of these mutations, there is a minimal chance that the child will have CF; however, the child will be a carrier of the CF gene.

Geake J, Tay G, Callaway L, Bell SC. Pregnancy and cystic fibrosis: Approach to contemporary management. Obstet Med. 2014; 7:147–155.

22. C Dietary and lifestyle advice

This middle-aged man has a history suggestive of sleep-disordered breathing. He is obese (body mass index 35 kg/m^2) and has hypertension and diabetes. Obesity, especially upper body obesity (and collar size >43 cm [17"]), is a risk factor for obstructive sleep apnoea/hypopnoea syndrome (OSAHS). OSAHS is part of a spectrum, ranging from snoring at one end and complete obstruction of the upper airway with frequent nocturnal awakenings at the other, with significant sleep fragmentation and excessive daytime somnolence. The combination of OSA identified by a sleep study together with symptoms of excessive daytime somnolence leads to the diagnosis of obstructive sleep apnoea hypopnoea syndrome. OSAHS is increasingly recognised as a risk factor for hypertension, cardiovascular and cerebrovascular disease, and complications of the metabolic syndrome, and is a major contributing factor to a large proportion of road traffic accidents.

It is important to differentiate sleepiness – tendency to fall asleep due to inadequate sleep from tiredness – feelings of exhaustion that may be multifactorial but not associated with a tendency to fall asleep. The severity of sleepiness may be assessed using the Epworth Sleepiness Score (ESS). This is scored out of 24; 0–9 is considered normal and >9 excessively sleepy.

Sleep studies are performed to confirm the diagnosis. These studies may vary from simple overnight oximetry, to oximetry with some other modalities of monitoring, e.g. chest and abdominal wall movements and oronasal flow (limited sleep study), to full polysomnography with EEG, electro-oculography (EOG) and electromyography (EMG), to stage sleep physiology. This will depend on local availability and protocols.

The sleep study is used to determine the severity of OSA; however, the values may vary according to each sleep centre. Expertise is needed to grade the sleep studies according to the apnoea–hypopnoea index (AHI), i.e. the number of events per hour.

The cut offs to assess severity are arbitrary but as a guide:
AHI <5 = normal
AHI 5–14 = evidence of mild OSA – does not normally require treatment, advise conservative measures if symptomatic

AHI 10–14 = mild OSA may require CPAP if very symptomatic
AHI 15–30 = moderate OSA – advise trial of CPAP
AHI > 30 = severe OSA – advise referral for urgent CPAP
(CPAP = continuous positive airway pressure)

Not all patients need treatment. The evidence for significant treatment benefit rests on symptoms, which drive treatment, rather than the degree of OSA on a sleep study.

This patient is not excessively sleepy – ESS <9 and the sleep study demonstrates an AHI of 11.4, i.e. mild OSA. Conservative approaches such as weight loss, reduction in alcohol consumption, smoking cessation and trying to sleep in the decubitus rather than the supine position should be recommended.

Mandibular advancement devices may be of benefit to snorers with mild OSA, assuming adequate dentition. Severe OSA with evidence of CO_2 retention may require non-invasive ventilation. Bariatric surgery may be needed for significant weight loss in morbidly obese patients.

Johns MW. A new method for measuring daytime sleepiness: The Epworth Sleepiness Scale. Sleep 1991; 14:540–545.
Scottish Intercollegiate Guidelines Network. SIGN Guideline No. 73: Management of obstructive sleep apnoea/hypopnoea syndrome in adults. Edinburgh: SIGN, 2003.

23. B Malignancy

Initial pleural fluid analysis should include the assessment of:
- Pleural fluid appearance
- Biochemistry (protein and lactate dehydrogenase)
- Cytology (for malignant cells and differential cell count)
- Microbiology (Gram stain and microscopy, culture, acid-fast bacilli (AFB) and tuberculosis (TB) culture
- pH

Determining whether an effusion is a transudate or an exudate is helpful to narrow the differential diagnosis. Light's criteria should always be used to assess whether an effusion is a transudate or an exudate.

By Light's criteria an effusion is present if:
- The pleural fluid protein divided by the serum protein is greater than 0.5
- The pleural fluid LDH divided by the serum LDH is greater than 0.6
- The pleural fluid LDH is over two thirds of the upper limit of the normal value of serum LDH

The pleural effusion described is an exudate. Additional pleural fluid investigations include cholesterol, triglycerides, haematocrit, glucose and amylase in certain clinical circumstances.

Common causes of exudative effusions include: empyema, TB and other infections, oesophageal rupture, pancreatitis, other connective tissue diseases and autoimmune conditions, and post-cardiac injury (Dressler's syndrome). An exudative effusion in a patient in this age group is most likely to be malignant. The sensitivity for pleural fluid cytology is about 60%.

Table 10.3 Common causes of exudative effusions

Parapneumonic effusion	May complicate 40% of bacterial pneumonias – most common cause of exudates in young patients
Malignancy	Most common exudative effusion in patients >60 years
Mesothelioma	Pleural fluid cytology – low sensitivity
Pulmonary embolism	Haemorrhagic effusion
Rheumatoid arthritis	Low glucose in pleural fluid (often <1.6 mmol/L)

Pleural effusions are common after coronary artery bypass grafting or post-cardiac injury syndrome (Dressler's syndrome), and typically occur as small, left-sided effusions with most resolving spontaneously. It would be unusual for this effusion to occur after 1 year and an alternative diagnosis should be sought.

Meigs' syndrome is a unilateral (often right sided) or bilateral benign transudative pleural effusion which may occur in women with ascites and ovarian tumours.

Liver cirrhosis causes a transudative pleural effusion (hydrothorax).

Pulmonary changes, including pleural effusions, may be the first manifestation of rheumatoid arthritis; however, rheumatoid pleurisy is more common in men (70% male). The pleural fluid glucose is typically low (<1.6 mmol/L) and pH is typically reduced (<7.3). These effusions can persist for months to years, although duration may be several weeks.

Pleural Disease Guidelines 2010. British Thoracic Society Pleural Disease Guideline 2010. Thorax 2010; 65(2). Light RW. Pleural effusion. N Engl J Med 2002; 346:1971–1977.

24. C Desquamative interstitial pneumonia

Desquamative interstitial pneumonia (DIP) is rare and the majority of patients are smokers, although it may occur with passive smoking. It typically occurs in patients aged 30–50 and presents with gradual onset of breathlessness and cough over weeks to months. Finger clubbing is common. High-resolution CT (HRCT) of the thorax may show ground-glass opacities in the lower zones and peripheries, with mild reticulation and honey-combing. Bronchoalveolar lavage may reveal an increase in pigmented macrophages; however, surgical biopsy is necessary for diagnosis. Smoking cessation is essential and corticosteroids are often used; however, their efficacy has not been studied. With smoking cessation, the prognosis is usually good.

Acute interstitial pneumonitis is a rapidly progressive (over days) form of interstitial lung disease (ILD) characterised by diffuse alveolar damage – formerly known as Hamman–Rich syndrome. The mean age of onset is 50 years. It is often preceded by 'viral'-type illness. It rapidly leads to respiratory failure requiring ventilator support; immunosuppressive therapy should be considered. The overall mortality rate is at least 50%.

Cryptogenic organising pneumonia (COP) is a disease of unknown cause characterised by 'plugging' of alveolar spaces with granulation tissue which may extend into the bronchioles. It is more common in non-smokers, with a mean age of onset of 55. There is typically a short (<3 months) history of breathlessness and cough, with malaise, fever and weight loss. Chest X-ray and HRCT demonstrate patchy areas of subpleural consolidation with air bronchograms which may migrate – 'flitting changes'. Transbronchial biopsy may often confirm the diagnosis. The management is with steroids and the prognosis is generally good.

Respiratory bronchiolitis-associated interstitial lung disease (RB-ILD) may present similarly to DIP; however, HRCT may demonstrate centrilobular nodules, ground-glass changes, thick wall airways and centrilobular emphysema. Affected patients are almost exclusively smokers or recent ex-smokers. Surgical biopsy is necessary for diagnosis which will demonstrate accumulation of brown pigmented macrophages. Prognosis is good with smoking cessation.

Usual interstitial pneumonitis (UIP) is an ILD of unknown cause. It typically presents in older patients, mean age 67 years; its prevalence increases with age. HRCT typically demonstrates subpleural reticulation, with minimal ground-glass changes and progressive fibrotic change with honey-combing.

Wells AU. Interstitial lung disease guideline: the British Thoracic Society in collaboration with the Irish Thoracic Society, Thoracic Society of Australia and New Zealand. Thorax 2008; 63:v1–v58.

25. E Self-limiting viral illness

This patient presents with an acute cough (<3 weeks' duration). This is the most common presentation to general practice. An acute cough is usually self-limiting and as a result of a viral illness. Ninety-three per cent of patients with flu-like illnesses may experience cough symptoms. Pneumonia and/or the inhalation of a foreign body may also cause an acute cough but there are no features to point to these diagnoses in the scenario described.

A cough lasting more than 8 weeks is defined as chronic and may be reported by 10–20% of adults and is more common in obese females. A careful history alone may identify the cause of the cough; however, a chest X-ray should be performed in all adults presenting with chronic cough.

Common causes of cough with a normal chest X-ray include: smoking, gastro-oesophageal reflux, asthma, allergic rhinitis and angiotensin-converting enzyme inhibitor use.

Morice A H, McGarvey L, Pavord I. Recommendations for the management of cough in adults, on behalf of the British Thoracic Society Cough Guideline Group. Thorax 2006; 61(I):i1–i24.

26. E Parapneumonic effusion

This young man presented with the typical history and clinical features of community-acquired pneumonia (CAP) and was previously well with no past medical history of note. This patient was considered to have a low risk of mortality–CURB65 score 1/5 (respiratory rate >30 breaths per minute); however, the clinical decision was made to commence intravenous antibiotics. Some patients with CURB65 0–1 may be considered for oral antibiotics and discharged home. Patients who are initially prescribed intravenous antibiotics should be reviewed early and switched to oral antibiotics if appropriate, as indicated by clinical improvement in terms of resolution of fever for >24 hours. If patients fail to improve, then they should be reviewed and it may be necessary to seek further senior advice, review the history and examination, and/or repeat the chest X-ray, inflammatory markers and review microbiology results if available. Parapneumonic effusion may complicate 40% of cases of CAP and early thoracocentesis is recommended. Rarer complications of CAP may include lung abscess (which typically occurs later in the clinical course) or development of adult respiratory distress syndrome (may be associated with severe sepsis). An underlying lung pathology is less likely in a young, previously fit patient; however, patients with CAP should have a follow-up chest X-ray at 6 weeks to ensure that the consolidation has resolved.

British Thoracic Society Standards of Care Committee. The British Thoracic Society Guidelines for the management of community acquired pneumonia in adults. Thorax 2009; 64(III).

27. C Inform the DVLA and stop driving until he has received adequate treatment

The oximetry demonstrates repeated episodes of desaturation suggestive of sleep-disordered breathing/obstructive sleep apnoea (OSA) and the patient is subjectively very sleepy – a diagnosis of obstructive sleep apnoea/hypopnoea syndrome (OSAHS). He should be told that he must stop driving and inform the DVLA of his diagnosis. He should be referred for urgent CPAP (continuous positive airway pressure) and will need appropriate follow-up to ensure that his overnight desaturation has improved and his symptoms of excessive daytime somnolence have resolved on therapy. The DVLA medical advisors will review his case and advise when he may return to driving. As he is a heavy-goods vehicle driver specialist consideration and close follow-up will be required. However, if he has been successfully treated and demonstrated good compliance with treatment, he may be able to resume his work.

All patients with sleep-disordered breathing problems will benefit from lifestyle and dietary advice (if overweight/obese); however, as this patient has evidence of severe OSAHS he will need treatment with CPAP.

Modafinil is a central nervous system-stimulating drug that may be used to treat narcolepsy. It was previously used to treat patients with OSA who were still symptomatic despite CPAP therapy but its licence for this indication was withdrawn due to concerns of addiction to the medication.

Johns MW. A new method for measuring daytime sleepiness: The Epworth Sleepiness Scale. Sleep 1991; 14:540–545.
Scottish Intercollegiate Guidelines Network. SIGN Guideline No. 73: Management of obstructive sleep apnoea/hypopnoea syndrome in adults. Edinburgh: SIGN, 2003.

28. E Pulmonary arterial hypertension

Primary pulmonary arterial hypertension (PPH), as defined by resting mean pulmonary artery pressure >25 mmHg, in the absence of significant underlying respiratory, cardiac or connective tissue disease, may be either familial or sporadic. The chest X-ray may demonstrate enlargement of central pulmonary arteries, with 'pruning' of peripheral vessels.

Sporadic cases of PPH may be associated with certain drug exposures (including fenfluramine, cocaine and amphetamines), human immunodeficiency virus (HIV), human herpesvirus (HHV)-8 or portal hypertension.

HIV-related pulmonary arterial hypertension (HIV-PAH) is a rare complication of the disease of uncertain cause. Other causes of PPH should be excluded. HIV patients are at increased risk of thromboembolic disease. The chest X-ray may demonstrate asymmetrical pulmonary vascular markings, but a CT pulmonary angiogram is the gold standard for diagnosis. An atrial septal defect may give subtle clinical features of a fixed split second heart sound. *Pneumocystis jirovecii* pneumonia is an opportunistic infection with insidious onset of dyspnoea and dry cough, with perihilar shadowing progressing to diffuse interstitial infiltration on the chest X-ray associated with significant desaturation on exercise.

Cicalini S, Chinello P, Petrosillo N. HIV infection and pulmonary arterial hypertension. Expert Rev Respir Med 2011; 5(2):257–266.

29. E 90% chance of resolution of disease within 2 years

The chest X-ray demonstrates bilateral hilar lymphadenopathy (BHL). The history of fevers, arthralgia and erythema nodosum together with the chest X-ray finding of BHL in a white person is most likely to be due to a diagnosis of Löfgren's syndrome (acute sarcoidosis). Löfgren's syndrome typically occurs as a mild acute disease, which is usually non-progressive. It is common in Irish, Scandinavian and African women. The diagnosis may be found by taking a detailed clinical history alone; however it is important to exclude other causes of BHL (see **Table 10.4**). High-resolution CT of the chest and lymph node aspiration and/or biopsy may be needed. Histology will demonstrate non-caseating granulomas.It is important to assess the extent and severity of the disease and to look for extrapulmonary involvement. Baseline biochemistry (urea and electrolytes, liver function tests and bone profile), full blood count and serum angiotensin-converting enzyme should be measured in all patients, and patients should have pulmonary function testing and an ECG.

Table 10.4 Differential diagnosis of bilateral hilar lymphadenopathy on chest X-ray
Sarcoidosis
Tuberculosis
Lymphoma
Coccidioidomycosis and histoplasmosis
Berylliosis
Hypogammaglobulinaemia and recurrent infections

Löfgren's syndrome has a good prognosis and 90% experience complete disease resolution within 2 years. Löfgren's syndrome does not need any specific treatment; however, conservative approaches such as simple analgesia/non-steroidal anti-inflammatory drugs and rest may be needed for some patients. The average time for BHL to resolve is 8 months. Fifteen per cent of patients will suffer progressive lung infiltration.

Neurological involvement occurs in up to 20% of patients and can affect any part of the central or peripheral nervous system. Most common is facial nerve lower motor neuron involvement; mononeuritis multiplex is also recognised and some patients may present with less specific features and psychiatric illness. Renal involvement may occur in one-third of patients; however, progression to renal failure is rare. Hypercalcaemia may be a feature due to conversion of vitamin D_3 to active 1,25-dihydroxycholecalciferol in the granulomas and is more common in summer months.

Costabel U, Ohshimo S, Guzman J. Diagnosis of sarcoidosis. Curr Opin Pulm Med 2008; 14(5):455–461.

30. B IV co-amoxiclav, oral clarithromycin and oseltamivir 75 mg twice daily for 5 days

This patient has signs and symptoms of a viral pneumonia (CURB 65 score of zero), and symptoms of influenza in the context of a declared influenza pandemic.

All patients with bilateral chest infiltrates on chest X-ray indicating viral pneumonia during pandemic influenza should be treated as having a severe pneumonia regardless of CURB 65 score, and so patients should be treated with intravenous co-amoxiclav (or local microbiologist guided equivalent) and a macrolide.

During an influenza pandemic patients should be treated with antivirals if all three of the following factors are present:

- Temperature >38°C
- An influenza-like illness of acute onset
- Length of viral symptoms of 48 hours or less

Lim WS. Pandemic flu: clinical management of patients with an influenza like illness during an influenza pandemic. Provisional guidelines from the British Infection Society, British Thoracic Society, and Health Protection Agency in collaboration with the Department of Health. Thorax 2007; 62(Suppl 1):1–46.

31. E Usual interstitial pneumonitis

Usual interstitial pneumonitis (UIP) may be diagnosed with typical clinical findings and on high-resolution CT (HRCT) which demonstrates the typical features of bilateral, peripheral and subpleural reticulation with honey-combing, traction bronchiectasis and minimal or no ground-glass opacification. Lung biopsy is not normally required for diagnosis unless there are atypical features.

The cause of UIP is unknown. The mean age at presentation is 67 years. Patients typically present with progressive dyspnoea and cough with an average of 9 months' history prior to presentation. Examination will reveal fine late inspiratory ('Velcro') crackles, finger clubbing in 50%, and signs of cyanosis or cor pulmonale in severe disease. Pulmonary function tests will demonstrate a restrictive lung defect with reduced gas transfer and arterial blood gases may demonstrate type I respiratory failure.

Bronchiectasis should be suspected in cases of chronic cough with sputum production – typically purulent and daily. HRCT will confirm the diagnosis with airway dilatation and thickening and mucus plugging.

Congestive cardiac failure should be excluded by performing echocardiography and serum BNP (brain natriuretic peptide). HRCT may demonstrate bilateral pleural effusion and dependent changes of interstitial oedema.

ACE inhibitors (ACEIs) are a common cause of chronic dry cough (side effect noted in up to 10% of women taking ACEIs), because of accumulation of bradykinin in the lung. Interstitial pneumonitis and pulmonary infiltration with eosinophilia are extremely rare complications of ACEIs. The patient may benefit from switching the ACEI to an angiotension II receptor blocker.

Desquamative interstitial pneumonia (DIP) is a very rare condition that occurs in smokers, typically aged 30–50 years. The HRCT demonstrates ground-glass opacification (present in all cases); reticulation and honey-combing may also occur.

Wells AU, et al. Interstitial Lung Interstitial lung disease guideline: the British Thoracic Society in collaboration with the Irish Thoracic Society, Thoracic Society of Australia and New Zealand. Thorax 2008; 63; v1–v58.

32. D Pulmonary arteriovenous malformation

Pulmonary arteriovenous malformation (PAVM) consists of an abnormal connection directly between a pulmonary artery and vein. Patients with PAVMs often present with abnormal chest X-rays, typically demonstrating a smooth, rounded, intrapulmonary mass with draining or feeding vessels. Symptoms may include dyspnoea, haemoptysis and atypical chest pain. PAVMs may present with acute stroke or cerebral abscesses; between 13 and 55% of patients are asymptomatic. Clinical examination may reveal mild hypoxia (because of right-to-left shunt), orthodeoxia (hypoxia on standing due to increase in blood flow to dependent lung areas, as 83% of PAVMs are basal), finger clubbing and bruits audible to auscultation. Between 47 and 80% of PAVMs occur in patients with hereditary haemorrhagic telangiectasia (HHT) and patients with HHT and their families should be screened for PAVMs because of the associated potential for neurological sequelae. Patients with PAVMs should be referred to a specialist centre for further assessment and consideration of embolisation to prevent shunting, hypoxia and risk of embolic stroke.

Asbestos-related pleural plaques typically occur as calcified areas of pleural thickening or a characteristic 'holly-leaf' appearance and are asymptomatic. Lung abscesses present with symptoms of productive cough, fevers and a cavitating lesion on chest X-ray.

A patient may be at risk of developing a lung abscess following a stroke if it is complicated by dysphagia and aspiration pneumonia; however, this patient does not have symptoms suggesting an infective aetiology. Old tuberculosis may be found incidentally on a chest X-ray which may demonstrate a calcified granuloma (Ghon focus), typically in the upper zone.

Patients may be at increased risk of developing pulmonary emboli (PEs) following a period of reduced mobility and would be associated with sudden-onset pleuritic chest pain and hypoxia. Often the chest X-ray appearance will be normal or may demonstrate a small unilateral effusion. Pulmonary infarction secondary to PE may lead to a wedge-shaped opacity on a chest X-ray; a rounded opacity would not be a typical feature of PEs.

Khurshid I, Downie GH. Pulmonary arteriovenous malformation. Postgrad Med J 2002; 78:191–197.
Hsu CC, et al. Embolisation therapy for pulmonary arteriovenous malformations. Cochrane Database Syst Rev 2010; (5):CD008017.

33. E Tropical pulmonary eosinophilia

Tropical pulmonary eosinophilia is caused by hypersensitivity to the migrating larvae of filarial worms, *Wucheria bancrofti* and *Brugia malayi*. It occurs in the Indian subcontinent, south-east Asia and South Pacific islands, Africa and South America. It presents with gradual-onset (weeks to months) cough, wheeze, sputum, dyspnoea, chest pain and fever, weight loss and fatigue. Symptoms can be worse at night, due to pulmonary sequestration of eosinophils. Chest X-ray typically demonstrates diffuse patchy shadowing. Blood tests demonstrate significant eosinophilia, the erythrocyte sedimentation rate (ESR) is raised in 90% of cases, a raised IgE is seen, and filarial complement is positive. Sputum and bronchoalveolar lavage contain eosinophils.

Löffler's syndrome (simple pulmonary eosinophilia) is caused by parasitic infection, usually *Ascaris lumbricoides*, but also *Strongyloides* and *Ankylostoma* species. The passage of larvae through the lung causes an allergic reaction and may be asymptomatic or present with cough, malaise, anorexia, low-grade fevers and night sweats. The illness typically lasts for around 2 weeks. Chest X-ray may show transient bilateral perihilar shadowing and there is low-level blood eosinophilia.

Miliary tuberculosis (TB) is a more common presentation of disseminated TB in immunocompromised individuals. Chest X-ray demonstrates a typical 'miliary' or 'millet-seed' pattern of diffuse nodularity. Full blood count may demonstrate lymphopenia – eosinophilia would not be a typical feature.

Pneumocystis jirovecii pneumonia is an opportunistic infection in immunocompromised individuals. Patients present with progressive dyspnoea and dry cough. Hypoxia and desaturation on exertion are common features. Chest X-ray demonstrates bilateral perihilar infiltrates that progress to alveolar shadowing. Full blood count is often normal.

Churg–Strauss syndrome is characterised by asthma, blood eosinophilia and eosinophilic granulomatous inflammation of the respiratory tract. It is often associated with sinusitis and other systemic features including vasculitic neuropathy and skin involvement.

Mullerpattan JB, Udwadia ZF, Udwadia FK. Tropical Pulmonary Eosinophilia – A review. Indian. J Med Res 2013; 138: 295–302.
Campos LE, Pereira LF. Pulmonary eosinophilia. J Bras Pneumol 2009; 35(6):561–573.

34. E Refer to cardiothoracic surgeons

This patient has a history of chronic lung disease and presented with a large pneumothorax – secondary spontaneous pneumothorax (SSP). Patients presenting with SSP should be admitted for further management. Supplemental oxygen should be administered in accordance with the British Thoracic Society guidelines for the use of oxygen in adults. Most patients presenting with SSP will require a small-bore chest drain attached to an underwater seal and early opinion from a respiratory physician should be sought to guide further management. Suction should not be used routinely, but high-volume, low-pressure suction may be recommended in some circumstances to aid re-expansion of the collapsed lung. Ongoing bubbling or failure of re-expansion may suggest persistent air leak and these cases should be discussed with a thoracic surgeon at 48 hours. The thoracic surgeon may employ one of the following techniques:

- Open thoracotomy and pleurectomy
- Video-assisted thoracoscopic surgery (VATS) with pleurectomy and/or pleural abrasion
- Surgical chemical pleurodesis with talc

Patients with persistent SSP who are unfit for general anaesthesia and/or surgical intervention may be considered for talc pleurodesis via the chest tube or for domiciliary management with a Heimlich valve, which is a one-way valve that prevents air from travelling back up a chest drain. There is no strong evidence that large-bore chest tubes will offer benefit over small-bore tubes.

The chest drain is still bubbling profusely, therefore flushing is not indicated and potentially risks introducing infection. A bubbling chest drain should never be clamped as it may lead to tension pneumothorax.

British Thoracic Society. Pleural Disease guidelines 2010. Thorax 2010; 65(2).

35. B Admit to negative pressure room and send sputum samples for acid-fast bacilli and TB (tuberculosis) culture

The clinical history, risk factors (homelessness and alcohol abuse) and chest X-ray demonstrating significant consolidation with loss of volume in the right upper lobe are strongly suggestive of pulmonary TB. People with TB (pulmonary or non-pulmonary) should not be admitted to hospital for diagnostic tests or for care unless there is a clear clinical or socioeconomic need, such as homelessness. If hospital admission is necessary, patients should be managed in a negative pressure room and separated from immunocompromised patients. If the clinical signs and symptoms are strongly suggestive of TB, three early morning sputum samples for acid-fast bacilli and culture should be sent and treatment should be initiated early – this may be before culture results are available. The four-drug initiation regimen is recommended (rifampicin, isoniazid, pyrazinamide and ethambutol) for 2 months and then rifampicin and isoniazid for a further 4 months if the cultures demonstrate a fully sensitive organism. Directly observed therapy may be particularly useful to compliance in certain at-risk groups, including homeless people with active TB.

This patient is not overtly septic so it may be possible to wait for sputum acid-fast bacilli smear results and seek specialist respiratory opinion regarding commencing antituberculous therapy, rather than commencing empirical antibiotics for community-acquired pneumonia. A CT scan and bronchoscopy may not be necessary if the diagnosis is confirmed on sputum results – sputum induction with nebuliser saline and physiotherapy may increase the diagnostic rate.

National Institute for Health and Clinical Excellence (NICE). NICE guideline NG33: Tuberculosis. London: NICE, 2016.

36. D Omeprazole

Chronic cough (cough lasting longer than 8 weeks) is more likely to occur in middle-aged women. Gastro-oesophageal disorders, including reflux (GORD) and oesophageal dysmotility, may be the cause in up to 40% of cases of chronic cough and may occur in the absence of heartburn or typical reflux symptoms. Proton pump inhibitors (e.g. omeprazole 20 mg twice daily for at least 8 weeks) may help in 75–100% of cases and an empirical trial of treatment should be considered as first-line therapy. Prokinetic agents such as metoclopramide or erythromycin may help some patients, but due to side effects should only be used for a short period of time. All patients should be advised regarding conservative measures to reduce GORD including: weight loss; reducing caffeine and alcohol intake; taking their main meal at lunch time; and elevating the head of the bed by 5 cm.

Some patients with resistant symptoms may require referral for specialist review and investigation including gastroscopy, oesophageal ambulatory 24-hour pH measurement and/or oesophageal manometry, barium meal and gastric emptying studies. Selected patients may benefit from fundoplication.

Angiotensin-converting enzyme inhibitors cause cough in about 10% of patients (women > men) – these medications should be stopped. The cough may take up to 40 weeks to resolve.

The patient has a mild restrictive lung defect (probably related to body habitus) with normal gas transfer and normal chest X-ray. There are no features in the history to suggest an interstitial or suppurative pathology – referral for a high-resolution CT scan of the thorax would not be the first appropriate investigation. Similarly, there are no features to suggest asthma/atopic disease and prednisolone may exacerbate reflux symptoms.

Morice AH, McGarvey L, Pavord I. Recommendations for the management of cough in adults, on behalf of the British Thoracic Society Cough Guideline Group. Thorax 2006; 61(I):i1–i24.

37. D Lobectomy

The patient has T2N0M0 adenocarcinoma of the lung. The 2011 NICE guidelines recommend all patients with non-small cell lung cancer whose disease is suitable for treatment with curative intent and who are medically fit should be offered lobectomy as the first-choice treatment.

These recommendations are largely based on observational and retrospective studies and there have been no randomised controlled trials comparing surgery with no intervention. The Early Lung Cancer Action Project, a lung cancer screening study, reported that 92% of patients who had surgical treatment for stage 1 lung cancer survived for 5 years, with all 8 patients who did not undergo surgery dying within 5 years. A 1963 trial comparing radiotherapy and surgery in lung cancer demonstrated improved survival in patients with early stage disease (T1a-3, N0-1, M0) treated with surgery.

Radical radiotherapy should only be offered to those with early stage non-small cell lung cancer (NSCLC) whose risk of surgical complications is unacceptable. Chemo-radiotherapy is the treatment of choice for patients with a good performance status and locally advanced NSCLC who are not suitable for surgery. Wedge resection and other lung parenchymal sparing operations should be considered for patients with T1a-b,N0M0 NSCLC who have borderline fitness providing complete resection of the tumour is possible.

National Institute for Health and Care Excellence (NICE). Lung cancer: diagnosis and management. Clinical Guideline 121. London: NICE, 2011.
Lim E, Baldwin D, Beckles M, et al. Guidelines on the radical management of patients with lung cancer. Thorax 2010; 65(Suppl iii).

38. D *Streptococcus milleri*

The clinical history and pleural aspirate are strongly suggestive of empyema. Immunocompromised patients, including people with diabetes, those who abuse drugs and alcohol, and patients with recurrent aspiration are at increased risk of developing empyema.

A pleural tap should be performed if empyema is suspected and may demonstrate turbid fluid or frank pus, pleural fluid pH <7.2 and/or positive Gram stain on bacterial culture. All of these features are indicators for the insertion of a chest drain. Forty per cent of pleural infections are culture negative. Bacterial causes of empyemas are shown in **Table 10.5**.

Table 10.5 Bacterial causes of empyema			
Community-acquired infection (% of cases)		**Hospital-acquired infection (% of cases)**	
Streptococcus spp. including (most frequently S. milleri – 28% of cases overall)	52%	Meticillin-resistant S. aureus	27%
Anaerobes (including Bacteroides)	20%	Staphylococcus aureus	22%
		Enterobacteria	20%
Staphylococcus aureus	11%	Enterococci	12%
Other organisms: enterobacteria, Haemophila influenzae, Pseudomonas spp., TB, Nocardia spp.	17%	Other organisms: Streptococcus spp. Pseudomonas spp., anaerobes	19%

British Thoracic Society. Pleural Disease Guidelines 2010. Thorax 2010; 65(2).

39. B Cystic fibrosis

Patients with cystic fibrosis (CF) are usually diagnosed as neonates or in childhood; however, some patients may be diagnosed in adulthood and these patients usually have milder phenotypes. Some patients may be detected following screening for male infertility. Male CF patients may be infertile due to failure of the normal development or blockage of the vas deferens, seminal vesicle, ejaculatory duct or epididymis; however, in some patients fertility may be preserved.

Primary ciliary dyskinesia (PCD) is a rare genetic disorder causing chronic respiratory disease because of abnormal cilia and reduced mucociliary clearance, microbiological colonisation and chronic infection, and the development of bronchiectasis. PCD is also associated with infertility in men because of functional abnormalities of the ductus epididymis and reduced sperm motility because the sperm tails have the same morphological defect as the cilia and do not beat correctly.

Bronchiectasis has a number of other causes including genetic (two examples described above), postinfective (tuberculosis or pertussis) and postobstructive (e.g. distal to an inhaled foreign body). Many of these conditions are not associated with infertility.

Pulmonary fibrosis would be an unusual diagnosis in a patient of this age group with a long history of recurrent infections. Tuberculosis should be considered in patients from high-risk groups presenting with a chronic productive cough; however, this would not lead to the history as outlined above.

Davies J, et al. Clinical review. Cystic fibrosis. BMJ 2007; 335:1255–1259.

40. D Pseudochylothorax

A cloudy, milky effusion is suggestive of chylothorax or pseudochylothorax. If the milky fluid is passed through a centrifuge or left to rest on the laboratory bench for 1 hour and fails to clear, it is suggestive of a pseudochylothorax. This may be confirmed on further testing with the identification of rhomboid-shaped crystals of cholesterol and the presence of raised total cholesterol, but normal triglyceride, levels. Causes of a pseudochylothorax include chronic pleural inflammation relating to persistent tuberculous effusion or rheumatoid pleuritis.

Chylothorax may occur following disruption of the thoracic duct, and pleural fluid may appear turbid, milky, serous or blood stained. The presence of pleural fluid chylomicrons or pleural fluid triglyceride level >11 mg/L confirms the diagnosis. Causes include: malignancy (particularly lymphoma), trauma, following lobectomy and pulmonary lymphangioleiomyomatosis.

Pleuritis and pleural effusions are commonly associated with rheumatoid arthritis (up to 30% of patients). Pleural effusions are usually asymptomatic and the fluid is typically exudative and straw coloured, with a low glucose and low pH and typically lymphocytic. Malignancy should be considered in the differential diagnoses, especially in patients in this age group; however, a milky effusion, as described above, would not be typical of malignancy.

Hillerdal G. Chylothorax and pseudochylothorax. Eur Respir J 1997; 10:1157–1162.
British Thoracic Society. Pleural Disease Guidelines 2010. Thorax 2010; 65(2).

41. D Silicosis

Pneumoconioses are non-malignant respiratory disease caused by the reaction of the lung to the inhalation of mainly mineral or organic dusts. Tiny inhaled particles (<5 μm) can reach the terminal airways and alveoli where they are slowly cleared by macrophages or alveolar cells, leading to inflammatory reactions and characteristic patterns of disease and radiological features.

Silica is used in industries such as ceramics and stone masonry. Acute silicosis may occur within 1–2 months of working with the dust and presents as a dry cough and rapid-onset shortness of breath. Chest X-ray typically demonstrates patchy bilateral lower airspace shadowing. Chronic silicosis occurs with lower dust concentration and patients are often asymptomatic. The chest X-ray may demonstrate mid- and upper zone small nodules (between 2–10 mm in size and typically 2–5 mm) which will calcify after about 10 years and can be associated with calcified hilar lymphadenopathy.

Inhalation of asbestos may lead to asbestosis, which is a form of chronic interstitial fibrosis that is made worse with cigarette smoking. It typically presents with shortness of breath and dry cough but after a long latency period that is often decades after initial exposure. The chest X-ray may be normal in early disease but may later show bilateral reticulonodular shadowing, predominantly affecting the lower zones, which may progress to affect the mid- and upper zones.

Coal workers' pneumoconiosis is caused by the deposition of coal dust within the lung and the risk increases with the duration and amount of exposure. The disease is characterised by the formation of nodules in the alveoli. With progressive massive fibrosis these nodules can extend to the chest wall also. Symptoms typically consist of a slow onset of progressive dyspnoea and blackened sputum. The chest X-ray demonstrates nodules located in the upper zones which enlarge and become increasingly radiodense.

Kaolinosis is a form of pneumoconiosis acquired by inhaling china clay dust (kaolin), which is used in the production of paper, ceramics, soaps, toothpaste and some medicines. Stannosis is another rare pneumoconiosis associated with tin oxide.

Sirajuddin A, Kanne JP. Occupational lung disease. J Thorac Imaging 2009; 24(4):310–320.

42. D She may fly without the need for in-flight oxygen

If there is concern regarding a patient's fitness to fly because of medical conditions a flight assessment should be performed. This should be done when the patient is stable and has recovered from any recent exacerbations. This patient has recovered from an infective exacerbation and is back to baseline function so the assessment may be performed now.

Flight assessments are performed by conducting a hypoxic challenge test. The patient receives 15% oxygen for 20 minutes and then arterial blood gases are performed to determine recommendations for in-flight oxygen.

If PaO_2 >6.6 kPa (>50 mmHg) or oxygen saturation 85% then in-flight oxygen not required.

If PaO_2 <6.6 kPa (<50 mmHg) or oxygen saturation <85% then in-flight oxygen required at 2 L/min via nasal cannulae.

Lung volumes (forced expiratory volume1) and oxygen saturations using pulse oximetry may be useful indicators of disease severity; however, it is more difficult to predict patient outcomes during flight when the available oxygen may be reduced to 15%. A hypoxic challenge test performed for 20 minutes may not replicate the patient's experience of a long-haul flight and should be interpreted with caution.

Patients with infectious tuberculosis, pneumothorax, large-volume haemoptysis and respiratory failure requiring >4 L/min oxygen should be advised not to travel by air.

Shrikrishna D, Coker RK. Managing passengers with stable respiratory disease planning air travel: British Thoracic Society recommendations. Thorax 2011; 66:831–833.

43. A Pulmonary haemodynamics

Long-term oxygen therapy (LTOT) should be considered in patients with stable chronic obstructive pulmonary disease (COPD) who have a resting arterial PO_2 of 7.3 kPa or less, or who have a resting PO_2 of 8 kPa or less and polycythaemia (haematocrit over 55%), pulmonary hypertension or peripheral oedema.

LTOT in COPD has been shown in two randomised controlled trials, the Nocturnal Oxygen Therapy Trial and the Medical Research Council (MRC) domiciliary oxygen study, to provide a mortality benefit. In the MRC trial after 5 years of follow up 19/42 patients in the LTOT treatment group and 30/45 in the group without oxygen therapy had died. The mortality improvement seen in LTOT is greater in patients with hypercapnia, although 24-hour per day oxygen therapy has the potential to increase CO_2 levels.

LTOT has been shown to decrease mean pulmonary artery pressure, and to prevent an increase in pulmonary artery pressure (versus an increase in the control group of 0.4 kPa), although the effect on pulmonary haemodynamics is small. A decrease in pulmonary artery pressure may be related to survival.

Quality of life has not been shown to be improved by LTOT although mood and neuropsychological function have been shown to be improved. Hospital admissions were not affected by treatment with LTOT in the MRC trial.

British Thoracic Society (BTS) Home Oxygen Guideline Group. BTS guidelines for home oxygen use in adults, Thorax 2015; 70:i1–i43.

44. A Insert 14 Fr drain immediately above a rib margin in the scalene triangle

This patient presents with severe symptoms and a large pneumothorax on a background of emphysema. This is a secondary spontaneous pneumothorax (SSP). Patients with SSP may often be more symptomatic and suffer greater compromise than patients presenting with primary spontaneous pneumothoraces due to reduction in physiological reserve. SSPs are less likely to resolve spontaneously and most patients will need some form of intervention. Oxygen therapy should be used with caution in patients at risk of carbon dioxide retention. Needle aspiration may be considered in some cases to try to avoid chest drain insertion; however, most cases will require the insertion of a chest drain to adequately treat the pneumothorax. A small-bore drain (14 Fr) will generally be sufficient and there is no evidence that these drain are inferior to large-bore chest (e.g. 28 Fr) drains.

Chest drains and all other procedures should be performed immediately above a rib margin to reduce the risk of injury to the neurovascular bundle that is situated below a lower rib margin. Similarly, where possible, all procedures should be performed in the 'triangle of safety' – the scalene triangle to reduce risk of injury to other organs and reduce risk of bleeding from intercostal arteries.

MacDuff A, Arnold A, Harvey J. Management of spontaneous pneumothorax: British Thoracic Society pleural disease guideline 2010. Thorax 2010; 65(suppl 2):ii18–ii31.

45. E Occupational asthma

The history is very suggestive of occupational asthma. The symptoms have commenced since she started working in a bakery. Occupational asthma is due to specific workplace sensitisers and may account for 10% of adult-onset asthma and more than 300 work-related allergens are recognised. The diagnosis may be difficult to establish and it is important to take a careful history of exposure to all of the potentially irritant substances and to document the temporal relationship of contact with development of symptoms. Early diagnosis is important, as an earlier removal from the workplace in affected individuals leads to a better outcome. The symptoms improve away from work, but can take several days to settle. Serial peak flow measurements should be recorded every 2 hours from waking to sleep for 4 weeks, although there are no changes to treatment. Holidays and periods away from work should be documented. There may be associated rhinitis and urticaria. Smoking increases the risk of developing occupational asthma and smoking cessation should be encouraged.

Hypersensitivity pneumonitis is a group of lung diseases caused by inhalation of an organic antigen to which the patient has been previously sensitised. It may follow an 'acute' or 'chronic' course. Many different antigens have been reported, including 'farmers' lung' and 'bird-fanciers' lung'. The condition typically presents with breathlessness, dry cough and constitutional symptoms including fevers and weight loss.

British Thoracic Society (BTS) and Scottish Intercollegiate Guidelines Network (SIGN). SIGN 153. British guideline on the management of asthma – a national clinical guideline. London and Edinburgh: BTS and SIGN, 2016.

46. D Assess risk using Brock model

In a patient with a pulmonary nodule of 10 mm on CT the appropriate next management step is to assess the risk of malignancy using the Brock model. Patients who are assessed to be at <10% risk of malignancy should be followed up with CT surveillance. Those who have an ≥10% risk of malignancy should have a PET-CT and further risk assessment using the Herder model. Depending on their risk of malignancy following the Herder risk assessment, patients should then be entered in to CT surveillance (<10% risk of malignancy), be considered for image-guided or excision biopsy or CT surveillance (10–70% risk of malignancy), or be considered for excision (over 70% risk of malignancy).

When a solid nodule is <5 mm in diameter, or <80 mm^3 in volume, there are clear features of benign disease or the patient would be unfit for treatment then they should be discharged.

Patients with a solid nodule on CT of <8 mm in diameter or <300 mm^3 volume should enter CT surveillance without risk assessment.

British Thoracic Society Pulmonary Nodule Guideline Development Group. BTS Guidelines for the Investigation and Management of Pulmonary Nodules. Thorax 2015; 70(Suppl ii):ii1–ii54.

Chapter 11

Rheumatology

Questions

1. A 34-year-old woman presented with a deep vein thrombosis of the left femoral vein. Apart from a weekend break to Spain, she had not travelled recently. She was usually fit and active and swam at least twice a week. Apart from two miscarriages at 11 and 13 weeks' gestation, there was no past medical history of note.

    On examination she had a swollen, tender, left calf.

    What is the most useful diagnostic investigation?

    A   Activated protein C
    B   Anticardiolipin antibodies
    C   Anti-dsDNA antibodies
    D   Antithrombin III
    E   Homocysteine

2. A 70-year-old woman presented following a fall. Her past medical history included type 2 diabetes mellitus and hypothyroidism. She has not had any fractures previously. She is an ex-smoker and drinks less than 7 units of alcohol per week.

    On examination and plain radiography, no fracture was found on this occasion. In follow-up, a dual energy X-ray absorptiometry (DEXA) scan was undertaken and her T-score is –2.9.

    Investigations:

    > 25-OH-Cholecalciferol/1,25 vitamin D3: 80 nmol/L (45–90)
    > calcium (corrected): 2.50 mmol/L (2.2–2.6)

    What therapy is indicated?

    A   None
    B   Raloxifene
    C   Bisphosphonate
    D   Calcium and vitamin D supplements
    E   Strontium

3. A 65-year-old man presented with new-onset headache, tenderness over both of his temporal arteries and jaw claudication.

    Investigations:

    > haemoglobin 105 g/L (130–180)   creatine kinase 100 U/L (25–195)
    > erythrocyte sedimentation rate 110 mm/1st h
    > (0–20)

Which of the following does not apply to his diagnosis?

A   Colour duplex ultrasound can aid with diagnosis
B   He must have an urgent temporal artery biopsy before starting any treatment
C   His symptoms should settle within 2 weeks of starting steroids
D   It is closely associated with polymyalgia rheumatica
E   Temporal artery biopsy may be normal

4.   A 37-year-old woman presented with symptoms of severe Raynaud's phenomenon and arthralgia of the small joints of her hands. She had recently developed indigestion. She had no other relevant past medical history and her current medication was omeprazole 20 mg once daily.
      On examination, she had digital ulceration and swelling. On respiratory examination there were fine bi-basal crackles.

Investigations:

haemoglobin 112 g/L (115–165)	erythrocyte sedimentation rate 46 mm/1st h (0–30)
white cell count 4.3 × 10⁹/L (4–11)	C-reactive protein 10 mg/L (<10)
platelets 167 × 10⁹/L (150–400)	

Antinuclear antibody 1:160 (<1:80)
Rheumatoid factor 60 (<20)
Anti-dsDNA: negative
Anticentromere antibody: positive

What is the most likely diagnosis?

A   Diffuse cutaneous systemic sclerosis
B   Limited cutaneous systemic sclerosis
C   Mixed connective tissue disease
D   Rheumatoid arthritis
E   Systemic lupus erythematosus

5.   A 19-year-old woman presented with a 6-month history of fatigue. This had been associated with intermittent fevers, and migratory arthralgia in her small and large joints. She had noticed a pruritic rash on her face. She had no past medical history and took no medications.
      On examination, she had tenderness and mild swelling of her left knee and the distal interphalangeal joints of her right hand. There was an erythematous, maculopapular rash on her face affecting the forehead and cheeks.

Investigations:

haemoglobin 102 g/L (115–165)	platelets 136 × 10⁹/L (150–400)
white cell count 2.8 × 10⁹/L (4–11)	erythrocyte sedimentation rate 38 mm/1st h (0–30)

Antinuclear antibody 1:160 (<1:80)
Anti-dsDNA 1:160 (<1:80)
Anticentromere antibody: negative

What is the most likely diagnosis?

A   Mixed connective tissue disorder
B   Polymyositis
C   Rheumatoid arthritis
D   Systemic lupus erythematosus
E   Systemic sclerosis

6. A 24-year-old man presented with a 1-week history of fever, polyarthralgia, sore throat and skin rash. The rash was salmon-pink coloured and occurred with the fever, fading as the fever resolved. He had a temperature of 38.5°C, pulse 100 beats per minute, blood pressure 130/75 mmHg and oxygen saturation 99% on air.

On examination, he had a pericardial rub. Examination of both small and large joints was normal.

Investigations:

haemoglobin 119 g/L (130–180)	alanine aminotransferase 189 U/L (5–35)
white cell count 15.9 × 10⁹/L (13.0–18.0)	alkaline phosphatase 87 U/L (45–105)
neutrophils 9.7 × 10⁹/L (1.5–7.0)	erythrocyte sedimentation rate 89 mm/1st h (0–30)
platelets 608 × 10⁹/L (150–400)	C-reactive protein 54 mg/L (<5)
bilirubin 7 mmol/L (1–22)	ferritin 6030 g/L (15–300)
albumin 31 g/L (37–49)	

What is the most likely diagnosis?

A   Adult Still's disease
B   Churg–Strauss syndrome
C   Haemophagocytosis
D   Periodic fever syndrome
E   Wegener's granulomatosis

7. A 36-year-old woman was admitted with shortness of breath. She had progressive dyspnoea for the last 2 months and now could only walk up to 200 metres on the flat. She did not have chest pain. She had a cough which produced only white sputum. Over the last month she had had occasional bouts of fever. She also had weakness and pain in her left arm and numbness in the lateral part of her right thigh. She had a past history of recurrent rhinitis, sinusitis and asthma.

On examination, her temperature was 38.4°C, pulse 102 beats per minute, blood pressure 104/70 mmHg, respiratory rate 20 breaths per minute and oxygen saturation 94% on air. There were purpuric spots and a maculopapular rash over the extensor aspect of left forearm. She had a polyphonic wheeze. There was a gallop rhythm at the apex and a pericardial rub. There was a left wrist drop as well as sensory loss over the lateral cutaneous nerve of right thigh.

Investigations:

haemoglobin 112 g/L (115–165)	potassium 5 mmol/L (3.5–5.0)
mean corpuscular volume 84 fL (80–96)	urea 8 mmol/L (2.5–7.5)
white cell count 12 ×10⁹/L (4–11)	creatinine 134 µmol/L (45–90)
platelets 349 × 10⁹/L (150–400)	albumin 45 g/L (37–49)
neutrophils 6 × 10⁹/L (1.5 –7.0)	bilirubin 3 mmol/L (1–22)
lymphocytes 3 × 10⁹/L (1.5–4.0)	alanine transaminase 39 U/L (5–35)
eosinophils 3 × 10⁹/L (0.04–0.4)	alkaline phosphatase 102 U/L (45–105)
sodium 138 mmol/L (135–145)	

Urinalysis: protein 2+, blood 2+, leukocytes +, nitrites

Electrocardiogram: sinus tachycardia

Echocardiogram:
left ventricle was slightly enlarged with ejection fraction of 50%
small pericardial effusion

Chest X-ray: infiltrates in both the lower lobes of the lung

What is the most likely diagnosis?

A   Cardiac amyloidosis
B   Churg–Strauss syndrome
C   Goodpasture's syndrome
D   Loffler's syndrome
E   Sarcoidosis

8.   A 33-year-old woman presented with a 2-month history of pain and swelling in her hands and feet. She had no past medical history of note and was on no regular medication.
     General examination was normal with normal heart sounds.
     On examination of skin and joints there was obvious dactylitis in the fingers of both hands and arthropathy affecting the distal interphalangeal joints. Examination of her feet revealed tenderness over the calcaneus bilaterally with onycholysis of most of her toenails.

Investigations:

> Rheumatoid factor: negative
> Antinuclear antibody: negative
> Extractable nuclear antigen: negative
> Antineutrophil cytoplasmic antibody: negative
> Antiendomysial antibodies: negative
>
> erythrocyte sedimentation rate 78 mm/1st h (0–30)

What is the most likely diagnosis?

A   Enteropathic arthropathy
B   Jaccoud's arthropathy
C   Psoriatic arthropathy
D   Reiter's syndrome
E   Rheumatoid arthritis

9.   A 41-year-old woman presented with pain and colour change in her fingers related to cold temperatures. She was a non-smoker who exercised regularly. On systems review she also reported some dysphagia to liquids.
     On examination, she had thickening of the skin in her fingers with some oedema of the digits. There were tender, white nodules over some of her interphalangeal joints. Around her mouth there were some telangiectasias.

Investigations:

> Rheumatoid factor: negative
> Antinuclear antibody: negative
> Antineutrophil cytoplasmic antibody: negative
>
> erythrocyte sedimentation rate 89 mm/1st h (0–30)   C-reactive protein 14 mg/L (<10)

What is the most appropriate treatment for her presenting complaint?

A   Clopidogrel
B   Doxazosin
C   Losartan
D   Nifedipine
E   Sildenafil

10. A 19-year-old Irish woman was referred with recurrent fever occurring five to six times a year for the last 10 years. On each occasion the fever lasted for 7–8 days and could be accompanied by abdominal pain, arthralgia and intermittent macular eruptions. Investigations during each febrile episode had always proved negative. She was adopted and had no siblings.

She was currently apyrexial and systemic examination was normal.

Investigations:

IgG 18.9 g/L (6.0–13.0)	IgA 2.9 g/L (0.8–3.0)
IgM 4.1 g/L (0.4–2.5)	IgD 70 (range 0–80) (0.0–8.0)
Urinary porphobilinogen not detected	
MEFV mutation not detected	
TNFRSF1A mutation detected	

What is the most likely diagnosis?

A Acute intermittent porphyria (AIP)
B Familial hibernian fever or tumour necrosis factor (TNF) receptor-associated periodic syndrome (TRAPS)
C Familial Mediterranean fever (FMF)
D Hyperimmunoglobulinaemia D syndrome (HIDS)
E Systemic lupus erythematosus (SLE)

11. A 33-year-old woman presented with arthralgia in the small joints of both hands and myalgia. She had suffered from Raynaud's phenomenon for many years, and this had recently worsened. She had no other relevant past medical history and was not on any medication.

On examination, she looked well. There was tenderness of the distal interphalangeal joints of both hands, and swelling of her fingers bilaterally. Palpation of the muscles in her limbs revealed tenderness.

Investigations:

haemoglobin 113 g/L (115–165)	lymphocytes 1.2 × 10⁹/L (1.5–4.0)
white cell count 3.1 × 10⁹/L (4–11)	platelets 145 × 10⁹/L (150–400)
neutrophils 2.1 × 10⁹/L (1.5–7.0)	
Rheumatoid factor: negative	
Antinuclear antibody: 1/160	
Anti-dsDNA: negative	
Anti-U1-ribonucleoprotein: 1/1000	
Anticentromere: negative	

What is the most likely diagnosis?

A Mixed connective tissue disease (MCTD)
B Polymyositis
C Rheumatoid arthritis (RA)
D Scleroderma
E Systemic lupus erythematosus (SLE)

12. A 36-year-old woman presented with a 2-month history of arthralgia and a recurrent itchy rash over her trunk and limbs. She had started antihistamine therapy with no benefit.

On examination, there were urticarial lesions all over the trunk. Skin biopsy revealed leukocytoclastic vasculitis and a diagnosis of urticarial vasculitis was made.

What is the most appropriate next step in management?

A   Azathioprine
B   Dapsone
C   Hydroxychloroquine
D   Naproxen
E   Prednisolone

13. A 40-year-old woman with type 2 diabetes and a history of stage 3 chronic kidney disease presented with an acutely painful, swollen and hot left knee. There was no history of trauma and she did not have any joint prosthesis. She also complained of a swollen and painful left elbow.
    On examination, she was afebrile. Her left knee was swollen, red, hot and tender to touch. There was reduction in the range of movements. Her left elbow also seemed swollen and red with a reduced range of movements.

Which one of the following statements is most likely concerning her diagnosis?

A   Plain joint radiographs will be useful in the acute diagnosis
B   The absence of a fever makes septic arthritis unlikely
C   The most likely causative organism is group a β-haemolytic streptococcus
D   The presence of crystals in join aspirate allow differentiation between a septic arthritis and a crystal arthropathy
E   The involvement of more than one joint does not exclude septic arthritis

14. A 52-year-old man presented with painful joints. He complained of swelling and stiffness of his wrists, knees and ankles. He had also noticed a rash on his face. He felt generally weak and tired and thought that he may have lost some weight. There was a history of poorly controlled hypertension, for which he took amlodipine, doxazosin and hydralazine, and asthma, for which he had a salbutamol inhaler. He had a chest infection last month and had completed a course of amoxicillin.

Investigations:

haemoglobin 97 g/L (130–180)	erythrocyte sedimentation rate 70 mm/1st h (0–20)
Antinuclear antibody 1/160 Extractable nuclear antigen: negative	
C3 0.88 g/L (0.65–1.9)	C4 0.15 g/L (0.15-0.5)
Antihistone antibodies: positive	

Which drug is most likely to have caused his symptoms?

A   Amlodipine
B   Amoxicillin
C   Doxazosin
D   Hydralazine
E   Salbutamol

15. A 33-year-old man presented with pain and swelling in his wrists and elbows. He also gave a history of red eyes with blurred vision. He had one mouth ulcer and had recently had an episode of epididymitis. He had a history of intermittent diarrhoea. There was no significant family history, he took no regular medications and denied any recent sexual activity.

What is the most likely diagnosis?

A   Behçet's disease
B   Crohn's disease

    C   Reactive arthritis
    D   Rheumatoid arthritis
    E   Syphilis

16. A 58-year-old man presented with fever, weight loss of 6 kg over the past 2 months and generalised arthralgia.
        His blood pressure was 190/85 mmHg.

Investigations:

creatinine 285 µmol/L (males 60–110)	erythrocyte sedimentation rate 100 mm/1st h (0–20)
Urine dipstick: blood ++, protein ++	

    He proceeded to have a renal biopsy. Post-biopsy he had significant macroscopic haematuria and a drop in blood pressure raising the suspicion of a post-biopsy bleed.
        To investigate this further he had a renal angiogram (see **Figure 11.1**).

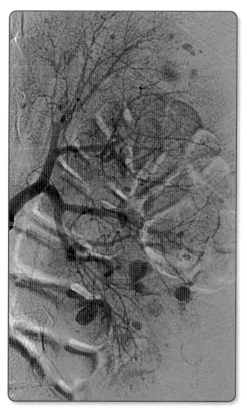

Figure 11.1

Which one of the following features is least likely to be associated with the underlying diagnosis?

    A   ANCA-associated vasculitis
    B   Elevated creatine kinase
    C   Hepatitis B viral infection

    D   Medium vessel vasculitis
    E   Presentation with hypertension and loin pain

17. A 64-year-old man presented with severe breathlessness and a non-productive cough. He had a past medical history of giant cell arteritis diagnosed by temporal artery biopsy 4 months previously. He smoked 20 cigarettes per day. His medication included prednisolone 20 mg daily and methotrexate 20 mg weekly.

    On examination, his oxygen saturation was 92% on air, respiratory rate 18 beats per minute and there were bi-basal, fine, end-inspiratory crackles.

Investigations:

haemoglobin 142 g/L (130–180)	creatinine 74 µmol/L (60–110)
white cell count 7.4 × 10⁹/L (4–11)	C-reactive protein 47 mg/L (<5)
HIV antibodies: negative	

    A CT of the chest was performed: see **Figure 11.2**.

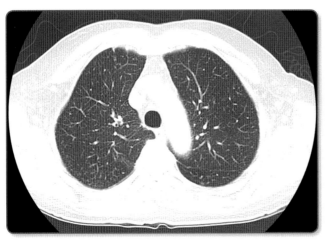

Figure 11.2

What is the most likely diagnosis?

    A   Aspergillosis
    B   Cardiac failure
    C   Methotrexate pneumonitis
    D   *Pneumocystis jirovecii* pneumonia
    E   Staphylococcal pneumonia

18. A 24-year-old man presented with a 10-day history of tender lumps over the shins, painful ankles, shortness of breath and lethargy. There was a preceding history of a mild coryzal-type illness.

    On examination, there were erythematous, subcutaneous nodules over the shins and synovitis of the ankles.

What is the most useful diagnostic investigation?

    A   Antinuclear antibodies
    B   C-reactive protein
    C   Chest X-ray
    D   Kveim's test
    E   Skin biopsy

19. A 57-year-old woman with rheumatoid arthritis was being considered for biological therapy with a tumour necrosis factor-α antagonist. She was currently well other than her arthritis, had a stable weight, and denied any cough, fevers or night sweats. She was born and grew up in the UK. She has never been treated for tuberculosis in the past.

    Examination was normal, with no respiratory signs and no adenopathy. There was a scar from a Bacillus Calmette–Guérin vaccine. Her chest X-ray was reported as normal.

    What is the next step in management?

    A   Tuberculin skin test
    B   Interferon-γ release assay
    C   Start infliximab
    D   Start rifampicin, isoniazid, pyrazinamide, ethambutol
    E   Start rifampicin and isoniazid

20. A 61-year-old woman was referred following an atraumatic vertebral fracture. She had a past medical history of an oesophageal pouch and gastro-oesophageal reflux for which she was taking omeprazole 40 mg. Two years ago, she was diagnosed with breast carcinoma for which she had a resection and remained on tamoxifen. She had no other medical problems and had received no previous corticosteroids.

    Investigations:

corrected calcium 2.35 mmol/L (2.2–2.6)
MRI: T12 crush fracture
Bone scan: no bony metastases
Dual-energy X-ray absorptiometry (DXA) scan: T-score –3.7 Z-score –1.3

    What is the most appropriate treatment?

    A   Alendronate
    B   Risedronate
    C   Raloxifene
    D   Strontium
    E   Teriparatide

21. A 64-year-old man presented with recurrent epistaxis and sinusitis.

    On examination he had painful red eyes and a purpuric rash on his lower limbs. Urine output was 50 mL/h.

    Investigations:

potassium 4.8 mmol/L (3.5–5.0) urea 25 mmol/L (2.5–7.5)	creatinine 452 µmol/L (males 60–110)
Antinuclear antibody: negative Antineutrophil cytoplasmic antibody: positive myeloperoxide <5 IU/L (<5)	proteinase 3 >100 IU/L (<5)
Anti-glomerular basement membrane (GBM): negative	
Urine dipstick: blood +++, protein ++++	
Chest X-ray: normal	

What is the most appropriate next step in management?

A   Broad-spectrum antibiotics
B   Haemodialysis
C   Plasma exchange
D   Prednisolone and cyclophosphamide
E   Prednisolone and methotrexate

22. A 29-year-old female student, originally from Korea, presented with a history of transient left arm weakness. She also gave a history of intermittent blurred vision for the last few months. She had lost 5 kg of weight over this period. She had no other significant past medical history, no relevant family history and took no regular medication. She was a non-smoker and did not drink alcohol.

    On examination, there was an audible bruit over her right carotid artery and her left radial pulse was absent. Her blood pressure was 110/80 mmHg in the left arm and, although difficult to auscultate, approximately 80/60 mmHg in the right arm.

Investigations:

haemoglobin 98 g/L (115–165)	erythrocyte sedimentation rate 90 mm/1st h (0–30)
Antinuclear antibody: negative	

What is the most likely diagnosis?

A   Atherosclerosis
B   Giant cell arteritis
C   Polyarteritis nodosa
D   Systemic lupus erythematosus (SLE)
E   Takayasu's arteritis

Answers

1. B Anticardiolipin antibodies

The diagnosis of antiphospholipid syndrome (APS) is based on the Sapporo classification criteria which uses clinical and laboratory criteria – patients need one of each:

A. Clinical:
- Evidence of vascular [deep vein (but not superficial vein), arterial or small vessel] thrombosis

or

- Pregnancy morbidity: unexplained fetal loss at ≥10 weeks' gestation, or one or more premature births ≤34 weeks' gestation due to pre-eclampsia, eclampsia or placental insufficiency, or three or more embryonic losses ≤10 weeks' gestation.

B. Laboratory: persistent presence in the serum of at least one type of antiphospholipid antibody (aPL) on two or more occasions at least 12 weeks apart and no more than 5 years before the manifestation of symptoms. The types of aPL can include IgG or IgM anticardiolipin antibodies, IgG or IgM β_2-glycoprotein I antibodies, or lupus anticoagulant antibodies.

Although not part of the diagnostic criteria, APS is associated with heart valve disease, livedo reticularis, thrombocytopenia, nephropathy and neurological manifestations such as stroke.

Activated protein C deficiency and antithrombin III deficiency are associated with venous thrombosis, but are not associated with a significant increase in pregnancy loss. Homocysteinaemia is associated with cerebrovascular accidents and myocardial infarction. Raised levels of anti-dsDNA are associated with systemic lupus erythematosus. This can be associated with APS, but this patient has no other diagnostic features of lupus, and therefore the diagnosis is most likely to be APS.

Espinosa G, Cervera R. Current treatment of antiphospholipid syndrome: lights and shadows. Nature Rev Rheum 2015; 11:586–596.

2. C Bisphosphonate

This woman has osteoporosis, as evidenced by her T score of greater than -2.5 standard deviations from the reference values (which were calculated based upon dual energy X-ray absorptiometry of the femoral neck for women aged 20–29 years). Her risk of developing osteoporotic fractures, including a hip fracture should be calculated as described in the NICE clinical guideline, using either the FRAX tool or the QFracture calculator. In this case, the 10-year risk of a hip fracture from the risk fractures described is in excess of 2%, and the 10-year risk of any osteoporotic fragility fracture is in excess of 8%. The NICE technology appraisal guidance for considering therapy for treating osteoporosis suggests that oral bisphosphonates (such as alendronic acid, risedronate or ibandronic acid) should be offered if the 10-year risk of an osteoporotic fragility fracture is >1%, and the intravenous bisphosphonates (zolendronic acid) should be considered if the risk is >10% or if oral bisphosphonates cannot be tolerated.

Prior to use of bisphosphonates, adequate calcium and vitamin D levels should be assured. If deficient they should be replaced, but in this case they were replete. Strontium is only indicated for those who have contraindications to bisphosphonates. Raloxifene is no longer recommended for primary prevention of fractures in postmenopausal women with osteoporosis.

National Institute for Health and Care Excellence (NICE). Technology Appraisal Guidance TA464. Bisphosphonates for treating osteoporosis. London: NICE, 2017.
National Institute for Health and Care Excellence (NICE). Clinical Guideline CG146. Osteoporosis: assessing the risk of fragility fracture. London: NICE, 2012.

3.   B He should have an urgent temporal artery biopsy before starting treatment

This patient has presented with giant cell arteritis (GCA), also known as temporal arteritis. The American College of Rheumatology criteria for diagnosis include:

- Age >50 years
- New-onset headache
- Abnormality of the temporal arteries
- ESR (erythrocyte sedimentation rate) >50 mm/1st h
- Positive temporal artery biopsy.

Three or more of these criteria will give the diagnosis with 97% sensitivity and 79% specificity. This patient has four of these criteria. Of patients with GCA, 95% will have an ESR >50 mm/1st h.

It is recognised that there is a strong association between polymyalgia rheumatica (PMR) and GCA, and some consider them to be part of the same disease spectrum. Of patients with GCA, 50% will also have symptoms of PMR and up to 15% of patients with PMR will have evidence of GCA on temporal artery biopsy.

The suspicion of GCA should prompt immediate treatment with high-dose corticosteroids (prednisolone 40–60 mg) to prevent the significant risk of blindness. Treatment should not be delayed by waiting for temporal artery biopsy. It is generally accepted that a temporal artery biopsy will still be useful up to 10–14 days after starting steroids.

Upon starting steroids, symptoms should quickly settle within 1–2 weeks. For those with PMR, the PMR symptoms will settle more quickly, within 2–3 days.

Temporal artery biopsy remains the gold standard for making the diagnosis, although colour duplex ultrasound is increasingly being used to complement this and may offer an alternative in the future. It has a negative predictive value of around 95%. A negative temporal artery biopsy does not exclude GCA as there may be skip lesions. It is accepted that a unilateral biopsy of at least 1 cm, but ideally 1.5–3.0 cm, in length will be around 85–90% sensitive. In the face of strong clinical suspicion steroids should be continued.

Buttgereit F, Dejaco C, Matteson EL, Dasgupta B. Polymyalgia rheumatica and giant cell arteritis: a systematic review. JAMA 2016; 315:2442–2458.

4.   B Limited cutaneous systemic sclerosis

Systemic sclerosis is a connective tissue disorder characterised by scleroderma (thickening and fibrosis of the skin) and a distinctive pattern of internal organ involvement. There are two recognised patterns of disease: limited cutaneous systemic sclerosis and diffuse cutaneous systemic sclerosis. In limited cutaneous systemic sclerosis fibrosis is mainly restricted to the hands, arms and face, with the onset of Raynaud's phenomenon occurring years before diagnosis and pulmonary hypertension usually present. Anticentromere antibodies are seen in 50–90% of patients. Diffuse cutaneous systemic sclerosis is usually rapidly progressive and affects a much larger area of skin, with one or more internal organs affected. It is associated with anti-topoisomerase I, anti-RNA polymerase and anti-fibrillin antibodies. Up to 99% of those with systemic sclerosis of either subclass will have Raynaud's phenomenon at some point in the disease. Common manifestations of systemic sclerosis are arthralgia, pulmonary fibrosis, sclerodermal renal crisis and gastrointestinal motility disorders. It is associated with a positive antinuclear antibody in 90% of cases and a positive rheumatoid factor in 30% of cases. Anticentromere antibodies are specific to limited cutaneous systemic sclerosis and are not associated with any of the other diagnoses. Mixed connective tissue disease is associated with a positive anti-U1-RNP.

Denton CP, Khanna D. Systemic sclerosis. Lancet 2017; 390:1685–1699.

5. D Systemic lupus erythematosus

Systemic lupus erythematosus (SLE) is a multisystem, autoimmune, connective tissue disorder with a wide spectrum of clinical presentations. It has a female:male ratio of 9:1 and its peak onset in women is in their late adolescence or early 40s. Its most common manifestations are constitutional symptoms of fatigue and fever, skin manifestations of a butterfly or photosensitivity rash, and musculoskeletal symptoms of arthralgia, arthritis and myositis. It can also manifest itself in a number of other systems: renal, haematological, neuropsychiatric, reticuloendothelial, gastrointestinal, respiratory and cardiac. The American College of Rheumatology diagnostic criteria for SLE are outlined below. To be diagnosed with SLE individuals need to fulfil at least four of the following criteria.

Manifestations:
- Oral ulcers
- Photosensitivity
- Malar rash
- Discoid rash
- Seronegative arthritis
- Evidence of serositis such as pleural effusion or pericarditis
- Renal involvement
- Neurological involvement
- Haematological involvement
- Positive for anti-dsDNA, anti-Sm, IgG or IgM anticardiolipin antibodies, or lupus anticoagulant
- Positive for antinuclear antibody (ANA).

Although the other conditions could have a similar presentation, antibodies to double-stranded DNA are highly specific for SLE.

Lisnevskaia L, et al. Systemic lupus erythematosus. Lancet 2014; 384:1878–1888.

6. A Adult Still's disease

This man presents with a systemic inflammatory condition with markedly high ferritin and a negative autoantibody screen. This is typical of adult Still's disease, a multisystem disease of unknown aetiology. In addition to the symptoms noted in this case pleuritis, weight loss and adenopathy can feature. The pathophysiology is driven by interleukins-1 and -6, interferon-γ, and tumour necrosis factor-α. There is no single diagnostic test for adult Still's disease, with diagnosis requiring exclusion of infectious, neoplastic and other autoimmune conditions. A leukocytosis, elevated acute phase reactants, a moderate transaminitis and, in particular, extremely elevated serum ferritin levels are suggestive of the diagnosis. Rheumatoid factor and antinuclear antibodies are usually absent. Treatment includes the use of non-steroidal anti-inflammatory drugs and corticosteroids in the first instance. Steroid-sparing immunosuppressants can then be introduced including methotrexate, azathioprine and ciclosporin. In refractory cases biologic agents including anakinra (an interleukin-1 receptor agonist) and etanercept (a tumour necrosis factor antagonist) have been successfully used. Prognosis actually tends to be more favourable when systemic symptoms predominate.

Haemophagocytosis is a multisystem disorder characterised by fever, hepatosplenomegaly, lymphadenopathy, jaundice and rash, with lymphocytosis, anaemia, neutropenia and thrombocytopenia, markedly elevated serum ferritin levels and abnormal liver enzymes. The absence of cytopenias or hyperbilirubinaemia makes this diagnosis less likely in this case. Churg–Strauss syndrome is a medium vessel vasculitis involving the lungs, gastrointestinal system, peripheral nerves and kidneys. Wegener's granulomatosis is a small vessel vasculitis that affects the nose, lungs and kidneys. Wegener's is closely associated with cytoplasmic antineutrophil cytoplasmic antibodies (cANCAs) and Churg–Strauss with pANCA (perinuclear ANCA). Periodic fever syndrome can also present in a similar way to this case and can have an associated leukocytosis and raised inflammatory markers. It is not commonly associated with the marked transaminitis or raised ferritin evident here.

Efthimiou P, et al. Diagnosis and management of adult onset Still's disease. Ann Rheum Dis 2006; 65(5):564–572.

7. B Churg–Strauss syndrome

The history of recurrent sinusitis, rhinitis, asthma and prominent eosinophilia should raise the suspicion of Churg–Strauss syndrome (CSS). The presence of mononeuritis multiplex, purpuric spots and rash should also raise suspicions of a vasculitis process. Additional clues to the presence of CSS is the cardiac and renal involvement. Presence of blood and protein in urine should raise suspicion of a glomerulonephritic process. Thus, the total picture is in keeping with CSS. Antineutrophil cytoplasmic antibodies (ANCAs) might be absent in more than 50% of cases. However, in the presence of renal involvement pANCA (perinuclear ANCA) is usually positive.

Cardiac amyloidosis usually does not present with a history of asthma, mononeuritis multiplex and vasculitis. Goodpasture's syndrome also has pulmonary and renal involvement, but eosinophilia and cardiac involvement are not present.

Sarcoidosis does not present with a vasculitic picture with purpuric rash, glomerulonephritic renal involvement and recurrent sinusitis.

CSS is an eosinophil-rich granulomatous vasculitis affecting small-to-medium arteries with involvement of the respiratory tract and gastrointestinal tract.

In CSS, an allergic rhinitis-like picture is the usual presentation along with recurrent sinusitis. Asthma usually manifests in the fourth decade and once a full vasculitic picture develops the asthma subsides. Pulmonary infiltrates are common; however, unlike Wegener's granulomatosis epistaxis and haemoptysis are not common.

Cardiac involvement can occur with myocardial infarction, conduction abnormalities, pericardial effusion and congestive cardiac failure, as in this patient. This is the usual cause of life-threatening complications.

Renal involvement usually takes the form of focal segmental glomerulonephritis or vasculitic manifestations.

The American College of Rheumatology criteria for diagnosis:
- Eosinophilia >10%
- Extravascular eosinophils seen on blood vessel biopsy
- Neuropathy (mono- or polyneuropathy)
- Asthma
- Non-fixed pulmonary infiltrates
- Paranasal sinus abnormality.

(Four criteria are needed for diagnosis.)

Treatment is with steroids – either oral prednisolone or intravenous methylprednisolone. Steroids can be combined with cyclophosphamide to induce remission in resistant cases. Once remission is achieved, azathioprine can be used instead of cyclophosphamide, or steroids alone can be used and then tapered.

Mahr A, et al. Eosinophilic granulomatosis with polyangiitis (Churg–Strauss): evolutions in classification, etiopathogenesis, assessment and management. Curr Opin Rheumatol 2014 ;26:16–23.

8. C Psoriatic arthropathy

This woman presents with a small joint arthropathy, dactylitis, a plantar fasciitis, psoriatic nail changes and a negative autoantibody screen – all consistent with a diagnosis of psoriatic arthropathy. Psoriatic arthropathy usually occurs in those with marked dermatological disease but can occur in those with any degree of psoriasis and affects 5% of those with the skin condition. Clinically five main categories of psoriatic arthritis are described:
- Asymmetrical: this category predominates representing 70% of psoriatic arthropathy and is generally mild. It usually involves fewer than three joints.
- Symmetrical: accounting for 25% of cases, joints on both sides of the body are affected and presentation is similar to rheumatoid arthritis.
- Arthritis mutilans: a severe, deforming progressive arthropathy. Arthritis mutilans has also been called chronic absorptive arthritis and a similar process can be seen in rheumatoid arthritis.
- Spondylitis: symptoms are predominated by spinal stiffness, but hand and foot involvement can occur as in the symmetrical arthritis form. May occur with or without sacroiliitis.

- Distal interphalangeal predominant: characterised by inflammation and stiffness in the distal interphalangeal joints. Nail changes are often marked.

Treatment is with non-steroidal anti-inflammatories and immunomodulatory agents. Methotrexate, leflunomide and azathioprine are often used and also improve the dermatological manifestations. Tumour necrosis factor-α inhibitors can be used in refractory cases.

Jaccoud's arthropathy is a chronic, non-erosive, rheumatoid-like deformity of the hands associated with rheumatic fever and systemic lupus erythematosus. The absence of valvular abnormalities makes rheumatic fever-associated Jaccoud's arthropathy unlikely, and the case does not fit with systemic lupus erythematosus. Enteropathic arthropathy (similar to psoriatic disease) is commonly associated with HLA-B27 but there is no history of enteric disease in this case. Reiter's disease is similarly associated with an antecedent infection, most commonly enteric or genitourinary, but in addition to the arthropathy evident in this case Reiter's disease manifests with conjunctivitis and urethritis.

Ritchlin CT, Colbert RA, Gladman DD. Psoriatic arthritis. N Engl J Med 2017; 376:957–970.

9. D Nifedipine

This woman is presenting with scleroderma (CREST syndrome – calcinosis, Raynaud's phenomenon, oesophageal dysmotility, sclerodactyly and telangiectasia). The question relates to her presenting complaint of Raynaud's phenomenon: episodes of digital pallor, cyanosis and rubor in response to cold or emotional stress. Colour changes are often accompanied by pain and paraesthesia and symptoms can last minutes to hours, but with an absence of symptoms between episodes. The mainstay of treatment is with calcium channel blockers. Short-acting agents are effective, but frequently associated with adverse effects (headache, flushing, oedema).

Use of angiotensin-converting enzyme inhibitors such as losartan (and angiotensin II receptor blockers) has no proven benefit over calcium channel blockers, but some evidence points to their utility in decreasing severity and frequency of episodes of vasospasm. Anti-platelet agents have had varied results in Raynaud's phenomenon, ticlopidine has shown benefits in one series but was ineffective in another study. Clopidogrel's effectiveness has not yet been studied in relation to Raynaud's phenomenon.

α-Adrenergic antagonists have provided some symptomatic relief in Raynaud's phenomenon. Physiological studies have shown that digital vasoconstriction is mainly mediated by adrenoceptors of the a_2-subtype rather than the a_1-adrenoceptors antagonised by doxazosin.

Phosphodiesterase inhibitors such as sildenafil have also been shown to be effective in Raynaud's phenomenon but should be used primarily as a second-line therapy.

Wigley FM, Flavahan NA. Raynaud's phenomenon. N Engl J Med 2016; 375:556–565.

10. B Familial hibernian fever or tumour necrosis factor (TNF) receptor-associated periodic syndrome (TRAPS)

This woman is presenting with a periodic fever syndrome, with the laboratory results indicating familial hibernian fever, also known as TNF receptor-associated periodic syndrome (TRAPS). There are a number periodic fever diseases described:

- TRAPS – characterised by episodes of fever, abdominal pain and painful, flitting, erythematous skin lesions. Attacks usually last for longer than 1 week and longer than in hyperimmunoglobulinaemia D syndrome and familial Mediterranean fever. It is caused by mutations in *TNFRSF1A*, detection of which is diagnostic. Suggestive laboratory results in a compatible clinical picture include polyclonal gammopathy as in this case. Treatment with non-steroidal anti-inflammatory drugs (NSAIDs) has been the mainstay of therapy but recently etanercept (an anti-TNF agent) has been shown to decrease the frequency, duration and severity of attacks.
- Familial Mediterranean fever (FMF) – caused by mutations in *MEFV*. The majority of patients have their first attack before 18 years of age, which is characterised by fever developing over 2–4 hours and lasting from 6 hours to 4 days. The metaraminol provocation test can be used

prior to genetic testing. NSAIDs are used for acute attacks and colchicine reduces attack frequency.

- Hyperimmunoglobulinaemia D syndrome (HIDS) – manifests as high fever, abdominal pain, vomiting and diarrhoea, and frequently joint pain. Diagnosis is with persistently high IgD levels.
- Muckle–Wells syndrome – a rare syndrome characterised by intermittent febrile episodes, progressive sensorineural deafness and AA amyloidosis with nephropathy.
- Familial cold autoinflammatory syndrome – a rare condition whereby cold exposure can produce a systemic inflammatory response involving fever, urticaria and arthralgia.

Acute intermittent porphyria is characterised by abdominal pain, neuropathies and constipation, but, unlike most types of porphyria, rashes are not part of the presentation. Although systemic lupus erythematosus can present with symptoms similar to those presented here and can manifest with a relapsing–remitting course, the overall recurrent but non-progressive clinical picture favours a periodic fever.

Cantarini L, et al. Tumour necrosis factor receptor-associated periodic syndrome (TRAPS): state of the art and future perspectives. Autoimmun Rev 2012; 12:38–43.

11. A Mixed connective tissue disease

Mixed connective tissue disease (MCTD) is an overlap syndrome with many features of systemic lupus erythematosus (SLE) and other connective tissue diseases. It most commonly presents with arthralgia or arthritis, with no particular pattern of distribution. Eighty-five per cent of those with MCTD suffer from Raynaud's phenomenon, and 66% have swollen fingers. MCTD had erroneously been thought to be the only cause of swollen fingers but they can occur in early scleroderma, eosinophilic fasciitis and anti-tRNA synthetase antibody overlap syndrome. The most concerning features of the disease are myositis, fibrosing alveolitis and pulmonary hypertension; patients should be routinely monitored for signs of these. Pulmonary hypertension is the most common cause of death. The presence of anti-U1-RNP antibodies in a high titre with negative antibodies to double-stranded DNA is diagnostic of MCTD. None of the other diagnoses given is associated with this antibody pattern, although SLE, scleroderma and rheumatoid arthritis could all present with similar clinical features.

Gunnarsson R, et al. Mixed connective tissue disease. Best Pract Res Clin Rheumatol 2016;30:95–111.

12. E Prednisolone

Urticarial vasculitis, also named hypocomplementaemic urticarial vasculitis, has a marked female predominance and may occur with other connective tissue disease including systemic lupus erythematosus, Sjögren's syndrome and cryoglobulinaemia. It presents with recurrent bouts of prolonged atypical urticaria, persisting for >24 hours and fading to leave brown pigmentation due to extravasation of red cells. Skin lesions tend to be painful and burn rather than itch.

Steroids should be used as first-line treatment to gain control of symptoms and the disease. Antimalarials, such as hydroxychloroquine, or dapsone may be used as second-line agents. Steroid-sparing agents such as azathioprine may also have a role in the long-term management but not in the acute setting. Non-steroidal anti-inflammatory drugs such as naproxen may help alleviate some discomfort, but will not resolve the lesions.

Venzor J, Lee WL, Huston DP. Urticarial vasculitis. Clin Rev Allergy Immunol 2002; 23(2):201–216.

13. E The involvement of more than one joint does not exclude septic arthritis

Any patient presenting with an acutely swollen, hot and red joint must be treated as an emergency and as having a septic arthritis until proven otherwise. The diagnosis is suspected clinically and confirmed with joint aspiration and culture. Diabetic patients, intravenous drug users and those with pre-existing joint disease or joint prosthesis are most at risk.

The most common causative organisms are Gram-positive cocci, the most common of which is *Staphylococcus aureus* [including MRSA (meticillin-resistant *S. aureus*)], followed by group A β-haemolytic streptococci. Unless specific risk factors are identified or the patient is immunocompromised there is no need to introduce empirical antibiotics against Gram-negative organisms, *Neisseria gonorrhoeae* (which has increasing prevalence in the USA and Australia) or *Haemophilus influenzae* type b, the incidence of which has dramatically reduced following introduction of vaccination.

Crystals and sepsis can coexist in a joint so the presence of crystals alone does not exclude a septic arthritis.

More than one joint is affected in up to 20% of patients with septic arthritis.

The presence or absence of a fever is not a reliable indicator as to whether a patient has a septic arthritis and 45% of patients with a septic arthritis will not present with a raised temperature.

Plain films of the affected joint may be useful as a baseline investigation in terms of assessing joint damage in the future, as well as for assessing for the presence of osteomyelitis. They may also show chondrocalcinosis, but they are not useful in the actual diagnosis of septic arthritis. Equally, a bone MRI will help distinguish between septic arthritis and osteoarthritis but will not differentiate between joint sepsis and inflammatory changes.

Coakley G, et al. BSR & BHPR, BOA, RCGP and BSAC guidelines for management of the hot swollen joint in adults. Rheumatology 2006; 45:1039–1041.

14. D Hydralazine

This patient has drug-induced lupus erythematosus (DILE). There is a list of around 80 drugs that have been recorded as being associated with this condition, but the five most common are hydralazine, minocycline, isoniazid, quinidine and procainamide. Others include angiotensin-converting enzyme inhibitors, anticonvulsants, antifungals and some of the biologic agents [interleukin, interferon and tumour necrosis factor (TNF)-α antagonists].

Drug-induced lupus has many similar presenting features to systemic lupus erythematosus (SLE), including presentation with arthralgia, myalgia, fever, rash, serositis and positive antinuclear antibodies. Central nervous system and renal involvement is rare in DILE. Although SLE is predominantly seen in younger women, DILE is typically seen in an older age group (aged 50–70 years) and has a roughly equal sex distribution. White people are affected more frequently than African–Caribbean patients. There are some laboratory differences that will help distinguish DILE from SLE including normal complements (which are often consumed in SLE), antihistone antibodies (which are typically positive in DILE) and anti-ssDNA (single-stranded DNA) antibodies being more common than anti-dsDNA antibodies (reverse in SLE).

Of the list of medications that this patient is on hydralazine is by far the most commonly associated with DILE. Although some antibiotics are associated, there are no reports with amoxicillin. Diltiazem has been reported as a causative agent but not amlodipine; there are no reports of salbutamol, and doxazosin has only very rarely been documented.

Anti-inflammatory drugs or steroids may have a short-term role in treating symptoms of DILE and symptoms should settle upon withdrawal of the causative drug. Autoantibodies may persist longer term.

Vedove CD, et al. Drug-induced lupus erythematosus. Arch Dermatol Res 2009; 301(1):99–105.

15. A Behçet's disease

Behçet's disease (or syndrome) is a chronic, relapsing, multi-system inflammatory disorder. It typically affects patients in their third and fourth decades and is more common in patients from the Middle East and Asia.

There are no particular clinical or lab findings specific to Behçet's disease and the International Study Group guidelines suggest that to make the diagnosis the patient must have oral aphthous ulcers (at least three times in 12 months) along with two out of the four of the following symptoms:
- Genital ulcers (including anal ulcers and swollen testicles or epididymitis)

- Ocular inflammation (including iritis and anterior or posterior uveitis)
- Cutaneous manifestations (erythema nodosum, folliculitis, acneiform lesions)
- Pathergy (papule >2 mm diameter 24–48 hours after needle prick).

Other symptoms recognised include diarrhoea, neurological involvement (rare), polyarthritis (commonly affecting the knees and ankles, elbows and wrists), superficial thrombophlebitis, cardiac involvement (coronary vasculitis, myocarditis, pericarditis) and lung involvement (pulmonary vasculitis, effusions, pulmonary hypertension).

Although this patient could have inflammatory bowel disease or rheumatoid arthritis, the spectrum of symptoms would be more clearly associated with Behçet's disease. Reactive arthritis would not explain his oral or ocular symptoms. Syphilis, which causes a primary chancre, and could account for his oral ulcers and arthralgia, is less likely based on the history.

Alpsoy E. Behçet's disease: A comprehensive review with a focus on epidemiology, etiology and clinical features, and management of mucocutaneous lesions. J Dermatol 2016; 43:620–632.

16. A ANCA-associated vasculitis

This patient's angiogram, done to look for a source of bleeding post-biopsy, shows multiple medium vessel aneurysms and is typical of classic polyarteritis nodosa (PAN). PAN is a rare necrotising arteritis which affects the medium vessels in the gut (presenting with abdominal pain and bloody diarrhoea), skin (causing livedo reticularis), nerves (manifesting as mononeuritis multiplex or peripheral neuropathy) and kidneys. Renal impairment results from ischaemic change or infarction and patients may be hypertensive as a result, or present with haematuria or loin pain from segmental infarcts. Vessels show transmural fibrinoid necrosis in medium-sized vessels. The antineutrophil cytoplasmic antibody (ANCA)-associated vasculitides affect small vessels and do not typically give this picture. They are often diagnosed by renal biopsy where you would expect a focal and segmental necrotising glomerulonephritis.

PAN may be associated with hepatitis B infection. Creatine kinase is elevated as a result of muscle injury. ANCA is negative.

Treatment centres on immunosuppression. This includes prednisolone with the addition of cyclophosphamide in the so-called 'high-risk' group (older patients with renal, gut or coronary involvement). With concomitant hepatitis B infection the evidence base for treatment is sparse but current opinion is that interferon treatment plus plasma exchange may also be required.

De Virgilio A. Polyarteritis nodosa: A contemporary overview. Autoimmun Rev 2016; 15:564–570.

17. C Methotrexate pneumonitis

Methotrexate pneumonitis is the most likely diagnosis in this situation. Pulmonary complications may be seen in 4–10% of patients treated with methotrexate. The chest X-ray or CT may demonstrate bilateral diffuse pulmonary infiltrates; pleural effusions may also be seen. Risk factors for developing methotrexate-induced lung disease include: diabetes; rheumatoid or other lung/pleural disease; daily rather than intermittent therapy; age >60 years; and smoking. It does not appear to be dose related and can occur at doses <20 mg per week. The condition may present acutely with interstitial pneumonitis, fever and eosinophilia, or in the more common subacute form within a year of treatment, presenting with dyspnoea, fever, cough, hypoxia and basal crackles. Treatment consists of drug withdrawal. The benefit of steroids is not proven.

Aspergillosis may be seen in patients with a history of longstanding, often poorly controlled asthma. It may present with a recurrent episodes of mucus plugging, fever and malaise, and expectoration of dark mucus plugs, sometimes as casts of the airways. The chest X-ray demonstrates flitting infiltration and the diagnosis may be supported by blood tests including positive IgG precipitins, positive IgE RAST (radioallergosorbent test) to *Aspergillus* species, raised total serum IgE and eosinophilia (may be suppressed if on steroids).

Patients receiving immunosuppressive therapy are at risk of developing opportunistic infections such as *Pneumocystis jirovecii* pneumonia (PCP – formoly *P. carinii* pneumonia). The condition may present with gradual onset breathlessness and dry cough with retrosternal tightness. Fever and tachypnoea may occur. Chest examination is typically normal. PCP may present with pneumothorax. The chest X-ray pattern demonstrates bilateral perihilar infiltrates that progress to alveolar shadowing. The chest X-ray may be normal in about 10% of cases.

The clinical presentation described above may be due to cardiac failure; however, it is a less likely cause in the absence of a previous cardiac history and, with the degree of chest X-ray changes, the patient is more likely to complain of a cough productive of frothy white sputum. A staphylococcal pneumonia is more likely to present with a lobar pneumonia and more pronounced inflammatory response. This patient may be more at risk of developing pneumonia as he is immunosuppressed; however, this is not the most likely diagnosis in this scenario.

Salliot C, van der Heijde D. Long-term safety of methotrexate monotherapy in patients with rheumatoid arthritis: a systematic literature research. Ann Rheum Dis 2009; 68(7):1100–1104.

18. C Chest X-ray

The clinical picture described is very suggestive of Löfgren's syndrome (acute sarcoidosis). This is a mild disease, which is usually non-progressive and presents with fevers, bilateral lymphadenopathy on chest X-ray, erythema nodosum (as described above) and arthralgia. It occurs particularly in white people. It has a good prognosis and resolves completely and spontaneously in 80% of patients within 1–2 years. Only a minority of patients may develop further lung disease. The typical history, as described above with a chest X-ray demonstrating bilateral hilar lymphadenopathy, is often sufficient to form the diagnosis without the need for further investigation. These patients should be advised to rest and take simple analgesia and non-steroidal anti-inflammatory drugs. The patients should be monitored and if there is diagnostic doubt further investigations may be necessary to exclude more serious causes of bilateral hilar lymphadenopathy including tuberculosis and lymphoma. Serum acetylcholinesterase levels may be raised; however, the level may also be normal in active sarcoid, following the trend of levels may be more useful in disease monitoring.

A skin biopsy may be useful to confirm the diagnosis if there is clinical doubt to confirm evidence of non-caseating granuloma. C-reactive protein may be elevated in many inflammatory conditions and has a poor specificity.

The Kveim test is no longer performed clinically because of the risks of transmissible disease. It involved injecting splenic tissue from a patient with known sarcoid to determine whether a granulomatous reaction occurred.

Valeyre D, et al. Sarcoidosis. Lancet 2014; 383:1155–1167.

19. B Interferon-γ release assay

This patient is about to start a biological agent (in this case an anti-TNF-α drug) and must therefore be assessed for the risk of latent infection which may reactivate upon starting this immunomodulatory agent. One of the key latent infections to be screened for is *Mycobacterium tuberculosis*.

The presence of the Bacillus Calmette–Guérin (BCG) scar in this case does not impart perfect immunity to the recipient, but does complicate diagnostics in the current investigation. Specifically, the history of a BCG vaccination means a tuberculin skin test is difficult to interpret in this case, and instead an interferon-γ release assay (such as the TB-Elispot or Quantiferon) should be used instead. This in vitro test is not affected by previous BCG vaccination, and should give a reliable result of whether the individual has ever been exposed to tuberculosis in the past, and therefore needs chemoprophylaxis (with 3 months of rifampicin and isoniazid dual therapy). The interferon-γ release assays can provide a false negative result, however, in the context of immunosuppression (which the patient has not yet started) or in the presence of active tuberculosis disease (which clinical assessment of this patient has indicated they do not have).

If there were clinical signs of active tuberculosis prior to commencing the biological agent, or which evolved during therapy with the biological agent (irrespective of whether tuberculosis chemoprophylaxis was administered prior to starting the therapy), urgent referral for investigation and management should be enacted.

Cantini F, et al. Guidance for the management of patients with latent tuberculosis infection requiring biologic therapy in rheumatology and dermatology clinical practice. Autoimmun Rev 2015; 14:503–509.

20. D Strontium

This woman has had a crush fracture and has a dual-energy X-ray absorptiometry scan consistent with osteoporosis. She therefore fits the NICE (National Institute for Health and Clinical Excellence) guidance for secondary prevention of further osteoporotic fractures in postmenopausal women. Strontium ranelate is indicated for use in those who cannot tolerate bisphosphonate therapy and has approval from NICE in these circumstances. It acts through decreasing bone resorption but also increasing new bone formation. Contraindications for use include chronic kidney disease and concomitant use of tetracycline antimicrobials, and care should be taken in those at increased risk of venous thromboembolic disease.

Alendronate is recommended for osteoporosis secondary prevention therapy when osteoporosis is confirmed (with a T-score ≥ -2.5) in postmenopausal women. As with most of the bisphosphonate class of agents, upper gastrointestinal side effects including dyspepsia are common. They should therefore be used with care in those with known oesophageal and gastric pathology. Selective oestrogen receptor modulators, such as raloxifene, aim to maximise the beneficial effects of oestrogen on bone without having a marked impact on endometrial or breast tissue. However, raloxifene is still contraindicated in those in whom there is either confirmed breast or uterine pathology or in whom there is symptomatology consistent with potential pathology (e.g. vaginal bleeding or breast lumps). In those who are unable to take bisphosphonates, strontium or raloxifene or in those who have had an unsatisfactory response to these agents a recombinant human parathyroid hormone, teriparatide, is available which has some effect in stimulating new bone formation.

National Institute for Health and Care Excellence (NICE). Technology Appraisal Guidance TA464. Bisphosphonates for treating osteoporosis. London: NICE, 2017.
National Institute for Health and Care Excellence (NICE). Clinical guideline CG146. Osteoporosis: assessing the risk of fragility fracture. London: NICE, 2012.

21. D Prednisolone and cyclophosphamide

This patient presents with typical symptoms and investigations suggesting a diagnosis of granulomatosis with polyangiitis (GPA – formerly Wegener's granulomatosis). GPA is a small vessel vasculitis characterised by ANCA (antineutrophil cytoplasmic antibody) positivity, typically proteinase 3 (PR 3 or cytoplasmic ANCA – cANCA). It is a rapidly fatal disease and, without treatment, 2-year mortality rate is around 90%. Upon diagnosis treatment to achieve remission should be initiated as soon as possible. There have been increasing numbers of trials over the last few years looking at the optimum agents and their duration both to achieve remission and for long-term maintenance. The current recommendations are that cyclophosphamide (oral or intravenous, varies among various renal units) and prednisolone (3 days of intravenous methylprednisolone then high-dose oral prednisolone) are the treatment of choice to achieve remission. Thereafter prednisolone and azathioprine are the usual maintenance agents. Rituximab may also be an option for inducing remission or treating relapse.

There are no indications in this case for haemodialysis. He is still passing reasonable volumes of urine and his potassium is safe. Methotrexate should not be used in renal impairment, particularly not if glomerular filtration rate <30 mL/min per 1.73 m². There is nothing in the history to suggest a focal infection so there is no reason to give broad-spectrum antibiotics.

Plasma exchange has been shown in trials to be of benefit if there is pulmonary haemorrhage, dialysis-requiring, rapidly progressive glomerulonephritis, creatinine >500 µmol/L or coexisting anti-glomerular basement membrane antibodies, none of which this patient has.

Pagnoux C, Guillevin L. Treatment of granulomatosis with polyangiitis (Wegener's). Exp Rev Clin Immunol 2015; 11:339–348.

22. E Takayasu's arteritis

Takayasu's arteritis (TA) is a rare large vessel vasculitis most commonly affecting women under the age of 40 years, and in particular those from Asia. The term TA is used to describe a granulomatous inflammation of the aorta and its major branches, and its symptoms reflect varying sites and stages of involvement. The aetiology is unknown. Patients present with constitutional symptoms, including headache, malaise and weight loss, vascular features, including bruits and absent distal pulses, and neurological features such as transient ischaemic attacks.

The American College of Rheumatology published a classification in 1990 for TA whereby the presence of factors diagnoses the disease with a sensitivity of 90.5% and a specificity of 97.8%. These factors include age at onset ($\geq$40 years), significant difference in systolic blood pressure in each arm (>10 mmHg), arteriographic changes suggesting aortic occlusion or branch occlusion, poor brachial pulse, subclavian/aortic bruits and distal claudication.

A diagnosis of atherosclerosis is unlikely as she is young and has no other significant risk factors. Equally she is not in the age group for giant cell arteritis which typically affects those over the age of 50 years. Although polyarteritis nodosa may present with general symptoms of malaise, headache and visual disturbance, it would not typically cause the absent pulses or discrepancy in blood pressures. Systemic lupus erythematosus should be considered in a young woman presenting with non-specific constitutional symptoms but again would not explain the vascular findings and one would expect antinuclear antibody to be positive.

Keser G, et al. Management of Takayasu arteritis: a systematic review. Rheumatology 2014; 53:793–801.

Chapter 12

Therapeutics and toxicology

Questions

1. A 25-year-old woman was brought to the emergency department in a stuporous state 3 hours after attempting suicide by ingesting around 100 mL of antifreeze.

    On examination, her Glasgow Coma Scale score was 12 (eyes 3, speech 4, motor 5). Her pulse was 72 beats per minute, blood pressure 125/89 mmHg, respiratory rate 20 breaths per minute and oxygen saturation 97% on air.

    Investigations:

Arterial blood gas on air:	sodium 140 mmol/L (135–145)
pH 7.32 (7.35–7.45)	potassium 5.1 mmol/L (3.5–5.0)
P_{CO_2} 3.1 kPa (4.7–6.0)	urea 6.4 mmol/L (2.5–7.5)
P_{O_2} 15.9 kPa (11.3–12.6)	creatinine 82 µmol/L (45–90)
bicarbonate 18.8 mmol/L (22–30)	glucose 5 mmol/L (3.0–6.0)
base excess –6 mmol/L (± 2)	lactate 4 mmol/L (0.6–1.8)
anion gap 17.5 mmol/L (8–16)	osmolar gap 18.1 (<10)

    What is the most appropriate management?

    A   Activated charcoal
    B   Fomepizole
    C   Gastric lavage
    D   Lorazepam
    D   Sodium bicarbonate

2. A 32-year-old woman with Crohn's disease wished to become pregnant. She had ileal Crohn's disease which was currently well controlled on budesonide 9 mg once daily and azathioprine 100 mg once daily. She had had perineal disease in the past, which had been successfully treated with infliximab infusions.

    Which one of the following treatments for Crohn's disease should always be discontinued during pregnancy?

    A   Azathioprine
    B   Budesonide
    C   Infliximab
    D   Mesalazine
    E   Methotrexate

3. A 47-year-old woman was referred with continuous headache. A clinical diagnosis of hemicrania continua was subsequently made.

    What is the most appropriate management?

    A   Aspirin with domperidone
    B   Ergotamine
    C   Indometacin
    D   Sumatriptan
    E   Verapamil

4. A 75-year-old woman was diagnosed with Alzheimer's dementia during an inpatient admission. Mini-Mental State Examination revealed a score of 9/30. Agitation was a prominent feature.

    What is the most appropriate pharmacological treatment?

    A   Donepezil
    B   Galantamine
    C   Memantine
    D   Rivastigmine
    E   None

5. A 27-year-old man presented with a 1-month history of fatigue, easy bruising and frequent epistaxis. He had no past medical history of note and was not taking any medications.
    Following investigation, he was diagnosed with immune thrombocytopenia [formerly known as idiopathic thrombocytopenic purpura (ITP)].

    Investigations:

haemoglobin 111 g/L (130–180)	international normalised ratio 1.1 (<1.4)
platelets 31 × 10⁹/L (150–400)	activated partial thromboplastin time 30 s (30–40)

    What is the most appropriate treatment?

    A   Corticosteroids
    B   Plasma exchange
    C   Platelet transfusion
    D   Rituximab (anti-CD20)
    E   Romiplostim

6. A 27-year-old man with a history of previous substance abuse had recently commenced treatment for pulmonary tuberculosis. His medications included rifampicin, isoniazid, pyrazinamide, ethambutol, pyridoxine and methadone. He was receiving directly observed therapy and was under close supervision from the drug rehabilitation team. He had been compliant with his medications, but was complaining of increasing symptoms of anxiety, insomnia and muscle aches.

    What is the most appropriate next step in management?

    A   Citalopram
    B   Diazepam
    C   Increase dose of methadone
    D   Increase dose of pyridoxine
    E   Stop all anti-tuberculous therapy and check liver function tests

7. A 24-year-old man presented in the early hours of the morning with confusion, headache and jaw pain. He had been at a nightclub and had taken two ecstasy pills prior to feeling unwell. He had no past medical history and took no prescribed medications.

On examination, he was disoriented in time and place. His temperature was 38.4°C, pulse 110 beats per minute and blood pressure 156/100 mmHg. Neurological examination revealed nystagmus and ataxia. The rest of his examination was normal.

Which of the following is not a recognised complication of 3,4-methylenedioxy-N-methylamphetamine (MDMA) ingestion?

A   Cerebral venous sinus thrombosis
B   Coronary vasospasm
C   Hyperpyrexia
D   Rhabdomyolysis
E   Serotonin syndrome

8. A 64-year-old woman was re-admitted with a high stoma output, dehydration and oedema, following a jejunostomy created 5 weeks previously for mesenteric infarction. She had lost 5 kg in weight and her stoma output was over 1.5 L per day. Parenteral nutrition was initiated shortly after her operation and then stopped 3 weeks prior to re-admission. She had been prescribed intravenous fluids, and was tolerating an oral diet.

On examination, she weighed 43 kg, and had bilateral peripheral oedema to her mid-thigh. Abdominal examination revealed a jejunostomy and midline laparotomy scar.

Investigations:

haemoglobin 124 g/L (115–165)	urea 4.6 mmol/L (2.5–7.5)
white cell count 5×10^9/L (4–11)	creatinine 96 µmol/L (45–90)
platelets 167×10^9/L (150–400)	magnesium 0.6 mmol/L (0.75–1.05)
sodium 138×10^9/L (150–400)	C-reactive protein 3 mg/L (<5)
potassium 3.6 mmol/L (3.5–5.0)	

What is the next most appropriate step in management?

A   Loperamide
B   Octreotide
C   Omeprazole
D   Low-fat, high-carbohydrate diet
E   Reduction of oral hypotonic fluids to less than 500 mL/day

9. A 73-year-old woman was referred because of an unpleasant 'crawling' sensation in her legs. It was worse in the evenings and was relieved by movement. She was unable to sit still for more than a couple of minutes without moving her legs. There was no past medical history of note. She did not drink alcohol.

Neurological examination was normal.

What is the most appropriate treatment?

A   Amitriptyline
B   Baclofen
C   Clonazepam
D   Dihydrocodeine
E   Ropinirole

10. A 24-year-old man was diagnosed with fully sensitive pulmonary tuberculosis. He was commenced on standard quadruple therapy (rifampicin, isoniazid, pyrazinamide and ethambutol).

What is the most likely mechanism of action of rifampicin in the treatment of mycobacterial infection?

A   Increases mycobacterial cell wall permeability
B   Inhibits mycobacterial protein synthesis

C   Inhibits mycobacterial RNA polymerase
D   Inhibits synthesis of mycobacterial fatty acids
E   Inhibits synthesis of mycolic acid in mycobacterial cell wall

11. A 31-year-old man presented with a 2-day history of flushing, vertiginous dizziness, diarrhoea
     and restlessness. Five days ago he was prescribed linezolid for a para-spinal lumbar abscess. He
     had a past medical history of depression and was taking the following medications: linezolid,
     tramadol, amitriptyline, citalopram and paracetamol.
          On examination, he had a pulse of 120 beats per minute and blood pressure 175/105 mmHg.
     Physical examination was normal.

     What is the most likely cause?

     A   Amitriptyline interaction with citalopram
     B   Amitriptyline interaction with linezolid
     C   Citalopram interaction with linezolid
     D   Inadvertent tramadol overdose
     E   Tramadol interaction with linezolid

12. A 36-year-old man presented to the emergency department with a 'staggered' paracetamol
     overdose over the course of 24 hours. He had a history of depression and deliberate self-harm. He
     took 32 × 500 mg paracetamol tablets in total. He had no other medical problems. He took regular
     venlafaxine, but no other medications.
          He was admitted, started on an *N*-acetylcysteine infusion and fluid resuscitation. Twenty-four
     hours after admission he became confused.

     Investigations:

haemoglobin 140 g/L (130–180)	urea 12 mmol/L (2.5–7.5)
white cell count 8 × 10⁹/L (4–11)	creatinine 346 µmol/L (60–110)
platelets 234 × 10⁹/L (150–400)	bilirubin 340 mmol/L (1–22)
prothrombin time 102 s (11.5–15.5)	alkaline phosphatase 184 U/L (45–105)
international normalised ratio 10 (< 1.4)	alanine transaminase 1342 U/L (5–35)
sodium 134 mmol/L (135–145)	albumin 32 g/L (37–49)
potassium 5 mmol/L (3.5–5.0)	
Arterial blood gas on air:	bicarbonate 12 mmol/L (22–30)
pH 7.18 (7.35–7.45)	base excess 8 mmol/L (± 2)
P_{O_2} 18 kPa (11.3–12.6)	lactate 2.8 mmol/L (0.6–1.8)
P_{CO_2} 2 kPa (4.7–6.0)	

     What is the one criterion that determines urgent liver transplantation referral?

     A   Bilirubin
     B   Creatinine
     C   Lactate
     D   pH
     E   Prothrombin time

13. A 20-year old man was referred because of excessive daytime somnolence, which was affecting
     his work and personal life. He had had this problem from childhood, and his academic
     performance at school had been affected. There was no previous medical or family history. He
     drank 15 units of alcohol per week but did not smoke or take any recreational drugs. Although his
     nightly sleep pattern was regular, he reported broken sleep with very vivid dreams. Occasionally,

on waking he would be unable to move for a few seconds. He reported no episodes of sudden collapse.

An overnight polysomnogram with multiple sleep latency testing confirmed the diagnosis. Unfortunately, his condition did not improve with a trial of methylphenidate.

Investigations:

haemoglobin 124 g/L (130–180)	urea 4.6 mmol/L (2.5–7.5)
white cell count 5 × 10⁹/L (4–11)	creatinine 96 µmol/L (45–90)
platelets 167 × 10⁹/L (150–400)	magnesium 0.6 mmol/L (0.75–1.05)
sodium 138 × 10⁹/L (150–400)	C-reactive protein 3 mg/L (<5)
potassium 3.6 mmol/L (3.5–5.0)	

What is the most appropriate treatment?

A   Clomethiazole
B   Ephedrine
C   Mephedrone
D   Modafinil
E   Promethazine

14. A 56-year-old man from Guinea Bissau presented with fever and all-over body pain. He was diagnosed with type 2 diabetes 5 years ago and started on oral medication. 3 years ago, he had had a non-ST segment myocardial infarction and was started on secondary preventive medications. Three months ago, after being found to have *Cryptosporidium* he had been diagnosed with HIV and commenced on antiretroviral therapy.

He was on a number of medications: aspirin, simvastatin, atenolol, ramipril, metformin, and Atripla (combination of efavirenz, emtricitabine and tenofovir).

On examination, he had tender muscle groups over his thighs and upper arms bilaterally.

Investigations:

sodium 138 mmol/L (135–145)	albumin 35 g/L (37–49)
potassium 4.0 mmol/L (3.5–5.0)	alanine transaminase 46 U/L (5–35)
urea 8.9 mmol/L (2.5–7.5)	alkaline phosphatase 103 U/L (45–105)
creatinine 136 µmol/L (60–110)	creatine kinase 13 780 U/L (25–195)
bilirubin 7 mmol/L (1–22)	lactate 1.2 mmol/L (0.6–1.8)

What is the most likely cause of his presentation?

A   Efavirenz-induced myositis
B   Metformin-induced lactic acidosis
C   Metformin-induced myositis
D   Statin-induced myositis
E   Tenofovir-induced lactic acidosis

15. A 34-year-old agricultural worker presented to the emergency department with a 2-hour history of confusion, tremor, blurred vision, diarrhoea and vomiting. He had been using pesticide earlier.

On examination, he had tearing eyes with pinpoint pupils, and was drooling excessively. His Glasgow Coma Scale score was 14 (eyes 4, speech 4, motor 6), pulse 48 beats per minute, blood pressure 90/54 mmHg, respiratory rate 10 breaths per minute and oxygen saturation 92% on air. Auscultation of the lungs revealed widespread wheeze. Heart sounds were normal. The abdomen was soft, with hyperactive bowel sounds. Neurological examination revealed extensive tremor and dystonia.

Apart from oxygen and fluid resuscitation, what is the next most appropriate step in management?

A   Adrenaline
B   Atropine
C   Diazepam
D   Glycopyrrolate
E   Pralidoxime

16. A 36-year-old man underwent investigation for secondary hypertension. His results showed elevated urinary catecholamine metabolites. A subsequent CT and MIBG (*meta-iodobenzylguanidine*) scan showed a 3 × 4 cm mass in the left adrenal gland, suggestive of a phaeochromocytoma.
    He was started on phenoxybenzamine 10 mg twice daily in preparation for tumour removal before being subsequently increased to 30 mg twice daily. At follow-up, his blood pressure was 150/100 mmHg.

What is the most appropriate antihypertensive agent to add next?

A   Atenolol
B   Bendroflumethiazide
C   Doxazosin
D   Furosemide
E   Spironolactone

17. A 58-year-old man with a renal transplant attended for review. He had good graft function with a creatinine of around 140 µmol/L. His immunosuppression comprised tacrolimus and azathioprine with a low dose of prednisolone. He had recently had an episode of gout and was started on allopurinol by his general practitioner. He had also had a lower respiratory infection and been given a course of amoxicillin and clarithromycin. He complained of tiredness and lethargy at clinic.

Investigations:

haemoglobin 63 g/L (130–180)	platelets 129 × 10⁹/L (150–400)
white cell count 1.5 × 10⁹/L (4–11)	

What is the most likely cause if his pancytopenia?

A   Allopurinol
B   Amoxicillin
C   Clarithromycin
D   Prednisolone
E   Tacrolimus

18. A 30-year-old woman attended the emergency department with a 7-day history of worsening headache. Over the course of the past day she had developed fever, nausea, photophobia and neck stiffness. She had been drowsy for the past few hours.
    On examination, her Glasgow Coma Scale score was 14 (eyes 3, verbal 5, motor 6). Her temperature was 39°C. There was no rash. Kernig's sign was positive

Investigations:

> MRI of the brain: mild hydrocephalus
>
> Cerebrospinal fluid: opening pressure 34 cmH$_2$O (5–18)
>
> ---
>
> white cell count 10 x 10^9/L (<5)   protein 0.8 g/L (0.15–0.45)
>
> 90% lymphocytes, 10% neutrophils   glucose 3 mmol/L (3.3–4.4)
>
> India ink stain of cerebrospinal fluid:
> encapsulated cells

What is the most appropriate treatment?

A   Intravenous amphotericin B and flucytosine
B   Intravenous caspofungin
C   Intrathecal fluconazole
D   Oral ketoconazole
E   Oral pyrimethamine, sulfadiazine and folinic acid

19. A 58-year-old man presented to the emergency department after a suspected bisoprolol overdose. He had a background of ischaemic cardiomyopathy and hypertension. On examination, his blood pressure was 70/40 mmHg, and his pulse was 35 beats per minute and regular. He was drowsy. The remainder of the examination was unremarkable.
    An EG showed sinus bradycardia, first-degree heart block, and a QRS duration of 160 ms.
    No response was seen after administering a bolus of intravenous crystalloid.

What is the most appropriate treatment?

A   Intravenous adrenaline
B   Nebulised salbutamol
C   Intravenous glucagon
D   Transvenous cardiac pacing
E   Intravenous sodium bicarbonate

20. A 58-year-old man with mild chronic obstructive pulmonary disease and epilepsy was referred to the smoking cessation clinic. He smoked 20 cigarettes per day and was keen to give up. He had failed to stop smoking with nicotine replacement therapy, and was attending group counselling sessions. The counsellor suggested that he might be a suitable candidate for pharmacotherapy.

What is the most appropriate treatment?

A   Acamprosate
B   Bupropion
C   Citalopram
D   Disulfiram
E   Varenicline

21. A 22-year-old man presented with pain in his elbows, shoulders and knees, 3 weeks after commencing quadruple therapy for pulmonary tuberculosis.

Investigations:

haemoglobin 123 g/L (130–180)	platelets 204 × 10⁹/L (150–400)
white cell count 7.2 × 10⁹/L (4–11)	erythrocyte sedimentation rate 32 mm/1st h (0–30)

Antinuclear antibody 1:40 (negative at 1:20 dilution)
Rheumatoid factor 38 kIU/L (<30)
Anticyclic citrullinated protein antibodies (anti-CCP) 15 (negative <20)

What is the most likely cause of his symptoms?

A   Ethambutol arthropathy
B   Isoniazid-induced systemic lupus erythematosus
C   Paradoxical reaction
D   Pyrazinamide-induced arthralgia
E   Rheumatoid arthritis

22. A 72-year-old man was admitted to hospital with an international normalised ratio (INR) of 9.2. He had been taking warfarin for atrial fibrillation (target INR 2–3), and his regular maintenance dose was 6 mg daily. Five days previously, he was found to have acute, severe prostatitis for which he had been started on ciprofloxacin.
      On examination, the patient was well and there was no evidence of bleeding.

What is the most appropriate management for this patient?

A   Halve the dose of warfarin and monitor INR daily
B   Omit warfarin for 2 days
C   Stop the ciprofloxacin and continue warfarin at 1 mg per day
D   Stop warfarin and prescribe 1 mg oral vitamin K
E   Stop warfarin and prescribe 1 unit of fresh frozen plasma

23. A 21-year-old woman with a history of complex partial seizures attended the neurology outpatient clinic for review. Despite complying with escalating doses of carbamazepine for the past 6 months, her seizure control remained poor. She was now keen to try an alternative medication.
      The plan was to switch to lamotrigine; however, she was concerned about side effects.

Which one of the following is a recognised side effect of lamotrigine?

A   Alopecia
B   Blurred vision
C   Menstrual irregularities
D   Skin rash
E   Tremor

24. A 43-year-old woman presented with fever and malaise for 1 month. Examination revealed a pansystolic murmur and splinter haemorrhages. She weighed 125 kg.
      Three sets of blood cultures grew α-haemolytic streptococcus, sensitive to penicillin and gentamicin. A transthoracic echocardiogram showed mobile vegetations on the mitral valve. She was commenced on benzylpenicillin 2.4 g every 4 hours and gentamicin 70 mg every 8 hours.
      After 24 hours her gentamicin levels were measured:

Investigations:

> Gentamicin: peak 1.2 mg/L (target 3–5 mg/L), trough <1 mg/L (target <1 mg/L)

What is the next most appropriate step in management?

A Decrease in frequency of gentamicin dosing
B Increase in frequency of gentamicin dosing
C Use of actual body weight to dose gentamicin
D Use of dose-determining weight to dose gentamicin
E Use of ideal body weight to dose gentamicin

25. A 46-year-old man with genotype 1a hepatitis C virus had a new outpatient appointment in the hepatology clinic to discuss treatment options for hepatitis C. He was treatment naïve and had been diagnosed 20 years ago but had been lost to follow up some years previously. He had been offered treatment in the past but had not wanted to be treated with pegylated interferon and ribavirin as friends had told him it made them feel terrible. He had injected heroin in his twenties and his current medications consisted of only methadone.

Investigations:

haemoglobin 137 g/L (130–180)	alkaline phosphatase 184 U/L (45–105)
white cell count 5.6 × 10⁹/L (4–11)	alanine transaminase 46 U/L (5–35)
platelets 198 × 10⁹/L (150–400)	albumin 40 g/L (37–49)
bilirubin 14 mmol/L (1–22)	hepatitis C virus RNA 894,000 copies/mL

Fibroscan: 7.2 kPa
Ultrasound scan of liver: smooth liver outline, normal size liver, normal size spleen, no hepatomegaly.

Which of the following statements is false regarding the treatment of chronic hepatitis C with new direct acting antivirals (DAAV)?

A. Sustained virological response rates with DAAV treatment for all genotypes of chronic hepatitis C virus, including in those with prior treatment failure and cirrhosis, are ≥90%
B. Hepatitis B virus reactivation can occur during treatment with DAAVs
C. After the introduction of DAAVs in England in 2014, liver transplants for hepatitis C virus reduced by 32% in the following year
D. Active injection drug use is a contraindication to treatment with DAAVs
E. Sustained viral response is defined as undetectable hepatitis C virus RNA at 12 weeks after treatment with DAAVs

26. A 55-year-old man presented with severe dysphagia, nausea and vomiting. He had a past medical history of hypertension and hypercholesterolaemia, and was taking amlodipine, bisoprolol, ramipril and atorvastatin.

   An oesophagogastroduodenoscopy showed severe oesophageal candidiasis. Oral fluconazole was started. A subsequent HIV test was positive, with a low CD4 count and high viral load. Antiretroviral treatment comprising tenofovir, emtricitabine and raltegravir was commenced. His nausea persisted, so metoclopramide and domperidone were prescribed on discharge.

   One week later, he suffered a cardiac arrest at work. The initial rhythm was *torsades de pointes*. Defibrillation was successful.

Which drug interaction is the most likely cause of the arrhythmia?

A   Metoclopramide and raltegravir
B   Fluconazole and domperidone
C   Atorvastatin and fluconazole
D   Raltegravir and bisoprolol
E   Tenofovir and atorvastatin

27. A previously fit and well 28-year-old man with a 1-week history of bleeding gums was found to have an excess of myeloid blast cells containing prominent granules and Auer rods on his blood film. Bone marrow biopsy showed an excess of promyelocytes. Cytogenetic studies confirmed the presence of a t(15:17) translocation.

He had no active bleeding points at presentation, but had stopped brushing his teeth because it was making his gums bleed for several hours afterwards.

Investigations:

haemoglobin 92 g/L (130–180)	international normalised ratio 1.2 (<1.4)
white cell count 27 × 10⁹/L (4–11)	activated partial thromboplastin time 35 s (30–40)
platelets 63 × 10⁹/L (150–400)	fibrinogen 3.1 g/L (1.8–5.4)

The most appropriate treatment for this patient is standard anthracycline-based induction chemotherapy for acute myeloid leukaemia (e.g. daunorubicin, idarubicin and cytosine)

What should this treatment be combined with?

A   All-trans-retinoic acid
B   Dexamethasone
C   Regular transfusions of fresh frozen plasma
D   Rituximab
E   Thalidomide

28. A 44-year-old woman presented to the emergency department with drowsiness, a persistent throbbing headache, nausea and vomiting. She had had difficulty concentrating at work and had noticed that she had been quite irritable recently. Her symptoms were worse in the morning, and were relieved when she was at work. She had recently moved house, and her cat had died shortly after this, so she had initially put her symptoms down to stress.

She had no past medical history, and took no medications.
Physical examination was unremarkable.

Investigations:

haemoglobin 130 g/L (115–165)	C-reactive protein 4 mg/L (<5)
white cell count 4.5 × 10⁹/L (4–11)	carboxyhaemoglobin 35% (non-smoker <2%, smoker 3–15%)
platelets 167 × 10⁹/L (150–400)	

What is the most important management step?

A   Administration of continuous positive airway pressure ventilation
B   Charcoal administration
C   Continuous veno–venous haemofiltration
D   High-flow oxygen therapy
E   Hyperbaric oxygen therapy

29. A 53-year-old man presented to the emergency department with headache, intraoral tingling, cramping abdominal pain and diarrhoea 15 minutes after eating tuna steak at a seafood restaurant.

    On examination, he was anxious with a flushed appearance. A blanching erythematous macular rash was noted predominantly over the trunk. His temperature was 37.4°C, pulse 110 beats per minute, blood pressure 98/54 mmHg, respiratory rate 22 breaths per minute and oxygen saturation 98% on room air. Cardiovascular, neurological and respiratory examinations were normal. There was some abdominal tenderness.

    What is the most likely cause?

    A   Botulinum toxin
    B   Ciguatera toxin
    C   Pectenotoxin
    D   Scombrotoxin
    E   Tetrodotoxin

30. A 78-year-old white woman was referred to the cardiology clinic with worsening shortness of breath. She had a previous history of ischaemic heart disease and had undergone coronary artery bypass surgery 15 years ago. She also had type 2 diabetes mellitus, hypertension and depression.

    She was taking gliclazide 40 mg twice daily, ramipril 10 mg once daily, simvastatin 40 mg once daily, aspirin 75 mg once daily, furosemide 80 mg twice daily, bisoprolol 7.5 mg once daily and citalopram 20 mg once daily. She had shortness of breath on walking 100 metres and used three pillows with occasional bouts of shortness of breath at night.

    On examination, her pulse was 50 beats per minute, blood pressure 130/68 mmHg, respiratory rate 18 breaths per minute, and oxygen saturation 96% on air. She had a 2/6 pansystolic murmur at the apex, radiating to the axilla. Lung fields were clear and there was no ankle swelling.

    Investigations:

sodium 138 mmol/L (135–145)	creatinine 78 µmol/L (45–90)
potassium 3.9 mmol/L (3.5–5.0)	

    Echocardiogram:
      dilated left ventricle with lateral akinesia and ejection fraction of 30%
      mild mitral regurgitation
      mild tricuspid regurgitation and pulmonary artery systolic pressure 30 mmHg
    Myocardial perfusion scan did not show any reversible ischaemia

    What is the most appropriate next step in management?

    A   Amiodarone
    B   Amlodipine
    C   Digoxin
    D   Isosorbide mononitrate
    E   Spironolactone

31. A 34-year-old woman presented with nausea and vomiting 4 hours after having taken an overdose of paracetamol. Her paracetamol level was above the treatment threshold and she was given intravenous *N*-acetylcysteine (NAC) in 5% dextrose.

    Two hours after starting the infusion the patient complained of feeling hot. On examination, she had obvious facial flushing. Her temperature was 37.5°C, pulse 90 beats per minute, blood pressure 110/65 mmHg, respiratory rate 20 breaths per minute and oxygen saturation 95% on air. There was no angio-oedema and her chest was clear.

What is the most appropriate next step in management?

A   Continue the NAC infusion at the same rate
B   Stop the NAC infusion and give oral methionine
C   Stop the NAC infusion and administer intravenous chlorpheniramine
D   Stop the NAC infusion and give oral NAC
E   Pause the NAC infusion and restart in 4 hours

32. A 19-year-old woman presented with fever, drowsiness and a rash. She had no past medical history and was not taking any medication.
    On examination, her Glasgow Coma Scale score was 14/15. There was a non-blanching petechial rash over her trunk and limbs. There was neck stiffness and photophobia but no focal neurological signs.

Investigations:

> Cerebrospinal fluid microscopy: Gram-negative diplococci

What is most appropriate treatment?

A   Ceftriaxone
B   Cefuroxime
C   Chloramphenicol
D   Ciprofloxacin
E   Vancomycin and high-dose dexamethasone

33. A 21-year-old woman presented with left heel pain radiating into her left calf, particularly on walking, and progressing in severity over the preceding 48 hours. She had a past medical history of partial thyroidectomy for a nodule and had recently been treated with several courses of oral antimicrobials by her general practitioner for a persistent urinary tract infection.
    On examination, the calf was soft and non-tender. There was focal tenderness over her heel with mild erythema but no oedema.
    Over the past 2 months she had been treated with levothyroxine, cephalexin, nitrofurantoin, co-amoxiclav and ciprofloxacin.

What is the most likely diagnosis?

A   Cephalosporin myopathy
B   Nitrofurantoin tendinopathy
C   Penicillin myopathy
D   Pretibial myxoedema
E   Quinolone tendinopathy

34. A 24-year-old man presented with a painful neck 24 hours after commencing olanzapine for paranoid schizophrenia.
    On examination, there was spasmodic torticollis.

Apart from stopping olanzapine, what is the most appropriate next step in management?

A   Intramuscular botulinum toxin
B   Intravenous dantrolene sodium
C   Intravenous procyclidine
D   Electroconvulsive therapy
E   Oral tizanidine

35. A 54-year-old woman presented to clinic with tiredness, abdominal and back pain, and constipation. She had a past medical history of a major depressive illness and started medication for this 1 year ago.

Examination was unremarkable.

Investigations:

corrected calcium 2.9 mmol/L (2.2–2.6)

phosphate 0.3 mmol/L (0.8–1.4)

alkaline phosphatase 577 U/L (45–105)

parathyroid hormone 8.5 pmol/L (0.9–5.4)

thyroid-stimulating hormone 0.1 mU/L (0.4–5.0)

free thyroxine 4 pmol/L (10–25)

What is the most likely cause?

A   Amitriptyline
B   Fluoxetine
C   Lithium
D   Mirtazapine
E   Venlafaxine

36. A 54-year-old woman presented with a 3-day history of breathlessness, fever and a cough productive of rusty-coloured sputum. She was oriented and gave a clear history of paroxysmal atrial fibrillation, treated with a beta-blocker and warfarin. She had not recently travelled and had no pets.

On examination, her temperature was 38.1°C, pulse 125 beats per minute, blood pressure 125/85 mmHg, respiratory rate 16 breaths per minute and oxygen saturation 93% on air. Auscultation of the chest revealed focal bronchial breathing at the left base.

Investigations:

haemoglobin 128 g/L (115–165)

white cell count 12.6 × 10⁹/L (4–11)

neutrophils 10.9 × 10⁹/L (1.5–7.0)

platelets 321 × 10⁹/L (150–400)

sodium 138 mmol/L (135–145)

potasssium 3.9 mmol/L (3.5–5.0)

urea 5.6 mmol/L (2.5–7.5)

creatinine 69 μmol/L (45–90)

C-reactive protein 127 mg/L (<5)

Chest X-ray: see **Figure 12.1**

What is the most appropriate therapy?

A   Amoxicillin
B   Amoxicillin and clarithromycin
C   Co-amoxiclav and clarithromycin
D   Doxycycline
E   Levofloxacin

Figure 12.1

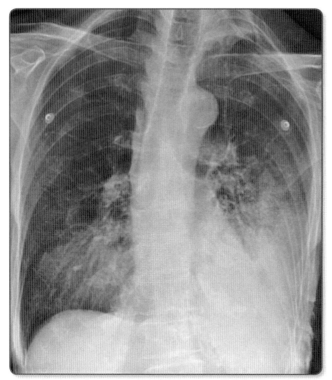

37. A 79-year-old woman presented with haematemesis. She had a past medical history of atrial fibrillation, osteoarthritis and hypertension. Her regular medications comprised bisoprolol, ramipril, and dabigatran. She had taken her last dose of dabigatran 14 hours before presentation.
    On initial assessment, she was drowsy and pale. Her blood pressure was 75/40 mmHg. She was peripherally vasoconstricted.

Investigations:

haemoglobin 65 g/L (115–165)	international normalised ratio 1.3 (<1.4)
platelets 530 × 10⁹/L (150–400)	activated partial thromboplastin time 32 s (30–40)
	thrombin time 30 s (15–20)

There was no change in her clinical state following a transfusion of two units of packed red cells.

Which additional treatment is indicated?

A   Abciximab
B   Fresh frozen plasma
C   Andexanet alfa
D   Idarucizumab
E   None of the above

38. A 28-year-old woman was admitted with a 36-hour history of flu-like illness during an epidemic of H1N1 influenza. She was 32 weeks' pregnant. She had been vaccinated against H1N1 influenza 6 weeks previously.

What is the most appropriate management?

A   Intravenous pooled human immunoglobulin
B   Intravenous zanamivir
C   Oral amoxicillin
D   Oral oseltamivir
E   Symptomatic treatment

39. A 45-year-old Lithuanian man was brought to the emergency department by his housemates in an acute confusional state. Earlier that evening he had been drinking home-made vodka. The patient did not speak English and was unable to give a history. His friends denied that he took drugs or other medication.

On examination, his Glasgow Coma Scale score was 12 (eyes 3, speech 4, motor 5). He was unkempt and smelled strongly of alcohol. His temperature was 37°C, pulse 104 beats per minute, blood pressure 90/58 mmHg, respiratory rate 28 breaths per minute and oxygen saturation 98% on air.

Cardiovascular, respiratory and abdominal examinations were normal. His pupils had normal and equal diameter but were slow to react to light. He could move all limbs. There was no neck stiffness, rash or marks on his skin.

Investigations:

sodium 131 mmol/L (135–145)	creatinine 102 μmol/L (60–110)
potassium 4.2 mmol/L (3.5–5.0)	chloride 104 mmol/L (95–107)
urea 8.6 mmol/L (2.5–7.5)	glucose 4.5 mmol/L (3.0–6.0)
Arterial blood gases (on air):	P_{O_2} 12.3 kPa (11.3–12.6)
pH 7.29 (7.35–7.45)	bicarbonate 13 mmol/L (22–30)
P_{CO_2} 3.0 kPa (4.7–6.0)	

The patient was initially treated with intravenous fluids, and an infusion of sodium bicarbonate.

What is the next most appropriate step in management?

A   Activated charcoal
B   Ethanol
C   Gastric lavage
D   Haemodialysis
E   Phenytoin

40. A 44-year-old man with a history of depression presented with nausea and vomiting, tinnitus and sweating after taking an overdose of an unknown substance a few hours earlier. He had no other past medical history.

On examination, he was sweating and anxious. His temperature was 38°C, pulse 100 beats per minute, blood pressure 132/96 mmHg and respiratory rate 36 breaths per minute. Physical examination was unremarkable.

Investigations:

Arterial blood gases on air:	PO_2 13 kPa (11.3–12.6)
pH 7.51 (7.35–7.45)	base excess −6 mmol/L (± 2)
P_{CO_2} 2.4 kPa (4.7–6.0)	bicarbonate 9 mmol/L (22–30)

What is the most likely diagnosis?

A   Ethylene glycol overdose
B   Methanol overdose
C   Organophosphate poisoning
D   Salicylate overdose
E   Tricyclic antidepressant overdose

41. An 18-year-old woman presented to the emergency department after an intentional overdose of an unknown quantity of ferrous sulphate. She complained of abdominal pain and vomiting. She was admitted for overnight observation. The following morning, she was feeling well and her symptoms had resolved.
    Her blood pressure was 112/68 mmHg, pulse 94 beats per minute, and respiratory rate was 24 breaths per minute.

Investigations:

haemoglobin 145 g/L (115–165)	creatinine 86 µmol/L (60–110)
platelets 340 × 10⁹/L (150–400)	chloride 99 mmol/L (95–107)
bilirubin 15 mmol/L (1–22)	bicarbonate 12 mmol/L (22–30)
alkaline phosphatase 97 U/L (45–105)	glucose 9.1 mmol/L (3.0–6.0)
alanine transaminase 22 U/L (5–35)	iron 26 µmol/L (12–30)
albumin 41 g/L (37–49)	total iron binding capacity 60 µmol/L (45–75)
	ferritin 120 µg/L (15–300)

What is the most appropriate treatment?

A   Gastric lavage
B   Activated charcoal
C   Intravenous desferrioxamine
D   Observe for a further 24 hours
E   No treatment indicated

42. A 25-year-old man presented to his general practitioner with a 7-month history of diarrhoea, urgency and crampy abdominal pain. The pain was worse after eating and associated with abdominal bloating. He reported no weight loss or rectal bleeding. He took no medications and had no family history of note.
    Physical examination was normal.

Investigations:

Full blood count, C-reactive protein and erythrocyte sedimentation rate: Normal
Tissue transglutaminase antibodies: negative

What is the most appropriate initial treatment?

A   Acupuncture
B   Amitriptyline
C   Hyoscine butylbromide
D   Cognitive–behavioural therapy
E   Mesalazine

43. A 25-year-old woman was brought to the emergency department by a friend, 2 hours after allegedly taking an amitriptyline overdose. She had a history of depression and attempted suicide. She denied taking any other medications. She complained of blurred vision and palpitations.

On examination, she was tearful and agitated. Her Glasgow Coma Scale score was 14 (eyes 3, speech 5, motor 6), temperature 37.4°C, pulse 130 beats per minute, blood pressure 95/52 mmHg, respiratory rate 10 breaths per minute and oxygen saturation 98% on air. Cardio-respiratory examination was normal but neurological examination revealed dilated pupils.

Investigations:

sodium 136 mmol/L (135–145)	creatinine 98 µmol/L (45–90)
potassium 3.4 mmol/L (3.5–5.0)	chloride 107 mmol/L (95–107)
urea 7.3 mmol/L (2.5–7.5)	
Arterial blood gases (on air):	Po_2 11.9 kPa (11.3–12.6)
pH 7.31 (7.35–7.45)	bicarbonate 16 mmol/L (22–30)
Pco_2 4.9 kPa (4.7–6.0)	lactate 3.9 mmol/L (0.6–1.8)

ECG: sinus tachycardia with a widened QRS complex (140 ms) and prolonged QT interval

Apart from fluid resuscitation, what is the most appropriate next step in management?

A   Diazepam
B   Gastric lavage
C   Glucagon
D   Hyperventilation
E   Sodium bicarbonate

Answers

1. B Fomepizole

This patient has ingested a potentially fatal dose of antifreeze. She is exhibiting features consistent with acute ethylene glycol intoxication, and her blood tests show that she has a raised osmolar gap. Although her arterial blood gases are not presently greatly deranged, they would be expected to deteriorate over the ensuing hours if no treatment is given. This is because ethylene glycol will be metabolised by alcohol dehydrogenase to glycoaldehyde, which in turn will be further metabolised to highly toxic entities including glycolic acid and subsequently oxalic acid; these cause a raised anion gap metabolic acidosis.

Therefore, the most appropriate step is to start treatment to prevent the metabolism of ethylene glycol (even though no serum ethylene glycol level has been recorded). This can be achieved by administering ethanol or fomepizole. Ethanol acts as a preferential substrate for alcohol dehydrogenase, thereby preventing the metabolism of ethylene glycol, whereas fomepizole is an inhibitor of alcohol dehydrogenase activity. Both prevent the formation of toxic ethylene glycol metabolites.

Unlike ethanol, fomepizole is not inebriating and does not require regular blood monitoring. Treatment should be continued until serum ethylene glycol falls below 50 mg/L.

Activated charcoal does not absorb ethylene glycol well. Gastric lavage is advised only if presentation is within 1 hour of ingestion. Intravenous lorazepam would be indicated if the patient were to develop frequent or prolonged seizures. Sodium bicarbonate may be indicated if severe metabolic acidosis develops. Haemodialysis is necessary in cases of severe poisoning, or if there is acute kidney injury.

Barceloux DG, et al. American Academy of Clinical Toxicology Practice Guidelines on the Treatment of Ethylene Glycol Poisoning. Ad Hoc Committee. J Toxicol Clin Toxicol 1999; 37(5):537.

2. E Methotrexate

Medical treatment for Crohn's disease, with the exception of methotrexate, should generally continue as the risks of stopping treatment usually outweigh the benefits. Methotrexate therapy has been shown to be teratogenic and embryotoxic in animal studies. It results in chromosomal damage and miscarriages and is contraindicated in pregnancy. Due to the long half-life of its metabolites it should be stopped at least 6 weeks before conception. Thiopurines are generally considered safe in pregnancy. In the USA, they have a Food and Drug Administration (FDA) rating of D, based on anecdotal reports of high abortion rates, but inflammatory bowel disease (IBD) follow-up studies of pregnancies during treatment with azathioprine and 6-mercaptopurine report normal deliveries and no excess rates of prematurity, low birth weight or chromosomal abnormalities. Studies of inhaled budesonide suggest that it is safe in pregnancy at the doses used, which are much higher than those used in IBD, so it is felt to be safe. There are no studies of oral budesonide in pregnancy. Infliximab use during pregnancy has been reported in 2 papers covering 92 pregnancies and no significantly increased risks of stillbirths, ectopic pregnancies, spontaneous abortions or low birth weight were found. Congenital abnormalities occurred in two pregnancies but this may have been related to the underlying increased risk in women with IBD. Mesalazine has been shown to be safe in pregnancy in doses of up to 3 g per day.

van Assche G, et al. The second European evidence-based consensus on the diagnosis and management of Crohn's disease: Special situations. Journal of Crohn's and Colitis 2010; 4:63–101.

3. C Indometacin

Most patients with hemicrania continua respond to indometacin, which is typically administered at 75–150 mg/day in divided doses. Absolute resolution of symptoms usually occurs within 2 or 3 days of commencing treatment (and failure to respond should raise doubts about the diagnosis). Unfortunately, high relapse rates are observed on cessation of treatment.

Clarke C, et al. Headache (Chapter 12). In: Neurology: A Queen Square Textbook, 2nd edn. Oxford: Wiley-Blackwell Publishing, 2016.

4. C Memantine

Alzheimer's disease is the most common form of dementia in the UK, affecting more than 350,000 people. Grading of severity is based on the Mini-Mental state examination score: mild (21–26), moderate (10–20) or severe (<10). Disease progression is insidious, and median survival is approximately 7 years from symptom onset.

Any one of the acetylcholinesterase inhibitors (donepezil, galantamine or rivastigmine) can be used in the treatment of mild or moderate Alzheimer's disease. In contrast, the only pharmacological treatment licensed for the treatment of severe Alzheimer's disease in the UK is memantine, a voltage-dependent, moderate affinity, competitive N-methyl-D-aspartate receptor antagonist. This drug has been deemed cost-effective in the treatment of severe Alzheimer's disease at an incremental cost-effectiveness ratio of £26 500 per quality-adjusted life year (QALY) gained (when compared with best supportive treatment). Memantine does not prevent disease progression (although it does a have a small but significant effect in delaying the need for nursing home care), but improves symptoms and is particularly useful in agitated patients.

National Institute for Health and Care Excellence. NICE Guidelines. Donepezil, galantamine, rivastigmine and memantine for the treatment of Alzheimer's disease (TA217). London: NICE, 2011.

5. A Corticosteroids

Treatment of immune thrombocytopenia is not usually indicated unless the platelet count is below 50 $\times 10^9$/L. First-line treatments include corticosteroids and intravenous immunoglobulin. Anti-D may also be an appropriate first-line treatment in patients who are rhesus D positive, with no evidence of autoimmune haemolytic anaemia. Second-line agents include steroid-sparing immunosuppressants and rituximab. Romiplostim is a thrombopoietin receptor agonist that has been approved by the National Institute for Health and Care Excellence for use in patients with chronic immune thrombocytopenic purpura (lasting more than 12 months) which has failed to respond to standard active treatments and rescue therapies, or in those who have severe disease and a significant risk of haemorrhage requiring frequent rescue therapies. Splenectomy may be indicated if medical therapies prove unsuccessful; however, approximately 14% of patients will not respond to this treatment and, of those who do, 20% will relapse in the fullness of time. Platelet transfusion would be indicated only if the patient were actively bleeding. Plasma exchange has no role as a treatment in isolation.

Immune thrombocytopenic purpura is discussed in more detail in Chapter 5.

Hoffbrand V, Moss P, Pettit J. Bleeding disorders (Chapter 23). In: Essential Haematology, 5th edn. Oxford: Blackwell Publishing, 2006.
Provan D, et al. International consensus report on the investigation and management of primary immune thrombocytopenia. Blood 2010; 115:168–186.

6. C Increase dose of methadone

Four drugs – rifampicin, isoniazid, pyrazinamide and ethambutol – are used together in the initial phase of tuberculosis treatment to reduce the bacterial population and reduce the risk of drug resistance. Rifampicin is generally well tolerated but may cause mild gastrointestinal upset and/or transient disturbance of liver function with elevated transaminases, which does not require interruption of therapy. Occasionally more serious liver toxicity may occur, requiring a change of treatment, particularly in those with pre-existing liver disease. Other major side effects include acute renal failure and thrombocytopenia. Patients should be warned that rifampicin will cause red discoloration of urine (useful for compliance monitoring) and other body fluids, and may discolour contact lenses.

Rifampicin induces hepatic enzymes, which accelerate the metabolism of several drugs including oestrogens, corticosteroids, phenytoin, sulphonlyureas, opiates and anticoagulants. His symptoms are suggestive of opiate withdrawal because of the increased metabolism of methadone, so the dose will need to be increased under close supervision. Similarly, in other patients taking concomitant medications, specific advice and monitoring may be necessary, e.g. in women taking hormonal contraceptives alternative family planning advice should be offered.

Isoniazid is well tolerated. The major side effect is age-dependent hepatitis and there is increased toxicity with chronic alcohol abuse. Peripheral neuropathy is uncommon; pyridoxine reduces the risk of this. There is an increased risk of peripheral neuropathy in diabetes, chronic alcohol abuse, HIV, malnutrition, and pregnancy, and an increased dose of pyridoxine should be prescribed.

Pyrazinamide also causes gastrointestinal upset and drug-induced hepatitis. Ethambutol very rarely causes optic neuritis, which presents with impairment of colour vision and/or loss of visual acuity.

Patients should receive appropriate counselling regarding the side effects associated with anti-tuberculous therapy, and informed to seek advice if they develop symptoms including abdominal pain, nausea, vomiting, rash and/or jaundice, so that appropriate action may be taken.

National Institute for Health and Care Excellence (NICE). NICE Guideline: Tuberculosis (NG32). London: NICE, 2016.

7. B Coronary vasospasm

MDMA (3,4-methylenedioxy-*N*-methylamphetamine) ingestion can cause a variety of clinical manifestations. Minor side effects, which are almost universal, include tachycardia, hypertension, mydriasis, dry mouth, sweating, confusion, ataxia and bruxism (teeth gnashing and jaw clenching). More severe adverse effects include hyperpyrexia with rhabdomyolysis and multi-organ failure, serotonin syndrome, long QT syndrome, acute liver failure and hyponatraemia, and cerebral oedema. In rare cases cerebral venous sinus thrombosis, cerebral haemorrhage and aplastic anaemia have been reported. Coronary vasospasm is not associated with MDMA ingestion, but is associated with cocaine.

Hall AP, Henry JA. Acute toxic effects of 'Ecstasy' (MDMA) and related compounds: overview of pathophysiology and clinical management. Br J Anaesth 2006; 96:678–685.

8. E Reduction of oral hypotonic fluids to less than 500 mL/day

The patient has short bowel syndrome secondary to her previous mesenteric infarction and subsequent surgery. This has been complicated by a high-output stoma. Management of a high-output stoma in small bowel syndrome is challenging. The primary driver for stomal fluid loss is oral intake, and hypotonic fluids cause high stomal losses, so treatment begins with the patient restricting their total oral hypotonic intake to less than 500 mL/day. Fluid requirements can be maintained by sipping a glucose/saline solution throughout the day, such as the modified WHO cholera rehydration solution. If there is marked sodium and water depletion then intravenous 0.9% saline may need to be given for 24–48 hours, while the patient is kept nil by mouth. Correcting electrolyte imbalances such as hypomagnesaemia is important, but correction of sodium and water depletion is an important first step in this process as it treats the secondary hyperaldosteronism caused by short bowel syndrome. Anti-motility drugs will reduce stoma output by 20–30% by increasing small intestinal transit time, and so are important in the management of high-output stoma, but reducing the high-output stoma drive is more important. Anti-secretory medications can be used when there is a net secretory output (more than 3 L in 24 hours) but absorption of energy, carbohydrate and lipids is not affected by proton pump inhibitors such as omeprazole and they do not reduce the severity of intestinal failure. Octreotide will reduce stomal output by 1–2 L in 24 hours but has no effect on energy, nitrogen or fat absorption, and should be used only in those with a net secretory output. Diet is important in the management of patients with short bowel and jejunostomy but the priority is correction of sodium and water imbalances.

Nightingale J, Woodward J M. Guidelines for management of patients with a short bowel. Gut 2006; 55(IV):iv1–iv12.

9. E Ropinirole

This patient has restless legs syndrome (RLS), a condition that can occur at any age. It tends to be more severe in older age, and affects women more frequently than men (2:1). It can occur as a primary disease, which has a familial tendency, or secondary to other factors (e.g. iron deficiency, renal failure, pregnancy, alcohol misuse). The diagnosis is clinical and requires the fulfilment of four criteria:
1. The presence of a compelling desire to move the lower limbs (often associated with an unpleasant dysaesthesia).
2. Motor restlessness (as movement tends to relieve, or improve, symptoms of dysaesthesia).
3. Worsening of symptoms at rest.
4. Circadian features, with symptoms being worse in the evening or at night.

Sleep disturbance and daytime fatigue are also common. Interestingly, patients diagnosed with RLS are often found to exhibit periodic limb movements of sleep (e.g. involuntary forceful dorsiflexion at the ankle) on polysomnography.
   First-line treatments include ropinirole, pergolide and gabapentin. Clonazepam may be helpful as a hypnotic treatment, but is otherwise not thought to be useful. There is insufficient evidence for the use of dihydrocodeine in the treatment of RLS, but opiates may have a role. Perhaps, somewhat surprisingly, RLS may develop secondary to amitriptyline use. Baclofen is not indicated.

Garcia-Borreguero, et al. European guidelines on management of restless legs syndrome. Eur J Neurol 2012:19:1385-1396.

10. C Inhibits mycobacterial RNA polymerase

Rifampicin is bactericidal and binds to the RNA polymerase deep within the RNA/DNA channel, preventing transcription to RNA and subsequent translation to proteins. It is lipophilic and is therefore a good agent in the treatment of tuberculous meningitis, which requires penetration through the blood–brain barrier. Isoniazid is bacteriostatic and inhibits synthesis of mycolic acids in mycobacterial cell walls.

11. C Citalopram interaction with linezolid

This man is presenting with a serotonin syndrome caused by the interaction of the new antimicrobial linezolid with the patient's longstanding selective serotonin reuptake inhibitor (SSRI). Linezolid itself is a weak monoamine oxidase inhibitor and combination with all serotonin active agents should be avoided. Serotonin syndrome is characterised by somatic, autonomic and cognitive effects, including hypo- and hypertension, tachycardia, sweating, excess bowel movements, hyperthermia, agitation, hallucinations, clonus and myotonia. There is no laboratory investigation to confirm the diagnosis but the clinical syndrome in the context of a relevant drug history is usually conclusive. Management is supportive: blood pressure can be controlled with a short-acting agent, hyperthermia and agitation with benzodiazepines (although intubation and sedation are required in severe cases); the most crucial management is withdrawal of the offending agent. SSRIs have long half-lives, but that of linezolid is relatively short, so symptoms should resolve within 24 hours.
   Tramadol itself does have some serotonergic activity, but it would be unlikely to cause a serotonin syndrome; amitriptyline also has serotonin activity and has been documented to cause serotonin syndrome both in overdose situations and in conjunction with linezolid and citalopram, but at a dose of 25 mg is unlikely to be the cause in this case.

Bernard L, et al. Serotonin syndrome after concomitant treatment with linezolid and citalopram. Clin Infect Dis 2003; 36(9):1197.

12. D pH

The King's College criteria for transplantation in acute liver failure following paracetamol overdose after 24 hours of treatment are:
>   Arterial pH <7.25

Or
>   All of the following:
>   Creatinine >300 mmol/L, PT (prothrombin time) >100 s and grade 3/4 encephalopathy.

The King's College Criteria have a very good specificity (96%) but a limited sensitivity, meaning that the criteria do not accurately predict all those who will die without liver transplantation.
    More recently the addition of a lactate of >3.5 on admission, or >3 after 24 hours of fluid resuscitation has been suggested to improve the sensitivity of the King's College criteria, but there has been discussion as to its utility. With the example given in the question, only pH <7.25 individually predicts the need for liver transplantation. The creatinine and prothrombin time (PT) are used in combination – on their own they are not sufficient for referral. The lactate value is not high enough to fulfil the predictive criteria, and bilirubin is not used as a factor to decide eligibility for liver transplantation.

O'Grady JG, et al. Early indicators of prognosis in fulminant hepatic failure. Gastroenterology 1989; 97:439.

13. D Modafinil

This patient has narcolepsy. Modafinil is the only medication in this list approved for treatment of narcolepsy in the UK. It is a novel wake-promoting agent, the precise mechanism of action of which remains unclear. Other agents used to treat narcolepsy are pitolisant, dexamfetamine, and sodium oxybate.
    Ephedrine is most commonly used as a nasal decongestant. Mephedrone is an illegal stimulant drug, known as 'miaow miaow', which has no medical uses. Clomethiazole is a prescription drug used to treat insomnia. Promethazine is a sedating antihistamine.

14. A Efavirenz-induced myositis

This man has a clinical and laboratory picture consistent with myositis and is on two agents likely to be the cause – simvastatin and efavirenz. The temporal drug history, with the statin having been introduced 3 years ago and the Atripla 3 months ago, makes efavirenz the likely cause. Simvastatin is metabolised via the cytochrome P450 3A4 (CYP3A4) isozymes and efavirenz is a mixed inducer and inhibitor of this pathway; however, co-administration of efavirenz and simvastatin actually decreases the plasma concentration of the statin and makes myositis from the statin less likely. Efavirenz itself does cause a myopathy and myositis in a small proportion of patients. Management is supportive, with removal of the offending agent, and fluids and renal support where necessary.
    Metformin can cause a metabolic acidosis and this can manifest with systemic disturbance, as exhibited in this case. The normal blood lactate excludes this, however. Metformin-inducing myositis is not described. Similarly, tenofovir can cause a lactic acidosis.

Klopstock T. Drug-induced myopathies. Curr Opin Neurol 2008; 21(5):590–595.

15. B Atropine

This patient is exhibiting signs of moderate-to-severe organophosphate poisoning, and needs to be treated aggressively. Organophosphates are frequently found in pesticides, and are a fairly common cause of intentional and unintentional poisoning worldwide, especially in poorer rural communities. Organophosphate poisoning can occur through ingestion, absorption through the skin, inhalation or injection. Organophosphates block the activity of acetylcholinesterase, preventing the degradation of acetylcholine within the nervous system. This, in turn, results in parasympathetic over-activation.

Atropine is the mainstay of treatment and should be started as early as possible. Many guidelines also advocate the combined early use of pralidoxime, a reactivator of phosphorylated acetylcholinesterase, but it should not be used without concomitant atropine because of possible worsening of symptoms through transient oxime-induced acetylcholinesterase inhibition.

Glycopyrrolate is an anticholinergic agent, but is not the first-line treatment. Intravenous diazepam would be appropriate should the patient develop seizures.

Eddleston M, et al. Management of acute organophosphorus pesticide poisoning. Lancet 2008; 371:597–607.
Peter JV, et al. Oxime therapy and outcomes in human organophosphate poisoning: an evaluation using meta-analytic techniques. Crit Care Med 2006 34:502–510.

16. A Atenolol

Most phaeochromocytomas secrete adrenaline or noradrenaline or occasionally both. For control of hypertension and symptoms initially α-adrenoreceptor blockade is needed.

If initial β blockade is used, the unopposed α- action could lead to a hypertensive crisis. After adequate α blockade, β blockade determines the drug of choice. Hence a cardioselective β-blocker such as atenolol or metoprolol would be preferred. Labetalol or carvedilol are not preferred as single agents because their α:β ratio is poor.

Calcium channel blockers such as amlodipine could be used but are not among the list of options.

Bendroflumethiazide, furosemide and spironolactone can make the volume depletion in phaeochromocytoma worse.

Pacak K. Pre-operative management of the phaeochromocytoma patient. J Clin Endocrinol Metab 2007; 92(11):4069–4079.

17. A Allopurinol

There are many interactions involving immunosuppressive medications and it is important to be aware of these when prescribing any other drugs. Azathioprine is a thiopurine that is metabolised to 6-mercaptopurine, the active metabolite of the drug. This inhibits purine synthesis. It is used in transplant recipients as well as in the treatment of many autoimmune conditions, including rheumatoid arthritis, pemphigus and inflammatory bowel disease.

Allopurinol is a xanthine oxidase inhibitor often used in the treatment of gout. Xanthine oxidase is involved in the metabolism of 6-mercaptopurine and, by inhibiting it, metabolism is pushed preferentially along the pathway that results in 6-thioguanine nucleotide formation, which is responsible for the majority of the immunosuppressant activity, but also bone marrow suppression.

The interaction between allopurinol and azathioprine is well known; deaths from bone marrow suppression have been recorded. In general, concomitant use should be avoided or, if deemed necessary, the dose of azathioprine should be significantly reduced (to around 25% of the starting dose) and full blood count should be monitored weekly. Recovery of cell counts is typically seen within 4–8 weeks of withdrawal of either drug.

Amoxicillin does not cause bone marrow suppression.

Clarithromycin should be used with caution, and preferably avoided, with calcineurin inhibitors (CNIs: tacrolimus or ciclosporin) as it interferes with the CYP3A4 enzyme (one of the cytochrome P450 enzymes) and will result in much higher levels of these drugs; this can cause toxicity, but not bone marrow suppression. If a macrolide is essential, the CNI dose should be pre-emptively reduced and levels monitored regularly.

Prednisolone does not cause bone marrow suppression. A high white blood cell count is usually seen in patients taking corticosteroids; this is mainly due to reduced margination of neutrophils.

Gearry RB, et al. Allopurinol and azathioprine: a two-edged interaction. J Gastroenterol Hepatol 2010; 25(4):653–655.
Venkat RG. Azathioprine and allopurinol: a potentially dangerous combination. J Intern Med 1990; 228(1):69–71.

18. A Intravenous amphotericin B and flucytosine

This is a case of cryptococcal meningitis. The yeast, *Cryptococcus neoformans*, is commonly found in soil and the excreta of pigeons. Transmission is usually by inhalation, with pulmonary colonisation and subsequent haematogenous spread to the meninges. A granulomatous meningoencephalitis results. Immunosuppressed patients (HIV, immunosuppressant medications or reticuloendothelial malignancy) are at greatest risk of infection; further investigation for such causes is necessary in this patient. Typical presenting features of cryptococcal meningitis include headache and fever. Meningism and drowsiness may also be present. Less commonly, focal neurological signs occur. MRI of the brain may be normal, or otherwise it may show hydrocephalus, meningeal enhancement, cryptococcomas or enlarged perivascular spaces (Virchow–Robin spaces), surrounding blood vessels for a short distance as they enter the brain. Lumbar puncture often reveals raised opening pressure, indicative of raised intracranial pressure. Cerebrospinal fluid analysis may reveal a mononuclear pleocytosis, raised protein and reduced glucose. Serum cryptococcal antigen is a useful screening test. The detection of *Cryptococcus* species on an India ink stain of the cerebrospinal fluid is diagnostic of the condition.

First-line treatment is with intravenous amphotericin B and flucytosine. This induction regimen is usually continued for at least 4 weeks in HIV-negative, non-transplant patients who do not have neurological complications and whose cerebrospinal fluid yeast culture is negative after 2 weeks of treatment. In those with neurological complications, the induction regimen is continued for a total of 6 weeks. Consolidation therapy, in the form of oral fluconazole (400 mg once daily), is usually given for 8 weeks. Maintenance therapy, with oral fluconazole 200 mg once daily, may be given for a further 6–12 months. In HIV-positive patients, the induction and consolidation regimen differs and oral fluconazole is normally used as life-long prophylaxis. Other treatment may include serial lumbar punctures to reduce cerebrospinal fluid opening pressure to within normal limits; however, persistent raised intracranial pressure may necessitate a ventriculoperitoneal shunt.

Caspofungin belongs to the echinocandin class of antifungal drugs. It is administered intravenously for the treatment of fungal infections, particularly in immunocompromised patients. It is most active against *Candida and Aspergillus species*.

Ketoconazole is inappropriate therapy as it does not readily cross the blood–brain barrier.

Oral pyrimethamine, sulfadiazine and folinic acid are used in the treatment of toxoplasmosis.

Perfect JR, et al. Clinical Practice Guidelines for the Management of Cryptococcal Disease: 2010 Update from the Infectious Diseases Society of America. Clin Infect Dis 2010; 50:291–322.

19. C Intravenous glucagon

Patients with impaired cardiac function are at higher risk of the toxic effects of beta-blocker overdose. The presence of hypotension and QRS prolongation in this patient indicates severe toxicity. In the absence of decompensated cardiac failure, the first stage of treatment is an intravenous fluid bolus. Of the options given, glucagon is the most appropriate next step in management. Glucagon has positive inotropic and chronotropic effects, and is often used to confirm as well as treat suspected beta-blocker toxicity. Atropine is an alternative agent for treating bradycardia, but it lacks the positive inotropic effects of glucagon, which directly acts on cardiac muscle. Intravenous insulin (with glucose supplementation) is an alternative agent which can also be used.

Transvenous pacing may be required if pharmacotherapy fails to restore cardiac output, but it would not be the first line strategy. Nebulised salbutamol would only be indicated if there were signs of bronchospasm. Adrenaline is an extremely potent α- and β- agonist; it can provoke ventricular arrhythmias and should only be used in a cardiac arrest situation. Sodium bicarbonate has no role in beta-blocker overdose. Other (rarer) complications of beta-blocker toxicity include hypoglycaemia, bronchospasm, hallucinations and seizures.

20. E Varenicline

Varenicline avidly binds to the $\alpha_4\beta_2$ neuronal nicotinic acetylcholine receptor. Its partial agonist action helps to reduce symptoms of nicotine withdrawal and craving, and reduces the satisfaction of smoking. Varenicline is prescribed as a 12-week course and patients are twice as likely to quit smoking than using willpower or nicotine replacement therapy. Side effects of the treatment include gastrointestinal disturbance, and it should be used with caution in patients with a history of psychiatric illness including depression. Patients should be counselled to stop treatment and seek advice if they notice a change in mood.

Bupropion has been used as an antidepressant and may be used to aid smoking cessation; its mode of action is not fully understood and may involve an effect on noradrenaline and dopamine neurotransmission. Bupropion is contraindicated in patients with a history of seizures, central nervous system tumours, cirrhosis, and acute alcohol and benzodiazepine withdrawal. It should be used with caution in patients taking other drugs that may lower seizure threshold or with a history of alcohol abuse, head injury or diabetes.

Acamprosate and disulfiram may be helpful in maintaining abstinence in alcohol-dependent patients. Citalopram is a selective serotonin reuptake inhibitor, which has no role in smoking cessation.

National Institute for Health and Care Excellence (NICE). Varenicline for smoking cessation. London: NICE, 2007.

21. D Pyrazinamide-induced arthralgia

Adverse reactions to tuberculosis (TB) treatment are common and occur in around 10% of patients, often requiring a change in medication. Reactions are more common in patients receiving non-standard treatment and in HIV-positive individuals. TB therapy should be managed by physicians with a specialist interest in the disease.

Side effects of pyrazinamide include arthralgia, affecting about 1 in 100 patients. Other side effects of standard TB treatment (rifampicin, isoniazid, pyrazinamide and ethambutol) include: drug-induced hepatitis (most frequently caused by pyrazinamide); rash and pruritus; gastrointestinal disturbance; dysuria; interstitial nephritis; malaise; and rarely fever.

Ethambutol rarely causes optic toxicity. Baseline visual acuity using a Snellen chart should be documented, and patients and care-givers should be informed to stop the medication and seek immediate medical attention if they develop new visual symptoms. Mild arthralgia has been very rarely reported with the use of ethambutol.

Isoniazid side effects include rash, abnormal liver function tests, hepatitis, sideroblastic anaemia, peripheral neuropathy, mild central nervous system (CNS) effects and drug interactions. Peripheral neuropathy and CNS effects are due to pyridoxine (vitamin B_6) depletion, but are uncommon at doses of 5 mg/kg. Patients with conditions in which neuropathy is common (e.g. diabetes, uraemia, alcoholism, malnutrition, HIV infection), as well as pregnant women, should be given pyridoxine (vitamin B6) supplementation (10–50 mg/day) with isoniazid. Isoniazid-induced systemic lupus erythromatosus has been rarely reported; however, the antinuclear antibody is negative so this diagnosis is not supported.

Paradoxical reactions are seen after commencing antituberculous therapy. The reaction may consist of increased size of lymphadenopathy or increased volume of pleural effusion/ascites. The diagnosis including HIV status, culture results, drug sensitivities and compliance should be checked and treatment should be continued. Oral corticosteroids may be given to support selected patients.

The rheumatoid factor is mildly positive, but this may be raised because of the underlying inflammatory process. Negative anticyclic citrullinated protein (anti-CCP) antibodies make the diagnosis of rheumatoid arthritis in this setting unlikely.

National Institute for Health and Care Excellence. NICE Guideline No. 117: Tuberculosis. Clinical diagnosis and management of tuberculosis, and measures for its prevention and control. London: NICE, 2011.

22. C Stop warfarin and prescribe 1 mg oral vitamin K

The British Society for Haematology guidelines recommend the cessation of warfarin and the prescription of 1–5 mg oral vitamin K in patients with an international normalised ratio (INR) >8.0 and no evidence of bleeding. The society recommends omitting one or two doses of warfarin in patients whose INR is 5.0–8.0, and in whom there is no evidence of bleeding. Fresh frozen plasma or factor IX complex is recommended in patients with elevated INR, in whom there is evidence of active bleeding.

Keeling, D et al. British Society for Haematology guidelines on oral anticoagulation with warfarin, 4th edition. Br J Haematol 2011; 154 (3):311–324.

23. D Skin rash

Lamotrigine is associated with the development of potentially life-threatening rashes. The patient should seek urgent medical attention if any rash appears. Typically, the rash will occur within the first 8 weeks of commencing the medication. In pre-marketing clinical trials for use of lamotrigine in epilepsy, serious rash with hospitalisation and discontinuation of lamotrigine occurred in 0.3% of adult patients. Skin reactions that have been reported include Stevens–Johnson syndrome, toxic epidermal necrolysis, angio-oedema and drug reaction with eosinophilia and systemic symptoms (DRESS). Other serious side effects include aseptic meningitis, blood dyscrasiae and suicidal ideation. Concomitant use of sodium valproate is associated with an increased risk of skin reactions.

Kanner, AM. Lamotrigine-induced rash: can we stop worrying? Epilepsy Curr 2005; 5(5):190–191.

24. D Use of dose-determining weight to dose gentamicin

This woman has streptococcal bacterial endocarditis. The UK guidelines for this recommend a 6-week course of penicillin (although ceftriaxone can also be used, particularly where outpatient antimicrobial therapy might be appropriate) with synergistic gentamicin for the first 2 weeks. Gentamicin should be dosed at 1 mg/kg three times daily. In overweight patients, the dose-determining weight should be used to arrive at the appropriate dose.

Use of actual body weight will lead to overdosing of the gentamicin and high peak and trough levels, with the potential for renal toxicity. Use of ideal body weight will result in under-dosing and inadequate peak levels, as in this case. This increases the likelihood of treatment failure and in case of bacterial endocarditis this can have serious sequelae.

The dose-determining weight is used in the context of obesity to arrive at a dose likely to achieve the necessary therapeutic target range. It is calculated as follows:

IBW + 0.3 × [ABW – IBW]

[IBW = ideal body weight; ABW = actual body weight.]

Obesity leads to altered pharmacokinetics and pharmacodynamics via various mechanisms: the volume of distribution of lipid-soluble drugs is increased; glomerular hyperfiltration and altered hepatic metabolism can also affect the half-life of many drugs.

Morrish G, et al. The effects of obesity on drug pharmacokinetics in humans. Expert Opin Drug Metab Toxicol 2011; 7(6):697–706.

25. D Active injection drug use is a contraindication to treatment with DAAVs

Direct acting anti-viral (DAAV) medications have revolutionised the treatment of chronic hepatitis C virus (HCV). Previously the only available treatment was pegylated interferon and ribavirin for 48 weeks (genotype 1 and 4 HCV) or 24 weeks (genotype 2 and 3 HCV) with sustained virologic response (SVR) rates of 40–50% or 80%, respectively. This treatment was poorly tolerated by many patients due to the side-effect profile including depression, flu-like symptoms and weight loss, and it could not be used in patients with decompensated cirrhosis due to the high mortality and morbidity associated with its use in these patients.

There are a number of different oral DAAV regimens for treatment of HCV. Following their introduction worldwide, in genotype 1 HCV the SVR rate has become over 95% regardless of disease stage or previous treatment status. The SVR rate in the now harder to treat genotype 3 is over 95% in treatment-naive, non-cirrhotic patients and 90% in cirrhotic and/or treatment-experienced patients. In England, for patients with advanced cirrhosis, liver transplants for HCV reduced by 32% between 2014 and 2015 with liver transplant registrations for HCV reducing by 42%, and deaths from HCV reducing by 8% in the same time period.

The majority of cases of HCV in the UK occur in people who have injected drugs, and treatment of this patient population is vital if eradication of HCV is to be achieved. Active injection drug use is not a contraindication to treatment.

SVR was previously defined as an undetectable HCV RNA 24 weeks after the end of treatment for HCV, and correlates with cure. However, in the trials of DAAVs SVR 12 was shown to be as accurate a predictor of cure as SVR 24, and so SVR 12 has been used in trials of DAAVs.

Hepatitis B reactivation can occur with treatment with DAAVs in patients who are HBsAg positive and in those who are HBV core antibody positive, although severe hepatitis appears to be rare.

Public Health England. Hepatitis C in England 2017 report. London: Public Health England, 2017.
Horsley-Silva JL, Vargas HE. New therapies for hepatitis C virus infection. Gastroenterol Hepatol 2017; 13:22–31.
Belperio PS, Shahoumian TA, Mole LA, Backus LI. Evaluation of hepatitis B reactivation among 62,920 veterans treated with oral hepatitis C antivirals. Hepatology 2017; 66:27–36.

26. B Fluconazole and domperidone

Both of these agents are well known causes of prolonged QT syndrome; their use in combination should generally be avoided. Prolonged QT syndrome predisposes to *torsades de pointes* via the 'R on T' phenomenon. *Torsades de pointes* is a life-threatening arrhythmia that can degenerate to ventricular tachycardia or fibrillation. Additional risk factors for it include female sex, electrolyte disturbance (hypokalaemia, hypomagnesaemia), congenital prolonged QT syndrome, bradycardia, and a history of heart disease. It is prudent to perform a baseline electrocardiogram in patients starting medications that can prolong the QT interval.

Many drugs can cause QT prolongation, but none of the other agents in this vignette are implicated. Sotalol is the only beta-blocker that causes QT prolongation. Among anti-retroviral agents, ritonavir is associated with cardiac conduction abnormalities, and should not be used in combination with domperidone. The combination of fluconazole with a statin can increase the risk of hepatotoxicity.

Schwarz PJ, Woosley RL. Predicting the unpredictable: drug-Induced QT prolongation and *torsades de pointes*. J Am Coll Cardiol 2016; 67:1639–1650.

27. A All-trans-retinoic acid

Acute promyelocytic leukaemia (AML-M3) is usually due to a t(15:17) translocation, resulting in abnormal fusion of the promyelocytic (*PML*) gene on chromosome 15 with the retinoic acid receptor α gene, *RARα*, on chromosome 17. The abnormal PML–RARα fusion protein acts as a transcriptional repressor, via its interaction with the retinoid X receptor (RXR), and prevents differentiation of promyelocytes. In contrast, RARα normally acts as an activator through its interaction with RXR. Treatment with high-dose all-trans-retinoic acid (ATRA) enables the abnormal promyelocytes, which are in a state of arrested development, to proceed with their normal differentiation into mature myeloid cells through its competitive agonism of RXR. Treatment with high-dose ATRA alone, however, will not eradicate the abnormal clone – hence, the need for standard chemotherapy. However, this may be complicated by ATRA syndrome, which is characterised by fever, pulmonary infiltrates, hypoxia and neutrophilia; this is usually treated with intravenous dexamethasone in the first instance.

It is important to note that patients with AML–M3 are at risk of disseminated intravascular coagulation and potentially fatal haemorrhage. They may, therefore, require regular transfusions with platelets and fresh frozen plasma if there is any suggestion of abnormal coagulation. Rituximab and thalidomide are not indicated in the treatment of AML–M3.

Sanz M, et al. Management of acute promyelocytic leukemia: recommendations from an expert panel on behalf of the European LeukemiaNet. Blood 2009; 113:1875–1891

28. D High-flow oxygen therapy

Carbon monoxide poisoning presents with insidious clinical symptoms and can be difficult to diagnose as it mimics many other illnesses. The most common symptom is headache, but it may also present with dyspnoea on exertion, fatigue and irritability, difficulty concentrating, dizziness, syncope, confusion, respiratory failure, seizures, coma or death. It should always be borne in mind as a differential diagnosis in patients who present with any of these symptoms. Important details in the history are whether other family members or pets have been affected, as pets will often be affected earlier and more severely because of their small size. Enquiries should also be made as to whether the patient feels better at work, or home, and when their boiler or heating system was last serviced. Carbon monoxide poisoning can be rapidly fatal as carbon monoxide has an affinity for haemoglobin of 250–300 times that of oxygen. The clinical sequelae of CO poisoning all result from tissue hypoxia. The management of CO poisoning is initially always high-flow oxygen. This reduces the half-life of CO from 240 minutes to 40–80 minutes. Hyperbaric oxygen is recommended in cases of severe CO poisoning, but there is debate as to what constitutes a severe case, and there is limited evidence to guide the use of hyperbaric oxygen. The recommendation is that hyperbaric oxygen should be given when there is a serum carboxyhaemoglobin concentration of over 40%.

Ilano AL, Raffin TA. Management of carbon monoxide poisoning. Chest 1990; 97:165–169.

29. D Scombrotoxin

Of the available answers scombrotoxin, ciguatera toxin and tetrodotoxin are most relevant to the ingestion of contaminated fish. Tetrodotoxin can be discounted since poisoning is usually associated with ingestion of the improperly prepared Japanese delicacy fugu (flesh of the Puffer fish); furthermore, it is a potent neurotoxin and its ingestion is often fatal. Scombrotoxin and ciguatera toxin poisoning can both be diagnosed clinically.

Scombrotoxin presents, as described above, with a self-limiting anaphylactoid response. Headache, flushing, tachycardia, palpitations, abdominal cramps and diarrhoea are common, as is blanching erythema, but weals are not typical. Wheezing can occur, but is said to occur more frequently in the context of existing asthma and histamine sensitivity. Management is supportive with intravenous fluids and antihistamines such as chlorpheniramine. Supplementary oxygen and bronchodilators may be necessary depending on respiratory involvement. Symptoms come on within 10 minutes to 2 hours of eating decaying fish, and usually resolve within 4–6 hours. The toxin forms when histidine is processed to histamine by bacterial decarboxylation; this occurs in the context of decay and is, obviously, associated with inappropriate storage of fish.

Ciguatera is the most common pathogenic marine toxin worldwide and is found principally in contaminated tropical reef fish. The affected individual typically presents within hours of ingestion of contaminated fish. There may be involvement of the gastrointestinal, neurological and cardiovascular systems. Abdominal pain, nausea, vomiting and diarrhoea are typical early features and may last for up to 2 days. Neurological involvement is variable, ranging from circumoral paraesthesia to reversal of temperature sensation, and from generalised weakness to respiratory paralysis and, rarely, coma. Cardiovascular involvement may include symptomatic bradycardia and hypotension. Management is supportive, and the prognosis is on the whole very good.

Botulism is, of course, principally associated with wound infection and ingestion of contaminated foodstuffs (typically canned foods). There are eight types of botulinum exotoxin which are produced by different strains of the anaerobe *Clostridium botulinum*. Types A and B are most common. Botulinum toxin is a neurotoxin that binds to the presynaptic membrane to prevent the release of acetylcholine at the neuromuscular junction. Ingestion of the heat-stable toxin or wound colonisation with *Clostridium botulinum* can be fatal.

Pectenotoxins are a group of toxins that have been implicated in diarrhoeal shellfish poisoning.

McLauchlin J, et al. Scombrotoxic fish poisoning. J Public Health 2006; 28:61–62.

30. E Spironolactone

This woman has New York Heart Association (NYHA) class III symptoms of heart failure.

The drugs that are proven to reduce mortality in heart failure are angiotensin-converting enzyme (ACE inhibitors), beta-blockers and spironolactone. Angiotensin receptor blockers (ARBs) also confer a mortality advantage – but are not given as an option in this question.

Non-dihydropyridine calcium channel blockers (e.g. amlodipine) can be used to treat concomitant hypertension or angina, but they do not affect mortality so this would not be the next agent to add; dihydropyridine agents (e.g. diltiazem, verapamil) should be avoided. Diuretics are used for the treating congestive cardiac failure or fluid overload, and have an important role in symptom management, but this patient has no signs of fluid overload; they also have no mortality benefit. Digoxin can be used for rate control in patients with permanent atrial fibrillation, which often gives symptomatic benefit; it also has a weak positive inotropic effect, so is an option as a third-line agent to treat severe heart failure (including patients with sinus rhythm).

Isosorbide mononitrate and other vasodilators are useful in heart failure, but as an alternative if ACE inhibitors/ARBs or aldosterone antagonists are not tolerated. This is especially true in those of African origin.

Although some patient with severe heart failure are at risk of life-threatening arrhythmias, amiodarone has not been found to be beneficial; rather implantable cardioverter defibrillators (ICD) are preferred to prevent sudden death in these patients. This person may qualify for an ICD.

Spironolactone confers a mortality advantage in patients with NYHA class III/IV heart failure and hence would be the next drug of choice in patients with preserved renal function and a safe potassium level (<5 mmol/L).

National Institute for Health and Care Excellence (NICE). NICE guidance: CG108. Chronic heart failure in adults: management. London: NICE, 2010.

31. A Continue the NAC infusion at the same rate

Paracetamol overdose is a common cause of intentional and unintentional overdose, and causes dose-dependent liver toxicity. A toxic metabolite of paracetamol, N-acetyl-p-benzoquinoneimine (NAPQI) causes the hepatotoxicity. NAPQI is detoxified by interaction with glutathione; if sufficient glutathione is present, the liver is protected. *N*-Acetylcysteine (NAC) prevents liver damage principally by restoring hepatic glutathione. 10–20% of patients can experience adverse effects when given NAC, which can vary from flushing to anaphylaxis.

Flushing itself is not an indication for stopping or slowing down the infusion. The development of angio-oedema or urticaria necessitates stopping the infusion and giving chlorpheniramine. Once the symptoms have abated, the infusion can continue. Those patients who also experience hypotension or respiratory symptoms should be switched to oral NAC. There is no convincing evidence that slowing the rate of the infusion reduces the risk of anaphylactoid reactions. Methionine is an alternative, but is used only if NAC is unavailable or cannot be tolerated.

Heard KJ. Acetylcysteine for acetaminophen poisoning. N Engl J Med 2008; 359:285–292.
Bailey B, McGuigan MA. Management of anaphylactoid reactions to intravenous N-acetylcysteine. Ann Emerg Med 1998; 31(6):710.

32. A Ceftriaxone

This patient has meningococcal meningitis (causative organism: *Neisseria meningitidis*). British Infection Association guidelines recommend ceftriaxone (2 g every 12 h) or cefotaxime (2 g every

6 h) as first-line intravenous antibiotics. Alternatives include benzylpenicillin or chloramphenicol. Of the options given, ceftriaxone (a third-generation cephalosporin) is the most appropriate.

High-dose dexamethasone before or at initiation of antibiotic treatment for pneumococcal or *Haemophilus influenzae* type b meningitis is associated with a better prognosis; however, to date there is no evidence to suggest that it improves outcomes in meningococcal meningitis. Regardless, some clinicians recommend the use of steroids in the treatment of all cases of community-acquired bacterial meningitis unless there is evidence of septic shock (irrespective of the causative bacteria). It should be borne in mind, however, that steroids may reduce central nervous system penetration of some antibiotics, such as vancomycin.

McGill F, et al. The UK joint specialist societies guideline on the diagnosis and management of acute meningitis and meningococcal sepsis in immunocompetent adults. J Inf 2016;72: 405–438.

33. E Quinolone tendinopathy

This patient presents with an Achilles tendonitis. Of the medications she has taken recently, ciprofloxacin is the most likely cause. Tendonitis is a well-described adverse effect of quinolone use and is related to cumulative dose; it can present some time from initial exposure: there are documented cases 6 months after the drug was taken. The Achilles tendon is commonly involved and bilateral tendinitis is common, unlike with other causes. The exact mechanism of action is unclear but matrix-degrading, toxic and ischaemic processes have all been proposed. Treatment is with rest, splinting where necessary and, in sites other than the Achilles tendon, peritendinous steroid injection. This should be avoided in the Achilles itself as tendon rupture has been documented.

Penicillin and cephalosporins are a frequent cause of rash, with up to 4% of the population developing this side effect, but only 0.04% exhibiting true anaphylaxis. Myopathy is rare and tendonitis has not been described. Nitrofurantoin can cause a peripheral neuropathy with prolonged use, and this is more common in the context of renal impairment; myopathy and tendonitis are rarely described. The case is not consistent with pretibial myxoedema.

van der Linden PD, et al. Increased risk of Achilles tendon rupture with quinolone antibacterial use, especially in elderly patients taking oral corticosteroids. Arch Intern Med 2003; 163(15):1801–1807.

34. C Intravenous procyclidine

Acute dystonic reactions, such as the one described here, are well-recognised complications of antipsychotic medications. After stopping the offending drug, the next most appropriate step is to promptly start treatment with a rapidly acting anticholinergic drug such as procyclidine or benztropine. These may be administered intravenously or intramuscularly. It is thought that the dopaminergic blockade caused by antipsychotic drugs (and other agents such as metoclopramide) results in relative cholinergic over-activity in the basal ganglia, resulting in acute dystonic reactions. The rationale of treatment with an anticholinergic is to restore the normal balance of dopaminergic and cholinergic activity.

Dantrolene sodium appears to act by disrupting the excitation–contraction coupling within skeletal muscle. It is thought that this is achieved through interference with the release of calcium from the sarcoplasmic reticulum of skeletal muscle cells. It may be used in the treatment of chronic spasticity resulting from upper motor neuron lesions. Additionally, it constitutes one of the pillars of management of malignant hyperthermia.

Electroconvulsive therapy has been approved by the National Institute for Health and Care Excellence for use in the treatment of severe depression, severe/prolonged mania, catatonia and some cases of schizophrenia. It is not used in the treatment of neuroleptic malignant syndrome itself.

Tizanidine is a centrally acting α_2-adrenergic agonist used for the treatment of spasticity resulting from multiple sclerosis or spinal cord injury.

Botox (OnabotulinumtoxinA, a form of botulinum toxin) is an injectable neurotoxin that acts at the neuromuscular junction by inhibiting the presynaptic release of acetylcholine. This, in turn, prevents muscular contraction. It has been approved in the UK for use in the treatment of a wide range of conditions including blepharospasm, hemifacial spasm, idiopathic cervical dystonia and focal limb spasticity. However, Botox would not be appropriate in this case, which almost certainly has a reversible cause.

Taylor D, Paton C, Kapur S. The Maudsley Prescribing Guidelines: 10th edn. The South London and Maudsley NHS Foundation Trust, Oxleas NHS Foundation Trust. London: Informa Healthcare, 2009.

35. C Lithium

The patient has biochemical and clinical evidence of hyperparathyroidism and hypothyroidism. The incidence of both of these disorders is increased in patients who take lithium. Hypothyroidism and hyperparathyroidism are not associated with any of the other medications listed. Another important side effect of lithium is nephrogenic diabetes insipidus; it may cause rashes or exacerbations of psoriasis.

McKnight RF, et al. Lithium toxicity profile: a systematic review and meta-analysis. Lancet 2012; 379:721–728.

36. A Amoxicillin

The patient in this vignette has community-acquired pneumonia and, given the rusty sputum and clinical and radiographic findings in keeping with lobar consolidation, this is most likely to be caused by *Streptococcus pneumoniae*. *S. pneumoniae* in the UK rarely exhibits penicillin resistance and hence β-lactam antimicrobials are the preferred choice. Although individual hospitals have differing antimicrobial policies based upon local resistance patterns and other issues, in the UK the National Institute for Health and Care Excellence has published guidelines and these are widely followed. This patient has a CURB65 score of 0; the guidelines suggest treatment with amoxicillin 500 mg po three times daily. The CURB65 score is a prognostication tool utilised predominantly to delineate whether admission is indicated in cases of community-acquired pneumonia. The criteria are: confusion, urea >7 mmol/L, respiratory rate >30 breaths per minute, systolic blood pressure <90 mmHg or diastolic <60 mmHg and age >65 years. A score of 2 or more warrants admission and those with a score of 1 or less can be considered for home-based treatment.

In penicillin-allergic patients, doxycycline or clarithromycin are appropriate alternatives, although empirical use of these must be with care as in some areas of the UK macrolide resistance approaches 15%. In this patient, there is additional need to avoid macrolides and quinolones as these are known to interact with warfarin.

National Institute for Health and Care Excellence (NICE). NICE guideline 191. Pneumonia in adults: diagnosis and management. London: NICE, 2014.

37. D Idarucizumab

The benefits of direct-acting oral anticoagulants (DOACs) over warfarin are that they do not require therapeutic monitoring, and there are fewer drug interactions. The drawbacks are that it is difficult to measure their effect using standard clotting studies, and most have no specific reversal agent (the exception being dabigatran).

Dabigatran is a direct thrombin inhibitor with a half-life of 12–17 hours. It has variable effects on the activated partial thromboplastin time (APTT) and international normalised ratio (INR), however the thrombin time (TT) is highly sensitive to its effects, so a normal TT reliably excludes presence of the drug.

Idarucizumab, a monoclonal antibody fragment that binds to dabigatran and rapidly reverses its action, is used in severe or life-threatening bleeding, or if emergency surgery is required. There is no randomised controlled trial evidence for its use, but a study reported rapid and complete reversal of anticoagulation (as measured using the TT) in most patients. It carries a small risk of inducing thrombosis, but this clearly has to be accepted in the case described.

If idarucizumab is not available, prothrombin complex concentrates can be used to mitigate the effects of DOACs, but fresh frozen plasma is not recommended. Andexanet alfa is a recombinant factor Xa decoy protein with emerging evidence in the reversal of factor Xa inhibitors (rivaroxaban, apixaban), but it is not licensed in the UK at the time of writing. Abciximab is a glycoprotein IIb/IIIa receptor antagonist that inhibits platelet aggregation; it would certainly not be indicated in this situation.

Pollack C et al. Idarucizumab for dabigatran reversal – full cohort analysis. N Engl J Med 2017; 377:431–441.
Connolly T et al. Andexanet alfa for acute major bleeding associated with factor Xa inhibitors. N Engl J Med 2017; 375:1131–1141.
National Institute for Health and Care Excellence (NICE). NICE evidence summary. Reversal of the anticoagulant effect of dabigatran: idarucizumab. London: NICE, 2016.

38. D Oral oseltamivir

Pregnant women are considered as a high-risk group during influenza outbreaks and should be advised to seek early advice to reduce the chance of complications. Pregnant patients presenting with flu-like symptoms during an influenza outbreak should be offered either oseltamivir or zanamivir (neuraminidase inhibitors active against influenza A and B viruses). This treatment should be started as soon as possible within the first 48 hours of symptoms. Oseltamivir is an oral preparation. Zanamivir is delivered by an inhaler (not intravenous).

There is no clear medical evidence that intravenous pooled human immunoglobulins improve outcome in H1N1 in pregnant women and it should not be given routinely. These patients are high risk and symptomatic treatment alone would not be the best advice in the scenario described. Amoxicillin would not be the agent of choice, unless there was super-added bacterial infection.

National Institute for Health and Care Excellence. NICE guidance: TA168. Amantadine, oseltamivir and zanamivir for the treatment of influenza. London: NICE, 2009.

39. B Ethanol

The patient has a metabolic acidosis with high anion gap and is most likely suffering from methanol poisoning. He has probably been consuming impure homemade vodka, and is exhibiting symptoms of toxicity. Some of these symptoms may mimic a 'hangover' from ethanol intoxication, but the abdominal pain and confusion are indicative of methanol toxicity. The sluggish pupillary responses, wide anion gap with metabolic acidosis, tachypnoea, tachycardia and hypotension add further weight to the clinical diagnosis. Blurred vision is also often associated with methanol toxicity.

Bicarbonate should be given to reverse the acidosis and reduce the amount of active formic acid. Methanol is first metabolised to formaldehyde by alcohol dehydrogenase, and this is subsequently metabolised by formaldehyde dehydrogenase to the toxic metabolite formic acid. Ethanol acts as a preferential substrate for alcohol dehydrogenase, preventing metabolism of methanol. This prevents the formation of toxic methanol metabolites and is continued until the intact methanol has been eliminated from the system.

There is no shortage of evidence to support the use of fomepizole, an alcohol dehydrogenase inhibitor, in the treatment of methanol poisoning.

Activated charcoal is not indicated, as it is relatively ineffective against methanol. Gastric lavage would not be beneficial: ingestion was some hours earlier, and methanol is rapidly absorbed. Phenytoin would not be indicated unless the patient was to develop seizures.

Haemodialysis is necessary if there is end-organ damage (e.g. acute kidney injury) or severe acid–base abnormalities that do not respond to medical management.

Barceloux DG, et al. American Academy of Clinical Toxicology Practice Guidelines on the Treatment of Methanol Poisoning. Clin Tox 2002; 40(4):415–446.
Brent J, et al. Fomepizole for the treatment of methanol poisoning. N Engl J Med 2001; 344:424–429.

40. D Salicylate overdose

Salicylate overdose can present with vomiting, dehydration, vertigo, tinnitus, deafness, sweating and hyperventilation. It classically causes a mixed respiratory alkalosis and metabolic acidosis, as in this case. It should be managed with activated charcoal if the patient presents within 1 hour of ingestion of more than 250 mg/kg. Elimination of salicylate can be improved by urinary alkalinisation with 1.26% sodium bicarbonate. Haemodialysis is used in severe cases. Tricyclic antidepressant, ethylene glycol and methanol overdose all cause a metabolic acidosis.

Organophosphate poisoning can cause respiratory distress and sweating but it does not commonly cause a respiratory alkalosis.

Dargan PI, Wallace CI, Jones AL. An evidence based flowchart to guide the management of acute salicylate (aspirin) overdose. Emerg Med J 2002; 19:206–209.

41. C Intravenous desferrioxamine

Iron causes toxicity by forming free radicals, which are harmful to tissues with high metabolic activity: the gastrointestinal tract, liver and heart are most susceptible. The toxodrome has five phases: the gastrointestinal toxicity phase (within hours) includes abdominal pain, vomiting, haematemesis and malaena; a latent phase follows (6–24 hours), in which patients are relatively stable, but may have subtle signs of acidosis or hypovolaemia (as in this case); overt shock and metabolic acidosis may then develop (hours to days), and multi-organ failure can ensue; hepatotoxicity, a consequence of high iron concentration in the portal circulation, can evolve (1–2 days); finally, gastrointestinal scarring (2–4 weeks) can cause gastrointestinal tract obstruction (most commonly pyloric stenosis).

Mild cases of poisoning result in gastrointestinal disturbance only, but it is important not to miss a patient in the latent phase, which may portend critical deterioration. A profound raised anion gap acidosis results from the generation of three hydrogen ions from every ferric ion (Fe^{3+}).

In general, serum iron concentrations greater than 90 µmol/L are associated with severe toxicity, but do not be falsely reassured by the normal level in this case: serum concentration peaks four to six hours after ingestion, then falls as it enters cells (where the damage occurs). Other features of toxicity include hyperglycaemia, seizure, coma, and coagulopathy.

It is too late for gastric lavage in this case, and activated charcoal does not bind iron well. Desferrioxamine binds circulating iron to form ferrioxamine, which is excreted in the urine. Alternative treatments for severe poisoning include haemodialysis and exchange transfusion.

Tenenbein M. Toxicokinetics and toxicodynamincs of iron poisonining. Toxicol Lett 1998; 102-103:653–656.

42. C Hyoscine butylbromide (Buscopan)

The diagnosis is irritable bowel syndrome (IBS). This should be suspected in people who present with abdominal pain that is associated with altered bowel frequency or stool form, or relieved by defecation, and accompanied by at least two of the following symptoms: altered stool passage; abdominal bloating, distension, tension or hardness; symptoms made worse by eating; or passage of mucus. First-line management of IBS includes diet and lifestyle management, and antispasmodic agents such as hyoscine butylbromide. Tricyclic antidepressants are second-line agents that can be used after 6 months. Acupuncture and mesalazine are not recommended in IBS, and cognitive–behavioural therapy is third-line management.

National Institute for Health and Care Excellence (NICE). NICE guidelines. Irritable bowel syndrome in adults: Diagnosis and management. London: NICE, 2008 (updated 2017).

43. E Sodium bicarbonate

This patient is symptomatic from a tricyclic antidepressant overdose. The presence of a metabolic acidosis and myocardial instability (widened QRS on ECG) indicate severe toxicity. Aggressive correction of the acidosis with intravenous sodium bicarbonate is indicated. Hyperventilation is not appropriate therapy. Gastric lavage is appropriate only if performed within 1 hour of a life-threatening overdose. Intravenous diazepam would not be appropriate unless the patient were to develop seizures. Intravenous glucagon may have a role in treatment of myocardial depression and hypotension, but the first line treatment is with sodium bicarbonate.

Body R, et al. Guidelines in Emergency Medicine Network (GEMNet): guideline for the management of tricyclic antidepressant overdose. Emerg Med J 2011; 28:347–368.